W9-DBI-240

ULTRASONOGRAPHY:

AN INTRODUCTION TO NORMAL STRUCTURE AND FUNCTIONAL ANATOMY

ULTRASONOGRAPHY:
AN INTRODUCTION TO NORMAL STRUCTURE AND FUNCTIONAL ANATOMY

REVA ARNEZ CURRY, PhD, RT(R), RDMS
Assistant Professor and Program Coordinator
Diagnostic Medical Sonography
Department of Diagnostic Imaging
Thomas Jefferson University College of Allied Health Sciences
Philadelphia, Pennsylvania

BETTY BATES TEMPKIN, BA, RT(R), RDMS
Ultrasound Consultant
Formerly, Clinical Director
Diagnostic Medical Sonography Program
Hillsborough Community College
Tampa, Florida

W.B. SAUNDERS COMPANY
A Division of Harcourt Brace & Company
Philadelphia, London, Toronto, Montreal, Sydney, Tokyo

W.B. SAUNDERS COMPANY
A Division of Harcourt Brace & Company

The Curtis Center
Independence Square West
Philadelphia, PA 19106

Library of Congress Cataloging-in-Publication Data

Ultrasonography : an introduction to normal structure and functional
anatomy / [edited by] Reva A. Curry, Betty Bates Tempkin. — 1st ed.
        p.   cm.
    ISBN 0-7216-4585-2
    1. Ultrasonic imaging.   2. Human anatomy.   I. Curry, Reva A.
II. Tempkin, Betty Bates.
    [DNLM: 1. Ultrasonography.   2. Anatomy.   WN 200 U47 1995]
QM25.U48   1995
616.17′543 — dc20
DNLM/DLC   93-26475

ULTRASONOGRAPHY: An Introduction to Normal
                   Structure and Functional Anatomy   ISBN 0-7216-4585-2

Printed in the United States of America.

Last digit is the print number: 9   8   7   6   5   4   3   2   1

This textbook is dedicated to my Lord and Savior Jesus Christ, for from Him, through Him, and to Him are all things.

My efforts with this textbook would not have been possible without the love and support of my family: Dwight, Tiana, and Serena. I love you.

R.A.C.

To David, for your good heart and good humor. Thanks for a great life! And to Mother and Dad, Cathy and Jim, Kitt, and Shannon for your interest and good spirits!

B.B.T.

CONTRIBUTORS

REVA ARNEZ CURRY, PhD, RT(R), RDMS

Assistant Professor and Program Coordinator, Diagnostic Medical Sonography, Department of Diagnostic Imaging, Thomas Jefferson University College of Allied Health Sciences, Philadelphia, Pennsylvania

The Pancreas; The Urinary System; Appendices: Ultrasound Documents Related to Patient Examination; Patient Chart Information: Medical/Surgical Assembly Order

MARILYN DICKERSON, BS, RDMS

Instructor and Program Director, Diagnostic Medical Sonography Program, Emory University School of Medicine, Atlanta, Georgia

The Liver; The Gastrointestinal System

MICHAEL C. FOSS, MEd, RDMS, RVT

Associate Professor of Allied Health Sciences, Director, Sonography Program, Department of Allied Health Sciences, Rochester Institute of Technology College of Science, Rochester, New York

The Biliary System; The Pancreas

DANIEL HAGAN, RT(R), RDMS

Program Director, El Paso Community College, El Paso, Texas

Body Systems

FELICIA M. JONES, BS, RDMS, RVT

Program Director, Diagnostic Medical Sonography, Tidewater Community College, Virginia Beach, Virginia

The Spleen; Breast Sonography; Introduction to Ultrasound of Human Disease

MICHAEL J. KAMMERMEIER, BSRT, RDMS, RVT

Sonographer, Pennsylvania Hospital, Philadelphia, Pennsylvania

The Male Pelvis

ALEXANDER LANE, PhD

Coordinator of Anatomy and Physiology, Triton College, River Grove, Illinois

Anatomy Layering and Sectional Anatomy

WAYNE C. LEONHARDT, BA, RT, RDMS, RVT

Staff Sonographer and Clinical Instructor, Summit Medical Center, Oakland; Faculty, Foothill College, Los Altos; Ultrasound Program; Consultant for Ultrasound Education Program Development, Los Altos, California

Thyroid and Parathyroid Glands

HEATHER LEVY, BS, RT(R)

Sonographer/Radiographer, Memorial Sloan-Kettering Cancer Center, New York, New York

Appendices: Ultrasound Documents Related to Patient Examination; Ultrasound Instrumentation; Film Processing; Patient Chart Information: Medical/Surgical Assembly Order

MAUREEN E. McDONALD, BS, RDMS, RDCS

Instructor of Echocardiography, Ultrasound Diagnostic School, Philadelphia; Staff Echocardiographer, Thomas Jefferson University Hospital, Philadelphia, Pennsylvania

Adult Echocardiography

VIVIE M. MILLER, BA, BS, RDMS, RDCS

Clinical Instructor, Department of Pediatrics, Section of Pediatric Cardiology, Medical College of Georgia, Augusta, Georgia

Pediatric Echocardiography

MARSHA M. NEUMYER, BS, RVT

Instructor of Surgery, Pennsylvania State University College of Medicine, Hershey; Technical Director, Vascular Studies Section, Department of Surgery, The Milton S. Hershey Medical Center, Hershey, Pennsylvania

Vascular Technology

JERRY PEARSON, MSA, RDMS

Director of Diagnostic Radiology, University Hospital, Oregon Health Sciences University, Portland, Oregon

The Abdominal Aorta; The Inferior Vena Cava; The Portal Venous System

M. NATHAN PINKNEY, BS

Imaging Consultant, Sonicor Inc., West Point, Pennsylvania; Clinical Instructor, Diagnostic Medical Sonography, Department of Diagnostic Imaging, Thomas Jefferson University College of Allied Health Sciences, Philadelphia, Pennsylvania

Physics; Instrumentation

BRIAN A. SCHLOSSER, BS, RDMS

Staff Sonographer, Children's Hospital of the King's Daughters, Norfolk, Virginia

The Neonatal Brain

G. WILLIAM SHEPHERD, PhD, RDMS, RVT

Clinical Instructor and Staff Ultrasonographer, Frankford Hospital, Philadelphia, Pennsylvania

The Urinary System; First Trimester Obstetrics; Second and Third Trimester Obstetrics; Obstetric Sonography/Special Situations

BETTY BATES TEMPKIN, BA, RT(R), RDMS

Ultrasound Consultant; Formerly Clinical Director Diagnostic Medical Sonography Program, Hillsborough Community College, Tampa, Florida

Anatomy Layering and Sectional Anatomy; The Pancreas; The Urinary System

DEBORAH D. WERNEBURG, MBA, RDMS

Lecturer in Diagnostic Medical Sonography, Department of Diagnostic Imaging, College of Allied Health Sciences, Thomas Jefferson University Hospital, Philadelphia, Pennsylvania

The Female Pelvis

PREFACE

We wrote this textbook for the novice sonographer. As the beginner learns to scan, it is important that she or he understand not only the anatomy of the organs or the structures that will be examined, but it is also essential that the sonographer know the anatomy that surrounds the area of interest. Which structures are anterior to what is to be visualized? Which structures are medial to it? Superior to it? A working knowledge of relational anatomy will assist the sonographer in finding and documenting the area of interest and its surrounding structure and is one of the first steps in learning sonography.

The sonographer must also know how the organ or structure functions. This is necessary before she or he can learn what happens when the body does not work correctly (i.e., in disease). A sonographer who understands anatomy and physiology is better able to make decisions in the examining room. Do the patient's symptoms match the organ or structure which the referring clinician has requested be examined? Should additional views be taken? Have the acquired images answered the referring clinician's question? The ability of the sonographer to problem-solve in the examining room results in more accurate information being relayed to the sonologist and ensures a complete study.

Therefore, we present anatomy and physiology in the first half of each chapter relating to an organ or body system. This gives the reader the opportunity to learn organ structure and function before viewing sonographic images. Next we present normal ultrasound images in the second half of each chapter. We have included many normal sonograms to increase the reader's comfort level with normal ultrasound anatomy, and most images are accompanied by a labeled diagram and a detailed legend.

To assist the novice further, we list key words and objectives in the beginning of each chapter. The key words are the medical terminology which is used in the chapter. It may be new to the beginner, and we encourage our readers to become comfortable with the terminology. The objectives are meant to focus the reader's attention when studying the chapter.

At the end of most chapters, we've included several reference charts to assist the reader: laboratory values and other diagnostic tests used for the organ or structure under discussion, and a list of physicians associated with the organ or structure of interest. We hope these listings will assist the novice to integrate sonography and other medical specialties.

References and a bibliography complete most chapters. When applicable, multiple references give the reader a broader scope of information. Selected bibliographies provide additional information sources to study.

We begin this textbook with chapters on physics principles and instrumentation to give the reader an introduction to the nature of sound waves and how sonographic images are produced on the scanning instrument. A chapter on body systems gives the reader a general overview of the organs and structures which will be discussed and how they interrelate. A sectional/layering anatomy chapter introduces the novice to the concept of viewing sectional anatomy, in which we explain how the anatomy is layered in the body and why it looks the way it does on sectional images.

The next section consists of chapters on the abdominal organs, and vessels, male and female pelvis, obstetrics, and small parts (thyroid and breast). These chapters are designed to begin the learner's study of general sonography.

Next we grouped introductory chapters to other ultrasound specialties, including chapters on vascular technology, adult echocardiography, pediatric echocardiography, and neurosonology. A single chapter on each of these specialties cannot give the topic the in-depth coverage it deserves. However, these chapters do serve the reader as a general overview and primer for continued studies in the specialty.

An introduction to ultrasound in pathology concludes the chapters of this textbook and serves as a bridge to a third book coming from Saunders, ULTRASOUND OF HUMAN DISEASE. (The first book in the series is Betty Bates Tempkin's ULTRA-SOUND SCANNING: PRINCIPLES AND PROTOCOLS.)

In the appendices of this textbook the student can review documents related to an ultrasound examination, learn about ultrasound system controls and how to operate them, and become familiar with the steps of film processing. This section also includes the information found in the patient chart.

As a companion to this book, there is a student workbook which includes unlabeled layering and sectional diagrams, unlabeled anatomic diagrams, review questions and answers, and images with accompanying unlabeled diagrams. We developed this to further assist the reader in identifying normal sonographic anatomy and understanding physics. The workbook also includes "Your First Scanning Experience" to assist the student with a step-by-step approach to scanning.

And, in an effort to meet the needs of the educator in fitting these books into classroom work, we created an instructor's manual. It contains chapter questions and answers and sections that we believe will be especially valuable to educators:

How to develop a course syllabus (including a sample)
How to develop tests

In summary, this text is designed to be the first book that the novice uses in her or his sonography education. The student should read and study it before she or he attempts clinical scanning and the identification of pathology. Most of the chapters use the same format to facilitate easier reading, studying, and testing. It is our hope that we have successfully built a text addressing the need in the sonography profession for a textbook designed for the beginner; a textbook which allows in-depth study of normal anatomy and physiology; a textbook that serves as a bridge to the vascular technology, adult echocardiography, pediatric echocardiography, and neurosonology specialties. Your comments on how to improve it will be anxiously awaited and gratefully received.

A very special thanks to our contributors. Your committment and hard work are greatly appreciated. Thanks also to Marsha Jessup and the staff of the Robert Wood Johnson Medical School. The artwork is exceptional and exemplary.

Best wishes for your sonography career.

REVA ARNEZ CURRY
BETTY BATES TEMPKIN

CONTENTS

SECTION I

PHYSICS

Chapter 1

PHYSICS

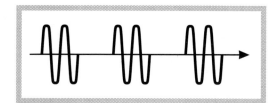

M. NATHAN PINKNEY

Objectives:

Define sound energy.

Describe the piezoelectric effect.

Describe the properties of ultrasound waves.

Describe the decibel and attenuation.

Describe sound speed, reflection, and transmission.

Describe axial and lateral resolution.

Describe the categories of bioeffects.

Define the key words.

Pulse-echo
Pulse repetition frequency
Pulse repetition period
Rarefaction
Reflected angle
Refraction
Resolution
Resonant frequency
Sidelobes

Spatial pulse length
Specular interface
Stiffness
Transducer
Transmitted angle
Ultrasound
Velocity
Wavelength

Key Words:

Acoustic impedance
Attenuation
Audible sound
Axial resolution
Barium titanate
Beam width
Bioeffects
Cavitation
Condensation
Continuous wave
Curie point
Damping
Density
Decibel
Dipole
Doppler
Duty factor
Elasticity

Energy
Focusing
Frequency
Hertz
Huygen's principle
Infrasound
Lateral resolution
Lead zirconate
 titanate
Longitudinal waves
Matter
Nonspecular interface
Period
Piezoelectric effect
Point source
Polarization
Propagation
Pulse duration

BASIC PRINCIPLES OF ULTRASOUND

Ultrasound is sound whose frequency is above the range of human hearing. Ultrasound is widely used in medical imaging for the evaluation of a patient's internal organs. Ultrasound energy is transmitted into the patient; then, because the various internal structures reflect and scatter sound differently, returning echoes can be used to form an image of a structure.

Sound Energy

Sound waves consist of mechanical variations containing **condensations** and **rarefactions** that are transmitted through a medium. Unlike x-rays, sound is not electromagnetic. Matter must be present for sound to travel, which explains why sound cannot propagate through a vacuum. **Propagation** of sound is the transfer of **energy** —not **matter**—from one place to another.

2   Chapter title illustration was adapted from Kremkau, F: Diagnostic Ultrasound: Principles, Instruments, and Exercises, 3rd ed. Philadelphia, WB Saunders Co., 1989, p. 69.

Categories of Sound

Sound is categorized according to its **frequency**. Frequency describes the number of mechanical variations or vibrations that occur per unit time. **Infrasound** is subsonic sound with a frequency below 20 **hertz**, where each hertz (Hz) represents one cycle per second. **Audible sounds** have frequencies that range from 20 Hz to 20,000 Hz. Sounds that have frequencies above 20,000 Hz (20 kHz) are **ultrasonic**. When ultrasound is used for **medical diagnostic** applications, operating frequencies **above one million hertz (1 megahertz; MHz)** are used.

Propagation Speed

Sound waves propagate through matter by causing molecules to vibrate successively along the sound path. **Stiffness, elasticity**, and **density** properties of a material determine the **velocity** of sound propagation. Normally, the velocity of sound is significantly higher in materials that are very stiff. (See Table 1–1.)

Piezoelectric Effect

High-frequency **transducers** are used to generate the ultrasonic energy. The major component of an ultrasound transducer is the **piezoelectric** element. Piezoelectric materials are capable of converting one form of energy into another.

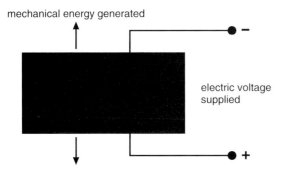

Piezoelectric effect: Electrical energy into mechanical energy. (Adapted from Pinkney N: A Review of Concepts of Ultrasound Physics and Instrumentation. 4th ed. Sonicor, Inc., 1992. Reproduced with permission.)

TABLE 1–1. Sound Velocities

MATERIAL	METERS PER SECOND
Air	330
Pure water	1430
Metal	5000
Fat	1450
Soft tissue	*1540*
Liver	1550
Blood	1570
Muscle	1585
Bone	4080

From Pinkney N: A Review of Concepts of Ultrasound Physics and Instrumentation. 4th ed. Sonicor, Inc., 1992. Reproduced with permission.

A voltage supplied to a piezoelectric element initiates vibrations at the element's **resonant** (operating) **frequency**. The resonant frequency is related to the element's **thickness**. The thinner the element, the higher the resonant frequency of the transducer.

Another function of the piezoelectric element is to receive echoes that return from the object being studied.

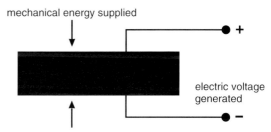

Piezoelectric effect: Mechanical energy into electrical energy. (Adapted from Pinkney N: A Review of Concepts of Ultrasound Physics and Instrumentation. 4th ed. Sonicor, Inc., 1992. Reproduced with permission.)

When the mechanical energy is received, the piezoelectric element converts it into an electrical voltage, which forms a visual image of the studied structure. Although a single piezoelectric element is capable of either transmitting or receiving, it cannot be used to perform both functions simultaneously.

Medical diagnostic ultrasound transducers use **ceramic** materials for piezoelectric elements. In order to make a ceramic material piezoelectric, it is necessary to heat it above a certain temperature, called the **Curie point**. It is at this temperature that a material's dipoles move freely and will align themselves with an electric field. An electrical potential is applied and the material is then cooled to room temperature while the voltage remains. This **polarization** of the ceramic material remains as long as the temperature of the material is kept below the Curie point. Ceramic materials typically used are **lead zirconate titanate** and **barium titanate**.

There are two basic modes of transducer operation that are used in medical diagnostic applications: **continuous** and **pulsed**. (Refer to Figure 1–1.)

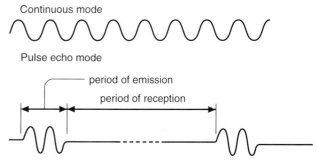

Figure 1–1. Graphs of continuous mode and pulse-echo mode in ultrasound. (Adapted from Pinkney D: A Review of Concepts of Ultrasound Physics and Instrumentation. 4th ed. Sonicor, Inc., 1992. Reproduced with permission.)

The continuous mode or continuous wave (CW) is used in some **Doppler** ultrasound systems. Separate elements are required for continuous sending and receiving. Doppler is used to detect blood flow through vessels. The Doppler technique detects not only the presence of blood flow but also the direction of flow by measuring the difference in the frequency of the reflected sound compared to the transmitted sound.

Pulsed transducers can use the same piezoelectric elements for sending and receiving because separate time intervals are provided for emission and reception.

Pulse-Echo Ultrasound

Pulse-echo ultrasound transducers operate by periodically sending short bursts of sound energy into the area being studied. Echoes are produced when changes in the characteristic of the material are encountered. When these echoes return to the transducer, they are converted into electrical signals. After processing, the information received forms an image of the studied area. The ultrasound system measures the **time** that it takes to receive the echoes after each transmitted pulse. By keeping track of the time between transmitted pulses and the returning echoes, the ultrasound system can determine the distances to the various reflectors. Most diagnostic ultrasound systems are calibrated for a velocity of **1540 meters per second** (1.54 millimeters per microsecond), which is the average velocity of sound through human soft tissue. Large propagation speed errors will result in improper positioning of echoes on a display.

Shock excitation is used to generate sound energy in pulse-echo ultrasound systems.

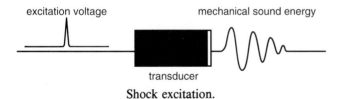

Shock excitation is used to generate sound energy in pulse-echo systems

Shock excitation.

The excitation is normally several hundred volts. The frequency of the excitation, which is the **pulse repetition frequency** (PRF), is normally greater than 1000 pulses per second (1 kHz). The **pulse repetition period**, which is the reciprocal of the PRF, decreases as the PRF is increased. Shorter pulse repetition periods may be used only when structures that are not very deep are being examined. This is because an ultrasound transducer should not be permitted to send out a pulse until sufficient time has been allowed to receive all returning echoes that are the result of the previous pulse.

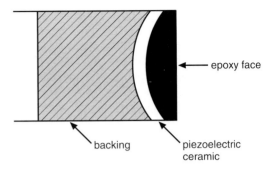

Single-element transducer.

Backing materials are present in pulse-echo transducers to provide **damping** of the piezoelectric element so that each transmitted sound pulse consists of only a few cycles to ensure a very short period of emission compared to a longer period of reception.

The relationship between the period of emission and the period of reception is called the **duty factor**, or duty cycle.

The duty factor of pulse-echo ultrasound instruments is very small, usually less than 1 percent. Continuous wave Doppler systems operate with duty factors of 100 percent because they are capable of sending and receiving at the same time. (Refer to Figure 1–2.)

Ultrasound Beam Generation

Any sound source creates waves from individual **point sources**. **Huygen's principle** demonstrates how these multiple single-point sources produce spherical secondary **wavelets**. Successive wavefronts will be present in areas of **tangency** to the secondary wavelets. (See Figure 1–3.)

Normally, the waves emanating from a piezoelectric element follow a defined beam path, but occasionally undesirable extraneous energy components are produced. These energy components, which are not in the primary direction of the ultrasound beam, are called **sidelobes**.

Each cycle from an expanding and contracting piezoelectric element results in condensation and rarefaction. The condensations and rarefactions of the molecules

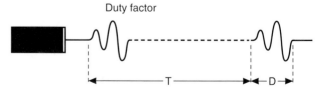

Duty factor

T = pulse repetition period
D = pulse duration

Figure 1–2. Graph of duty factor. (Adapted from Pinkney N: A Review of Concepts of Ultrasound Physics and Instrumentation. 4th ed. Sonicor, Inc., 1992. Reproduced with permission.)

Single-point source

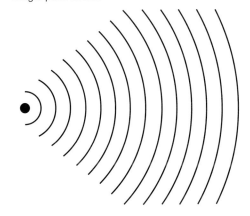

A

Multiple single-point sources
on a single-element transducer

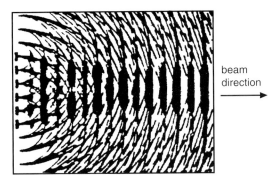

beam
direction

B

Figure 1–3. *A,* single-point source. *B,* beam formation due to Huygen's principle. (Adapted from Pinkney N: A Review of Concepts of Ultrasound Physics and Instrumentation. 4th ed. Sonicor, Inc., 1992. Reproduced with permission.)

produce **longitudinal** sound waves. (See Figure 1–4.) Longitudinal sound waves have particle motion that is back and forth along the direction of propagation. Longitudinal waves are very useful in medical diagnostic ultrasound.

A graph of ultrasound waves may represent a scale of **time.** The time required to produce each cycle depends on the operating frequency of the transducer. This time

condensation   rarefaction

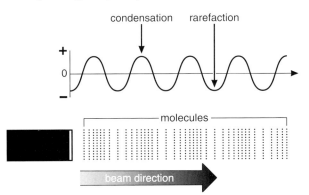

molecules

beam direction

Figure 1–4. Graph representing longitudinal waves. (Adapted from Pinkney N: A Review of Concepts of Ultrasound Physics and Instrumentation. 4th ed. Sonicor, Inc., 1992. Reproduced with permission.)

TABLE 1–2. Frequency vs. Period

EXAMPLES
Period of a 1 MHz wave is 1 microsecond
Period of a 2 MHz wave is 0.5 microsecond
Period of a 3 MHz wave is 0.33 microsecond
Period of a 5 MHz wave is 0.2 microsecond

interval is the **period** of the wave. The period of a diagnostic ultrasound cycle is typically less than a microsecond. (Refer to Table 1–2.) The total time of each sound pulse is the period multiplied by the number of cycles in each pulse. This time interval, which is the **pulse duration**, decreases along with the period when higher-frequency transducers are used. It is the pulse duration divided by the pulse repetition period that gives the duty factor. The following figure shows a graph of period and pulse duration.

Wave parameters
period
T

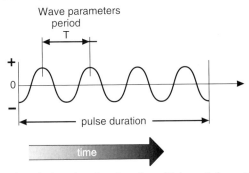

pulse duration

time

Graph of period and pulse duration. (Adapted from Pinkney N: A Review of Concepts of Ultrasound Physics and Instrumentation. 4th ed. Sonicor, Inc., 1992. Reproduced with permission.)

A graph of ultrasound waves may also represent a scale of **distance.** The distance occupied by each cycle depends on the operating frequency of the transducer and the velocity of the sound. This distance interval is the **wavelength** of the cycle. The wavelength of a diagnostic ultrasound cycle is typically less than a millimeter. (Refer to table 1–3.)

The total distance occupied by a sound pulse is the wavelength multiplied by the number of cycles in the pulse. This distance, which is the **spatial pulse length**, decreases along with the wavelength when higher-frequency transducers are used. (See Figure 1–5.)

wavelength λ

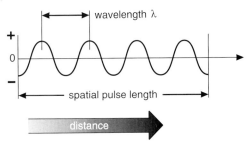

spatial pulse length

distance

Figure 1–5. Graph of wavelength and spatial pulse length. (Adapted from Pinkney N: A Review of Concepts of Ultrasound Physics and Instrumentation. 4th ed. Sonicor, Inc., 1992. Reproduced with permission.)

TABLE 1–3. Frequency vs. Wavelength

EXAMPLES FOR A VELOCITY OF 1540 M/SEC
Wavelength for 1 MHz is 1.54 mm
Wavelength for 2 MHz is 0.77 mm
Wavelength for 3 MHz is 0.51 mm

From Pinkney N: A Review of Concepts of Ultrasound Physics and Instrumentation. 4th ed. Sonicor, Inc., 1992. Reproduced with permission.

Sound Reflection

Sound reflection occurs at an **acoustic interface**, which is the boundary between two media of different **acoustic impedance**. The acoustic impedance (measured in rayls) of a material is the product of the material's **density** and the velocity of sound in the material. (See Table 1–4.)

The difference in the acoustic impedance of the two materials determines the amount of sound energy transmitted and reflected at a boundary. The greater the difference in the acoustic impedance, the higher the reflection and the lower the transmission through the interface. As a general rule, medical diagnostic ultrasound energy will not travel through air. (Refer to Table 1–5.) This is why acoustic couplants (water, oil, or gel) are needed. Acoustic couplants are used to provide a good sound path between the transducer and the skin.

TABLE 1–4. Typical Acoustic Impedance Values

MATERIAL	Z
Air	400
Fat	1,380,000
Water	1,430,000
Tissue	1,630,000
Muscle	1,700,000
Bone	7,800,000

From Pinkney N: A Review of Concepts of Ultrasound Physics and Instrumentation. 4th ed. Sonicor, Inc., 1992. Reproduced with permission.

TABLE 1–5. Typical Reflection Percentages (Approximate)

INTERFACE	% REFLECTION
Fat-muscle	1%
Fat-bone	50%
Tissue-air	100%

From Pinkney N: A Review of Concepts of Ultrasound Physics and Instrumentation. 4th ed. Sonicor, Inc., 1992. Reproduced with permission.

Reflections most frequently received are those that occurred at **normal** (perpendicular) incidence. The **angle of reflection** is usually equal to the **angle of incidence**. This is true at most **specular interfaces**, where the boundary of the interface is smooth and where the dimensions of the interface are larger than the wavelength. (See Figure 1–6.) Examples of specular interfaces include the diaphragm, the walls of vessels and anechoic structures, and the boundaries of many organs.

Sound that is not reflected is **transmitted** through the interface. **Refraction** can occur if the incident angle is not zero and if the velocities of sound in the two materials forming the boundary are not equal. Refraction is a change in **direction** of sound as it passes through a boundary. The transmitted angle will be **larger** or

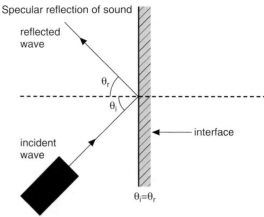

Figure 1–6. Specular reflection at an interface. (Adapted from Pinkney N: A Review of Concepts of Ultrasound Physics and Instrumentation. 4th ed. Sonicor, Inc., 1992. Reproduced with permission.)

smaller than the angle of incidence in proportion to an **increase** or **decrease** in the respective velocity. Refraction can result in improper placement of displayed echoes. (See Figure 1–7.)

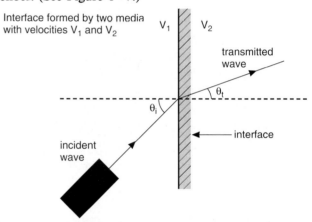

Figure 1–7. Refraction. (Adapted from Pinkney N: A Review of Concepts of Ultrasound Physics and Instrumentation. 4th ed. Sonicor, Inc., 1992. Reproduced with permission.)

Interfaces that are either smaller than the wavelength or not smooth are **nonspecular**. Scattering of the sound occurs at nonspecular interfaces. (See Figure 1–8.) Examples of nonspecular interfaces include red blood cells, liver parenchyma, and other materials representing the tissue characteristics of an organ.

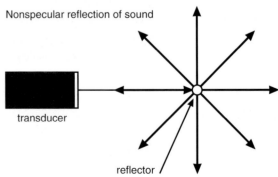

Figure 1–8. Scatter at a nonspecular interface. (Adapted from Pinkney N: A Review of Concepts of Ultrasound Physics and Instrumentation. 4th ed. Sonicor, Inc., 1992. Reproduced with permission.)

Resolution

Resolution is the minimum reflector separation required to produce separate reflections in a **pulse-echo** system.

Axial resolution is the minimum reflector separation **along the sound path** required to produce separate echoes.

The axial resolution, which does not vary with depth, is improved by using short **spatial pulse lengths**. High-frequency, highly damped transducers produce shorter spatial pulse lengths. See Figure 1–9, depicting good and poor axial resolution. **Lateral resolution** is the minimum reflector separation **perpendicular to the sound path** required to produce separate echoes. Lateral resolution, which is the **beam width**, can change with depth. Lateral resolution is affected by the **diameter** of the piezoelectric element and transducer **focusing**. Focusing creates a beam pattern with a smaller cross-sectional area. Lateral resolution is also improved when high-frequency transducers are used. See Figure 1–10, illustrating good and poor lateral resolution.

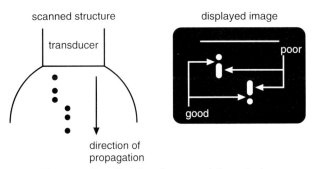

Figure 1–9. Good and poor axial resolution.

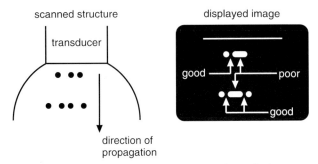

Figure 1–10. Good and poor lateral resolution.

Attenuation

Although higher-frequency transducers provide improved axial and lateral resolution, there is increased **attenuation**. Increased attenuation results in less penetration through the medium. Attenuation is the decrease in energy as a wave travels through a medium. Attenuation is caused by absorption, reflection, beam divergence, and scattering. Scattering increases with an increase in frequency. In human soft tissue, sound is attenuated at the rate of **0.5 decibel per centimeter per million hertz.** In bone, attenuation is greater and is more frequency-dependent, but in water, it is very low.

> NOTE: The decibel (dB) is a relative measure and is used to compare the relative intensities of two ultrasound beams. The dB is a function of the logarithm of the ratio of the two intensities. (Refer to Table 1–6A and B.)

TABLE 1–6A. Intensity Ratio vs. Decibel Value

INTENSITY RATIO	dB
1	0
2	3
4	6
8	9
1,000,000	60
0.50	−3
0.25	−6

From Pinkney N: A Review of Concepts of Ultrasound Physics and Instrumentation. 4th ed. Sonicor, Inc., 1992. Reproduced with permission.

TABLE 1–6B. Typical Transducer Frequencies

1.9 MHz		2.25 MHz
3.0 MHz		3.5 MHz
5.0 MHz	7.5 MHz	10.0 MHz

The lower frequencies are used for large patients or for any study that requires imaging at great depths.

Transducers in the 3.0 MHz or 3.5 MHz range are used for general-purpose imaging.

For studies of thin patients or small parts, higher frequencies may be used.

From Pinkney N: A Review of Concepts of Ultrasound Physics and Instrumentation. 4th ed. Sonicor, Inc., 1992. Reproduced with permission.

BIOEFFECTS

Bioeffects (biological effects) are the effects of ultrasound on tissue. The categories of bioeffects are **(1) heat, (2) cavitation,** and **(3) other.** Heat is the effect created by the motion of the vibrating molecules. Any heating is negligible when pulse ultrasound is used for diagnostic purposes. Cavitation results in the production of gas bubbles. Cavitation is possible when pulsed ultrasound with very high intensity is used. Cavitation can eventually result in damage to cell walls. The "other" category includes various minor mechanical effects that are not related to heat or cavitation.

Bioeffects have not been confirmed for pulsed ultrasound intensities below **100 milliwatts per square centimeter, SPTA.**

> NOTE: SPTA refers to a method often used to measure ultrasound intensities, where SP (spatial peak) is intensity measured at the center of a beam. TA (temporal average) indicates that the intensity is the average value during the periods of emission and reception.

Chapter 2

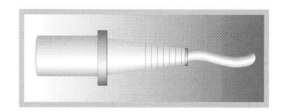

INSTRUMENTATION

M. NATHAN PINKNEY

BASIC PULSE-ECHO INSTRUMENTATION

A basic **pulse-echo** ultrasound system contains a **transducer** which, depending on its configuration, can contain one or more piezoelectric elements. The energy within a pulse-echo system is electrical but the energy in the pa-

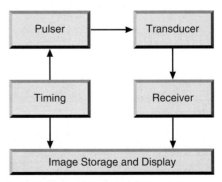

(Adapted from Pinkney N: A Review of Concepts of Ultrasound Physics and Instrumentation. 4th ed. Sonicor, Inc., 1992. Reproduced with permission.)

Chapter title illustration was adapted from Kremkau, F. Diagnostic Ultrasound-Principles, Instruments, and Exercises, 3rd ed. Philadelphia, WB Saunders Co., 1989, p. 69.

tient's body is sound, which is mechanical. The function of the transducer is to convert electrical energy into mechanical energy during transmission and to convert mechanical energy back into electrical energy during reception.

The **pulser** section of a pulse-echo system provides the shock excitation to the transducer. The excitation voltage from the pulser can be varied in some ultrasound systems. Varying the transducer's excitation voltage affects the amount of energy leaving the transducer. Typical controls that affect the pulser's voltage could be labeled:

TRANSMITTER
OUTPUT
ACOUSTIC POWER
PULSER POWER
ENERGY OUTPUT

A **receiver** is used to provide the initial processing of the received echo information. **Time gain compensation** (TGC), or **swept gain**, is a receiver function used to equalize differences in received echo amplitudes due to reflector depth. TGC provides gradually increasing **amplification** with depth. Amplification is the increasing of smaller voltages to larger ones. The TGC control is just one of the receiver-associated controls that affect the amplification of echoes. The actual names of the various controls will vary with each manufacturer. Typical controls that affect the amplification of echoes could be labeled:

NEAR GAIN
TGC DELAY
SLOPE (TGC)
FAR GAIN
OVERALL GAIN

Many manufacturers incorporate a group of sliding potentiometers to control the amplification of received echoes. Each potentiometer in the group is programmed

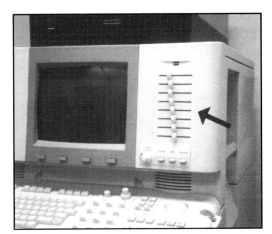

TGC Potentiometers.

to affect echoes returning from a specific depth. Some ultrasound displays include a **TGC curve**, which is a graphic display of the settings of the receiver's gain controls. Figure 2–1 shows image examples of abnormal and normal TGC settings.

Another receiver function is **dynamic range**, which is the ratio of the largest signal to the smallest signal that a system can handle. A wider dynamic range, which is often expressed in decibels (dB), ensures a wider range of displayed gray levels. **Compression** is a related function that *decreases* the difference between small and large amplitude signals. Compression effectively reduces the dynamic range of the receiver. Figure 2–2 is an image that shows narrow and wide dynamic range settings. Controls that permit the operator of an ultrasound system to vary the dynamic range could include:

DYNAMIC RANGE
COMPRESSION
LOG COMPRESSION

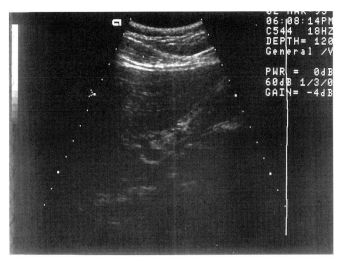

A. Without TGC

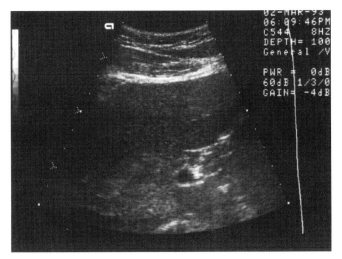

B. With TGC

Figure 2–1. Images with abnormal and normal TGC settings.

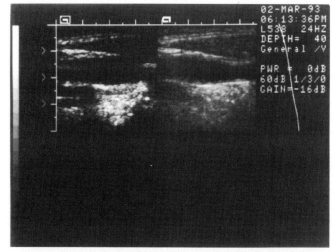

Left: Narrow dynamic range   Right: Wide dynamic range

Figure 2-2. Images with narrow and wide dynamic ranges.

The **timing** section of a pulse-echo system provides synchronization so that the returning echo information can be stored and then displayed with proper axial positions.

DISPLAY MODES

There are two basic display modes for returning echo information: A mode and B mode. (See Figure 2-3.)

A mode (A scan) provides an amplitude-modulated display. The escalation of the displayed spikes is a relative indication of the strength of returning echoes. The distance from the reference spike ("main bang") to other spikes along the baseline is an indication of the relative distances to the various reflectors.

B mode provides a brightness-modulated display where there is a change in spot brightness for each echo received by the transducer.

M mode (TM mode) is a graphic B mode display that is a single-dimension time display which represents the

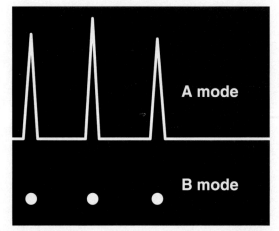

Figure 2-3. A mode and B mode. (Adapted from Pinkney N: A Review of Concepts of Ultrasound Physics and Instrumentation. 4th ed. Sonicor, Inc., 1992. Reproduced with permission.)

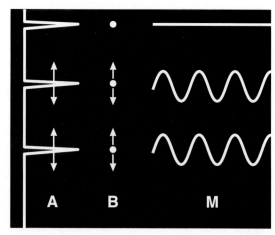

Figure 2-4. A mode, B mode, M mode. (Adapted from Pinkney N: A Review of Concepts of Ultrasound Physics and Instrumentation. 4th ed. Sonicor, Inc., 1992. Reproduced with permission.)

motion of various reflectors. M mode, which is commonly used during echocardiographic studies, is often provided as an option on general purpose ultrasound systems. Figure 2-4 shows examples of A mode, B mode, and M mode.

B scans are B mode displays that provide cross-sections of objects through scanning planes. The term *B scan* applies to both the older static and the newer **real-time** imaging systems. See Figure 2-5 for an image example of B scan, A mode, and M mode. Most static B scan systems were of the contact type. Contact scanners produced images with wide fields of view.

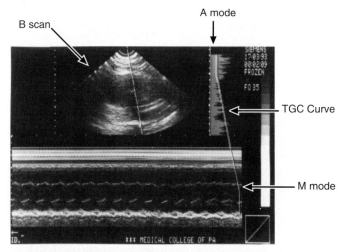

Figure 2-5. Image of A mode and M mode with real time sector B scanning.

CROSS-SECTIONAL IMAGE DISPLAY PATTERNS

The two basic real-time scanning formats for cross sectional imaging are **linear** and **sector**.

The linear format provides a rectangular field of view.

Linear scanning pattern.

The sector format provides either a pie-shaped or a trapezoidal field of view.

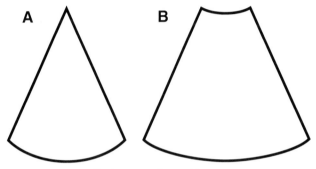

Sector scanning patterns.

The linear format displays a large field of view for structures close to the transducer. The linear format also provides greater accuracy when horizontal digital caliper measurements are made. However, the parallel acoustic beam format of the linear pattern often makes it difficult to obtain images of structures located beneath other anatomical areas. Moreover, it is often difficult to maintain complete skin contact with the large scanning surface of a linear transducer. Ultrasound scanners that produce sector images have overcome this primary disadvantage of the large linear transducer.

TRANSDUCER CONFIGURATIONS

A transducer typically used to provide a linear (rectangular) scanning pattern is a **linear array** transducer. The term *linear array* normally refers to a flat sequenced array, which contains a number of linearly arranged piezoelectric elements that are pulsed sequentially, in groups. Figure 2–6 gives examples of flat linear array transducers.

Each group of elements, when pulsed, generates an **acoustic line**; the same group waits for returning echoes before the next group is pulsed. The acoustic line from each group of elements of a flat sequenced array is parallel to the other acoustic lines produced. See Figure 2–7 for a drawing of sequenced linear array firing, and Figure 2–8 for an image produced with flat sequenced array.

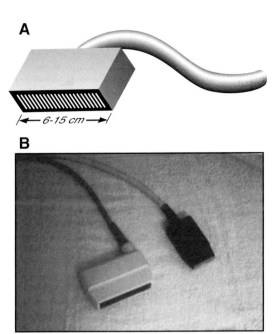

Figure 2–6. Flat linear array transducers. (Adapted from Pinkney N: A Review of Concepts of Ultrasound Physics and Instrumentation. 4th ed. Sonicor, Inc., 1992. Reproduced with permission.)

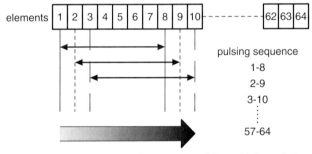

Figure 2–7. Sequenced linear array firing. (Adapted from Pinkney N: A Review of Concepts of Ultrasound Physics and Instrumentation. 4th ed. Sonicor, Inc., 1992. Reproduced with permission.)

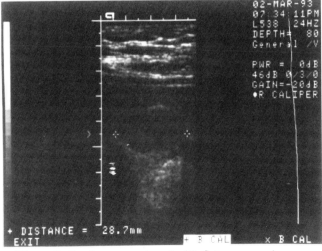

Figure 2–8. Image produced with flat sequenced array.

Another sequenced array transducer is the **curved linear array**, which is often termed **convex array**. Figure 2–9 depicts examples of curved linear array transducers.

Similar to the flat sequenced array, a curved linear array also contains a number of piezoelectric elements that are pulsed sequentially, in groups. The curved scanning surface of this transducer produces a sector cross-sectional image. (See Figure 2–10.)

A

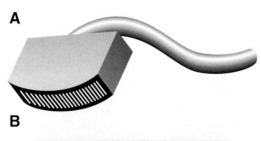

B

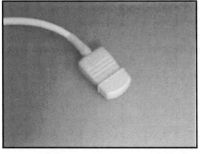

Figure 2–9. Curved linear array transducers. (From Pinkney N: A Review of Concepts of Ultrasound Physics and Instrumentation. 4th ed. Sonicor, Inc., 1992. Reproduced with permission.)

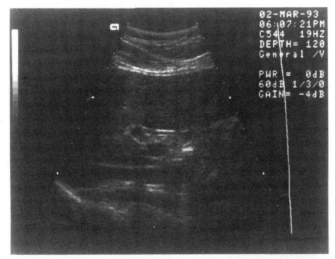

Figure 2–10. Image produced with curved linear array.

A **phased array** transducer contains a number of piezoelectric elements along a small scanning surface. Figure 2–11 gives examples of phased array transducers.

Each acoustic line from a phased array transducer is steered by pulsing all of the elements as one group, but with small time (phase) differences between them. (See Figure 2–12.)

A

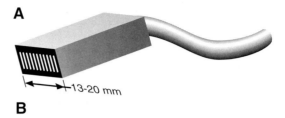

←13–20 mm→

B

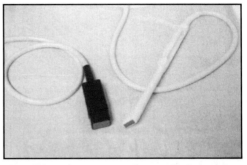

Figure 2–11. Phased array transducers. (Adapted from Pinkney N: A Review of Concepts of Ultrasound Physics and Instrumentation. 4th ed. Sonicor, Inc., 1992. Reproduced with permission.)

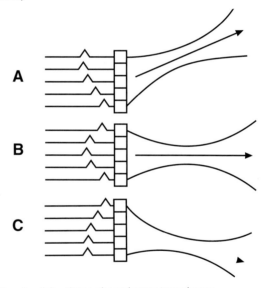

(For simplicity, these phased array transducers have been drawn with only 5 elements each)

Figure 2–12. Phased array beam steering. (Adapted from Pinkney N: A Review of Concepts of Ultrasound Physics and Instrumentation. 4th ed. Sonicor, Inc., 1992. Reproduced with permission.)

The phased array transducer produces a sector image; however, compared with the curved linear array, the skin contact area is much smaller and the pie-shaped sector image produced has a limited field of view of structures located near the skin surface. Figure 2–13 shows an image produced with a phased array transducer.

Recent developments in transducer technology have combined sequenced array and phased array techniques to produce a trapezoidal imaging format. This is accomplished by adding a sector field of view to both sides of a rectangular linear image.

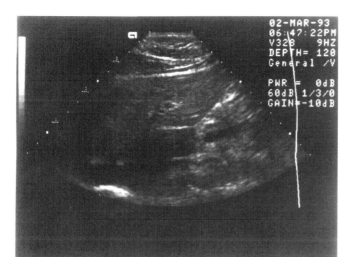

Figure 2–13. Image produced with phased array transducer.

Flat linear array, curved linear array, and phased array transducers have no moving parts. The electronics in the systems using these transducers can rapidly switch between different modes of operation to provide simultaneous display modes. The simultaneous display modes could include real time, M mode, or Doppler. Additionally, transducers containing arrays have electronic beam **focusing** capability. Electronic beam focusing is accomplished by varying the delays of the excitation voltages applied to an array's individual piezoelectric elements. This allows control of the width of each acoustic line to provide an improvement in the lateral resolution of the image.

A **mechanically steered** ultrasound transducer uses a motor to sweep or rotate one or more piezoelectric elements through a sector angle. Figure 2–14 provides examples of mechanically steered transducers.

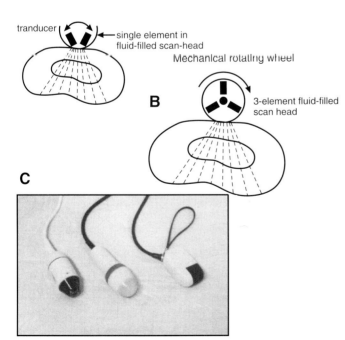

A Mechanical "wobbler"

tranducer ⟶ single element in fluid-filled scan-head

Mechanical rotating wheel

B 3-element fluid-filled scan head

C

Figure 2–14. Mechanically steered sector transducers.

A sector scanning pattern is produced when each excitation voltage produces a new acoustic line that travels at a slightly different angle from the previous acoustic line. Figure 2–15 shows an image produced with a mechanically steered transducer.

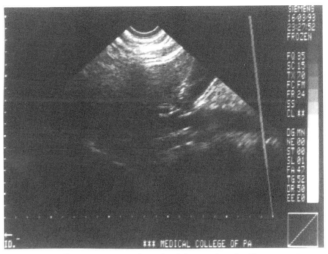

Figure 2–15. Image produced with mechanically steered sector transducer.

Some mechanically steered transducers contain **annular arrays**. An annular array is a group of ring-shaped elements that are arranged concentrically. (See Figure 2–16.)

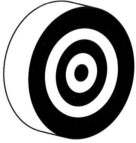

Figure 2–16. Annular array. (Adapted from Pinkney N: A Review of Concepts of Ultrasound Physics and Instrumentation. 4th ed. Sonicor, Inc., 1992. Reproduced with permission.)

Each acoustic line from an annular array can be electronically focused to achieve narrow beam widths throughout an area of interest to optimize the resolution of the image. Figure 2–17 shows a comparison of acoustic beam from conventional single element and acoustic beam from annular array.

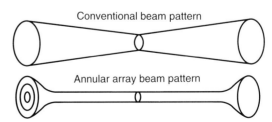

Conventional beam pattern

Annular array beam pattern

Figure 2–17. Conventional vs. annular array beam pattern. Comparison of acoustic beam from conventional single-element transducer and acoustic beam from annular array.

REAL-TIME FRAME RATES

A real-time ultrasound image is updated every fraction of a second to produce a live display. The **frame rate** represents how often the updating occurs. Generally, higher frame rates are useful for imaging rapidly moving structures, while lower frame rates improve image quality by increasing the number of acoustic lines that make up the image. Higher **pulse repetition frequencies** (PRFs) can also increase the number of acoustic lines, but high PRFs can limit the maximum depth that can be accurately imaged. Depending on the system, frame rates can be fixed or operator selectable, or can vary automatically. Frame rates that vary automatically often depend on the transducer frequency or the field of view size chosen by the operator.

IMAGE STORAGE AND DISPLAY

The signal that passes through the receiver of a pulse-echo system represents both echo-amplitude information and echo-position information. This information is normally **analog**, which means that it does not represent discrete values. A **scan converter** is used to convert the information from its original format into a signal format that can be fed to a standard **TV monitor**. (Refer to Figure 2–18.)

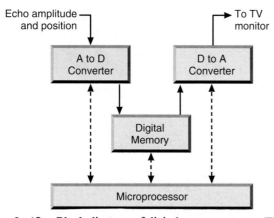

Figure 2–18. Block diagram of digital scan converter. (From Pinkney N: A Review of Concepts of Ultrasound Physics and Instrumentation. 4th ed. Sonicor, Inc., 1992. Reproduced with permission.)

The same TV signal can be fed to various image recording devices. During the conversion process, the information is temporarily stored in the scan converter's **digital memory**. The digital memory is an electronic device that stores discrete signals. Because the echo information is analog, it must first enter the digital scan converter's **analog-to-digital** (A-to-D) converter. One function of the A-to-D converter is to assign discrete

shades of gray to the incoming echo amplitudes. This process is called **preprocessing**. Figure 2–19 shows preprocessing assignments.

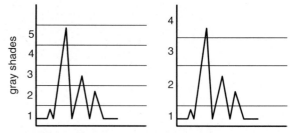

Figure 2–19. Preprocessing assignments. (Adapted from Pinkney N: A Review of Concepts of Ultrasound Physics and Instrumentation. 4th ed. Sonicor, Inc., 1992. Reproduced with permission.)

Selectable preprocessing permits the operator to vary the texture of the displayed image. Because preprocessing occurs prior to the digital memory, changing the selection will not affect any image information once it is stored. See Figure 2–20 for image examples of different preprocessing settings.

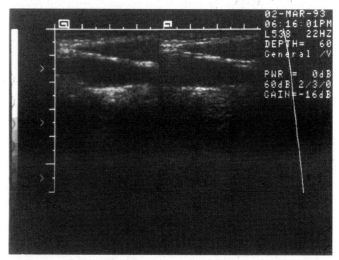

Figure 2–20. Images produced with different preprocessing settings.

Another image processing function that occurs prior to the digital memory is **write-magnification**. Selectable write-magnification permits the operator to electronically change the size of the displayed image prior to storage in the digital memory. Controls often associated with write-magnification include:

SCALE
FIELD OF VIEW
DEPTH
RES

Figure 2–21 shows images produced with different fields of view.

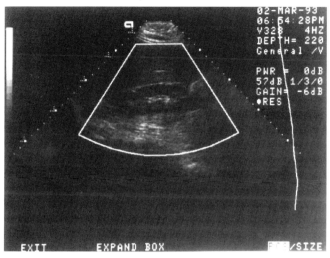 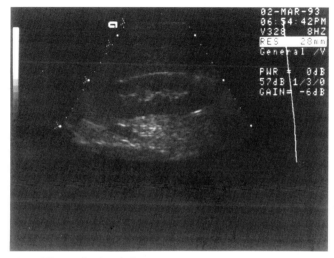

Figure 2–21. Images produced with different fields of view.

A typical digital memory is configured with an image-matrix memory size of **512 × 512**, which represents the number of rows and columns of digital picture elements, or **pixels**. Each pixel in a 512 × 512 matrix represents one of 262,144 discrete horizontal-vertical echo locations, which will be displayed as a specific shade of gray. (Refer to Figure 2–22.)

The maximum number of possible **gray scale** levels depends on the number of **bits** (binary digits) of information that can be stored and displayed for each horizontal-vertical location. Typical bit values are **4, 5, 6, 7, and 8** to provide **16, 32, 64, 128, or 256** gray scale levels, respectively. Because a TV monitor is designed to display analog information, the information stored in the scan converter's digital memory must be fed to a **digital-to-analog** (D-to-A) converter. One function of the D-to-A converter is to determine the brightness level that will be displayed for each gray scale level. This function is called **postprocessing**. Selectable postprocessing permits the operator to vary the emphasis given to various

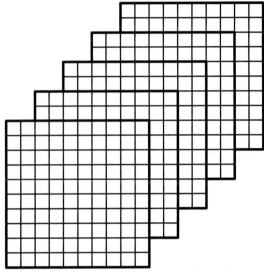

A typical pixel (picture element) matrix with a 5 bit memory (32 gray levels).

Figure 2–22. (Adapted from Pinkney N: A Review of Concepts of Ultrasound Physics and Instrumentation. 4th ed. Sonicor, Inc., 1992. Reproduced with permission.)

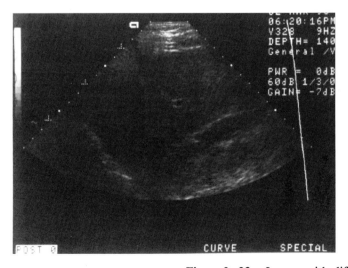 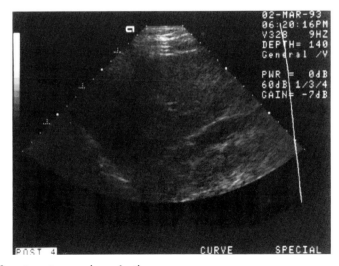

Figure 2–23. Images with different postprocessing selections.

gray scale ranges. Since postprocessing occurs after the digital memory, it can affect stored and live images. See Figure 2–23 for image examples of different postprocessing selections.

Another image processing function that occurs after the digital memory is **read-magnification**. Selectable read-magnification permits an operator to enlarge a selected area of the display by enlarging each pixel. By enlarging each pixel, fewer pixels are present on the display. Images magnified in this manner are coarse when compared to images that are magnified using write-magnification techniques. (See Figure 2–24.)

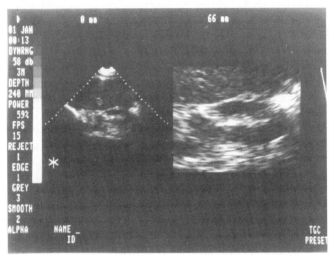

Left: Without read magnification   Right: With read magnification

Figure 2–24. Images without and with read magnification.

The TV monitors used in diagnostic ultrasound systems are designed to operate according to National Television Standards Committee (NTSC) specifications. Complete television pictures or frames are displayed on the cathode ray tube (CRT) **30** times every second. Each frame contains **525** horizontal scan lines. The frame's odd-numbered scan lines are produced first by an electron beam that illuminates the CRT's phosphor* by starting at the top and moving from left to right. The beam then turns off, drops down to the next odd-line position at the left, and moves again from left to right. This process repeats for every odd-line position down to the bottom of the CRT, producing **262½** lines. When the last odd line is finished, the electron beam shuts off and

returns to the top of the screen at the position of the first even line, and repeats the process from the top to the bottom of the CRT for all of the even lines. This process of "interlacing" an odd and even field every ¹⁄₆₀ second into one frame repeats end-on-end for successive ¹⁄₃₀ second frames. In addition to the horizontal and vertical placement of the CRT's electron beam, the aspect that determines a displayed pixel's brightness is the electron beam's intensity. This aspect is referred to as **luminance**.

DOPPLER INSTRUMENTATION

The **Doppler shift** is a change in frequency of a reflected wave due to relative motion between the reflector and the transducer's beam. The change in frequency is proportional to the velocity of the moving reflector. The higher the original (transmitted) frequency, the greater the shift in frequency for a given reflector velocity. The returning frequency increases if the reflector is moving toward the transducer and decreases if the reflector is moving away from the transducer. The Doppler effect produces the shift that is the reflected frequency minus the transmitted frequency. (See Figure 2–25.)

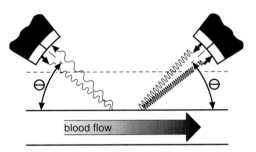

blood flow

Figure 2–25. Doppler shifts from blood vessel. *Left,* Flow away from the beam causes a shift to a lower frequency. *Right,* Flow toward the beam causes a shift to a higher frequency. (Adapted from Pinkney N: A Review of Concepts of Ultrasound Physics and Instrumentation. 4th ed. Sonicor, Inc., 1992. Reproduced with permission.)

A Doppler shift can only occur if the angle between the transducer's beam and the direction of movement of reflector (red blood cells) is *not* 90 degrees. The maximum Doppler shift occurs if the angle is zero. A basic **continuous wave** (CW) Doppler system contains a transducer with two piezoelectric elements, one for sending, and one for receiving. Figure 2–26 shows a diagram of a CW Doppler system.

The sending or source element is energized by a voltage generator that oscillates at the transducer's resonant frequency. When the reflected sound returns to the receiving element, it is converted into an electrical voltage, which is fed to a receiver. The receiver also receives a voltage with a frequency that was supplied to the source

---

*NOTE: A cathode ray tube (CRT) is an ultrasound system's display device. It is constructed of glass and encloses a vacuum. An electron gun at the rear of the CRT produces a narrow beam of electrons that travel through the cathode ray tube until it strikes the tube's face, which has a phosphor coating. When the electrons strike the phosphor, light is produced. Before reaching the phosphor, the electron beam passes through a changing magnetic field and is deflected to illuminated various areas of the phosphor. The beam's intensity is varied as it is being deflected to produce the various gray shades that are displayed.

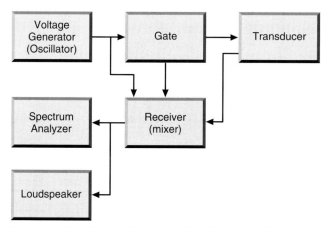

Figure 2–26. Block diagram of continuous wave Doppler system. (Adapted from Pinkney N: A Review of Concepts of Ultrasound Physics and Instrumentation. 4th ed. Sonicor, Inc., 1992. Reproduced with permission.)

element. The receiver electronically "mixes" the two voltages and produces, at its output, a voltage having a frequency representing the Doppler shift. The voltage can be fed to a loudspeaker to produce an audible sound or to a **spectrum analyzer** to provide a visual representation of the shift frequencies. CW Doppler is capable of detecting a wide range of shift frequencies that are caused by high blood flow velocities. A disadvantage of CW Doppler is that it detects all movement in the path of the beam and cannot selectively detect Doppler shifts from specific depths.

A **pulsed Doppler** or **gated Doppler** system is depth selective. Figure 2–27 shows a diagram of a pulsed Doppler system.

Figure 2–27. Block diagram of pulsed Doppler system. (Adapted from Pinkney N: A Review of Concepts of Ultrasound Physics and Instrumentation. 4th ed. Sonicor, Inc., 1992. Reproduced with permission.)

The **gate** section of the system controls the timing of the oscillation voltage that is periodically supplied to the transducer. Another function of the gate is to synchronize the receiver of the pulsed Doppler system. This synchronization results in information from the loudspeaker or spectrum analyzer that represents only the Doppler shifts from selected depths. A cursor can be superimposed over a cross-sectional B mode image to select the direction from which Doppler shift frequencies

are to be sampled. For pulsed Doppler operation, the cursor's gate is positioned to select the desired depth for Doppler frequency shift detection. A drawback of pulsed Doppler is the possibility of **aliasing**, which occurs when high blood flow velocities are present. Aliasing, which does not occur with CW Doppler, results in the display of incorrect Doppler shift information. It occurs when the Doppler shift exceeds the **Nyquist limit**. The Nyquist limit, which represents the maximum accurately detectable Doppler shift, is equal to one-half the Doppler pulse repetition frequency (PRF). The PRF of a pulse Doppler system represents intervals of transducer excitation controlled by the gate's timing function. Increasing the PRF raises the Nyquist limit, which increases the possibility of detecting greater velocities without aliasing. A high PRF may also result in **depth ambiguity**. Depth ambiguity reduces the maximum depth from which the location of a Doppler shift can be accurately detected. Other methods that can reduce the chances for aliasing include using a lower-frequency transducer or a steeper Doppler angle.

Conventional Doppler ultrasound systems are designed only to measure and indicate frequency shifts. Many systems also provide indications of blood flow velocity. Blood flow velocity is not measured, but calculated. The operator must position an "angle-correction" cursor parallel with the blood flow to ensure an accurate velocity calculation. Figure 2–28 is an image showing simultaneous real-time and Doppler displays. A **duplex**

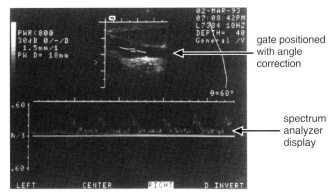

gate positioned with angle correction

spectrum analyzer display

Figure 2–28. Image showing simultaneous real-time and Doppler displays.

ultrasound system makes imaging and Doppler possible with the same transducer. A "true" duplex system is capable of providing "simultaneous" Doppler and real-time imaging from a single probe. Most linear array and electronically steered phased array imaging systems are capable of simultaneous Doppler and real-time imaging. In these systems, the same piezoelectric elements can be rapidly switched to permit their nearly simultaneous use for both functions. A mechanically steered probe requires separate piezoelectric elements for simultaneous Doppler and real-time imaging. (See Figure 2–29.)

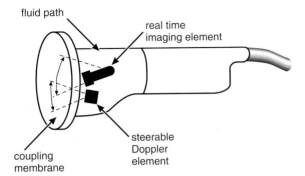

Figure 2–29. Mechanically steered duplex transducer. (Adapted from Pinkney N: A Review of Concepts of Ultrasound Physics and Instrumentation. 4th ed. Sonicor, Inc., 1992. Reproduced with permission.)

Color flow Doppler permits instantaneous global detection of the Doppler shift frequencies by superimposing colors over the normal white and black cross-sectional image. The displayed colors, with hues which normally range from red to blue, are used to indicate the direction of blood flow relative to the selected angle of Doppler detection. See Figure 2–30 for an image with color flow Doppler.

IMAGE RECORDING DEVICES

Ultrasound images may be recorded using various methods.

Photographic methods are routinely used to provide permanent **hard copies** by capturing images directly from TV monitors supplied with video signals from ultrasound system scan converters. Polaroid film makes it possible to make **hard-copy recordings** in black and white or color. Some Polaroid photographic devices are self-contained with built-in TV monitors.

Multi-image cameras are self-contained photographic devices with built-in TV monitors that can record multiple images on single sheets of film or photographic paper. The multiple recording positions are produced by moving lenses, multiple lenses, moving film cassettes, or combinations of techniques. The exposed film or paper is normally developed in an x-ray film processor to provide transparent or opaque hard-copy images.

Laser imagers also produce multiple images on single sheets of film using nonphotographic techniques. Laser imagers operate by capturing video frames in digital memories. The stored digital information is then used to

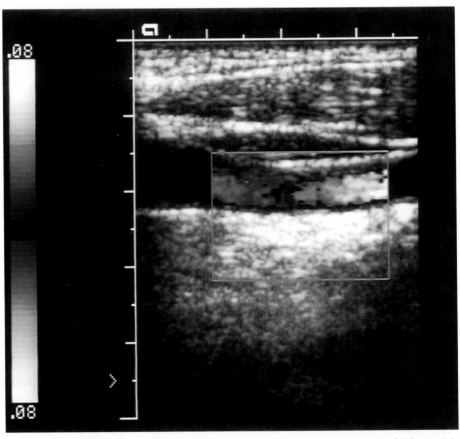

Figure 2–30. Color flow Doppler image. (See Color Plate 1 at the back of this book.)

control the intensity of a laser beam that exposes the film, using a sequential scanning technique.

Other nonphotographic hard-copy devices use thermal recording techniques. Black and white thermal printers use heat-sensitive paper as a recording medium. The image recorded on the paper is the result of the paper's passing over a multielement thermal head. The temperatures of the various elements are controlled by the TV signal information fed to the printer from the ultrasound system. A color thermal printer produces a hard-copy color image by using a thermal head to melt portions of a multicolored ribbon onto a sheet of paper.

Video tape recorders and disk recorders store TV image information using a magnetic medium. A video tape recorder can store live or frozen images. Disk recorders are designed to record frozen images. Because playback equipment is required for viewing the recorded information, the recordings themselves are not considered to be hard copies.

SECTION II

SONOGRAPHIC APPROACH TO UNDERSTANDING ANATOMY

Chapter 3

BODY SYSTEMS

DANIEL HAGAN

Objectives:

Describe the function of the musculoskeletal system.

Explain the motor, storage, and support capabilities provided by the musculoskeletal system.

Describe the function of the circulatory system.

Describe an artery and a vein, noting their differences.

Describe the function of the urinary system.

Trace the production of urine from the kidney to the urethra.

Describe the function of the digestive system.

Explain the digestive process from oral cavity to anus.

Describe the function of the respiratory system.

List the organs used in breathing.

Describe the function of the reproductive system.

Explain the normal menstrual cycle.

Describe male and female gamete production.

Describe the function of the endocrine system.

Explain the interrelationship of the various hormone-producing organs.

Describe the function of the central nervous system.

Explain how nerve impulses are transmitted.

Define the key words.

Key Words:

Abdomino-pelvic cavity	Endocrine
Alveoli	Epidermis
Anastomose	Estrogen
Apex	Follicle stimulating
Arteries	hormone
Autonomic system	Gametes
Base	Homeostasis
Bone marrow	Hormone
Collaterals	Human chorionic
Compact bone	gonadotropin
Convection	Hypodermis
Corpus luteum cyst	Involuntary muscles
Cranial cavity	Kidneys
Dermis	Large intestine
Diaphragm	Ligaments
Diastolic	Luteinizing hormone
Dorsal cavity	Lymph

Metabolism	Spinal cavity
Nephron	Spermatozoa
Neurons	Spongy bone
Ovum	Suprarenal glands
Peripheral system	Sweat glands
Peritoneal	Systolic
Phagocytes	Tendons
Pleura	Thoracic cavity
Renal pelvis	Trachea
Retroperitoneal	Tunica media
Rugae	Ureter
Sebaceous glands	Urinary bladder
Sequelae	Veins
Small intestine	Voluntary muscles

INTRODUCTION

Although the importance of having a thorough understanding of the specific anatomic organs and areas within the body will be stressed throughout this textbook, a general knowledge of body systems and their relationship(s) to one another is equally important. A general comprehension not only enables the sonographer to determine underlying events, but may also be the determining factor guiding him or her to further investigate other areas or body systems during a sonographic examination. Throughout this chapter on body systems, comparisons will be made as often as possible to everyday objects in order to provide a visual image.

One of the most important concepts a sonographer can master is the interdependence within the body. The sonographer is the equivalent of a detective: review evidence (laboratory values and patient history), interrogate the witness (scan body organs and vessels), and track clues (changes in normal appearance or flow) to identify the culprit (the area of origin).

Human Development

During embryo-fetal development, molecules form specific specialized cells determined by deoxyribonucleic acid (DNA). These cells unite to form organs that work together to form a system (eg, several anatomic organs form the digestive system). Each organ has a specialized function, or possibly multiple functions that it must carry out (eg, ovaries are both endocrine and exocrine organs) based on the type of tissue cells that were formed as a group. There are a multitude of cell and tissue types that have specific functions (eg, nephrons within the

kidneys, neurons within the brain). These systems work together to control the body's **metabolism** (build-up and breakdown of various chemicals) in order to maintain **homeostasis** (equilibrium).

Body Cavities

The body has several natural "vaults" that contain organs within a region. (See Figure 3–1.) A brief list is presented below; details will be provided in upcoming chapters.

The **ventral cavity** is composed of the following cavities:

Abdominopelvic Cavity. Cavity whose boundaries are the pubic bone inferiorly and the diaphragm superiorly.

Thoracic Cavity. Enclosed area that basically corresponds to the rib cage. It is separated from the abdominal cavity by its inferior boundary, the diaphragm.

Peritoneal. Anterior area of the abdominopelvic cavity within the peritoneal lining.

Retroperitoneal. Posterior area of the abdominopelvic cavity, located posterior to the peritoneal lining.

The **dorsal cavity** is composed of the following cavities:

Cranial Cavity. Containing the brain (calvarium).

Spinal Cavity. Containing the spinal cord.

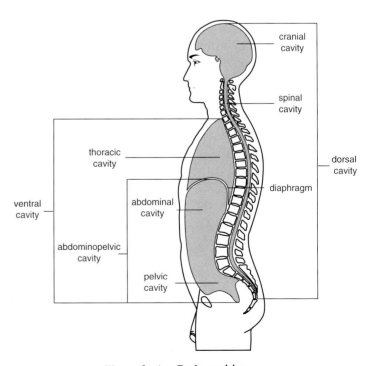

Figure 3–1. Body cavities.

MUSCULOSKELETAL SYSTEM

Function

The musculoskeletal system (see Figure 3–2A and B) is a support system best compared to a high-rise building. Similar to the framework of a building, the bones enable other systems to attach and provide a means to counteract gravity. This system has several basic functions.

Ligaments attach bones to one another; **tendons** attach muscle to bone, allowing for movement. Both the bony skeleton and the muscles themselves unite to perform movement. The bones provide areas for muscle attachment via the tendons; with articulation areas, movement is now possible through contraction and relaxation. Various joint types (ball and socket, hinge, and others) allow movement.

Both bone and muscle provide protection from external forces. Although there are many other protective mechanisms within the body, as described elsewhere in this book, bone and muscle combine to form a protective covering for the vital organs. The brain and heart are excellent examples. The brain is encased in the bony protective calvarium, while the heart and lungs are surrounded by a bony cage (the rib cage).

Blood cell production occurs within the bone marrow and plays a vital role. Blood cells usually function for only 120 days at most before wearing out, at which time they break down into amino acids and other proteins.

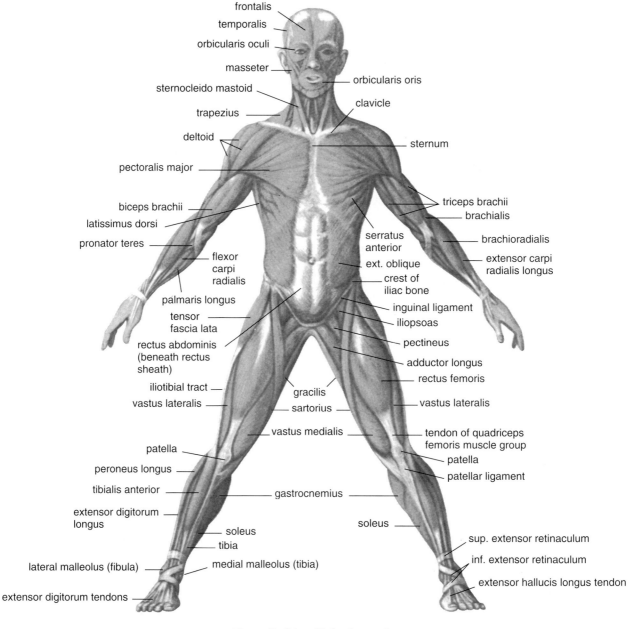

Figure 3–2A. Skeletal muscles.

Should the marrow cease to function appropriately as in leukemia or severe radiation damage, death is certain due to the inability to replace dying blood cells. One mechanism which affects red blood cell (RBC) production is erythropoietin (a hormone) produced in the kidneys. Major functions are often "controlled" by completely dissimilar systems, a type of protective measure in case the primary system fails due to disease processes.

There is decreased venous pressure in the lower limbs due to the effects of gravity. Muscle contraction moves blood up through the veins assisted by valves that prevent the blood from returning downward after each contraction. Normal contraction and relaxation cycles occur when one walks.

The bones contain minerals including calcium, sodium, and potassium. These chemicals are mobilized and transported by the blood stream to any part of the body as needed. This is accomplished via the release of specific hormones and chemicals that break down bone.

Each bone is composed of a hard outer shell termed **compact bone** and a softer inner core, the **bone marrow.** Between the hard outer core and the soft marrow is a honeycomb type of bone structure termed **spongy bone.** This is similar to aircraft wings, which are made of a hard outer shell and a honeycomb inner carbon material. This construction permits moderate flexing without causing stress fractures. (See Figure 3–3.)

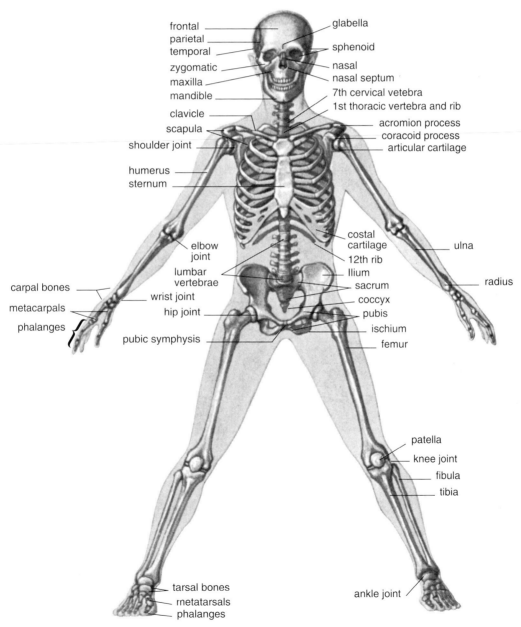

Figure 3–2B. Skeletal bones.

Muscle Types

Muscles fall into two categories: The **voluntary muscles** are those in which flexion and extension are controlled by the person. **Involuntary muscles** are those in which muscle action is controlled by the autonomic nervous system (cardiac and visceral). Involuntary muscles control various body activities without our thinking about them (the heartbeat and digestion are examples).

CIRCULATORY SYSTEM

Function

The circulartory system is a network of tubes and tubules responsible for transporting blood, oxygen, and nutrients throughout the body and getting rid of waste. This system relies on a single pump, the heart.

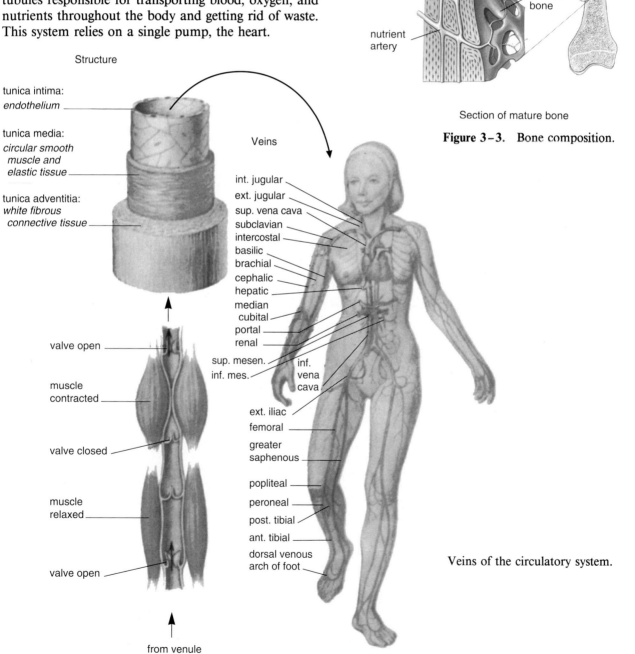

Figure 3–3. Bone composition.

Veins of the circulatory system.

Composition of Arteries and Veins

The circulatory system is composed of arteries, arterioles, veins, venules, and capillary beds. There are differences in structure, mainly related to the thickness of the musculature area (the **tunica media**) within an artery or vein. (See Figure 3–4.) The difference in structure is directly related to the pressures that are maintained within those vessels. Arteries must withstand higher pressures than veins; thus their muscular layers are proportionately thicker.

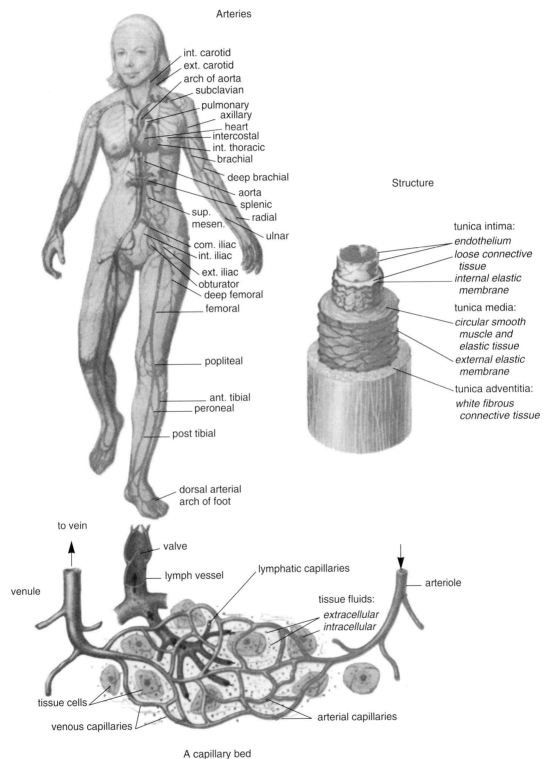

Arteries of the circulatory system, and a capillary bed.

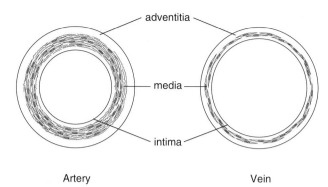

Figure 3-4. Structure of arteries and veins.

The difference in structure is an asset in renal dialysis procedures. An artery is connected to a vein in the forearm, forcing the vein to expand; a tube inserted within the vein sustains this distended state. As a result, the patient can undergo dialysis several times per week with much less likelihood of rupture of the vein.

Blood Flow Throughout the Body

The left side of the heart and the arterial system are under high pressure (**systolic**) whereas the right side of the heart and venous vessels are under low pressure (**diastolic**). Generally, the **arteries** carry oxygenated blood, and the **veins** transport deoxygenated blood. There are two exceptions as follows: During fetal circulation the umbilical vein carries oxygenated blood; the umbilical arteries carry deoxygenated blood. Also, the pulmonary artery and pulmonary veins are functionally reversed: the artery carries deoxygenated and the veins carry oxygenated blood.

As previously described, blood in the legs would stagnate were it not for the presence of valves within the veins, along with muscular contraction. Arteries do not contain valves, the exception being the pulmonic and aortic valves. The thick muscular wall in the arteries squeezes the blood forward. (Refer to Figure 3-4.)

Special Situations

There are two body areas in which the blood flow is unique—the liver and the kidney. In most organs blood flow is as follows:

Artery→Arteriole→Capillary→Venule→Vein
(Refer to Figure 3-8.)

Blood enters the liver via the hepatic artery. In the liver the hepatic artery conveys blood to the liver cells to provide nourishment and energy. The unusual circumstance is that there is simultaneously free mixing of portal venous and hepatic arterial blood (deoxygenated with oxygenated). Blood is carried away from the liver via the hepatic veins, which drain into the inferior vena cava. Note: Mixing of oxygenated and deoxygenated blood

within the liver is possible due to the close proximity of the heart.

Also, the kidney contains two sets of capillary beds rather than a single set (as is the case in all other areas). This additional set enables the kidney to maintain a state of blood pressure equilibrium, a safety feature that maintains blood pressure even when systemic pressure changes occur. (See Figure 3-5.)

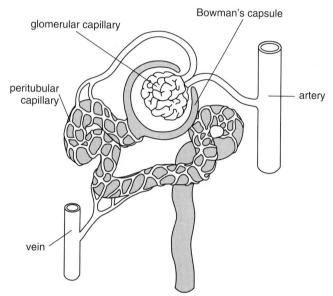

Figure 3-5. The two capillary beds of the kidney.

Conditions Due to Prolonged Venous Hypertension

Veins under constant pressure begin to expand. We might compare this body with the plumbing in a house. If pressure in the plumbing is increased excessively, the result is a burst pipe. In humans the result is an increase in the size of a vein or organ. One of two things then happens: (1) A nearby organ might begin to enlarge (eg, hepatomegaly, splenomegaly). The cause of such dilation can be determined by tracking its point of origin. (2) If there is no organ near the area of expansion collaterals may develop. **Collaterals** are analogous to detours due to roadwork. The vessel under pressure will seek assistance from nearby vessels and **anastomose** (create an additional connection) to those vessels.

Lymphatic System

The lymphatic system has two major functions, the first being to transport excess fluid out of the tissues and back to the bloodstream, and the second being to attack harmful bacteria and foreign substances through phagocytes within the lymph nodes. (The special function of phagocytes is to destroy foreign substances). Without this transport capability excess fluid in the tissues would develop (called edema).

When harmful bacteria are destroyed an immune response may occur in which a foreign substance is recognized as hostile and is destroyed by white blood cells (WBC). In an infection, macrophages (large phagocytes) are created in such large numbers within the lymph nodes that the lymph node increases in size.

The lymphatic system is similar to the circulatory system, the only major differences being that the lymphatic system lacks a pump; lymph travels in only one direction, and the lymphatic system contains lymph nodes. (See Figure 3–6.) Lymphatic vessels throughout the body course along with the circulatory system. During blood exchange in the capillary beds, some fluid (**lymph**) remains within the tissues and must be eliminated. The excess fluid is transported via the lymphatic vessels and is filtered through the lymph nodes as the lymph courses toward the thorax. Lymphatic flow is identical to venous flow via muscle contraction. Lymph nodes along the lymphatic system (groin, axilla, neck, and periaortic area), are "stations" that the lymph must pass through on its way toward the chest, being filtered in the process. Once in the chest, lymph reenters the bloodstream which is essential in maintaining the correct level of fluid within the blood. The spleen is part of the lymphatic system; its function is to eliminate wornout blood cells from the circulatory system.

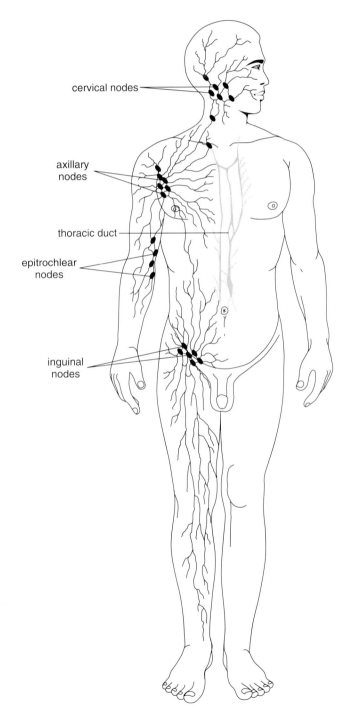

cervical nodes

axillary nodes

thoracic duct

epitrochlear nodes

inguinal nodes

Figure 3–6. The lymphatic system.

URINARY SYSTEM

Function

The basic function of the urinary system is to filter out waste products such as urea, uric acid, and creatinine, while maintaining a state of equilibrium within the body. When blood is filtered in the kidneys, wastes are removed but much of the water and other substances required by the body is reabsorbed and becomes part of the general circulation. Additional functions of the kidney include producing substances that influence blood pressure, producing erythrocytes (red blood cells), and maintaining serum levels of phosphate and calcium.

Anatomy

The urinary system is made up of paired kidneys and ureters (one on each side of the body), as well as a bladder and urethra. On the superior medial surface of each kidney is an adrenal gland, discussed in the endocrine system section of this chapter. (See Figure 3–7.)

Each kidney has its own artery, vein, and ureter emanating from the renal hilum. As noted earlier, there is a slight variation in the circulation of blood within the kidney related to the existence of an additional capillary bed not commonly found in other areas (blood pressure regulators).

The functional structure of the kidney is the **nephron.** There are over a million microscopic nephrons in each kidney. A nephron is shown in Figure 3–8; note that its major components are a glomerulus and tubules. Each glomerulus is a cluster of capillaries derived from the afferent arteriole.

Figure 3–7. The urinary system. The **kidneys** are bean-shaped organs situated in the posterior part of the abdomen at about the height of the elbows. Each kidney functions independently. The **renal pelvis** is a funnel-shaped reservoir that collects urine from all parts of the kidney. Urine leaves the kidney by way of the **ureter** and passes to the **bladder,** where it is temporarily stored. Urine is excreted from the bladder through the **urethra.** Although the **suprarenal glands** (also called adrenal glands) are located one above each kidney, they are not part of the urinary system. The adrenal glands are endocrine glands that secrete several hormones.

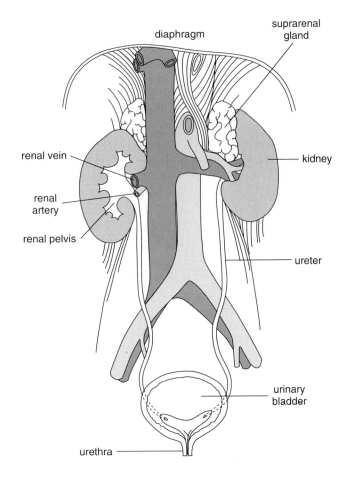

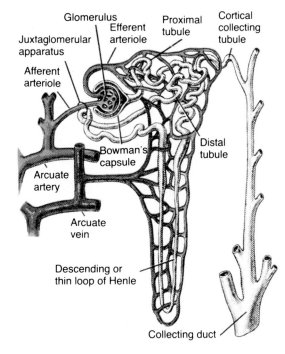

Figure 3–8. A nephron and surrounding capillaries. (From Guyton AC: Textbook of Medical Physiology, 6th ed. Philadelphia, W. B. Saunders, 1981.)

Filtration

Within the renal cortex, the glomeruli inside Bowman's capsule act to filter the blood passing through. (Refer to Figure 3–8.) An analogy for this action is to compare the kidneys to a washing machine. Cells within Bowman's capsule have "slits" that allow smaller molecules to pass, while keeping larger molecules from passing through. In a washing machine, waste products are removed by size much in the same way. Laundry is spun allowing water to run through the small holes (waste) yet keeping the clothes (blood cells) where they belong. Damage to the kidneys would be the equivalent of in-creasing the hole size and letting unwanted substances such as blood cells pass through (ie, gross hematuria).

Urine Flow

Utilizing gravity, urine leaves the renal pyramids toward the renal pelvis via the major and minor calyces, one drop at a time. Urine leaves the renal pelvis, descends the ureter, and enters the urinary bladder in streams termed "jets" that are commonly seen on ultrasound. The bladder temporarily stores the urine until it is excreted from the body via the urethra.

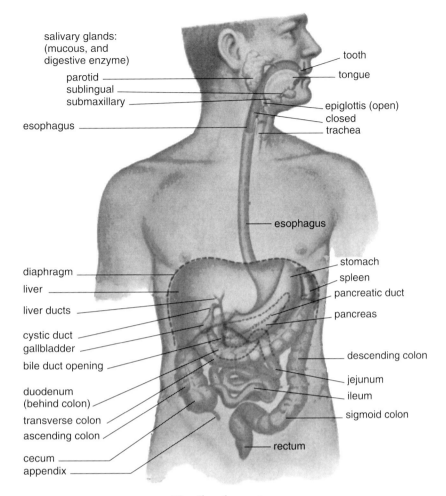

salivary glands:
(mucous, and
digestive enzyme)
parotid
sublingual
submaxillary
esophagus

tooth
tongue
epiglottis (open)
closed
trachea

esophagus

diaphragm
liver
liver ducts
cystic duct
gallbladder
bile duct opening
duodenum
(behind colon)
transverse colon
ascending colon
cecum
appendix

stomach
spleen
pancreatic duct
pancreas
descending colon
jejunum
ileum
sigmoid colon
rectum

The digestive system.

DIGESTIVE SYSTEM

Function

The function of the digestive system is to convert ingested food into substances the body uses to maintain metabolism. The mouth, esophagus, stomach, small intestine, colon, liver, and pancreas work together in the breakdown and absorption process. The gallbladder also participates by storing and releasing bile that is produced in the liver when chyme (semidigested material) is detected.

Anatomy

From the oral cavity to the anus, the digestive canal is one long unbroken tube. The stomach consists of folds call **rugae** that allow expansion and contraction. Between the rugae are glands that secrete acid and mucus.

The **small intestine** consists of villi, finger-like projections that add to the overall surface volume of the intestine and function to absorb substances such as nutrients and minerals from digested food. (See Figure 3–9.) In

addition to producing enzymes capable of digesting lipids (fats), carbohydrates, and proteins, the small intestine receives enzymes from the common bile duct and pancreatic duct to aid in digestion.

The **large intestine** transports unabsorbed material to the sigmoid colon and anus to be expelled. A note of importance to the sonographer is the vermiform appendix (part of the cecum of the intestine), which can become inflamed, and is demonstrable on ultrasound.

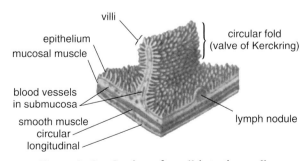

villi
epithelium
mucosal muscle
circular fold
(valve of Kerckring)
blood vessels
in submucosa
smooth muscle
circular
longitudinal
lymph nodule

Figure 3–9. Section of small intestine wall.

RESPIRATORY SYSTEM

Function

The respiratory system provides a means of supplying oxygen to the body while eliminating carbon dioxide, which is a natural bioproduct of cellular activity.

Anatomy

Air enters the body via the **trachea,** which subdivides into bronchi, bronchioles, alveolar ducts, and alveoli. The **alveoli** are small sacs with a very thin tissue lining, which facilitates the exchange of gases (oxygen and carbon dioxide). (See Figure 3–10A and B.)

The lungs, contained within the thoracic cavity, are

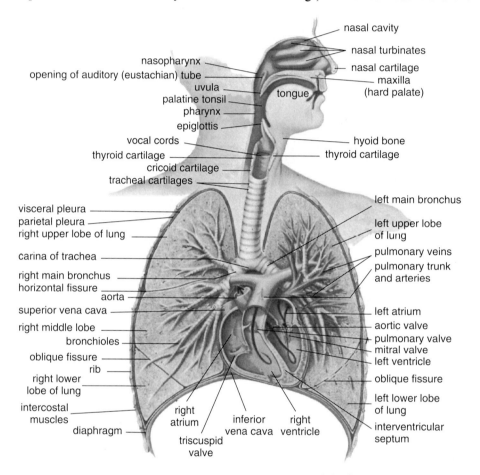

Figure 3–10A. The respiratory system and the heart.

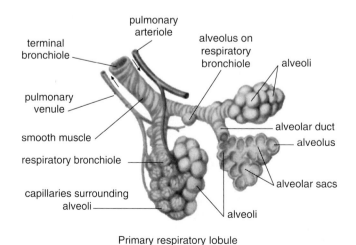

Primary respiratory lobule

Figure 3–10B. Alveoli.

somewhat triangular in shape with their **apex** superior and **base** inferior. The lungs are separated from the abdominal cavity by the muscular diaphragm located at the base of the lungs. They are divided into lobes with the right having three lobes and the left only two. The lungs are surrounded by a double-walled sac called the **pleura** (visceral and parietal pleura). These two sacs, with pleural fluid between them, enable the lung to expand and contract without adhering to the walls. Pressure within the lungs is below atmospheric pressure, which causes the lungs to remain partially inflated at all times. Diaphragmatic movement enables inhalation and exhalation. In the fetus, the pressure within the lungs is not less than the atmospheric pressure, which results in the fetal lungs maintaining a collapsed state until birth. The lungs receive their blood supply from the descending aorta.

REPRODUCTIVE SYSTEM

Function

The reproductive system provides a means to perpetuate the species. The male and female reproductive systems differ from the previously described systems in that they do nothing directly to contribute to the survival of the human body such as breathing, blood flow, and digestion.

Male spermatozoa and a female ovum (called **gametes** or germ cells) must combine in order for fertilization to occur. Fertilization normally occurs within the fallopian tube with implantation occurring by the seventh day after ovulation.

Male Gamete Production

Spermatozoa are produced in the testes and mature in the epididymis. The vas deferens transports the sperma-

tozoa from the epididymis and is joined by the seminal vesicle prior to becoming the ejaculatory duct. The ejaculatory duct courses through the prostate, joining the prostatic urethra, and exits the penis via the urethra. The scrotum is capable of protraction and retraction which aids in spermatozoa production and maintenance. The scrotum actually moves away from the body if the temperature is too high and closer to the body if the temperature is too low.

Female Gamete Production and Fertilization

Following is the process involved in ovulation and attempted fertilization from the beginning of the menstrual cycle:

1. **Follicle-stimulating hormone** (FSH) is released by the pituitary gland, which stimulates the ovaries to produce follicles.

2. **Estrogen** is released by ovarian tissue during the FSH release in order to prepare the endometrium lining the uterus for possible implantation.

3. **Luteinizing hormone** (LH) is released on approximately the fourteenth day of the menstrual cycle, which stimulates the follicle to burst and release its ovum. The empty follicle becomes a corpus luteum cyst, which is maintained by LH release. The ovum enters the fallopian tube, moving toward the endometrial canal of the uterus.

4. The **corpus luteum cyst** releases both estrogen and progesterone.

5. The detection of progesterone released by the corpus luteum cyst causes LH to stop being released. This disrupts maintenance of the corpus luteum cyst and subsequent menstruation.

If pregnancy occurs, the corpus luteum cyst is maintained. No other follicles are stimulated during the re-

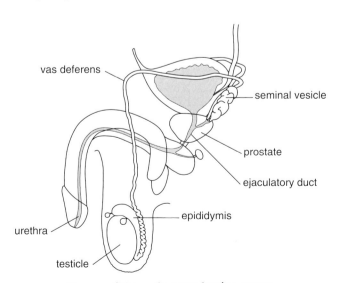

Organs of the male reproductive system.

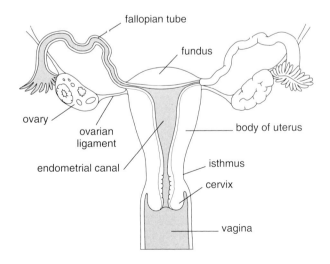

Organs of the female reproductive system.

maining months of the pregnancy. Below are the differences that occur in the presence of fertilization:

1. The blastocyst (embryonic cell) releases an enzyme prior to implantation which "loosens" the implantation site, enabling it to bury itself deep into the endometrium.

2. A second release from the blastocyst prevents the endometrium from being shed and maintains the corpus luteum, thus suppressing menstruation. The hormone BhCG or **human chorionic gonadotropin** can now be detected via blood or urine for pregnancy testing.

Union of the spermatozoa and ovum usually occurs within the fallopian tube. The cells undergo several cell divisions prior to implantation within the uterus. Twins develop due to either the fertilization of two separate ova or division of the embryo prior to implantation (refer to Chapter 18 for diamniotic and dichorionic definitions). Embryonic division beyond the twelfth day after fertilization results in the development of Siamese twins (conjoined).

ENDOCRINE SYSTEM

Function

The endocrine system regulates other body systems based on nerve impulse information and direct blood level information performed by the body. It is regulated by the hypothalamus of the brain.

The endocrine system is composed of eight glands that may be considered the body's messengers. (See Figure 3–11.) Chemicals released from the various organs may act on a specific tissue type or several tissues in general. The term **endocrine** means ductless. The released substance enters directly into the bloodstream. These chemical substances are called hormones.

Target areas within the brain monitor the levels of many chemicals within the body. These receptors are said to control whether a releasing or inhibiting chemical is released, which acts directly upon the pituitary gland.

The effect of each hormone on the body varies. The term **hormone** is a general classification. For example, the hormone insulin has a different function from the reproductive or thyroid hormones.

Glands of the Endocrine System

The following lists each endocrine gland, some of the hormones each produces, and its general function.

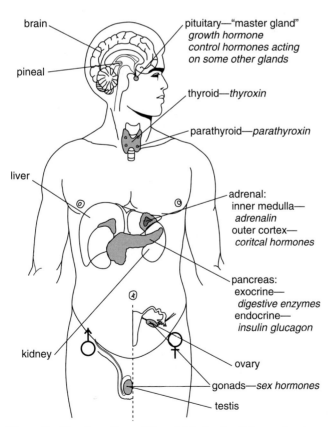

Figure 3–11. Location of the eight glands of the endocrine system.

Pituitary Gland

Follicle stimulating hormone (FSH)	Assists in ovarian follicle development in females
Luteinizing hormone (LH)	and sperm maturation in males
Thyrotropin (TSH)	Thyroid-stimulating hormone
Adrenocorticotropin (ACTH)	Adrenal stimulating hormone
Growth hormone (GH)	Stimulates growth in general.
Prolactin	Initiates and maintains milk secretion in females.

Thyroid Gland

Thyroxine (T_4) Triiodothyronine (T_3) Note: The number in parentheses indicates the number of attached iodine cells (eg, thyroxine + 4 iodine cells)	Responsible for assisting in metabolism of lipids, proteins, and carbohydrates. Their presence can increase the body's need for oxygen. This leads to increased heat production (body temperature elevation) that will influence most tissues.
Calcitonin	Responsible for removing calcium via absorption. This causes calcium to be removed from the blood and sent to the bones for storage.

Parathyroid Glands

Parathyroid hormone (PTH)	Basic antagonist for calcitonin. PTH sends a signal causing bone reabsorption. If the body is low in calcium, it will take what it needs from the bones, adding calcium to the bloodstream.

Adrenal Glands

Epinephrine	Causes blood glucose levels to elevate. The heart races and major vessels dilate. It also causes ACTH to be released from the pituitary.
Norepinephrine	Causes diastolic and systolic blood pressure to increase. It is also a vasoconstrictor, and causes peripheral vessels to constrict. It makes sense to keep the blood flow where needed in the heart, lungs, and voluntary muscles—for running.
Mineralocorticoids	Control sodium and potassium levels.
Glucocorticoids	Control glucose use by conserving consumption (ACTH controlled).

Pancreas

Insulin	Controls the uptake/use of glucose to prevent glycogen breakdown within the liver; it is responsible for decreasing the blood sugar level. Glucagon antagonist to glucocorticoids; it increases the blood sugar level.

Ovaries

Estrogen	Responsible for female secondary sex characteristics. Released during the menstrual cycle to prepare the uterus for possible implantation.
Progesterone	Released during the menstrual cycle to prepare the uterus for possible implantation.

Testes

Testosterone	Responsible for male sex characteristics.

CENTRAL NERVOUS SYSTEM

Function

The central nervous system is the body's "computer." It is responsible for processing input data from all areas of the body. **Neurons** (nerve cells) transmit messages to and from the brain, controlling everything from pain sensation to coordination, from high-level cognitive processing to the endocrine-regulating hypothalamus.

Anatomy

The brain and spinal cord are the main components of the central nervous system. They are well protected by bone, the cranial vault and the spinal column which surrounds these structures like protective armor.

The central nervous system is classified into peripheral and autonomic nervous systems, also referred to as voluntary and involuntary control. The **peripheral system** is responsible for voluntary actions such as walking. The **autonomic system** controls involuntary actions of the heart, endocrine glands, and other internal organs.

The brain receives blood via two carotid arteries and two vertebral arteries. Although relatively small, these vessels receive approximately 20 percent of the total blood flow. Blood exits the cranium via the jugular veins. Because of its blood supply requirements, the brain is susceptible to severe perfusion **sequelae** (conditions associated with changes in blood flow).

Neuron

A neuron is a nerve cell, responsible for transmitting impulses much the same way that a wire carries an electric charge. Most nerve cells are covered by a myelin sheath, which is analogous to the plastic covering or insulation of a wire or cord. When neurons are damaged, other neurons often attempt to compensate by assuming additional tasks.

Special Sensory Organs: The Ear and the Eye

The ear is composed of three parts: outer, middle, and inner. The outer ear (the pinna or auricle) focuses sound toward the middle ear. The middle ear consists of the tympanic membrane and the three smallest bones of the body—malleus, incus, and stapes. Their function is to conduct sound to the inner ear, which is composed of the cochlea and semilunar canals. The inner ear is responsible for both balance and conversion of physical sound waves to electrical impulses that the brain can recognize. This is similar to a reverse piezoelectric effect (see Chapter 1).

The eye functions like a camera. Light is focused toward the back of the eye, to be recorded or converted into a signal recognizable by the brain. The eye focuses on thousands of objects every day. It is estimated that 12 video cameras would be required to match the recording capabilities that the eye performs in a single day.

The cornea of the eye serves to refract (bend) light through the iris and lens toward the retina at the back for processing. Problems with the lens and/or cornea cause light to be refracted to the back of the eye, but not toward the retina. In this case, glasses are needed to correct the refraction problem.

The eyelids shield the eye from debris and impact. They also clean the surface of the eyes—similarly to the action of windshield wipers.

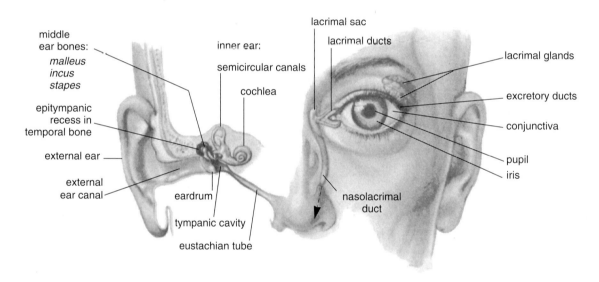

1. The ear; the eye.

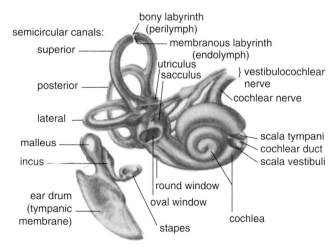

2. The middle ear and the inner ear.

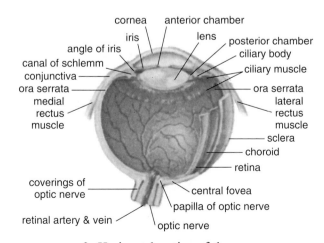

3. Horizontal section of the eye.

SUMMARY

The body has many specialized cells and tissues having highly specific functions. These cells and tissues allow the body to maintain a state of equilibrium (balance) by performing their individual duties and working together. Body compartments (cavities) separate many of these systems from one another.

Muscles and bones afford physical protection and work together in movement. Bones are a reservoir for calcium and produce blood cells within the marrow. Muscles are subgrouped into those that the individual controls (voluntary) and those that are not under the individual's control (involuntary).

The circulatory system (blood and lymph) carries vital nutrients to the tissues and removes excess fluid. Lymph in the capillaries is filtered as it passes through the lymph nodes to remove foreign bodies. Both the circulatory system and the lymphatic system depend on muscle contraction for transport.

The urinary system filters waste from the blood and helps maintain the body's equilibrium. Blood is filtered through the nephrons of the kidney which also serve to reabsorb water and other substances that the body can utilize. The kidneys also influence blood pressure, the production of red blood cells, and serum levels of phosphate and calcium.

The digestive system metabolizes ingested food. Starting at the oral cavity, mastication (chewing) and saliva begin the initial breakdown of food. The stomach is the organ in which gastric acids begin to further break down the food so that it may enter the small intestine. At the duodenum, both pancreatic enzymes and hepatic bile aid in breaking down lipids and proteins, illuminating the importance of both the pancreas and liver as accessory organs to the digestive system. The small intestine also absorbs essential nutrients and then passes the chyme on to the large intestine for expulsion at the anus.

Oxygen and carbon dioxide are exchanged across a thin alveolar membrane during inhalation and exhalation assisted by the diaphragm. Although the lungs are not routinely evaluated by ultrasound, excess fluid in the pleural sac (pleural effusion) and infectious pus pockets (empyema) may be demonstrated.

Reproduction of the species is very intricate as demonstrated by the number of hormones required to prepare for and maintain a pregnancy. Equally important is the capability of protraction and retraction of the scrotum to aid in spermatozoa maintenance.

The endocrine system enables the body to regulate a multitude of functions by detecting changes in blood chemistry. Release of hormones directly into the bloodstream ensures immediate response to the hypothalamus's signal regulating blood pressure, blood sugar, calcium levels, and other body functions.

The brain controls all actions within the body via both voluntary and involuntary muscle signaling. Additional functions of the brain include control of sensory areas (sight, hearing, smelling, and touch) and regulatory areas (hypothalamus and pituitary control of the endocrine system).

General comprehension of body systems and how they interrelate is essential to ultrasound evaluation of the body. Coming chapters describe specific organs and vessels to facilitate instruction. However, it is essential to keep in mind the interdependency of specific organs and vessels. Knowledge of this interaction not only enables the sonographer to determine underlying events, but may also be the determining factor leading to investigation of other areas or body systems during a sonographic evaluation.

Bibliography

Larson, D: Mayo Clinic Family Healthbook. New York, William Morrison, 1990.

Rothenberg, D: The New Lexicon Illustrated Medical Encyclopedia and Guide to Family Health. New York, Lexicon Publishing, 1988.

Spence, A: Basic Human Anatomy. Massachusetts, Benjamin/Cummings, 1982.

Stedman's Medical Dictionary 24th ed. Baltimore, William & Wilkins, 1982.

Chapter 4

ANATOMY LAYERING AND SECTIONAL ANATOMY

ALEXANDER LANE
BETTY BATES TEMPKIN

Objectives:

Define the directional terminology used in sonography.

Describe how the body is divided.

Classify body layers (anatomical tissue layers) into four classes and describe each briefly.

Describe the visceral layers (including muscles and blood vessels) of the abdomen and pelvis.

Describe body planes and sonographic scanning planes and their interpretation.

Describe the positional orientation of body structures.

Define the significance of describing the relationship of adjacent body structures.

Describe the similarities and differences among body structures as they appear in cadaver sections and ultrasound image sections.

Describe the sonographic appearance of body structures.

Define the key words.

Key Words:

Abdominal cavity
Anechoic
Anterior
Contralateral
Coronal plane
Crura of the diaphragm
Deep
Diaphragm
Distal
Dorsal cavity
Echogenicity
Extravisceral layers
False pelvis
Foramen of Winslow
Greater sac
Homogeneous
Hyperechoic
Hypoechoic
Inferior

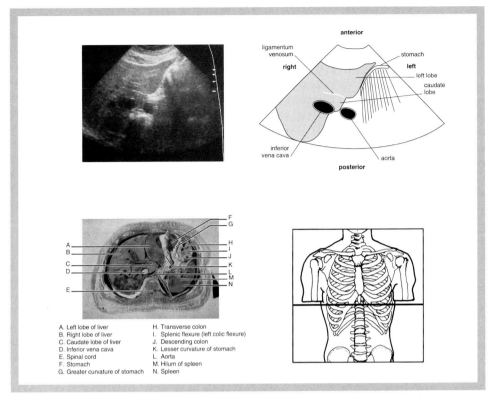

ligamentum
venosum

right

anterior

stomach

left

left lobe

caudate
lobe

inferior
vena cava

aorta

posterior

A. Left lobe of liver
B. Right lobe of liver
C. Caudate lobe of liver
D. Inferior vena cava
E. Spinal cord
F. Stomach
G. Greater curvature of stomach

H. Transverse colon
I. Splenic flexure (left colic flexure)
J. Descending colon
K. Lesser curvature of stomach
L. Aorta
M. Hilum of spleen
N. Spleen

Cadaver section and ultrasound image section. See Figure 4–14, p. 58, for more details.

Intraperitoneal
Intravisceral luminal layers
Intravisceral nonluminal layers
Ipsilateral
Isosonic
Lateral
Lesser sac
Medial
Mesentery
Omentum
Parietal peritoneum
Pelvic cavity
Pelvic inlet
Peritoneal cavity
Peritoneal membrane
Posterior
Proximal
Retroperitoneal
Sagittal plane
Somatic layers
Superficial
Superior
Transverse plane
True pelvis

Ventral cavity
Visceral peritoneum

This chapter relates to the methodology for learning sectional anatomy.[1,2] Recent advances and expansions in the field of radiologic diagnostic medicine have demanded an update in the teaching of human anatomy. Thus, a new methodology is formulated. This methodology is guided by computer imaging modalities. Each computer imaging modality, including ultrasound, depicts the body in sections in various views, layer by layer. Therefore, an analysis of body sections is essential in the diagnostic process.

The guidelines for the sonographic study of sectional anatomy can be standardized and are outlined below. These guidelines utilize a systematic search pattern for the accurate identification and description of layered anatomy, sectional anatomy, cadaver sections, and clinical images. These eight orientation guidelines for sectional anatomy follow:

1. Understanding the *directional terminology* that sonographers use is the key to accurate description and

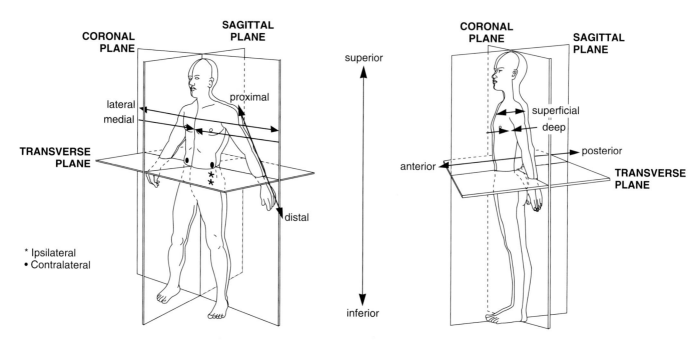

Figure 4–1. View of the body in the anatomic position (standing erect, arms at the sides, face and palms directed forward)[3,4] with body planes (sagittal, coronal, transverse) and directional terms.

to communication. Table 4–1 defines those terms and Figure 4–1 demonstrates them.

2. The ***divisions of the body*** are the next consideration in this approach. It is important that sonographers be able to differentiate the natural cavities and spaces of the body, not only because of the bulk of structures they contain but because of the potential abnormalities that can invade them. A brief list of all the body cavities is covered in Chapter 3. The peritoneal cavity is the primary focus of this section.

The human body consists of two main cavities: **ventral** and **dorsal**, one situated on the anterior (ventral) area, the other on the posterior (dorsal) area. Each of these cavities, in turn, is divided into smaller cavities. The ventral cavity is separated by the **diaphragm** (a muscular partition which assists inspiration) into the thoracic cavity and the peritoneal cavity. The **peritoneal cavity** is the largest body cavity, as it encompasses the abdomen and pelvis.[3–6]

The peritoneal cavity is lined by the **peritoneal membrane**, a thin sheet of tissue which secretes serous fluid; the fluid acts as a lubricant and facilitates free movement between organs. The peritoneum is classified as **parietal**, the portion of peritoneum lining the cavity, and **visceral**, the portion of peritoneum covering the organs.[3,4,6] The parietal peritoneum forms a closed sac, except in females, in whom a portion of the fallopian tubes opens into it. The enclosed, or **intraperitoneal**, structures include the liver (except for a bare area posterior to the dome), gallbladder, spleen (except for its hilum), stomach, the majority of the intestines, and the ovaries. The

intraperitoneal abdominal organs are connected to the cavity wall by the **mesentery**, a double fold of peritoneum.

Retroperitoneal structures are located posterior to the sac and are covered anteriorly with peritoneum. This applies to the kidneys, ureters, adrenal glands, pancreas, aorta, inferior vena cava, urinary bladder, uterus, and prostate gland. The ascending colon, descending colon, and most of the duodenum are also situated in the retroperitoneum, as are the abdominal lymph nodes and somatic nerves.[4,6,7]

The abdominal portion of the peritoneal cavity can be divided further into two peritoneal compartments: the greater sac and the lesser sac. The **greater sac** extends from the diaphragm to the pelvis and covers the width of the abdomen. The **lesser sac**, or omental bursa, is a diverticulum of the greater sac located posterior to the stomach. The neck, or area of communication between the sacs, is termed epiploic foramen or **foramen of Winslow**.[4–7] Table 4–2 summarizes several additional peritoneal cavity spaces created by the complex arrangement of the peritoneum. These spaces are particularly appreciated sonographically when filled with free fluid.

The **omentum** is a double layer of peritoneum which extends from the stomach to adjacent abdominal organs.[3–6] It is classified into the greater omentum, which attaches to the anterior surface of the transverse colon, and the lesser omentum, which joins the lesser curvature of the stomach and the first part of the duodenum to the porta hepatis (area of the liver where the hepatic artery and main portal vein enter the liver and the biliary ducts

TABLE 4-1. Directional Terminology[3-5]

TERM	DEFINITION	EXAMPLES	TERM	DEFINITION	EXAMPLES
Anterior (ventral)	Situated at or directed toward the front. A structure in front of another structure.	The liver is situated anteriorly in the body. The head of the pancreas is anterior to the inferior vena cava.	*Lateral*	Situated at, on, or toward the side. To the right or left of the middle or the midline of the body.	The spleen is situated left laterally in the body. The carotid arteries are lateral to the thyroid.
Posterior (dorsal)	Situated at or directed toward the back. A structure behind another structure.	The kidneys are situated posteriorly in the body. The inferior vena cava is posterior to the head of the pancreas.	*Ipsilateral*	Situated on or affecting the same side.	The spleen and left kidney are ipsilateral.
			Contralateral	Situated on or affecting the opposite side.	The ovaries are contralateral.
Superior (cranial)	Situated above or directed upward. Toward the head. A structure higher than another structure.	The lungs are situated superiorly in the body. The diaphragm is superior to the liver.	*Proximal*	Situated closest to the point of origin or attachment.	The common hepatic duct is proximal to the common bile duct.
Inferior (caudal)	Situated below or directed downward. Toward the feet. A structure lower than another structure.	The uterus is situated inferiorly in the body. The superior mesenteric artery is inferior to the celiac axis.	*Distal*	Situated farthest from the point of origin or attachment.	The abdominal aorta is distal to the thoracic aorta.
			Superficial	Situated on or toward the surface. External.	The testicles are superficial structures.
Medial	Situated at, on, or toward the middle or midline of the body.	The spine is situated medially in the body. The aorta is medial to the left kidney.	*Deep*	Situated away from the surface. Internal.	The pancreas is a deep structure.

TABLE 4-2. Peritoneal Cavity Spaces[2,4,5,9]

SPACE	LOCATION	SPACE	LOCATION
Supracolic compartment (supramesocolic space)	The area above the transverse colon constitutes the supracolic compartment, which includes the right subhepatic space, left subhepatic space, right subphrenic space, and left subphrenic space.		and the descending colon. The gutter to the right of the mesentery is a space between the mesentery and the ascending colon. The gutter to the left of the mesentery is a space between the mesentery and the descending colon.
Subhepatic spaces	Classified as right and left as they are respectively located posterior to the right and left lobes of the liver. The right subhepatic space includes Morrison's pouch, which lies between the superior pole of the right kidney and the posterior aspect of the right lobe of the liver. The left subhepatic space includes the lesser sac.	*Perirenal space*	An area located around the kidney, adrenal gland, and fat, surrounded by fascia (Gerota's fascia).
Subphrenic spaces	Classified as right and left as they are respectively located on each side of the falciform ligament. The spaces lie between the diaphragm and the anterior portion of the right and left lobes of the liver.	*Pararenal space*	Classified as anterior and posterior. The anterior pararenal space is located between the anterior surface of the renal fascia (Gerota's fascia) and the posterior portion of the peritoneum. The posterior pararenal space is located between the posterior surface of the renal fascia and the transversalis fascia.
Infracolic compartment (inframesocolic space)	The area inferior to the transverse colon constitutes the infracolic compartment, which includes the right paracolic gutter, left paracolic gutter, the gutter to the right of the mesentery, and the gutter to the left of the mesentery.	*Posterior cul-de-sac (pouch of Douglas or rectouterine pouch)*	The most posterior and dependent portion of the peritoneal sac. A space located between the urinary bladder and rectum in the male and the rectouterine pouch in the female.
Paracolic gutters	The right paracolic gutter is located between the right lateral abdominal wall and the ascending colon. The left paracolic gutter is between the left lateral abdominal wall	*Anterior cul-de-sac (vesicouterine pouch)*	A shallow space located between the anterior wall of the uterus and the urinary bladder. This space all but disappears as the urinary bladder fills with urine. This space does not exist in the male.

leave).[3] In some instances, there are folds of peritoneum running from one organ to another, called ligaments. The names of the ligaments are directly related to the organs to which they are attached.[4,5]

The abdominal portion of the peritoneal cavity, or **abdominal cavity**, excluding the retroperitoneum and the pelvis, is bounded superiorly by the diaphragm, anteriorly by the abdominal wall muscles, and posteriorly by the vertebral column, ribs, and iliac fossa.[4,6,7] It is continuous with the pelvic cavity inferiorly through the pelvic inlet.[5] The abdominal contents include the liver, gallbladder and biliary tract, pancreas, adrenal glands, kidneys, ureters, spleen, stomach, intestines, and lymph nodes. Also included is the abdominal aorta and its branches, which supply blood to these structures, and the inferior vena cava and the main portal vein, which receive and remove blood from them.[4,6,7] The left and right **crura of the diaphragm** (muscular bands that arise from the lumbar vertebrae and insert into the diaphragm) are also within the abdominal cavity.[2,3,6]

The peritoneal cavity is routinely described as nine regions and four quadrants. Sonographers use these divisions to accurately describe the location of abdominal structures. Figure 4–2 demonstrates those divisions and also the surface landmarks used to describe the abdominal wall.

The pelvic portion of the peritoneal cavity, or **pelvic cavity**, is bounded anteriorly and laterally by the hip bones and posteriorly by the sacrum and coccyx.[3,6,7] It extends superiorly from the iliac crests to the pelvic diaphragm inferiorly. Deep to this bony framework lie the muscles which line the pelvic cavity. The pelvic contents include the distal portion of the ureters, urinary bladder, urethra, the distal portion of the ileum, the cecum, appendix, sigmoid colon, rectum, lymph nodes, and the iliac vessels. Additionally, the female pelvis includes the uterus, fallopian tubes, and ovaries, and the male pelvis contains the prostate gland and seminal vesicles.[4,6,7]

The pelvis is divided into the false and the true pelves by an oblique plane circumscribing the following features: the sacral promontorium, ala of the sacrum, arcuate line of the ilium, pectineal line of the pubis, the pubic crest, and the upper edge of the pubic symphysis. The circumference of this plane is the **pelvic inlet**. The **false pelvis** (greater pelvis or pelvis major) forms the walls of the most superior portion of the pelvic cavity. It is situated superior to the pelvic inlet. The **true pelvis** (lesser pelvis or pelvis minor) is shorter than the false pelvis, with considerably greater depth on its posterior wall than on its anterior wall. It is situated inferior to the pelvic inlet and contains the bladder, the distal portion of the ileum, the cecum, appendix, sigmoid, rectum, and some of the reproductive organs.[6]

The pelvic portion of the peritoneal cavity is described as three regions: right iliac, hypogastric, and left iliac. These regions are subdivisions of the hypogastrium.[2]

(See Figure 4–2, *top left*). Sonographers use these regions to accurately describe the location of the pelvic viscera. For example, the right iliac region includes the cecum and appendix. The hypogastric region contains structures such as the distal end of the ileum, urinary bladder, uterus (nonpregnant), and prostate. The sigmoid colon, distal end of the left ureter, and left ovary are found in the left iliac region.[2,6]

3. *Tissue layers (anatomical layers)* are classified based upon location into four classes: (1) Somatic layers, (2) Extravisceral layers (visceral layers), (3) Intravisceral luminal layers, and (4) Intravisceral nonluminal layers. The **somatic layers** include the multilayers found on each body region from skin to cavity. In a region where no cavity exists, the somatic tissue layers consist of the whole region from peripheral to deep. The **extravisceral layers (visceral layers)** indicates the serial sequence of viscera (internal organs), blood vessels, and spaces between each organ within each cavity. **Intravisceral luminal layers** are found within the walls of organs with a lumen, such as the stomach. **Intravisceral nonluminal layers** involves organs without a prominent lumen. An excellent example of an intravisceral nonluminal organ is the adrenal glands.[8]

The **extravisceral layers (visceral layers)** of the abdomen and pelvis are outlined and discussed, going from deep to superficial. Each **visceral** layer (organ layers including muscles and blood vessels) from posterior to anterior is named and discussed. For example, the stomach is anterior to the pancreas. This layering approach is the best method for clarifying the intricate relationships of adjacent body structures regardless of body plane or scanning plane. For further information on the layering concept and visceral unit layers of the abdominal and pelvic regions refer to Figure 4–3,[9] which illustrates the layers of the abdomen, and Figure 4–4,[4,6,7] which illustrates the layers of the pelvis.

4. *Classification of the structures* in cadaver and ultrasound sections into four anatomic units follows mastery of the anatomic layers. The four units are the musculoskeletal, vascular, visceral, and enclosing units. In the musculoskeletal unit the skeletal muscles in the body wall are specified. In the vascular unit, origin and distribution of the vessels are noted. In the visceral unit, the location and course are discussed. The structures of the enclosing unit include membranes, fossae, spaces, depressions, and recesses. (See the layering figures, Figures 4–3 and 4–4, to assist in classifying structures.)

5. The next step in this approach is determining the *positional orientation of structures within the body*. Note, in the layering illustrations, that some structures lie in a vertical position (inferior vena cava), and some are vertical oblique (portal vein, kidneys). Other body structures lie transversely (renal arteries and veins) or transverse oblique (pancreas), and some vary in position (gallbladder). Figure 4–5 illustrates these examples.

Text continued on page 51

REGIONAL DIVISIONS OF THE ABDOMEN

QUADRANT DIVISIONS OF THE ABDOMEN

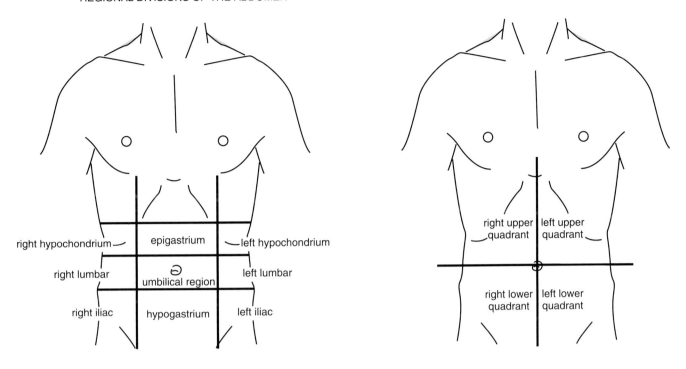

SURFACE LANDMARKS OF THE ABDOMINAL WALL

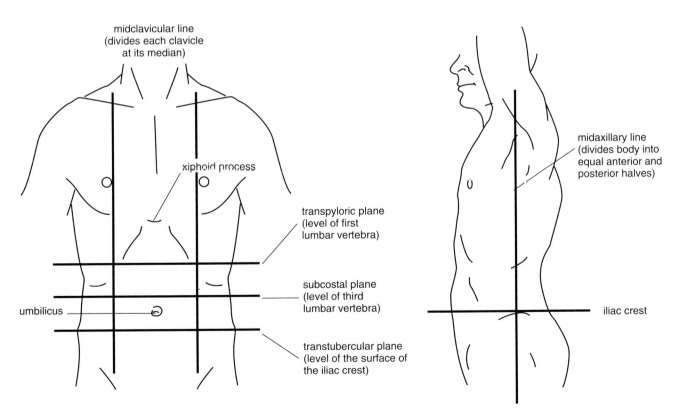

Figure 4–2. Divisions of the peritoneal cavity and surface landmarks.

Figure 4-3. The anatomic layers of the abdomen. The layering approach is the best method for clarifying the intricate relationships of adjacent body structures regardless of body plane or scanning plane.

A, The posterior muscle layer is the most dorsal layer of the abdomen which includes the lumbar spine, psoas major muscle, and the quadratus lumborum muscle. The *psoas major muscle* is a somewhat triangular, bilateral muscle that originates from the lower thoracic and the lumbar vertebrae.[6] It courses slightly anterior and slightly lateral as it descends through the lower abdomen immediately lateral to the spine. Near the fifth lumbar vertebra the psoas major separates from the spine and courses more laterally on its descent to the iliac crests. This separation creates a space between the vertebral column and psoas major through which the iliac vessels run.[4] The *quadratus lumborum muscle* is also a bilateral muscle tissue that extends from the iliolumbar ligament, the adjacent portion of the iliac crest, and the transverse processes of the lower lumbar vertebrae.[3] The muscle courses upward, lateral to the psoas major muscle, until it reaches the twelfth rib.

B, This layer includes the *kidneys* and *adrenal glands.* The kidneys are retroperitoneal organs that lie on each side of the spine in the area between the twelfth thoracic and fourth lumbar vertebrae. The adrenals are located superior, anterior, and slightly medial to each kidney. The kidneys and adrenal glands lie just anterior to the quadratus lumborum and psoas major muscles; however, the largest portion of the psoas muscle is located more medially.

C, The *inferior vena cava* originates at the junction of the two common iliac veins anterior to the body of the fifth lumbar vertebrae.[6,7] It ascends the retroperitoneum anterior to the spine and psoas major muscle and passes through the diaphragm to enter the right atrium of the heart. Note the location and transverse lie of the *renal vein* tributaries. Also note the location of the *hepatic vein* tributaries.

D, The *aorta* originates at the left ventricle of the heart, then descends (thoracic aorta) posterior to the diaphragm into the retroperitoneum of the abdominal cavity (abdominal aorta). The aorta continues to descend, anterior to the spine and psoas major muscle, then bifurcates into the common iliac arteries at the level of the fourth lumbar vertebra.[6,7] Note the anterior branches of the abdominal aorta: the celiac axis and the superior mesenteric artery. The *celiac axis* has three branches: the *splenic artery,* which courses left laterally toward the spleen; the *hepatic artery,* which courses right laterally toward the liver; and the *left gastric artery,* which travels superiorly, then left laterally toward the stomach and esophagus. Note the *gastroduodenal artery,* a branch of the hepatic artery which travels inferiorly toward the head of the pancreas. The *superior mesenteric artery* runs anterior and parallel to the aorta. Note the layers and the left renal vein passing right between the aorta and superior mesenteric artery as it traverses the body from the left kidney to the inferior vena cava. Note that both *renal arteries* lie just posterior to the renal veins. Also, the right renal artery runs just posterior to the inferior vena cava on its course to the right kidney.

E, This layer includes the *portal venous system,* which supplies blood to the liver for metabolic processes. This blood originates from the stomach, small intestine, large intestine, and spleen. The *splenic vein* courses laterally to medially, adjacent and inferior to the splenic artery. Note that it passes just anterior to the *superior mesenteric artery.* The splenic vein terminates posterior to the neck of the pancreas as it unites with the superior mesenteric vein to form the *portal vein.* Note that the superior mesenteric vein and inferior mesenteric vein tributaries course from inferior to superior. Also note the proximity of the superior mesenteric vein and superior mesenteric artery. Note that after the main portal vein forms it courses superiorly approximately 5 to 6 cm, then bifurcates into right and left branches.[6] Note that the hepatic artery is anterior to the portal vein.

Legend continued on page 46.

THE LAYERS OF THE ABDOMEN

A. POSTERIOR MUSCLES

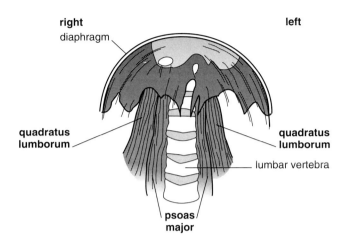

B. KIDNEYS AND ADRENAL GLANDS

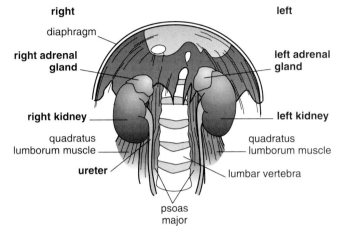

C. VENA CAVA

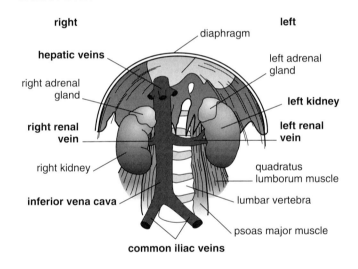

D. AORTA

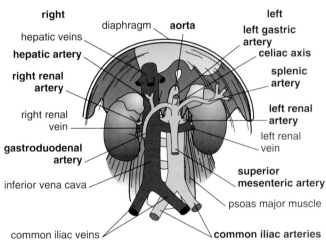

E. PORTAL VENOUS SYSTEM

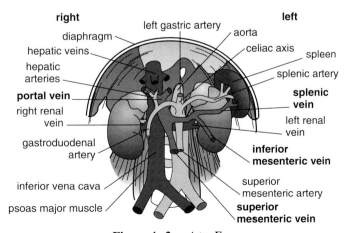

Figure 4–3. *A* to *E*

Figure 4–3. *continued*

F, The *pancreas* is a retroperitoneal organ that traverses the body from the hilum of the spleen to the duodenum. The *head* of the pancreas lies to the right of the superior mesenteric vein and immediately anterior to the inferior vena cava. Note that the head lies slightly inferior to the body and tail. Also note the gastroduodenal artery that lies on the anterolateral surface of the head. The *uncinate process* is a medial projection of the head that lies just posterior to the superior mesenteric vein. Because it varies in size, it may extend to lie between the superior mesenteric artery and the aorta. The pancreatic *neck* is immediately anterior to the superior mesenteric vein and slightly superior to that level it lies anterior to the formation of the portal vein.[4] The *body* of the pancreas lies to the left of the pancreatic neck, immediately anterior to the splenic vein. Note the layers as the splenic vein is then anterior to the superior mesenteric artery, which branches anteriorly from the aorta. The pancreatic body extends left laterally to the tail of the pancreas. The *tail*, like the body, lies just anterior to the splenic vein. The tail of the pancreas extends left lateral to the hilum of the spleen. Note that the body and tail of the pancreas are inferior to the splenic artery.

G, This layer includes the intraperitoneal *gallbladder* and the *biliary tract*. The position of the gallbladder is variable but it is common to see the fundus anterior to the superior pole of the right kidney and/or the head of the pancreas. The gallbladder neck is fixed in its position. Note that the cystic duct is immediately superior to the gallbladder neck. The *common hepatic duct* courses inferomedially and meets the cystic duct to form the common bile duct. Note that the common hepatic duct is anterior to the portal vein. The *common bile duct* also courses inferomedially, running behind the duodenum on its way to the head of the pancreas. Note the layers, in that the common bile duct is anterior to the portal vein and hepatic artery at certain levels. Also note that at other levels the common bile duct is right lateral to the hepatic artery.

H, In this layer the *gastrointestinal (GI) tract* consists of the stomach and duodenum. Note the anterior lie of this portion of the GI tract and the numerous structures it covers. The anterior surface of the *stomach* is in contact with the diaphragm, the thoracic wall formed on the left by the seventh, eighth, and ninth ribs, the left lobe of the liver, and the anterior abdominal wall.[11] The posterior surface of the stomach is related to the diaphragm, spleen, left adrenal gland, the superior pole of the left kidney, the anterior surface of the pancreas, and the splenic flexure of the colon.[12] The course of the *duodenum* presents a remarkable curve, somewhat in the shape of an imperfect circle, so that its termination is not far removed from its starting point.[6] The first portion of the duodenum begins at the pylorus of the stomach and ends at the neck of the gallbladder. This portion is usually posterior to the gallbladder and anterior to the gastroduodenal artery, head of the pancreas, common bile duct, common hepatic artery, and portal vein (note the layers).[6,11,13] It then takes a sharp curve and descends along the right margin of the head of the pancreas for a variable distance, usually to the level of the superior edge of the fourth lumbar vertebra.[6] Now it curves again, passing from right to left with a slight inclination upward, anterior to the inferior vena cava, aorta, and vertebral column. The duodenum ends opposite the second lumbar vertebra at the jejunum.[6]

I, The *liver* is the most anterior visceral organ of the peritoneal cavity and is intraperitoneal except for a bare area that is posterior to its dome.[6,7] It occupies the right upper quadrant and often extends past the midline into the left upper quadrant. The superior and lateral surfaces of the liver border the diaphragm. The left lobe is just anterior to the stomach and body of the pancreas. The right lobe is immediately anterior to the gallbladder, right kidney (primarily the superior pole), right adrenal gland, and head of the pancreas.

J, The most anterior layer of the abdomen is the *abdominal wall*, which extends from the xiphoid process of the sternum to the pelvic bones. It consists of subcutaneous tissue and muscles. The subcutaneous tissue contains fat, fibrous tissue, fascia, small vessels, and nerves.[4-6] The *rectus abdominis muscle* is an anterior, bilateral muscle immediately lateral to the linea alba (a white line of connective tissue in the median of the abdomen).[2] This muscle originates at the pubis, then ascends to insert at the xiphoid process and costal cartilages of the fifth, sixth, and seventh ribs.[3] The *rectus sheath* encloses the rectus abdominis muscle. The *external oblique muscle* is a bilateral muscle tissue that originates from the outer surface of the lower eight ribs, then fans out to insert into the xiphoid process, linea alba, pubic bones, and anterior iliac crest.[2,4,6] The *internal oblique muscle* is also a bilateral muscle immediately deep to the external oblique muscle. Its muscle fibers run at right angles to those of the external oblique.[2,4]

F. PANCREAS

right   left

diaphragm
hepatic veins
hepatic artery
portal vein
right renal vein
gastroduodenal artery
psoas major muscle
inferior vena cava

left gastric artery
aorta
celiac axis
spleen
splenic artery
pancreas
left renal vein
inferior mesenteric vein
superior mesenteric artery
superior mesenteric vein

neck
body
tail
head

G. GALLBLADDER AND BILIARY TRACT

right   left

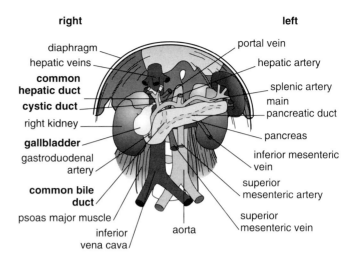

diaphragm
hepatic veins
common hepatic duct
cystic duct
right kidney
gallbladder
gastroduodenal artery
common bile duct
psoas major muscle
inferior vena cava

portal vein
hepatic artery
splenic artery
main pancreatic duct
pancreas
inferior mesenteric vein
superior mesenteric artery
superior mesenteric vein
aorta

H. GASTROINTESTINAL TRACT

right   left

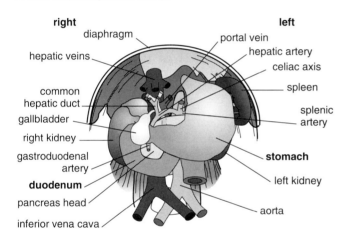

diaphragm
hepatic veins
common hepatic duct
gallbladder
right kidney
gastroduodenal artery
duodenum
pancreas head
inferior vena cava

portal vein
hepatic artery
celiac axis
spleen
splenic artery
stomach
left kidney
aorta

I. LIVER

right   left

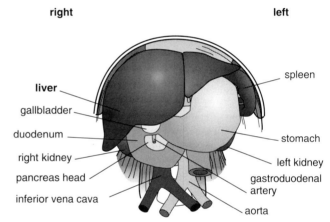

liver
gallbladder
duodenum
right kidney
pancreas head
inferior vena cava

spleen
stomach
left kidney
gastroduodenal artery
aorta

J. ANTERIOR MUSCLES

right   left

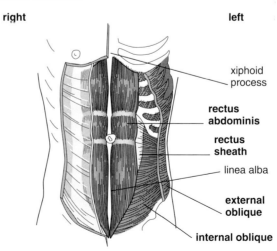

xiphoid process
rectus abdominis
rectus sheath
linea alba
external oblique
internal oblique

Figure 4–3. *F to J*

Figure 4–4. The anatomic layers of the pelvis. The layering approach is the best method for clarifying the intricate relationship of adjacent body structures regardless of body plane or scanning plane.

A, The true pelvis muscle layer is the deepest layer of the pelvis. The muscles of this layer include the obturator internus, piriformis, coccygeus, iliococcygeus, and pubococcygeus. The *obturator internus muscle* is a triangular, bilateral muscle tissue that originates at the pelvic brim. It courses parallel and adjacent to the lateral pelvic wall, narrowing inferiorly to pass through the lesser sciatic foramen to the greater trochanter of the femur. It is lateral to the pelvic viscera.[2,4,6] The *piriformis muscle* is also a triangular, bilateral muscle that arises from the sacrum. It extends laterally, narrowing to pass through the greater sciatic foramen to the greater trochanter of the femur.[3,4,6] The pubococcygeus, iliococcygeus, and coccygeus muscles are a group referred to as the pelvic diaphragm. This muscle group lines the floor of the true pelvis. The pubococcygeus, puborectalis, and iliococcygeus muscles form the hammock-like portion of the pelvic floor and together are termed the levator ani muscles. The *pubococcygeus muscles* course from the pubic bone to the coccyx. There is a separation in a section of the muscle termed the genital hiatus, which allows the passage of the urethra, vagina, and rectum (as demonstrated here).[6,7] A section of the puborectalis muscle embraces the sides of the prostate. This portion is called the levator prostate and the pubovaginalis in females.[6] The pubococcygeus muscle pair are the most medial and anterior muscles of the pelvic diaphragm. The *iliococcygeus muscles* extend from the ischial spine to the coccyx.[6] They lie just lateral to the pubococcygeus muscles. The *coccygeus muscles* also course from the ischial spine to the coccyx.[6] They are the most posterior muscle pair of the pelvic diaphragm.

B, Muscles of the posterior body wall and false pelvis include the quadratus lumborum, psoas major, iliacus, and iliopsoas. The *quadratus lumborum muscle* is a bilateral muscle tissue that extends from the iliolumbar ligament, the adjacent portion of the iliac crest, and the transverse processes of the lower lumbar vertebrae.[3] It courses upward, lateral to the psoas major muscle, until it reaches the twelfth rib. The *psoas major muscle* is a somewhat triangular, bilateral muscle that originates from the lower thoracic and lumbar vertebrae.[6] It courses slightly anteriorly and slightly laterally as it descends through the lower abdomen immediately lateral to the spine. Near the fifth lumbar vertebra, the psoas major separates from the spine and courses more laterally on its descent to the iliac crests. This separation creates a space between the vertebral column and the psoas major through which the iliac vessels run.[4] At the level of the iliac crests, the psoas major muscles join the iliacus muscles to form the iliopsoas muscles. The *iliacus muscles* arise from the iliac fossa and the base of the sacrum and extend to meet the psoas major. The *iliopsoas muscles* continue a lateral descent, passing over the pelvic inlet to insert into the lesser trochanter of the femur.

C, This layer includes the rectum and a portion of the colon. The *descending colon* passes downward through the abdominal cavity along the lateral border of the left kidney. It curves medially at the inferior pole of the kidney toward the lateral border of the psoas major muscle, then descends in the angle between the psoas major and quadratus lumborum muscle to the iliac crest.[6,7] The distal portion (iliac colon) begins at the iliac crest and runs just anterior to the psoas major and iliacus muscle to the sigmoid portion of the colon.[6] The *sigmoid colon* is continuous with the descending colon and passes transversely, anterior to the sacrum to the right side of the pelvis. It then curves toward the left to reach the midline of the pelvis where it bends downward and ends at the rectum. The sigmoid colon is anterior to the external iliac vessels and the left piriformis muscle.[6] The *rectum* is continuous with the sigmoid colon above and ends in the anal canal below. It courses inferiorly, anterior to the coccyx, where it bends back sharply into the anal canal. This inferior portion lies directly anterior on the sacrum and coccyx, and levator ani muscle.[6,7]

D, The anatomy of the female pelvis and the urinary bladder are appreciated at this layer. Note that a large portion of the bladder has not been drawn, to facilitate the location of the organs just adjacent to it. The organs of the female pelvis include the uterus, vagina, fallopian tubes, and ovaries. The nonpregnant *uterus* is located in the true pelvis, anterior to the rectum and posterior to the bladder. There are spaces posterior and anterior to the uterus not demonstrated here that are referred to as the posterior cul-de-sac (pouch of Douglas or rectouterine pouch) and anterior cul-de-sac formed by the peritoneum. The fundus is the superior, anteriorly tilted part of the uterus. The body is the vertical, oblique portion between the fundus and the cervix. The cervix is inferior to the body of the uterus and adjacent to the vagina.[2] The *vagina* is a vertically elongated structure located just anterior to the rectum and posterior to the bladder (trigone) and urethra. Note that the distal portion of the ureters is lateral to the vagina. The *fallopian tubes* lie in the superior part of the broad ligament and extend laterally toward the ovaries. The broad ligament is actually a double fold of peritoneum covering the anterior surface of all of the pelvic viscera except for the *ovaries*, which are located on the posterior portion of the broad ligament and entirely inside the peritoneal sac. For this reason the ovaries are not demonstrated here, because while "attached" laterally to the uterus by the fallopian tubes and broad ligament, they are posterior to both structures. The ovary is also immediately anterior to a portion of the ureter and internal iliac vessels. The *urinary bladder* is situated in a vertical and oblique position in the anterior pelvis. The superior portion is anterior to the inferior part.[2]

E, The organs of the male pelvis appreciated at this layer are the prostate gland, seminal vesicles, and urinary bladder. The *prostate gland* is retroperitoneal. The prostate is anterior to the rectum and inferior to the bladder. The lateral surfaces are in close proximity to the levator prostate muscles, which are separated from the gland by a plexus of veins. Not demonstrated here but important to note is that the prostate is perforated by the urethra and ejaculatory duct.[6] The *seminal vesicles* lie superior to the prostate and posterior to the bladder. The *urinary bladder* is situated in a vertical and oblique position in the anterior pelvis. The superior portion is anterior to the inferior part.[2] It is immediately anterior to the rectum.

F, The most anterior muscle of the pelvis is the *rectus abdominis muscle,* a bilateral muscle tissue immediately lateral to the linea alba (a white line of connective tissue in the median of the abdomen).[2] It originates at the pubis, then ascends to insert at the xiphoid process and costal cartilages of the fifth, sixth, and seventh ribs.[3]

THE LAYERS OF THE PELVIS

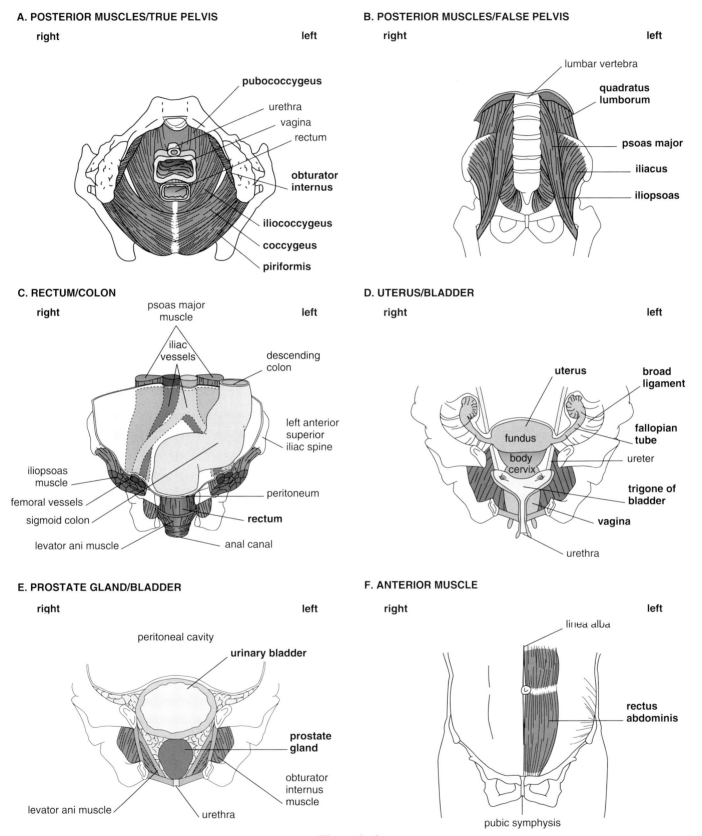

A. POSTERIOR MUSCLES/TRUE PELVIS

right   left

pubococcygeus
urethra
vagina
rectum
obturator internus
iliococcygeus
coccygeus
piriformis

B. POSTERIOR MUSCLES/FALSE PELVIS

right   left

lumbar vertebra
quadratus lumborum
psoas major
iliacus
iliopsoas

C. RECTUM/COLON

right   left

psoas major muscle
iliac vessels
descending colon
left anterior superior iliac spine
iliopsoas muscle
femoral vessels
sigmoid colon
peritoneum
rectum
levator ani muscle
anal canal

D. UTERUS/BLADDER

right   left

uterus
broad ligament
fundus
fallopian tube
ureter
body
cervix
trigone of bladder
vagina
urethra

E. PROSTATE GLAND/BLADDER

right   left

peritoneal cavity
urinary bladder
prostate gland
obturator internus muscle
levator ani muscle
urethra

F. ANTERIOR MUSCLE

right   left

linea alba
rectus abdominis
pubic symphysis

Figure 4–4.

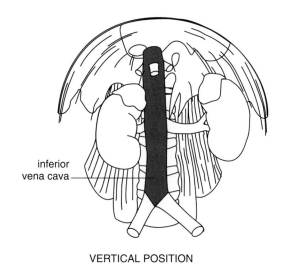

VERTICAL POSITION

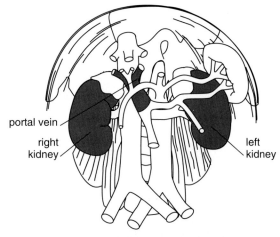

VERTICAL OBLIQUE POSITION
(the superior pole of the kidneys is medial to the inferior pole —
the portal vein's inferior portion is medial to its superior portion)

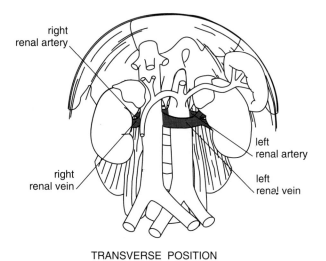

TRANSVERSE POSITION

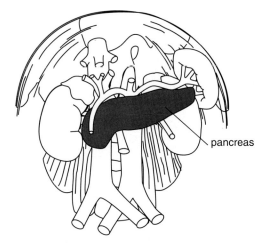

TRANSVERSE OBLIQUE POSITION
(the lateral end of the pancreas is slightly more superior than the
medial end)

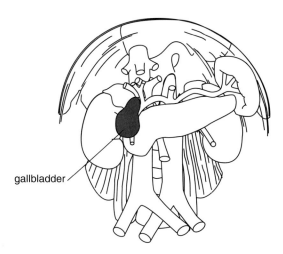

VARIABLE POSITION
(the variable position of the gallbladder is dependent on the amount of bile it contains
and/or the length of its mesenteric attachment)

Figure 4-5. Positional orientations of structures within the body.

Knowledge of the specific position of body structures makes their identification more recognizable on cadaver and ultrasound sections.

6. *Sectional planes.* The classic anatomic planes are the transverse, sagittal, and coronal. (See Figure 4–1.) The **transverse plane** divides the body into unequal superior and inferior sections perpendicular to the long axis of the body. The **sagittal plane** divides the body into unequal right and left sections parallel to the long axis of the body. Equal right and left sections are described as being from the midsagittal plane. The **coronal plane** divides the body into unequal anterior and posterior sections perpendicular to the sagittal planes and parallel to the long axis of the body. Equal anterior and posterior body sections at the midaxillary line are described as being from the midcoronal plane. The scanning planes used in sonography are the same as anatomic body planes while their interpretations are dependent on the location of the transducer and the sound wave approach. Positional orientation of the transducer and its location on the body determine the scanning plane viewed. Generally, positional orientation is set by the manufacturer of the transducer. Sagittal plane orientation, for example, is usually indicated when a notch or raised portion of the transducer appears on the top surface. Rotating the transducer 90 degrees changes the scanning plane. Figures 4–6 and 4–7 demonstrate standard scanning plane interpretations. The endovaginal and endorectal scanning plane interpretations are shown in Figure 4–8. Figure 4–9 demonstrates how to interpret neurosonography (sonography of the brain) scanning planes.

7. *Describing the relationship of adjacent body structures* is the best way to accurately classify specific anatomy. Currently, most ultrasound is performed with real-time sector scanners. This results in ultrasound images of isolated sections of the body that may or may not contain major body structures such as the spine for locational reference. For this reason, the specific area of the body being imaged, patient position (scanning approach), and scanning plane must be clarified on the image for accurate interpretation. With clarification of the above specifics and determination of the relationship of adjacent structures, the anatomy in an image section can be classified. This is a critical discipline for the sonographer to adopt because errors can occur when structures are identified solely on the basis of their expected standard location and sonographic appearance. Too many normal variants exist to rely strictly on memorization as to where a structure "ought" to be or what its sonographic appearance "should" be. Consideration must also be given to disease processes that can affect the standard location of body structures and most certainly their sonographic appearance. Because of these variables and the fact that ultrasound images are isolated sections, classifying anatomy according to the relationship of adjacent structures is the most accurate form of interpreta-

tion. For example, in a sagittal section the target organ or area of interest is related to a structure immediately anterior to it, posterior to it, superior to it, and inferior to it. (See Figure 4–10.) In a coronal section the target organ or area of interest is related to a structure immediately lateral (right or left) to it, medial to it, superior to it, and inferior to it. (See Figure 4–11.) In a transverse section taken from either an anterior or a posterior approach (transducer position), the target organ or area of interest is related to a structure immediately anterior to it, posterior to it, right lateral to it, and left lateral to it. (See Figure 4–12.) In a transverse section taken from either a right or left lateral approach, the target organ or area of interest is related to a structure immediately lateral (right or left) to it, medial to it, anterior to it, and posterior to it. (See Figure 4–13.)

8. The final guideline is *the comparison of structures of cadaver sections and ultrasound image sections.* It is immediately apparent that the size, shape, and relationship of adjacent structures, positional orientation, and location of body structures do not change in regard to cadaver sections and ultrasound images. (See Figure 4–14.) The single difference is the sonographic appearance of the structures. It is important to note that the standard sonographic appearance of body structures is not dependent on the scanning plane from which they are imaged. An understanding of the normal appearance provides the baseline against which to recognize variations and abnormalities.[4] Each structural characteristic varies in sonographic appearance, as follows.

Organ parenchyma, muscles, placenta, and abdominopelvic wall tissues are described in terms of echo textures. The normal echo texture of organ parenchymas, muscles, and tissues is described as **homogeneous** (uniform composition or structure throughout) with ranges in **echogenicity** (echos produced or reflections of the sound beam). For example, the liver may be described as homogeneous and moderately echogenic.[10] (See Figure 4–15.) In the same respect, the echogenic textures of organs are commonly compared to one another. In the case of the liver, it may be **isosonic** or isogenic (same relative echodensity) to the renal parenchyma or slightly more echogenic. (See Figure 4–16.) It is usually isosonic to the pancreas or slightly less echogenic.[10] (See Figure 4–17.) Another example of the sonographic appearance of organ parenchyma is the myometrium of the uterus. It may be described as homogeneous with low to moderate echogenicity. (See Figure 4–18.) Other considerations in describing organ parenchyma depend on an organ's density, vascular components, normal variations, and the presence of disease processes.

Muscle echo texture appears homogeneous with low echogenicity. (See Figure 4–19.) Muscles are usually less echogenic than the organ(s) they are adjacent to. Normal variations and the presence of disease processes are other factors to consider when describing muscle texture.

Text continued on page 64

A. ANTERIOR APPROACH/SAGITTAL PLANE

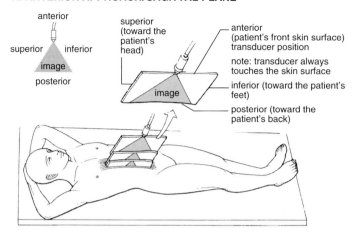

B. POSTERIOR APPROACH/SAGITTAL PLANE

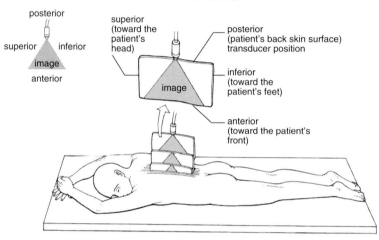

C. ANTERIOR APPROACH/TRANSVERSE PLANE

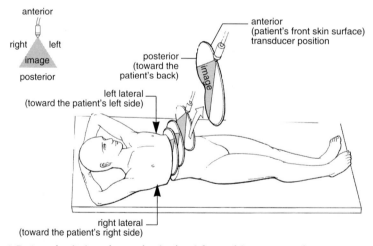

Figure 4–6. *A,B,* A sagittal plane image is obtained from either an anterior or a posterior scanning surface approach. From either approach the interpretation includes the following specific anatomic areas as seen on the ultrasound image: anterior, posterior, superior, and inferior.

C,D,E, A transverse plane image is obtained from either an anterior, a posterior, or a lateral scanning surface approach.

C,D, From the anterior or posterior approach the interpretation includes the following anatomic areas: anterior, posterior, right, and left. E, From the right or left lateral approach the interpretation includes the following anatomical areas: lateral (right or left), medial, anterior, and posterior. (From Tempkin BB: Ultrasound Scanning: Principles and Protocols. Philadelphia, WB Saunders, 1993.)

D. POSTERIOR APPROACH/TRANSVERSE PLANE

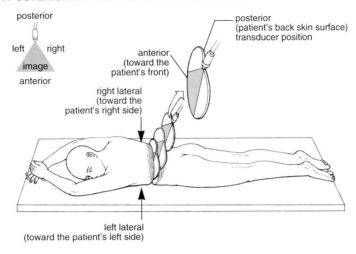

E. LATERAL APPROACH/TRANSVERSE PLANE

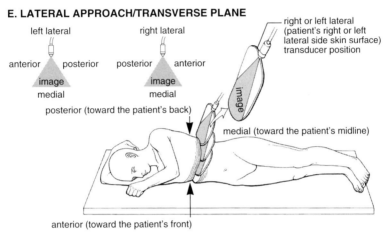

F. LATERAL APPROACH/CORONAL PLANE

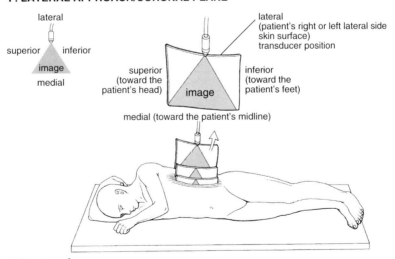

Figure 4–6. *Continued*
F, A coronal plane image is obtained from either a right or a left lateral scanning surface approach. From either approach the interpretation includes the following anatomic areas: lateral (right or left), medial, superior, and inferior. (From Tempkin BB: Ultrasound Scanning: Principles and Protocols. Philadelphia, WB Saunders, 1993.)

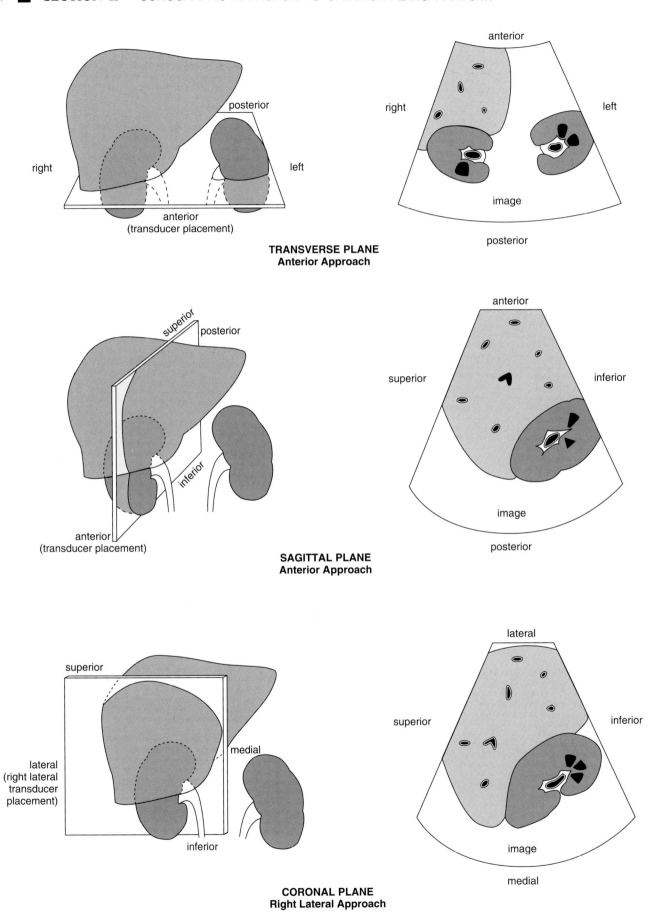

Figure 4–7. Transverse, sagittal, and coronal planes through the liver and kidneys.

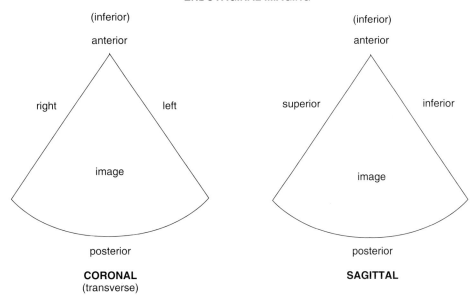

ENDOVAGINAL IMAGING

(inferior)
anterior

right   left

image

posterior

CORONAL
(transverse)

(inferior)
anterior

superior   inferior

image

posterior

SAGITTAL

ENDORECTAL IMAGING

anterior

right   image   left

posterior
(rectum)

CORONAL
(transverse)

anterior

superior   image   inferior

posterior
(rectum)

SAGITTAL

Figure 4–8. Endovaginal imaging and endorectal imaging are obtained from an inferior endocavital approach, which is technically organ-oriented. Image orientation still varies among authors and textbooks; however, the scanning plane interpretations shown here are currently being used by many institutions.

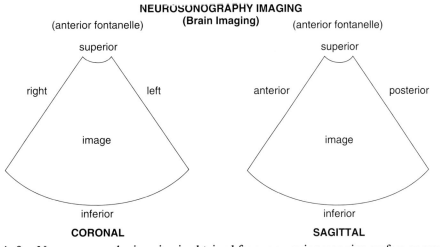

NEUROSONOGRAPHY IMAGING
(Brain Imaging)

(anterior fontanelle)
superior

right   left

image

inferior

CORONAL

(anterior fontanelle)
superior

anterior   posterior

image

inferior

SAGITTAL

Figure 4–9. Neurosonography imaging is obtained from a superior scanning surface approach in which the transducer is placed on the head. Coronal and sagittal views are standard.

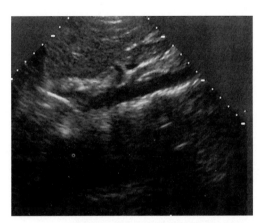 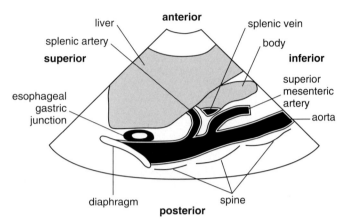

Figure 4–10. In this sagittal section the area of interest is the body of the pancreas. Note that the liver is just anterior to the pancreas and the splenic vein and superior mesenteric artery are posterior to it. Also, note that the pancreatic body lies just inferior to the splenic artery. (From Tempkin BB: Ultrasound Scanning: Principles and Protocols. Philadelphia, WB Saunders, 1993.)

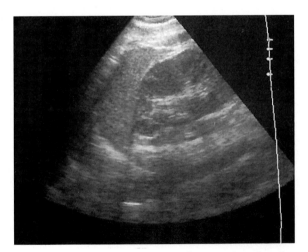 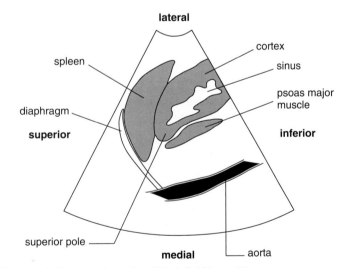

Figure 4–11. In this coronal section the area of interest is the superior pole of the left kidney. Note the spleen just lateral and superior to the left kidney. Also note the psoas muscle and aorta medial to the kidney. (From Tempkin BB: Ultrasound Scanning: Principles and Protocols. Philadelphia, WB Saunders, 1993.)

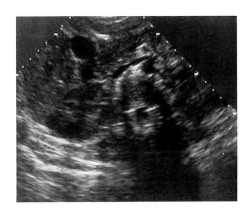
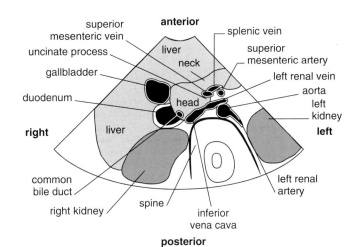

Figure 4–12. In this transverse section the area of interest is the head of the pancreas. Note the liver just anterior to the pancreas head and the inferior vena cava immediately posterior to it. Also note the duodenum and gallbladder right lateral to the pancreas, and the superior mesenteric vein left lateral. (From Tempkin BB: Ultrasound Scanning: Principles and Protocols. Philadelphia, WB Saunders, 1993.)

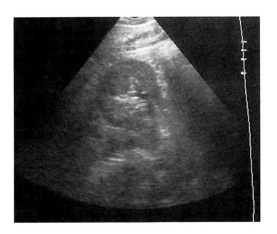
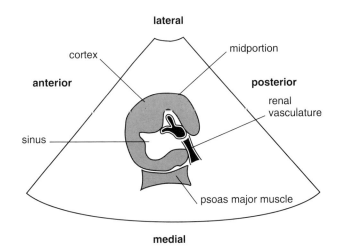

Figure 4–13. In this transverse section the area of interest is the midportion of the left kidney. Note the psoas major muscle and vasculature just medial to the kidney. (From Tempkin BB: Ultrasound Scanning: Principles and Protocols. Philadelphia, WB Saunders, 1993.)

A

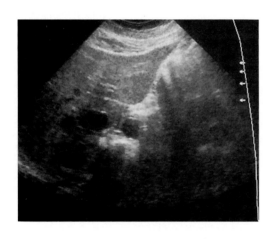

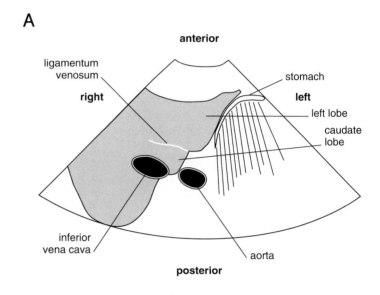

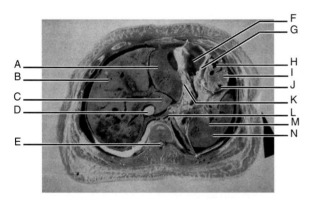

A. Left lobe of liver
B. Right lobe of liver
C. Caudate lobe of liver
D. Inferior vena cava
E. Spinal cord
F. Stomach
G. Greater curvature of stomach

H. Transverse colon
I. Splenic flexure (left colic flexure)
J. Descending colon
K. Lesser curvature of stomach
L. Aorta
M. Hilum of spleen
N. Spleen

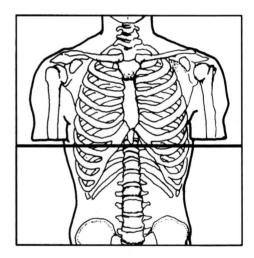

Figure 4-14. Comparison of structures of cadaver sections and ultrasound image sections.

A, In this comparison of cadaver section and ultrasound image at the level of the tenth thoracic vertebra, it is apparent that the size, shape, positional orientation, and location of the left lobe and caudate lobe of the liver are the same. Note the location and adjacent relationships of the inferior vena cava, aorta, and stomach.

Illustration continued on following page.

B

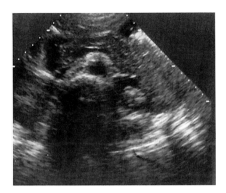

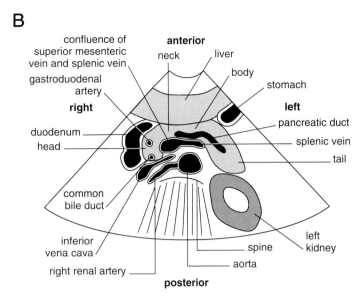

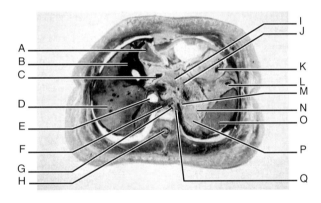

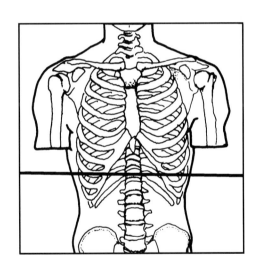

A. Stomach
B. Gallbladder
C. Descending duodenum (second segment of duodenum)
D. Right lobe of liver
E. Inferior vena cava
F. Right crus of diaphragm
G. Aorta
H. Spinal cord

I. Head of pancreas
J. Body of pancreas
K. Colon
L. Colon
M. Left suprarenal (adrenal) gland
N. Tail of pancreas
O. Spleen
P. Left kidney
Q. Left crus of diaphragm

Figure 4–14. *Continued*
B, Comparing this cadaver section and ultrasound image at the level of the twelfth thoracic vertebra, it is apparent that the size, shape, positional orientation, and location of the pancreas and adjacent structures are the same. Note that the head of the pancreas rests against the duodenum and sits immediately anterior to the inferior vena cava. Also note the location and adjacent relationships of the aorta, tail of the pancreas, and left kidney.

Illustration continued on following page.

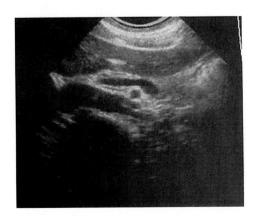

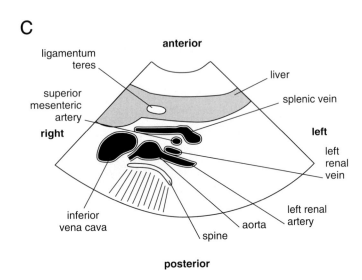

C

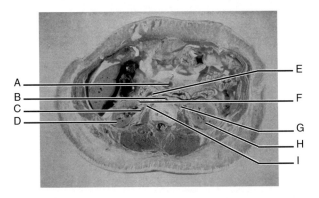

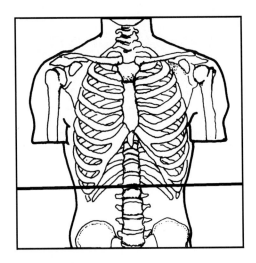

A. Superior mesenteric artery
B. Descending abdominal aorta
C. Right renal artery
D. Right kidney
E. Inferior vena cava

F. Right renal vein
G. Left sympathetic nerve trunk
   · (sympathetic chain)
H. Left kidney
I. Right sympathetic nerve trunk

Figure 4–14. *Continued*
C, This cadaver and ultrasound section are at the level of the second lumbar vertebra. Compare the identical size, location, and positional orientation of the superior mesenteric artery and aorta. Note the comparable relationship of the right renal artery and inferior vena cava. Note the adjacent relationship of the kidneys on the cadaver section.

Illustration continued on following page.

D

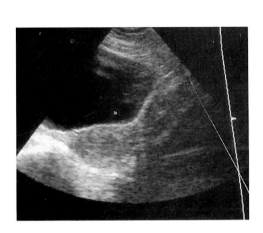

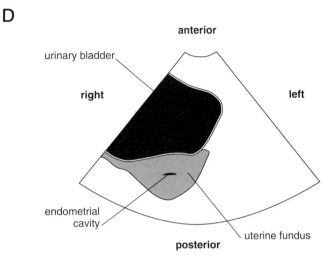

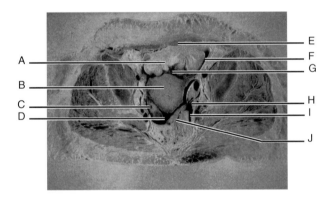

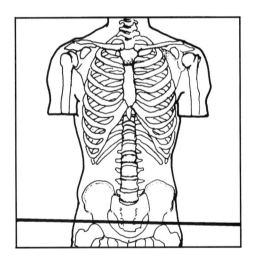

A. Urinary bladder
B. Uterus (womb)
C. Ovary
D. Rectouterine pouch
   (posterior cul-de-sac)
E. Retropubic space

F. Paravesical fossa
G Uterovesical (vesicouterine) pouch
   (anterior cul-de-sac)
H. Ureter
I. Pararectal fossa
J. Rectum

Figure 4–14. *Continued*
D, In this comparison of cadaver section and ultrasound image at the level of the fifth vertebra of the sacrum, it is obvious that the size, shape, and positional orientation of the uterus are the same on both sections. Note the comparable locations of the urinary bladder. Also note the location and adjacent relationships of the rectum, rectouterine pouch (posterior cul-de-sac), and ovary as indicated on the cadaver section. (From Tempkin BB: Ultrasound Scanning; Principles and Protocols, Philadelphia, WB Saunders, 1993; and Lane A, Sharfaei H: Modern Sectional Anatomy. Philadelphia, WB Saunders, 1992.)

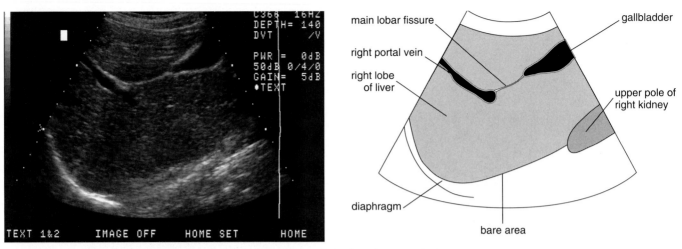

Figure 4–15. The sonographic appearance of the liver is normally homogeneous and moderately echogenic.

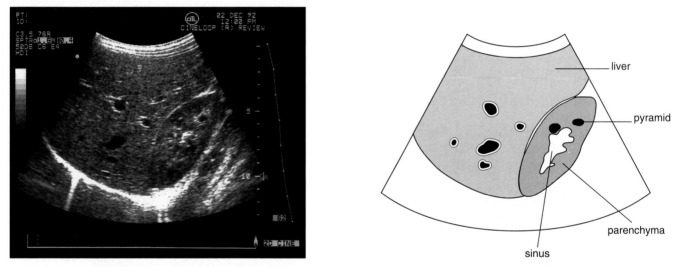

Figure 4–16. In this comparison of the sonographic appearance of liver and renal parenchyma, the liver may be described as being more echogenic than the kidney.

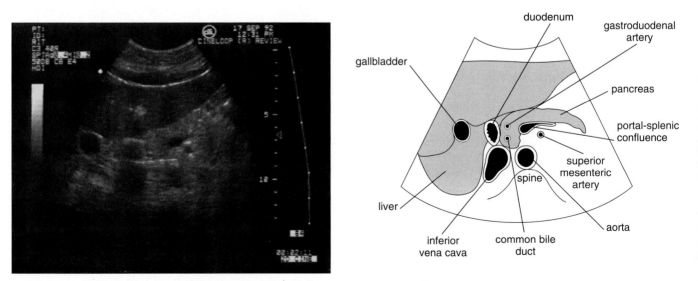

Figure 4–17. In this comparison of the sonographic appearance of liver and pancreatic parenchyma, the liver may be described as being less echogenic than the pancreas.

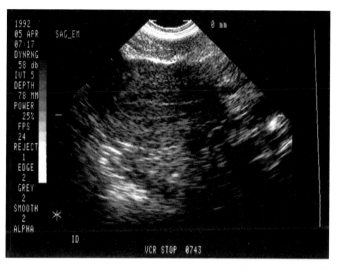
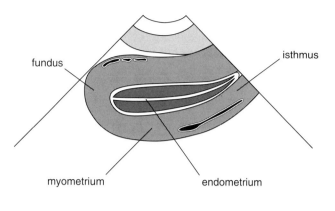

Figure 4–18. The sonographic appearance of the myometrium of the uterus is normally homogeneous, with low to moderate echogenicity.

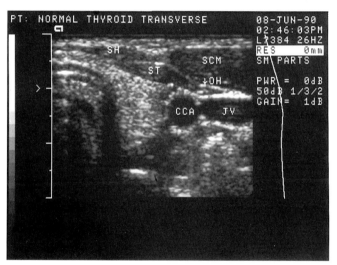
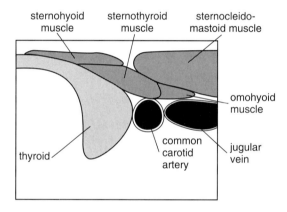

Figure 4–19. The sonographic appearance of muscles is normally homogeneous, with low echogenicity. Note that the muscles are less echogenic than the thyroid.

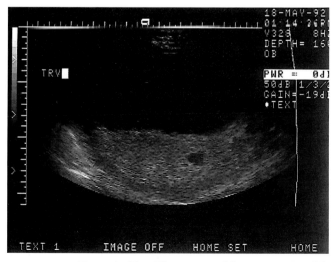
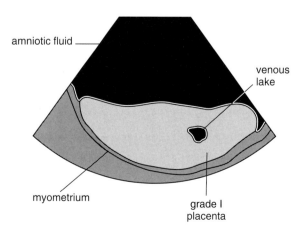

Figure 4–20. The sonographic appearance of the placenta is normally homogeneous, with moderate to high echogenicity. Note that the placenta is more echogenic than the myometrium.

The echo texture of the placenta varies throughout a pregnancy and can be described as homogeneous with moderate to high echogenicity. (See Figure 4–20.) The otherwise-homogeneous texture may be interrupted by vascular components termed venous pools or lakes. Comparatively, the placenta is more echogenic than the adjacent myometrium of the uterus. Other considerations in describing the placenta would depend on any disease or abnormal processes that may be present.

Tissue echo texture, specifically the distinguishable abdominopelvic subcutaneous tissue layers anterior to the muscles, appears homogeneous with moderate echogenicity and strongly reflective borders. (See Figure 4–21.) Description would also depend on any disease or abnormal processes present.

Any fluid-filled structure such as blood vessels, ducts, umbilical cord, and amniotic sac, as well as the ventricles of the heart and brain, ovarian follicles, the urine-filled medullary pyramids and urinary bladder, and the bile-filled gallbladder, for example, are all described as having **anechoic** (echo free) lumens and highly echogenic walls. (See Figure 4–22.) Sound waves readily pass through these fluid-filled structures into surrounding tissues. The sonographic appearance of this through transmission or acoustic enhancement of the surrounding structures is an increase in echogenicity. (See Figure 4–23.) Other considerations in description depend on normal variations and the existence of disease processes.

The *gastrointestinal (GI) tract* is described as having generally **hypoechoic** (echoes not as bright as surrounding tissues) thin walls, though they may appear **hyperechoic** (echoes brighter than surrounding tissues) de-pending on the amount of fat surrounding them. The sonographic appearance of the GI tract lumen depends on its contents. Therefore, the appearance of the lumen varies from anechoic (fluid), to highly echogenic (gas, air, or collapsed lumen), to a mixed pattern (fluid, gas, air, digested food, or feces). (See Figure 4–24.) The GI lumen containing gas or air may cast a shadow because gas and air reflect the sound beam, preventing through transmission. When the bowel is empty and collapsed it is described as having a bull's-eye appearance because of the highly echogenic collapsed lumen and hypoechoic walls. Other considerations in description depend on normal variations and disease processes that may be present.

Bone, fat, air, fissures, ligaments, and the diaphragm are described as echogenic. The degree of echogenicity depends on the density of the structure, its distance from the sound beam, and the angle at which the beam strikes the structure. In most cases these structures are hyperechoic to adjacent tissues. (See Figure 4–25.) Bone, for example, is so dense that it absorbs or attenuates the sound beam, preventing through transmission. This attenuation means that the surface of the bone is generally all that is seen. It appears highly echogenic, with a shadow cast behind it. (See Figure 4–26.) Other considerations in description depend on normal variations and any existing disease processes.

Structures not routinely imaged by sonography include normal lymph nodes, nerves, normal fallopian tubes, normal ureters, and second-order vascular branches. However, with the advancement of ultrasound technology it may become possible to sonographically evaluate these structures.

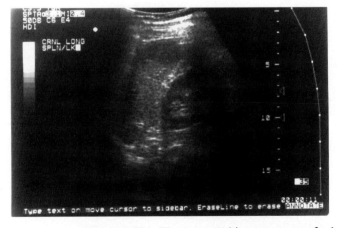

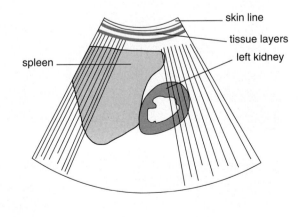

Figure 4–21. The sonographic appearance of subcutaneous tissue layers is normally homogeneous with moderate echogenicity. Note the highly reflective borders.

A

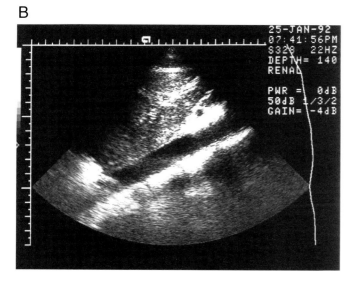
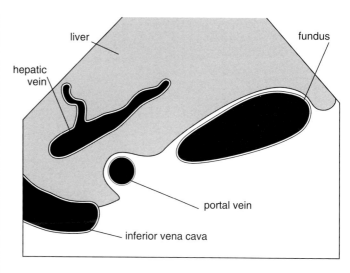

B

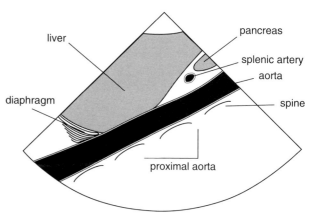

C

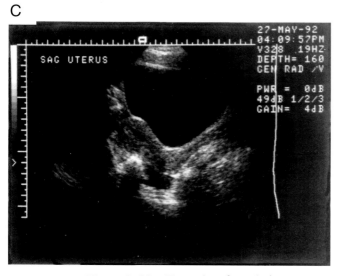
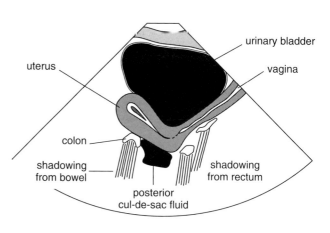

Figure 4–22. Examples of anechoic structures. *A*, The gallbladder, portal vein, inferior vena cava, and hepatic vein. *B*, The aorta and splenic artery. *C*, The urinary bladder. Note the anechoic free fluid in the posterior cul de sac.

Illustration continued on following page.

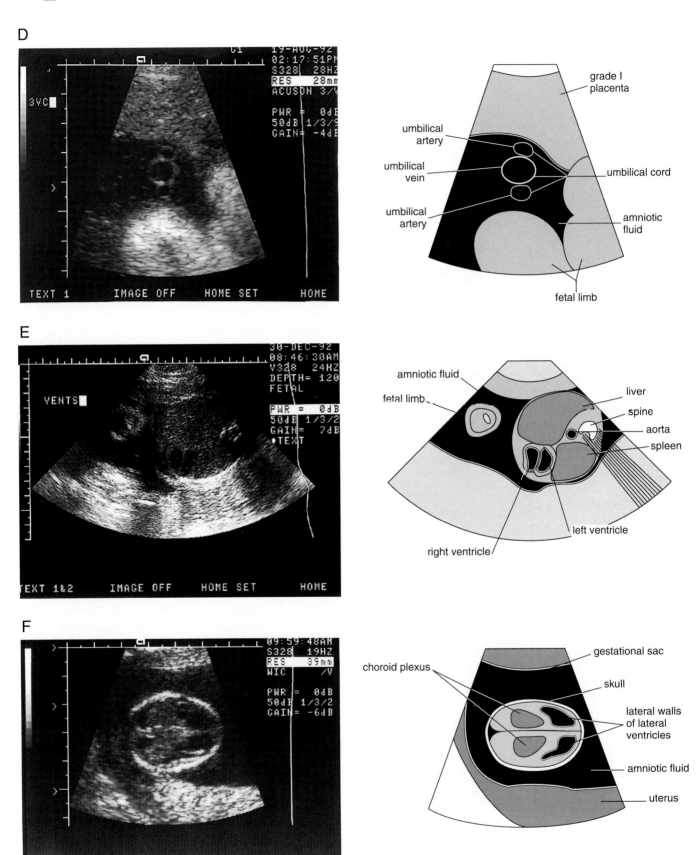

Figure 4–22. *Continued*
D, The umbilical cord surrounded by anechoic amniotic fluid. *E*, The ventricles of the fetal heart, the fetal aorta. Note the surrounding anechoic amniotic fluid. *F*, The ventricles of the fetal brain. Note the surrounding anechoic amniotic fluid.

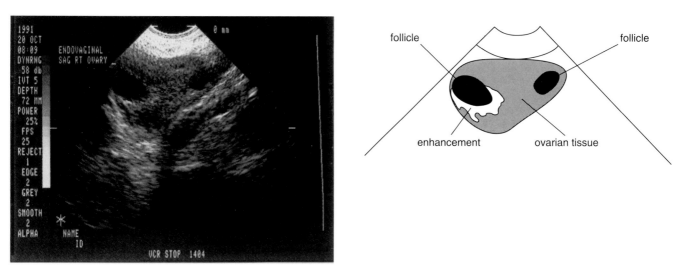

Figure 4-23. The sonographic appearance of acoustic enhancement is increased echogenicity.

A

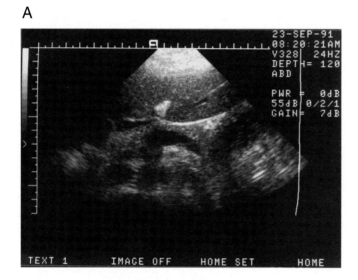
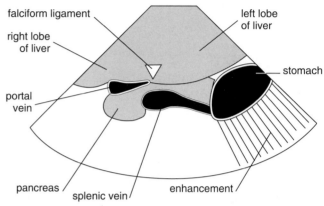

B

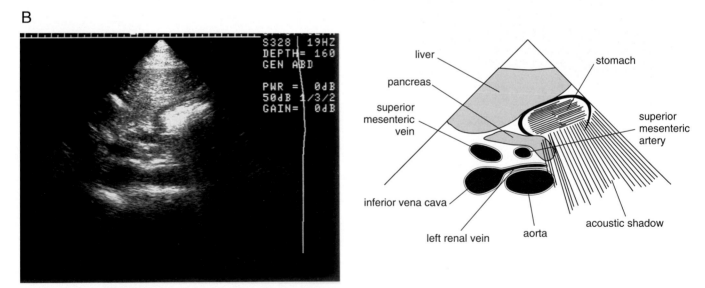

Figure 4–24. The sonographic appearance of the GI tract depends on its contents. *A,* The stomach is fluid filled and appears anechoic. Note the posterior acoustic enhancement. *B,* The stomach lumen appears highly echogenic from either gas or air (its size is too large to be collapsed). Note the hypoechoic appearance and size of the stomach wall. Also note the shadow cast posteriorly.

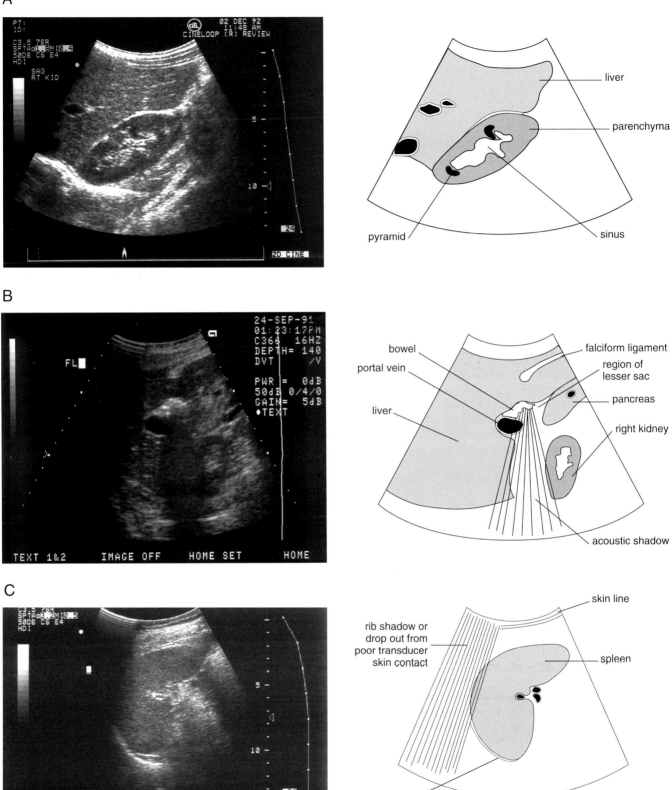

Figure 4–25. Fat, ligaments, and the diaphragm are some of the highly echogenic structures in the body. Note how hyperechoic they are to adjacent structures. *A*, The renal sinus is composed primarily of fat, which causes this highly echogenic appearance. Note how hyperechoic the sinus is to the adjacent renal cortex. *B*, Ligaments are composed of either folds of peritoneum or fibrous cording, which cause this highly echogenic appearance. Note the hyperechoic appearance of the falciform ligament compared to the surrounding liver. *C*, The diaphragm is a very thick, highly echogenic section of muscle. Note its hyperechoic appearance compared to the adjacent spleen.

A

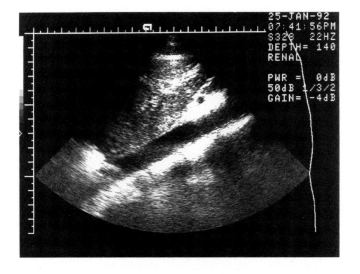

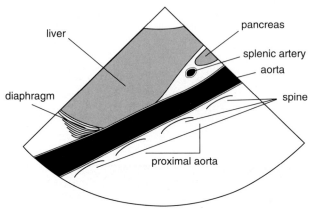

B

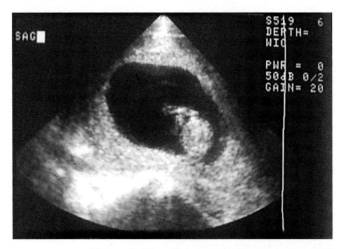

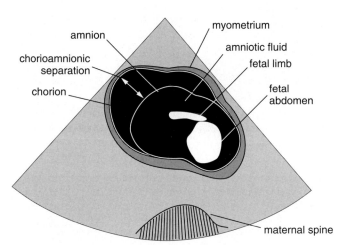

Figure 4–26. The sonographic appearance of bone. *A*, A longitudinal section of the spine showing its highly reflective surface. *B*, A transverse section of the maternal spine demonstrating its reflective surface and the shadow it casts.

Illustration continued on following page.

C

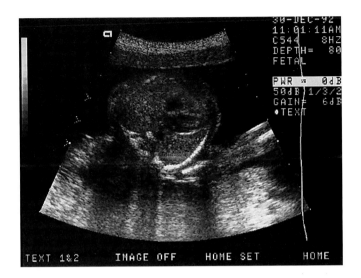

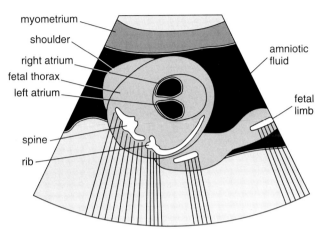

D

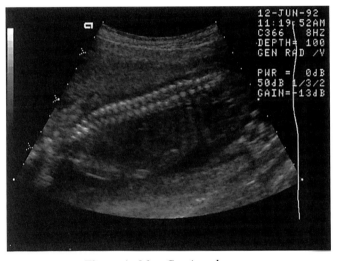

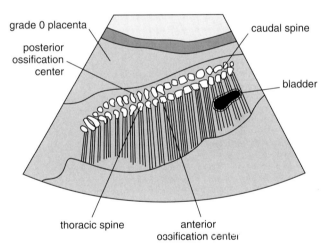

Figure 4–26. *Continued*
C, In the fetus, the bones are easily recognized because of their highly echogenic appearance and characteristic shadowing. *D,* The echogenic fetal spine and the shadow it casts.

References

1. Lane A: Sectional anatomy: Standardized methodology. J Int Soc Plastination 4:16, 1990.
2. Lane A, Sharfaei H: Modern Sectional Anatomy. Philadelphia, WB Saunders, 1992.
3. Dorland's Pocket Medical Dictionary, 24th ed. Philadelphia, WB Saunders, 1982.
4. Kawamura DM: Diagnostic Medical Sonography, vol 3. Philadelphia, JB Lippincott, 1992.
5. Hagen-Ansert SL: Textbook of Diagnostic Ultrasonography, 3rd ed. St. Louis, CV Mosby, 1989.
6. Gray H: Anatomy of the Human Body, 27th ed. Philadelphia, Lea & Febiger, 1965.
7. Grant JCB: An Atlas of Anatomy, 6th ed. Baltimore, Williams & Wilkins, 1972.
8. Lane A: Using plasinated specimens to teach the body layering concept correlated with ultrasound scans. J Int Soc Plastination 19, No. 2, 1994.
9. Heap SW: Cross sectional anatomy of the vessels and ducts of the upper abdomen. Austral Radiol 24:32, 1980.
10. Mittelstaedt CA: Abdominal Ultrasound. New York, Churchill Livingstone, 1987.
11. Gray H: Anatomy, Descriptive and Surgical, 15th ed. New York, Crown Publishers, 1977.
12. Jones B, Braver JM: Essentials of Gastrointestinal Radiology. Philadelphia, WB Saunders, 1982.
13. April EW: Anatomy. Media, PA, Harwal, 1984.

SECTION III

ABDOMINAL SONOGRAPHY

Chapter 5

THE LIVER

MARILYN DICKERSON

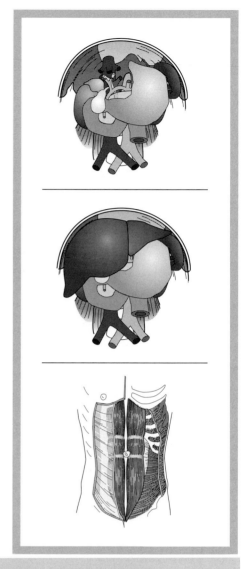

The liver and surrounding anatomic layers. See Figure 4-3 H, I, J, pp. 46-47, for more details.

Objectives:

Identify the functions of the liver.

Describe the location of the liver.

Describe the size of the liver.

Describe and identify the vasculature of the liver.

Identify the ligaments, segments, and fissures of the liver.

Describe the sonographic appearance of the liver.

Describe the associated physicians, diagnostic tests, and laboratory values related to the liver.

Define the key words.

Key Words:

Albumin	Ductus venosus
Bare area	Falciform ligament
Caudate lobe	Fibrinogen
Cholesterol	Gastrohepatic ligament
Coronary ligament	Glisson's capsule
Diverticulum	Hemopoiesis

Hepatic segments	Porta hepatis
Hepatocytes	Portal confluence
Hepatoduodenal ligament	Portal triad
	Prothrombin
Hilus	Quadrate lobe
Left hepatic vein	Reidel's lobe
Left intersegmental tissue	Right hepatic vein
	Right triangular ligament
Left triangular ligament	Round ligament
Lesser omentum	(ligamentum teres)
Ligamentum venosum	Septum transversum
Main lobar fissure	Subhepatic
Main portal vein	Subphrenic
Middle hepatic vein	(subdiaphragmatic)
Papillary process	Transverse fissure

INTRODUCTION

The liver is a powerhouse among abdominal organs, the largest parenchymal organ in the body. Its bulky mass displaces gas-filled components of the digestive system and provides an acoustic window for visualization of upper abdominal and upper retroperitoneal structures.[1]

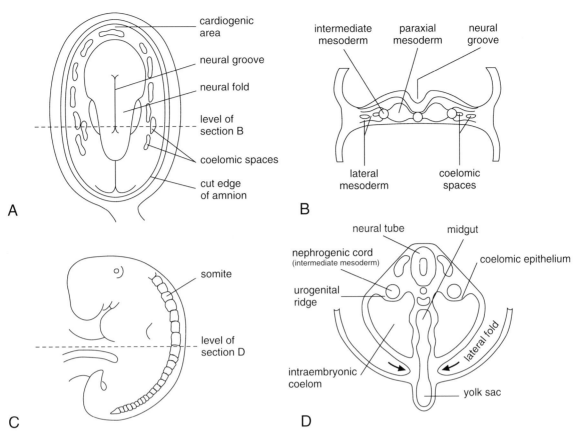

Figure 5-1. Median section of an embryo outlining primitive gut.

Liver structures include the portal veins; the hepatic veins, arteries, and ducts; and the hepatic ligaments and fissures. On ultrasound images, many of these structures help divide the liver into easily identifiable segments.

PRENATAL DEVELOPMENT

The primitive gut is formed during the fourth week of embryonic life and is composed of three parts: a foregut, a midgut, and a hindgut. The liver develops from the foregut.[2] (See Figure 5-1.)

The distal or caudal foregut outpouches between the layers of the ventral mesentery. The head of the outpouch demonstrates a superior diverticulum (a circumscribed sac), also known as the extrahepatic biliary ducts.[2,3] The diverticulum invades the septum transversum and divides to form the right and left hepatic lobes.[3]

The endodermal cells of the diverticulum give rise to the liver parenchymal cells, the **hepatocytes.** These cells become arranged in a series of branching and anastomosing plates.[2] Hepatic cells are corded within and join the blood sinuses of the umbilical and vitelline veins to complete the formation of hepatic parenchyma.[3] The parenchyma is composed of hepatocytes interspersed with Küpffer cells and organized into lobules approxi-

mately 1 by 2 mm in size.[1] Typically, some one million lobules are found in the liver. Peripherally, around each lobule are several portal triads, each containing portal venules, bile ductules, and hepatic arterioles.[1]

The **septum transversum** is a mesodermal structure and becomes the connective tissue of the liver.[3] The Küpffer cells and the fibrous and hematopoietic tissue are derived from the splanchnic mesenchyme of the septum transversum.[2]

The liver grows rapidly and bulges into the midportion of the abdominal cavity. **Hemopoiesis** — the formation and development of blood cells — begins during the sixth week of embryonic life and is primarily responsible for the liver's large size.[2]

The inferior portion of the hepatic diverticulum enlarges to form the gallbladder.[2,3] The common bile duct is derived from the stalk, which connects the hepatic and cystic ducts to the duodenum.[2]

Anomalies of the liver include the left-sided liver (situs inversus), congenital cysts, congenital hemangioma, and intrahepatic biliary duct atresia or stenosis.[3]

LOCATION

The liver occupies a major portion of the right hypochondrium. Normally it extends inferiorly into the epi-

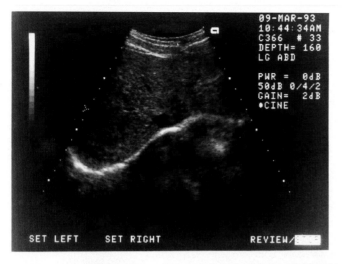

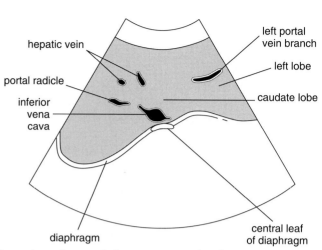

Figure 5-2. Transverse view of the diaphragmatic undersurface and the posterosuperior liver surface.

gastrium and laterally into the left hypochondrium. Superiorly, it reaches the dome of the diaphragm and posteriorly it borders the bony lumbar region of the

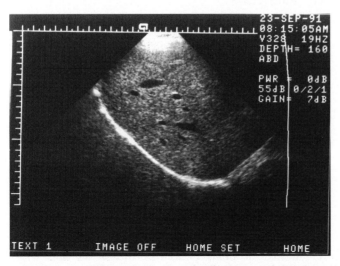

Figure 5-3. Depiction of anterior liver surface.

muscular posterior abdominal wall. The bulk of the liver lies beneath the right costal margin.[3-5] (See Figure 5-2.)

The superior surface, anterior surface, and a portion of the posterior surface of the liver are in contact with the diaphragm.[6] The inferior or visceral surface of the liver rests upon the upper abdominal organs.[4] (See Figure 5-3.)

The right lobe of the liver lies close to the anterolateral abdominal wall. Its square, convex right lateral surface is the base of its pyramid. (See Figure 5-4.) The right lobe is related to the right lateral undersurface of the diaphragm along the right midaxillary line from the seventh to the eleventh ribs.[3] On the lateral right side, the liver is related to the diaphragmatic recess and the descending fibers of the diaphragm.

The left lobe of the liver is closely related to the undersurface of the diaphragm. The smallest lobe, the **caudate,** is related to the lumbar region of the porterior abdominal wall and to the lower posterior thoracic wall.[3] The

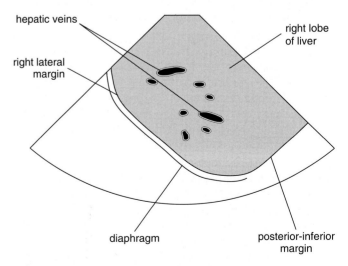

Figure 5-4. Longitudinal scan of right lateral margin of liver illustrating base of liver pyramid.

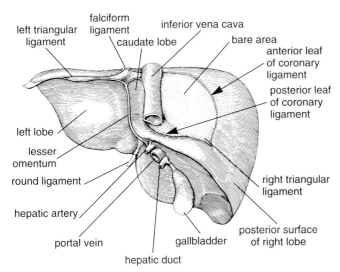

Figure 5-5. Depiction of posterior surface outlining boundaries of bare area of liver.

anterior boundary of the caudate lobe is marked by the posterior surface of the left portal vein and the posterior boundary is the inferior vena cava.[7] The lateral margin projects into the superior recess of the lesser sac, and the caudal border forms the cephalad margin of the epiploic foramen of Winslow.[7]

The inferior vena cava courses through the **bare area** of the liver, which lies between the leaflets of the anterior inferior and posterior superior coronary ligaments.[8] The right kidney and right adrenal gland lie near the bare area laterally and inferiorly. The boundaries of the bare area include the falciform ligament, right anterior inferior and right posterior superior coronary ligaments, right triangular ligament, gastrohepatic ligament, left anterior and left posterior coronary ligaments, and the left triangular ligament.[8] (See Figure 5-5.)

The major relations of the right posterosuperior surface are the right posterior fibers of the diaphragm, the upper posterior abdominal wall, the right kidney, and the right adrenal gland.[3] The inferior segment of this surface below the inferior leaf of the coronary ligament communicates with the upper end of the right lumbar paracolic gutter and the visceral surface of the liver.[3]

The posterior surface of the liver is protected by the bony and muscular posterior abdominal wall. The border between the anterior aspect of the liver and the visceral surface is the inferior margin.[4]

The inferior surface of the liver is marked by indentations from organs in contact with its surface. Right-sided inferior indentations occur at the right hepatic flexure of the colon, the right kidney and adrenal gland, the first part of the duodenum, and the gallbladder.[3,5] The left side of the inferior surface contains a gastric indentation, and the posterior surface is marked by the groove which surrounds the inferior vena cava.[5] (See Figure 5-6.)

The inferior (visceral) surface is related to the gallbladder, pylorus, duodenum, right colon, right hepatic flexure of the colon, right third of the transverse colon, right adrenal, and right kidney.[3] The anterior midportion of the inferior surface is the medial portion of the left lobe of the liver. This portion is also referred to as the **quadrate lobe** of the liver. The left lateral boundary of this portion is the falciform ligament, noted just to the right of the midline. (See Figure 5-7.)

The posterior midportion of the inferior surface, below the porta hepatis, marks the location of the **caudate lobe**. The posterior portions of the left and caudate lobes forms a portion of the anterior boundary of the lesser sac.[9] The lesser sac lies anterior to the pancreas and posterior to the stomach.[10]

The left hepatic lobe varies in size and shape and may extend deeply into the left upper quadrant.[9,11] The free

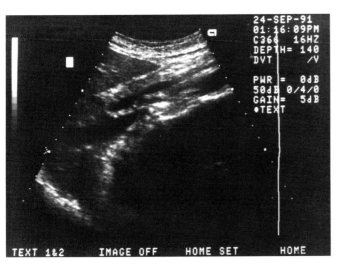

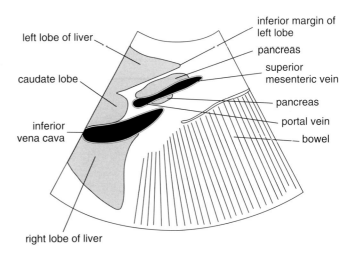

Figure 5-6. Longitudinal image of left inferior margin of left hepatic lobe. Note the superior mesenteric vein merging into the portal confluence, and the emerging main portal vein anterior to the inferior vena cava.

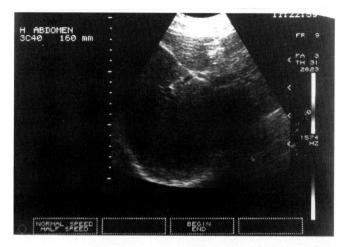

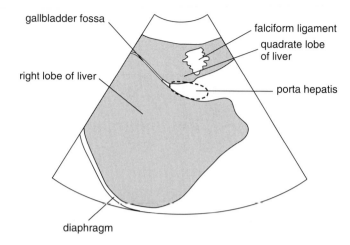

Figure 5–7. Transverse scan of liver. The falciform ligament appears as a bright echogenic focus demarcating the lateral border of the quadrate lobe.

inferior margin of the left lobe is closely related to the gastric body and antrum of the stomach. It frequently lies anterior to the body of the pancreas, the splenic vein, and the splenic artery.[9]

SIZE

In the adult male the liver weighs between 1400 and 1800 g; in the adult female, between 1200 and 1400 g.[3]

The contours of the liver are determined by the length of the right lobe and the size of the lateral segment of the left lobe.[11]

The right lobe is larger than the left, containing approximately two thirds of the parenchymal tissue.[12] Along the midclavicular line, the normal longitudinal measurement of the right lobe is less than or equal to 13 cm.[13] This measurement has also been stated to be 15 to 17 cm.[14]

The left lobe is more varied in size.[12] It may be atrophic if interference with the left portal venous supply arises as the ductus venosus closes at birth.[11] A larger left lobe helps in visualization of the pancreas and left upper quadrant.[11,12]

GROSS ANATOMY

The liver is divided into three lobes; a right lobe, a left lobe, and a caudate lobe. The right and left lobes are subdivided into four segments, anterior and posterior segments on the right, and lateral and medial segments on the left.[16] The **caudate lobe** is a midline structure on the posterior aspect of the liver which separates a portion of each of the right and left hepatic lobes.[7] The caudate lobe is separated from the left hepatic lobe by the proximal portion of the left hepatic vein and the fissure for the ligamentum venosum.[1] This fissure contains the

ligamentum venosum and a portion of the lesser omentum.[17]

The anterior midportion of the inferior surface of the liver is sometimes called the **quadrate lobe.** It is not an anatomically distinct lobe, but is more correctly identified as the medial segment of the left lobe.[1] The **left intersegmental fissure** divides the medial and lateral segments of the left hepatic lobe.[1]

The hepatic veins drain blood from the segments and lobes of the liver.[1] They are interlobar and intersegmental.[16] The **right hepatic vein** separates and drains the anterior and posterior segments of the right lobe. The **left hepatic vein** separates and drains the medial and lateral segments of the left lobe of the liver. The **middle hepatic vein** separates and drains the right and the medial left liver lobes.[18,19] (See Figures 5–8 and 5–9.) The hepatic veins subdivide into superior and inferior groups. The smaller inferior veins drain the caudate lobe and the posteromedial portion of the right lobe.[20]

The portal veins course within and supply the hepatic lobes and segments.[16] Although the hepatic veins usually divide the liver segments, the left portal vein serves as an intersegmental boundary between the medial and lateral segments of the left lobe on caudal transverse scans of the left hepatic lobe.[19]

The portal system supplies 75 percent of total blood flow to the liver and has three main tributaries to its **confluence:** the splenic vein, the superior mesenteric vein, and the inferior mesenteric vein, which may join the splenic vein on its course to the portal confluence.

The main portal vein enters the porta hepatis and divides into left and right branches. These veins then branch into medial and lateral divisions on the left and anterior and posterior divisions on the right, and become intrasegmental.[11] The main and right portal veins traverse and supply the bulk of the liver centrally. The left portal vein ascends anteriorly, proximal to the falciform ligament. In patients with severe portal hypertension, the

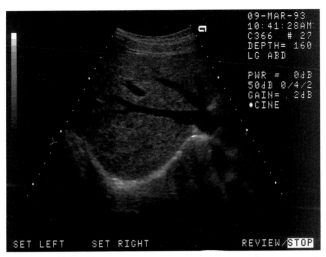
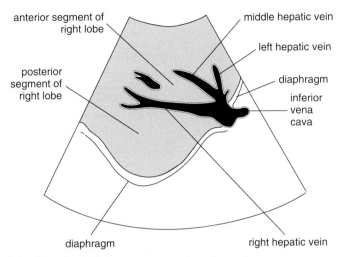

Figure 5–8. Transverse scan of hepatic veins draining into the inferior vena cava. Anterior and posterior segments of the right hepatic lobe are prominently displayed.

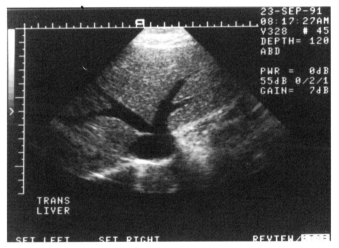
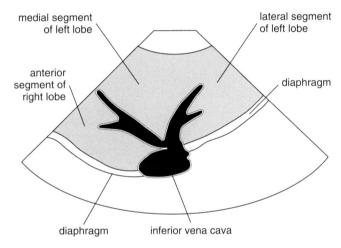

Figure 5–9. Transverse scan of liver showing hepatic veins in the "bunny sign."

left portal vein enters the falciform ligament and communicates with the umbilical vein.[16,21] The caudate lobe is supplied with blood from both the right and left portal veins. (See Figures 5–10 to 5–13.)

The anterosuperior surface of the liver fits snugly into the dome of the diaphragm, separated from the overlying pleural cavities and pericardium.[3] On the right, on full expiration it rises to the level of the fourth rib interspace. On full expiration the thin edge of the superior surface of the left lobe reaches the level of the fifth rib. The anterosuperior surface runs superiorly, then posteriorly, to the anterior leaf of the coronary ligaments on the right. On the left, it runs posteriorly to the left triangular ligament. The right anterosuperior surface of the liver is closest to the anterolateral abdominal wall and is palpable most often when the organ is enlarged.[3]

The liver is enclosed by a tight, fibrous capsule known as **Glisson's capsule,** and is largely covered by the peritoneum of the greater sac. The caudate lobe is covered by the peritoneum of the lesser sac.[3] To the left of the midline, the posterosuperior surface of the liver is covered by the peritoneum of the greater sac. A portion of the posterior surface of the liver is without a peritoneal covering and is called the **bare area.** This is in direct contact with the diaphragm.[6]

Peritoneal ligaments connect the liver to upper abdominal structures. The **coronary ligament** connects the posterosuperior surface of the liver to the diaphragm at the margins of the bare area.[5] The bare area separates and lies between the right posterior subphrenic space above from the posterior **subhepatic space** (Morrison's pouch) below.[3,10] (See Figure 5–14.) The upper layer of the coronary ligament extends from the superior liver surface to the inferior surface of the diaphragm. The

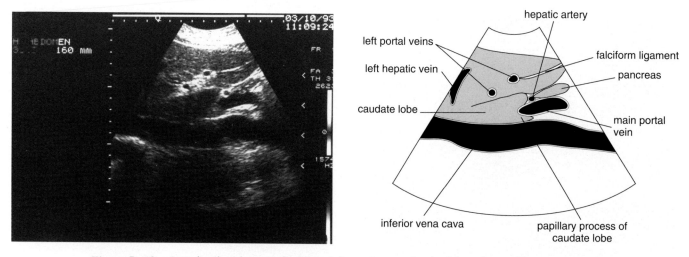

Figure 5–10. Longitudinal image of origin of the main portal vein. Note the papillary process of the caudate lobe.

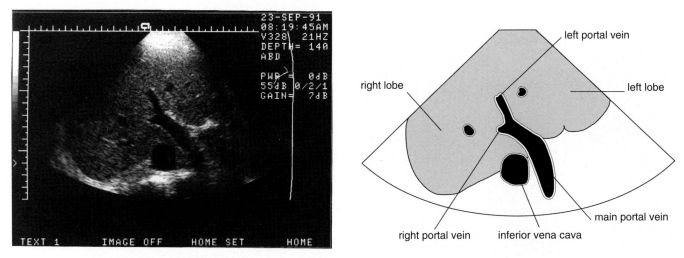

Figure 5–11. Main portal vein entering the porta hepatis just anterior to the IVC and dividing into right and left branches.

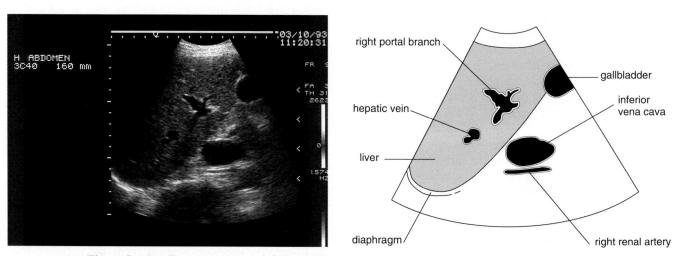

Figure 5–12. Transverse scan of right portal vein. Note the right renal artery coursing linearly posterior to the short-axis IVC.

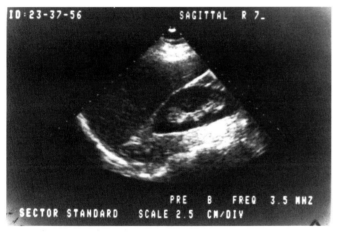

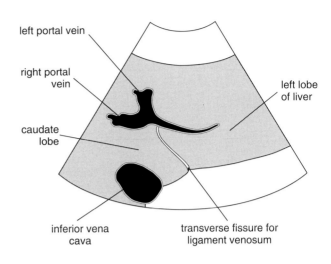

Figure 5–13. Transverse scan of the portal vein branches at the level of the porta hepatis. Note the caudate lobe anterior to the IVC and posterior to the left portal vein (LPV) at this level.

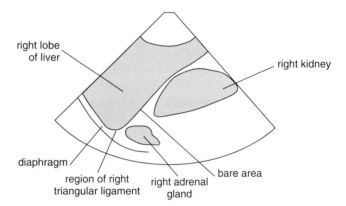

Figure 5–14. Longitudinal scan of the right kidney and the right adrenal gland in contact with the bare area of the liver.

lower layer extends from the posterior surface of the right lobe of the liver to the right kidney, the right adrenal gland, and the inferior vena cava.[3]

The **right triangular ligament** is formed by an extension of the coronary ligament inferiorly to the right.[5] It begins at the right margin of the bare area and connects the posterior surface of the right lobe to the right undersurface of the diaphragm.[5] The posterior subphrenic and posterior subhepatic spaces, separated by the bare area medially, become continuous, lateral to the right triangular ligament.[10]

The **left triangular ligament** is an extension of the falciform ligament to the left. As the falciform ligament passes over the liver dome, it divides into two leaflets. The left leaflet forms a portion of the left triangular ligament.[3] The right leaflet merges with the coronary ligament.[3] It connects the posterior surface of the left lobe to the left aspect of the diaphragm. The triangular

and coronary ligaments are not normally visualized on ultrasound examinations.

The **falciform ligament** connects the liver to the anterior abdominal wall and to the diaphragm. The attachment extends from the superior surface of the liver at the umbilical notch to the inferior surface at the porta hepatis.[3] (See Figure 5–15.) The right, anterior, and superior surfaces unite to form the convex upper surface of the liver. The posterior surface is a continuation of that surface.[5]

The **lesser omentum** is a mesentery or double layer of peritoneum that joins the lesser curvature of the stomach and the proximal duodenum to the liver.[22] The lesser omentum contains the gastrohepatic and hepatoduodenal ligaments.

The **gastrohepatic ligament** is that portion of the lesser omentum which extends across the **transverse fissure** (fissure for the ligamentum venosum) of the liver at the

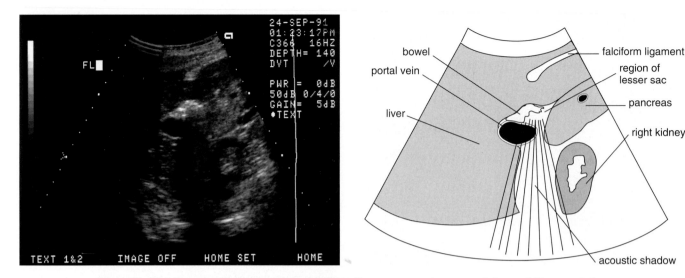

Figure 5–15. Longitudinal scan of the falciform ligament coursing toward the umbilicus and the anterior abdominal wall. Note the characteristic sickle shape.

porta hepatis to the lesser curvature of the stomach.[3] The lesser omentum separates the lesser sac from the gastrohepatic recess.[10]

The **ligamentum venosum** marks the left anterolateral border of the caudate lobe.[3] The lateral segment of the left lobe is separated from the caudate lobe by the fissure for the ligamentum venosum. The ligamentum venosum is a remnant of the fetal **ductus venosus,** which shunted oxygenated blood from the umbilical vein to the inferior vena cava.[19] (See Figure 5–16.) The fissure for the ligamentum venosum contains the gastrohepatic ligament.

The **hepatoduodenal ligament** is that portion of the lesser omentum which extends as the right free border of the gastrohepatic ligament to the proximal duodenum

and the right hepatic flexure of the colon.[3] The hepatoduodenal ligament marks the right ventral border of the lesser omentum. Portions of the common bile duct and the hepatic artery are often visualized on transverse scans at the level of the hepatoduodenal ligament, just cephalad to the head of the pancreas and adjacent to the porta hepatis.[9] The **porta hepatis** is the opening of the liver through which the portal veins and hepatic arteries enter and through which the hepatic ducts exit. The common bile duct and hepatic artery course anterior to the portal vein in the **portal triad** at this level. The common bile duct is the anterolateral vessel. It then passes posterior to the duodenum and enters the pancreas. (See Figure 5–17.)

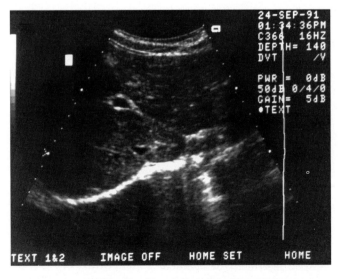

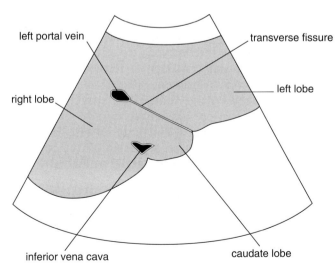

Figure 5–16. Transverse scan of the caudate lobe. The transverse fissure courses toward the left portal vein, marking the anterior border of the caudate.

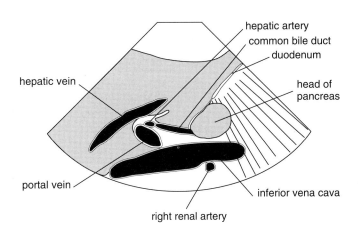

Figure 5-17. Longitudinal scan of the common bile duct coursing toward the head of the pancreas at the level of the hepatoduodenal ligament.

PHYSIOLOGY

The liver is a primary center of metabolism, supporting multiple body systems and activities.

In support of the digestive and excretory systems, the liver metabolizes fats, carbohydrates, and proteins and forms bile and urea.[4]

The liver absorbs blood received from the portal veins. The blood contains products of digestion such as amino acids and glucose. The liver uses glucose to metabolize carbohydrates. For carbohydrate metabolism, the liver breaks down, stores, and manufactures simple sugars.[15] It metabolizes amino acids into proteins.[4] The liver synthesizes the blood proteins **albumin, fibrinogen,** prothrombin, and globulins.[15] Fat is absorbed from fatty acids and desaturated in the liver. Fat metabolism results in the formation of cholesterol and phospholipids. **Cholesterol** is a major component of the bile which is secreted by the liver and which serves to emulsify fats.[4] Approximately 1 pint of bile is secreted each day.[15]

The liver is a contributor to the lymphatic system by the formation of lymph fluid.

The liver also stores vitamins and other metabolic substances, detoxifies harmful chemicals, regulates blood volume, and is a major source of body heat.

SONOGRAPHIC APPEARANCE

The liver should be homogeneous and moderately echogenic throughout.[16,23]

A boundary between the left and right hepatic lobes can be imagined along a line coursing posteriorly from the gallbladder fossa to the groove for the inferior vena cava. This line is the **main lobar fissure.**[3,5] This fissure is identified on most sonograms along the right oblique plane and extends a varying and short distance between the long axis neck of the gallbladder and a cross-section of the main portal vein. The fissure does not extend cephalad to the plane of the right portal vein.[19] The reflection is hyperechoic and appears as a thin line connecting the gallbladder neck to the portal vein. (See Figure 5-18.)

Many landmark structures are visible on a longitudinal scan through the long axis of the inferior vena cava. Cephalad (superiorly) to caudad (inferiorly), one should see, anterior to the inferior vena cava, the following structures: the right atrium, the central leaf of the diaphragm superior to the left hepatic lobe, the middle hepatic vein as it enters the vena cava, the caudate lobe of the liver separated from the lateral left lobe by the ligamentum venosum, the extrahepatic main portal vein in cross-section, and the head of the pancreas.[21] The superior mesenteric vein may be seen coursing toward its junction with the splenic vein at the portal confluence. The left portal vein may be visualized on its c-shaped superior course, proximal to the falciform ligament.

Ligaments and fissures are demonstrated as highly echogenic because of the presence of collagen and fat within and around these structures.[9] The attachment of the **falciform ligament** from the upper surfaces of the liver to the diaphragm and the upper abdominal wall appears to divide the right and left lobes.[3] It represents the lower margin of peritoneum surrounding the ligamentum teres, or round ligament, of the liver. The falciform ligament is highly echogenic on both longitudinal and transverse scans, appearing sickle shaped on longitudinal scans and pyramidal on transverse scans. (See Figure 5-19.)

The **round ligament** (ligamentum teres) is the obliterated umbilical vein, a fibrous cord which extends upward from the diaphragm to the anterior abdominal wall.[3] On transverse scan it most often is identifiable coursing within the lower margin of the falciform liga-

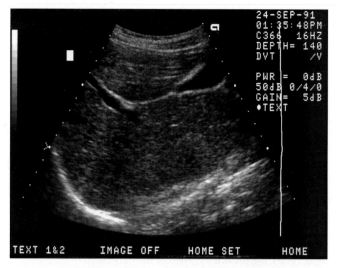
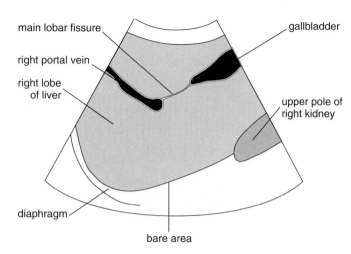

Figure 5–18. Longitudinal scan of the main lobar fissure seen as an echogenic line connecting the neck of the gallbladder to the right portal vein.

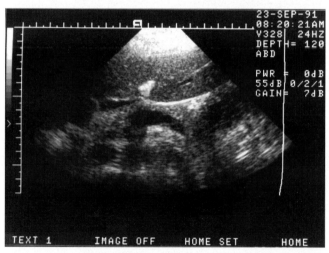
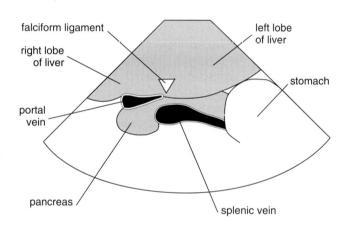

Figure 5–19. Transverse scan of the falciform ligament. Note its characteristic pyramidal shape. The echogenic focus is also referred to as the round ligament or ligamentum teres at this level.

ment. These structures lie close to the anterior midline surface of the body and within the near field of the transducer. They are displayed on the upper midportion of the screen.

The echogenic falciform ligament courses anteriorly and inferiorly from the left portal vein toward the umbilicus.[21] Transverse scans through the liver frequently demonstrate an echogenic focus in the area of the falciform ligament. This structure correlates the sonographic appearance of the falciform ligament with its appearance on computed tomography (CT) scan, although it may be prominent enough to raise the suspicion of a solid mass.[24] The presence of a recanalized umbilical vein within the falciform ligament should be looked for in cases of portal hypertension.[16,21]

The **main portal vein** is visualized at its origin, posteroinferior to the neck of the pancreas. Identification of

the porta hepatis is possible with visualization of the main portal vein lying anterior to the inferior vena cava. This point of contact is also an indicator for the **hilus** of the liver.[11,25] Once the main portal vein enters the porta hepatis, it divides into a smaller, more anterior and more superior left portal vein and a larger, more posterior and more inferior right portal vein.[11] Portal veins decrease in size as they approach the diaphragm.[25]

The junction of the right and left portal veins is noted on a superiorly angled transverse scan just inferior to the plane which demonstrates the convergence of the three hepatic veins on the inferior vena cava (IVC). This level identifies the location of the union of the left and right hepatic ducts to form the common hepatic duct. The right portal vein is followed medially to detect the common hepatic duct crossing linearly anterior to it. The common hepatic duct should be measured at this loca-

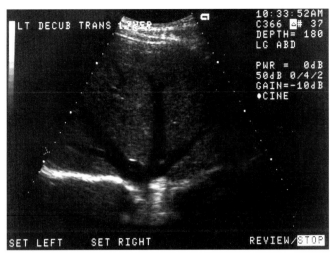

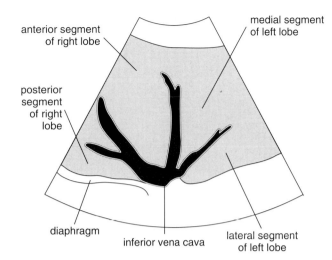

Figure 5-20. Transverse scan of hepatic veins draining into the IVC, providing for sonographic segmentation of hepatic lobes.

tion anterior to the right portal vein. Any measurement greater than 5 mm raises the possibility of biliary obstruction.

The hepatic veins increase in size as they drain toward the diaphragm and inferior vena cava.[25] Any large vein in the liver near the diaphragm may be considered a hepatic vein.[11] There are several features which distinguish hepatic veins from portal veins: Hepatic veins course between lobes and segments. Portal veins course within segments. Hepatic veins drain toward the right atrium and usually have anechoic borders, except near the IVC where the venous walls are more reflective.[11] The positions of the hepatic veins can therefore be used to identify the segments of the liver and provide precise descriptions of focal lesions.[20]

Identification of **hepatic segments** is important in localizing potentially resectable lesions of the liver.[21] Lesions of this type include primary hepatic neoplasms, single metastatic lesions, and some nonmalignant hepatic abnormalities.[9] (See Figure 5-20.)

Posterior to the inferior vena cava on parasagittal scans, the anechoic right renal artery is seen in short axis, anterior to the right linear crus of the diaphragm noted with midlevel echoes.[21] Any other solid-appearing mass posterior to the inferior vena cava and inferior to the liver should suggest the presence of enlarged lymph nodes or adrenal lesions.[21]

SONOGRAPHIC APPLICATIONS

Ultrasound examinations of the liver are indicated for suspected liver enlargement, hepatic or perihepatic masses, abscesses, and obstructive or metastatic lesions. Cystic, solid, and complex masses are readily identifiable because they distort the smooth contour of the liver. Abnormal lesions usually are increased or de-

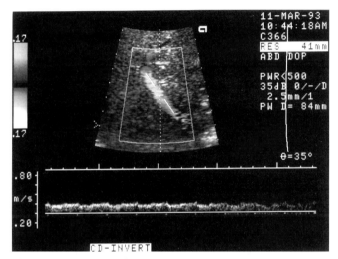

Figure 5-21. Color flow Doppler image showing the characteristic waveform of a normal portal vein. Note that the blood flow is in the direction of the liver toward the transducer. (See Color Plate 2 at the back of this book.)

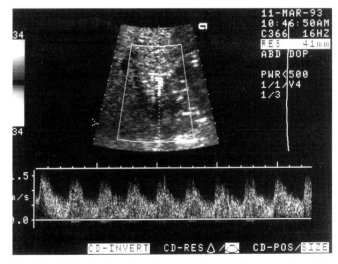

Figure 5-22. Color flow Doppler image demonstrating the characteristic arterial waveform of the normal hepatic artery. (See Color Plate 3 at the back of this book.)

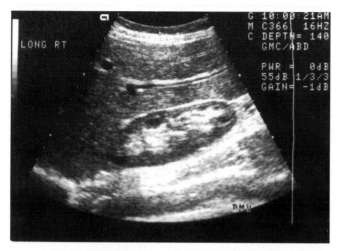
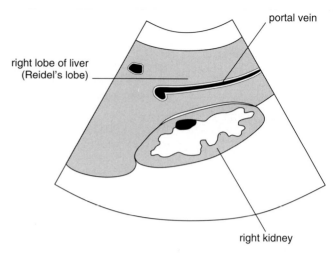

Figure 5-23. Longitudinal image in a woman with Reidel's lobe, a tongue-like extension. This lobe extends caudally to the iliac crest.

creased in echogenicity when compared to the moderate echo strength of the liver parenchymal reflectors. The liver parenchyma is normally homogeneous and should be carefully examined to exclude small focal lesions. Pleural effusions may be visualized in the **subdiaphragmatic** (subphrenic) region superior to the liver capsule. Ascites is identifiable when fluid collects in the subcapsular or intraperitoneal spaces surrounding the liver.

Vascular structures of the liver and porta hepatis are evaluated using duplex abdominal Doppler techniques and color flow Doppler techniques. (See Figures 5-21 and 5-22.) The presence, direction, and blood-flow velocity in a sample volume are assessed with these examinations.[26] The portal vein, the hepatic arteries and veins, and the splenic artery and vein are the upper abdominal vessels normally evaluated. The usual indications for sonography are cases of suspected portal hypertension, portal or hepatic vein thrombosis, and pre- and postoperative hepatic surgery.[26]

NORMAL VARIANTS

Reidel's lobe is a tongue-like inferior extension of the right lobe, as far caudally as the iliac crest.[11,14] (See Figure 5-23.) It has the same sonographic appearance as normal liver parenchyma. On ultrasound this variant can be identified when liver tissue extends well below the inferior pole of the right kidney during normal respiration.

The caudate lobe may have a distal **papillary process** which may be confused with an enlarged lymph node or another extrahepatic lesion.[7,27] This process appears as a rounded prominence on the anteroinferior aspect of the caudate lobe.[27] The papillary process may appear as a separate structure on both longitudinal and transverse sections.[27] It has the same sonographic appearance as normal liver parenchyma.

Another variation is an elongated left lobe with a tip which may extend laterally to the spleen.[1] Sonographic appearance is the same as the normal liver.

REFERENCE CHARTS

Associated Physicians

Gastroenterologist: Specializes in treating diseases of the gastrointestinal tract, including the stomach, small and large bowel, the gallbladder, and bile ducts.

Internist: Specializes in studying the physiology and pathology of internal organs and diagnosing and treating disorders of those organs.

Oncologist: Specializes in the study and treatment of tumors and malignancies.

Radiologist: Specializes in the diagnostic interpretation of imaging modalities that assess to liver.

Vascular specialist: Studies and treats disorders of blood vessels.

Surgeon: Utilizes operative procedures to treat diseases, trauma, and organ deformity.

Common Diagnostic Tests

Examination	Use
COMPUTED TOMOGRAPHY (CT)	Focal lesions Tumor masses Bone displacement Fluid accumulation Biopsy

This x-ray examination utilizes a narrow collimated beam of x-rays that rotate around the patient in a continuous 360° arc in order to image the body in cross-sectional slices. The image is created by a digital computer which calculates attenuation or tissue absorption of the x-ray beams. Very small differences in density of body structures may be demonstrated and are displayed on x-ray film. The examination is performed by radiologic technologists who specialize in computed tomography and is interpreted by radiologists.

Examination	Use
ANGIOGRAPHY	Focal lesions Myocardial infarction Vascular occlusion Portal hypertension Renal tumors Pulmonary emboli Mass characterization Vascular anatomy Therapy

This examination utilizes x-rays to visualize the internal structure of the heart and blood vessels after the injection of a contrast medium into an artery or vein. A catheter is used to insert the contrast material into a peripheral artery, and threaded through the vessel to a visceral site. Angiograms are performed by radiologists and assisted by radiologic technologists. The examination is interpreted by the radiologist.

Examination	Use
MAGNETIC RESONANCE IMAGING (MR, MRI)	Focal lesions Tumors Brain functions Body chemistry Heart disease 3-D imaging

The MR scanner surrounds the patient with powerful electromagnets which create a magnetic field. Hydrogen atoms in the patient's body are disturbed by this field. The atoms' protons become aligned in the direction of the magnetic field's poles. The computers process and measure the speed and volume with which the protons return to their normal state, and display a diagnostic image of striking clarity on a monitor. Intravenous contrast materials may be given to enhance image definition. MR produces cross-sectional and sagittal soft tissue images. The examinations are performed by registered radiologic technologists and interpreted by radiologists. Physicists assist radiologists in the MR laboratory because of the complexity of the MR equipment.

Examination	Use
RADIONUCLIDE SCINTIGRAPHY	Focal lesions Tumors Cysts Abscesses Vascular anatomy

Scintigraphy utilizes a gamma camera to detect radioactive substances given intravenously or by mouth. Scintigraphy commences when the radioisotope reaches optimum activity in the part being examined. For liver studies this begins immediately after injection. A technetium sulfur colloid is the radionuclide used in liver studies. Recording devices convert voltage impulses received from the scanner into a paper or x-ray film record of a series of dots which reflect the radiation intensities received. Abnormalities are indicated by an absence of activity. The examinations are performed by certified nuclear medicine technologists. They are interpreted by radiologists or nuclear physicians.

Laboratory Values

LIVER FUNCTION TESTS

Test	Normal	Increase	Decrease
Bilirubin-T[1]	0.2–1.0 mg/dl	Jaundice	
Bilirubin-C[2]	0–0.2 mg/dl		
Alkaline phosphatase (ALP)	1.5–4.5 BU/dl	Metastases	
	0.8–2.9 BLB	Obstruction	
	Unit	Lesions	
		Jaundice	
AST (SGOT)	5–30 U/L	Hepatitis	
		Liver injury	
		Jaundice	
		Cholestasis	
		Myocardial infarction	
		Muscle disease	
		Cirrhosis	
		Metastases	
		Fatty liver	
		Lymphoma	
ALT (SGPT)	6–37 U/L	Jaundice	
		Hepatitis	
Cholesterol[1]	140–200 mg/dl		Liver disease
			Cancer
Lactic dehydrogenase (LD)	100–225 U/L[3]	Liver disease	
	180–280 U/L[4]	Cancer	
Protein[1]	6.5–8.3 g/dl	Chronic liver disease	
Prothrombin			
Time (PTT)	11–15 seconds	Liver disease	

1 — Total
2 — Conjugated
3 — Forward
4 — Reverse

Normal Measurements

Nonapplicable.

Vasculature

ARTERIAL SYSTEM

Vessel	Branch of	Supplies
Common hepatic artery	Celiac artery	Liver
Proper hepatic artery	Common hepatic	Liver
Right hepatic artery	Proper hepatic	Right lobe Right caudate
Left hepatic artery	Proper hepatic (may arise from left gastric artery)	Left lobe Quadrate lobe Left caudate

VENOUS SYSTEM

Vessel	Tributary to	Drains
Central veins	Hepatic veins	Sinusoids
Right hepatic vein	Inferior vena cava	Right lobe
Middle hepatic vein	Inferior vena cava	Right lobe Caudate lobe
Left hepatic vein	Inferior vena cava	Left lobe Quadrate lobe

PORTAL SYSTEM

Vessel	Tributary to	Drains
Main portal vein		Gastrointestinal tract
Superior mesenteric vein	Portal vein	Gastrointestinal tract
Inferior mesenteric vein	Splenic vein	Gastrointestinal tract
Splenic vein	Portal vein	Spleen Pancreas

Affecting Chemicals

Nonapplicable.

References

1. Sarti DA: Diagnostic Ultrasound: Text and Cases, 2nd ed. Chicago, Year Book, 1987.
2. Moore KL: The Developing Human: Clinically Oriented Embryology, 4th ed. Philadelphia, WB Saunders, 1988.
3. Linder HH: Clinical Anatomy. Norwalk, CT, Appleton & Lange, 1989.
4. Netter FH: The CIBA Collection of Medical Illustrations, vol. 3, The Digestive System. Summit, NJ, CIBA Pharmaceutical, CIBA-Geigy, 1977.
5. Bockus HL: Gastroenterology, 2nd ed., vol. 3. Philadelphia, WB Saunders, 1965.
6. Basmajian JV, Slonecker, CE: Grant's Method of Anatomy, 11th ed. Baltimore, Williams & Wilkins, 1989.
7. Dodds WJ, Erickson SJ, Taylor AJ, et al: Caudate lobe of the liver: anatomy, embryology, and pathology. Am J Roentgenol 154:87–93, 1990.
8. April EW: Anatomy. Media, PA, Harwal, 1984.
9. Kane RA: Sonographic anatomy of the liver. Semin Ultrasound 2:190–196, 1981.
10. Rubenstein WA, Auh YH, Whalen JP, Kazam E: The perihepatic spaces: computed tomographic and ultrasound imaging. Radiology 149:231–239, 1983.
11. Marks WM, Filly RA, Callen PW: Ultrasonic anatomy of the liver: a review with new applications. J Clin Ultrasound 7:137–146, 1979.
12. Bartrum RJ, Crow HC: Real-time Ultrasound: A Manual for Physicians and Technical Personnel. Philadelphia, WB Saunders, 1983.
13. Bisset RA, Khan AN: Differential Diagnosis in Abdominal Ultrasound. London, Bailliere Tindall, 1990.
14. Mittelstaedt CA: Abdominal Ultrasound. New York, Churchill Livingstone, 1987.
15. Anderhub B: Manual of Abdominal Sonography. Baltimore, University Park Press, 1983.
16. Bernardino ME: The liver: anatomy and examination techniques. In Tavares JM, Ferruchi JT (eds.) Radiology: Diagnosis-Imaging-Intervention, vol. 4. Philadelphia, JB Lippincott, 1988, (ch. 60) pp. 1–8.
17. Parulekar SG: Ligaments and fissures of the liver: sonographic anatomy. Radiology 130:409–411, 1979.
18. Pagani JJ: Intrahepatic vascular territories shown by computed tomography (CT). Radiology 147:173–178, 1983.
19. Sexton CC, Zeman RK: Correlation of computed tomography, sonography, and gross anatomy of the liver. Am J Radiol 141:711–718, 1983.
20. Cosgrove DO, Arger PH, Coleman BG: Ultrasonic anatomy of hepatic veins. J Clin Ultrasound 15:231–235, 1987.
21. Cooperberg PL, Rowley VA: Abdominal sonographic examination technique. In Tavares JM, Ferruchi JT (eds.) Radiology: Diagnosis-Imaging-Intervention, vol. 4. Philadelphia, JB Lippincott, 1988 (ch. 56) pp. 1–11.
22. Applegate EJ: The Sectional Anatomy Learning System: Concepts. Philadelphia, WB Saunders, 1991.
23. Kane RA, Lavery M: Techniques of liver examination. Seminars Ultrasound 2:198–201, 1981.
24. Hillman BJ, D'Orsi CJ, Smith EH, Bartrum RJ: Ultrasonic appearance of the falciform ligament. Am J Radiol 132:205–206, 1979.
25. Carlsen EN, Filly RA: Newer ultrasonographic anatomy in the upper abdomen. I. The portal and hepatic venous anatomy. J Clin Ultrasound 4:85–90, 1976.
26. Becker CD, Cooperberg PL: Sonography of the hepatic vascular system. Am J Radiol 150:999–1005, 1988.
27. Donoso L, Martinez-Noguera A, Zidan A, Lora F: Papillary process of the caudate lobe of the liver: sonographic appearance. Radiology 173:631–633, 1989.

Chapter 6

THE BILIARY SYSTEM

MICHAEL C. FOSS

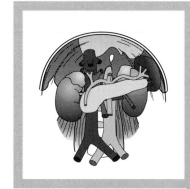
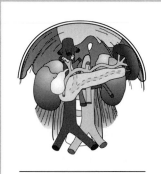
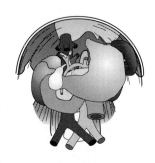
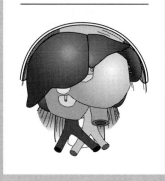

The biliary system and surrounding anatomic layers. See Figure 4-3 F, G, H, I, pages 46-47, for more details.

Objectives:

Describe the gross anatomy of the biliary system.
Describe the basic function of the biliary system.
Describe the ultrasound appearance of the biliary system.
Describe other imaging modalities that may be used to examine the biliary system.
Define the key words.

Key Words:

Ampulla of Vater	Gallbladder
Bilirubin	Hartmann's pouch
Cholecystectomy	Hepatic ducts
Cholecystitis	Hilum/hilus
Cholecystokinin	Infundibulum
Cholelithiasis	Intrahepatic
Common bile duct	Pancreatic duct
Common hepatic duct	Polyps
Cystic duct	Porta hepatis
Extrahepatic	Sludge
Fossa	Sphincter of Oddi
Fundus	Spiral valve of Heister

INTRODUCTION

The biliary system is intimately associated with the liver and pancreas. It consists of the **gallbladder**, acting as a reservoir for bile, and the ducts that drain the liver of bile. For our purpose, we will not include the pancreatic ducts as part of the biliary system, although in many people, the two do join to form the ampulla of Vater before opening into the duodenum.[1] The pancreas and associated ducts will be the focus of Chapter 7.

The basic function of the biliary system is to drain the liver of bile and to store the bile until it is needed to aid in the digestive process. As mentioned, the gallbladder acts as the storage receptacle for bile, and the various ducts provide a place to which the bile flows. The gallbladder concentrates the bile by secreting mucus and absorbing water. If you feel you need to review the process of bile production, reread Chapter 5, "The Liver," before continuing.

PRENATAL DEVELOPMENT

The liver, gallbladder, bile ducts, and part of the pancreas are formed by a ventral diverticulum, or sac, which turns into the septum transversum. This process begins at about 4 weeks or when the embryo is about 2.5 mm in length.[2] The gallbladder is present in the fetus and is often noted on sonography. It is nonfunctional until birth.[3]

LOCATION

Gallbladder

A **fossa** (or indentation) is located on the posterior and inferior portion of the right lobe of the liver where the gallbladder is situated. This fossa or bed is closely related to the main lobar fissure of the liver.[4] (See Figure 6–1.) Even though the gallbladder is typically not totally surrounded by hepatic tissue, it is possible for this to occur. An **intrahepatic** gallbladder will be totally (or almost totally) enclosed in liver tissue.

Following the main portal vein as it courses toward the right side of the body will usually reveal the gallbladder to be just inferior to the level of the right portal vein in longitudinal slices. In a transverse cut of the abdomen, finding the portal vein (or portal-splenic confluence) and following it to the right will reveal (in typical order of appearance) the portal vein, head of the pancreas, duodenum, liver, the gallbladder, and, again, liver. (See Figure 6–2.) The right kidney may also be typically noted on both transverse and longitudinal imaging with the gallbladder immediately anterior.

The gallbladder will change location as the patient changes position. A gallbladder found to be just at the inferior border of the right lobe of the liver with the patient supine, may then be found to have shifted closer to the midline when the patient is placed on the left side with the right side raised (LPO).

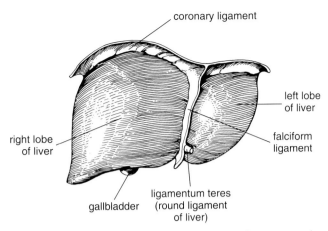

Figure 6–1. Location of gallbladder in relation to anterior view of the liver.

Some imagers believe that the location of the gallbladder may be estimated by simply bending the right arm at the elbow at 90 degrees and then placing that hand over the midline. The gallbladder will probably be very near the area of the wrist. This method is not particularly accurate, but it does give a rough idea of the location of the gallbladder.

Hepatic Ducts

Bile from the liver reaches the gallbladder through the hepatic and cystic ducts. The left and right **hepatic ducts** join at about the level of the liver **hilum** (also called the **porta hepatis** or doorway) to form the **common hepatic duct** (CHD). The common hepatic duct will eventually become the common bile duct (CBD), entering the duodenum near the head of the pancreas. (See Figure 6–3.)

The right and left hepatic ducts are considered **intra-**

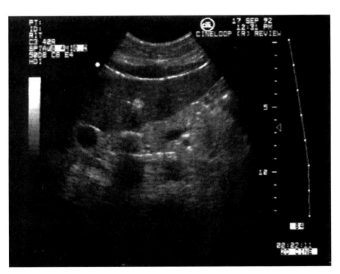

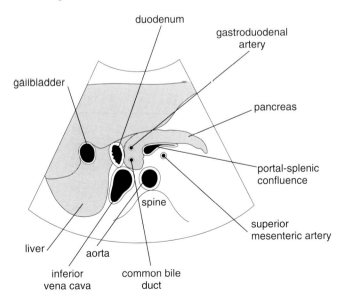

Figure 6–2. Relationship of gallbladder, duodenum, and pancreas. A transverse cut through the abdomen may reveal the above relationship. Note that the gallbladder is just lateral to the duodenum, which is just lateral to the head of the pancreas.

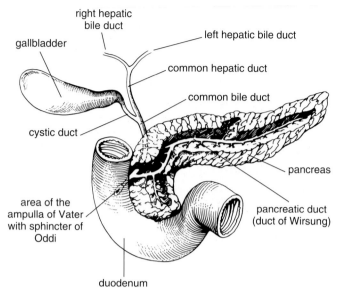

Figure 6-3. The biliary system, including the pancreas and pancreatic duct.

hepatic because they are completely enclosed by liver tissue. On longitudinal cuts of the cadaver abdomen, the common hepatic duct will most likely be located just anterior to the right portal vein. (See Figure 6-4.) It is often mistaken for the common bile duct, which is generally more closely associated with the main portal vein than the right branch. However, there are always variations, so it is possible to see the common bile duct and the right portal vein at the same time. To make matters more interesting, the cystic artery is also located near the portal veins and may appear as a bile duct. Careful

examination should reveal that the bile duct is usually more lateral to the portal vein, while the cystic artery is usually more medial.[5]

Cystic Duct

The **cystic duct** connects the gallbladder to the common hepatic duct. Bile flowing from the liver via the hepatic ducts must pass through the cystic duct to finally reach the gallbladder. It is sometimes difficult to distinguish a very short cystic duct from the neck of the gallbladder. Once the cystic duct joins the common hepatic duct at about the level of the gallbladder, the common hepatic duct is then called the common bile duct.

Common Bile Duct

The **common bile duct** extends from the point where the cystic duct joins the common hepatic duct all the way to the duodenum. It has a very close association with the main portal vein, being usually located slightly lateral and anterior to the main portal vein. The hepatic artery is usually found medial and also slightly anterior to the main portal vein. The portal vein, common bile duct, and hepatic artery form the portal triad which has become known as Mickey's sign when viewed in a transverse section. The portal vein is the "face" of the famous mouse, while the hepatic artery forms the left "ear," with the common bile duct forming the right "ear." (See Figure 6-5.)

When referring specifically to the common bile duct, anatomists use terms that relate its position to the duodenum. That part of the common bile duct superior to the duodenum is the supraduodenal section. As the

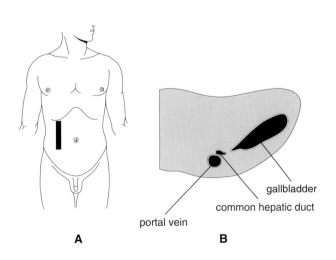

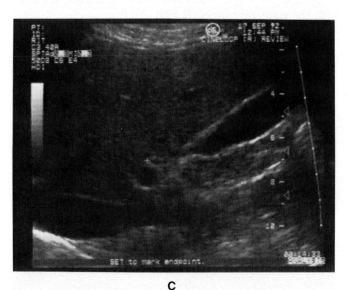

Figure 6-4. Common hepatic duct and portal vein relationship. Longitudinal diagram demonstrating the relationship between the right portal vein, common hepatic duct, and the gallbladder. The common hepatic duct is often mislabeled as the common bile duct, which is located more inferiorly and is more closely associated with the main portal vein. *A*, Position of transducer on patient. *B*, Diagram of relationship. *C*, Sonogram of common hepatic duct (cursor "+").

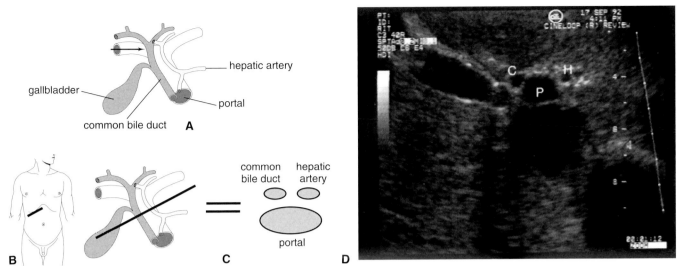

Figure 6–5. *A,* Relationship of the portal vein to the hepatic artery and common bile duct. Note that the common hepatic duct is just anterior to the right portal vein (arrow). *B,* Taking an image at about the angle of the solid line (approximately the same as the right costal margin angle) may produce the relationship demonstrated in *C.* The common bile duct and the hepatic artery are of about equal diameter. *D,* Sonogram of Mickey's sign (P = portal vein, H = hepatic artery, C = common bile duct).

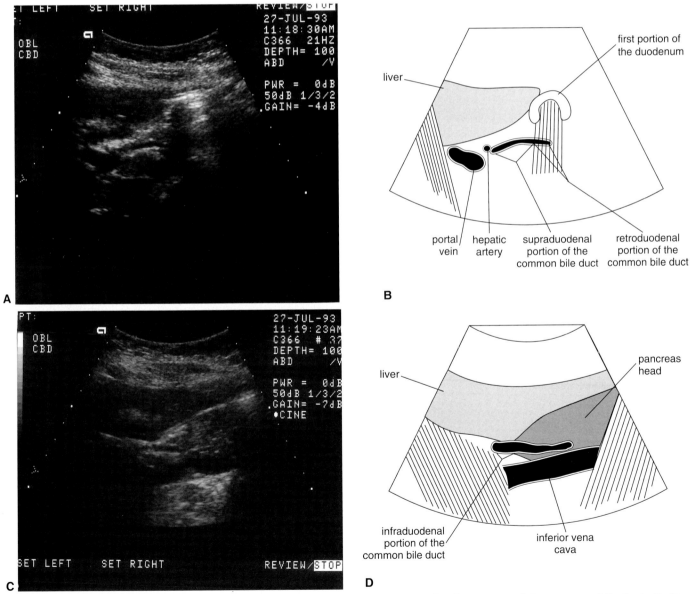

Figure 6–6. *A, B,* A longitudinal section of the supraduodenal and retroduodenal segments of the common bile duct. *C, D,* Longitudinal section of the infraduodenal segment of the common bile duct. (Ultrasound images courtesy of Jeanes Hospital, Philadelphia, PA.)

names imply, the portion posterior to the duodenum is the retroduodenal section; infraduodenal, inferior to the duodenum; and that part of the common bile duct within the duodenum, the intraduodenal portion.[6] (See Figure 6–6.) The infraduodenal portion of the common bile duct may lie within a groove on the head of the pancreas or may travel through an opening in the head. It continues on to enter the duodenum at the **ampulla of Vater**, sometimes called the hepatopancreatic ampulla.[2] A muscle sheath, the **sphincter of Oddi**, or Oddi's muscle, surrounds the common bile duct (joined at times by the **pancreatic duct**) at the ampulla of Vater. The sphincter of Oddi aids in regulating bile flow into the duodenum.[7]

SIZE

Gallbladder

The overall length of the normal gallbladder is highly variable, being dependent on the amount of bile within and the normal variants. There are times when the gallbladder is simply difficult to see, due, not to some structural variation, but to physiology. As an example, a patient who has fasted since midnight prior to an ultrasound examination may present with a full, easily visualized gallbladder. A patient who has eaten, smoked, chewed gum, or had coffee with cream and sugar (to name just a few examples) may present with a very small gallbladder or may even appear, at first, to completely lack a gallbladder. However, when the gallbladder is visualized it is found to have a length of about 8 to 9 cm in many cases, as measured from the neck to the fundus. It is about 3 cm in diameter and holds up to about 40 ml of fluid.[2,8,9] To give you some idea of the amount of fluid suggested, a teaspoon typically holds about 5 ml of fluid; therefore, the gallbladder would hold about 8 teaspoonfuls of fluid. Recall that 2.5 cm equals 1 inch; this will give you a better picture of the sizes involved when dealing with the biliary system. With experience, the sonographer will discover that the gallbladder has a wide variety of shapes, sizes, and locations.

Common Hepatic Duct

The length and inside diameter of the common hepatic duct are variable. Schwartz reports a common hepatic duct length of 3 cm to 4 cm.[7] A fairly widely accepted upper limit for the inner diameter of the common hepatic duct is 4 mm.[10] Cosgrove has reported the diameter to range from about 1 mm to 7 mm in the normal patient, depending on age, previous surgery, and gallbladder function or disease.[5] It is typical for an individual sonographic practice to set an acceptable upper limit on duct size based on criteria used by referring physicians, especially surgeons.

Cystic Duct

The diameter of the cystic duct is about 3 mm. The length is highly variable, ranging from 1.0 cm to 3.5 cm.[2] An average length of 4 cm has been reported at surgery.[7] The apparent large difference in these figures is common and holds little significance on sonography.

Common Bile Duct

The length of the common bile duct is also highly variable, being determined by the junction of the cystic duct and the common hepatic duct. A range in length of 8 cm to 11.5 cm has been suggested.[7] The diameter has been reported to be from 1 mm to 7 mm in the normal patient, and up to 10 mm in a patient following **cholecystectomy** (surgical removal of the gallbladder).[5,7,10] As before, individual practices will set an upper limit that is appropriate to their particular patient population.

GROSS ANATOMY

Gallbladder

The normal gallbladder appears a bit like a partially filled water balloon in that it is slightly more oval than round. A gallbladder that appears very round (spherical) may indicate the presence of disease, especially those conditions that cause obstruction of the lower portion of the biliary system. The shape of the gallbladder has also been likened to that of a pear, which has a narrow "neck" and a round "bottom."[1] The walls are generally only a few millimeters thick, only up to about 3 mm.[5,9] This wall thickness is important to note. Certain conditions, such as **cholecystitis** (inflammation of the gallbladder), may cause the walls to appear edematous and perhaps even greatly thickened. Localized thickening of the gallbladder wall may indicate the presence of a mass or other condition that would call for further investigation. As would be expected, the wall thickness will be slightly less when the gallbladder is full (the walls are stretched), as compared to an empty gallbladder, when the walls will be slightly thicker.

There are three distinct layers to the gallbladder wall. The inner layer is the mucosa, the middle is the fibromuscular layer, and the outer is the serous layer. Inside the gallbladder are many minute inward folds or rugae.[8] These folds aid in concentrating the bile through absorption of water and secretion of mucus.

The gallbladder may be divided into three major sections: fundus, body, and neck. The **fundus** is the "bottom" of the pouch. (See Figure 6–7.) It is important to notice the location of the fundus in relation to gravity. Gallstones and **sludge** (thick bile) may find their way to the fundus, but only if the fundus is closest to the center

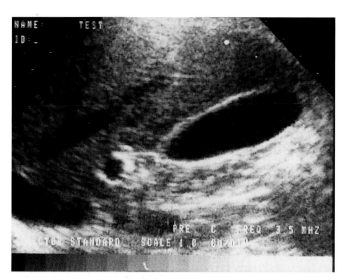

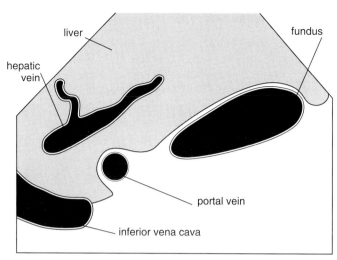

Figure 6–7. Longitudinal section of the gallbladder fundus.

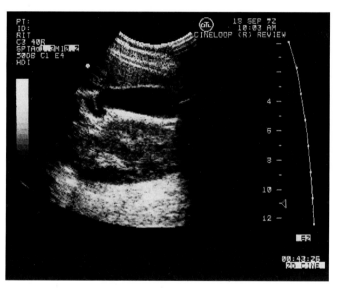

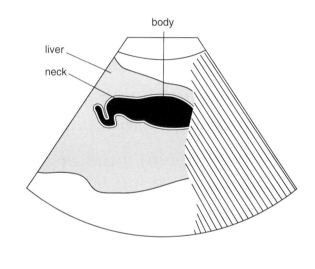

Figure 6–8. Longitudinal section of the gallbladder neck and body.

of the earth. The exception, of course, is "floating" stones. That part of the gallbladder that is closest to the center of the earth is called the dependent portion. The dependent portion will change with a change in the position of the patient.

The middle and main portion of the gallbladder is called the body while the more narrow area leading into the cystic duct is called the neck. (See Figure 6–8.) A small sacculation (outpouching) may be seen in some patients in the area of the gallbladder neck. This has been called **Hartmann's pouch** after Henri Hartmann, a French surgeon who lived from 1860 to 1952.[11] The term **infundibulum** is also applied to this dilatation of the gallbladder neck area.[7] The sacculation itself is considered as an abnormality by some and as an oddity by others. No matter: it must be carefully screened to detect coexisting abnormalities such as **cholelithiasis** (gallstones). (See Figure 6–9.)

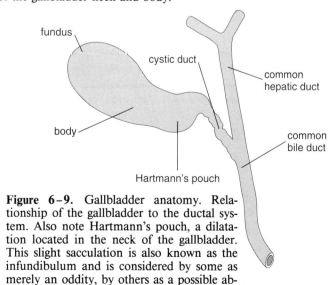

Figure 6–9. Gallbladder anatomy. Relationship of the gallbladder to the ductal system. Also note Hartmann's pouch, a dilatation located in the neck of the gallbladder. This slight sacculation is also known as the infundibulum and is considered by some as merely an oddity, by others as a possible abnormality. In either case, it should be examined carefully for related disease, such as gallstones.

Hepatic Ducts

The intrahepatic bile ducts run alongside portal veins and hepatic arteries in portal triads, surrounded by connective tissue and radiating through the lobes and segments of the liver.[12] The intrahepatic ducts join to form the right and left main hepatic ducts and, as previously mentioned, the right and left main hepatic ducts join at about the level of the porta hepatis to form the common hepatic duct.

Cystic Duct

You will recall that the cystic duct connects the gallbladder to the common hepatic duct, where the cystic duct and common hepatic duct join they form the common bile duct. The lumen of the cystic duct contains a series of mucosal folds, the **spiral valves of Heister**. Even though it is common to call this area of folds a valve, it is really misnamed. There does not seem to be any valve or flow control action; bile flows freely in both directions through the cystic duct. Pressure differences in the biliary system along with the stimulated contraction of the gallbladder seem to govern the flow of bile, while the spiral valves of Heister prevent the cystic duct from overdistending or collapsing.[5]

Common Bile Duct

Formed by the junction of the cystic duct and common hepatic duct, the common bile duct courses inferiorly along the right border of the lesser omentum, then along the hepatoduodenal ligament and posterior to the first part of the duodenum, passing on or through the head of the pancreas just anterior to the inferior vena cava.[12] The duct terminates at the posteromedial aspect of the descending portion of the duodenum. The common bile duct and the cystic duct and part of the common hepatic duct are **extrahepatic** (not enclosed by liver tissue) ducts. They are lined with subepithelial connective tissue and some smooth muscle fibers.[6,13]

PHYSIOLOGY

Bile is produced by the liver and carried to the gastrointestinal system by the biliary ducts. The sphincter of Oddi, located in the duodenum, regulates the passage of bile into the duodenum and at the same time prevents reflux of gastrointestinal fluids into the biliary system. When closed, the sphincter of Oddi forces the gallbladder to fill with bile. When fats and amino acids are ingested, the duodenal mucosa releases **cholecystokinin** (CCK), a peptide hormone. Cholecystokinin stimulates the gallbladder to contract, and the sphincter of Oddi to relax, and increases hepatic production of bile.[5,14] An injectable form of cholecystokinin has been used to stimulate the gallbladder during sonographic examination for a type of function test.

The gallbladder is actually more than just a storage area for bile. Related blood vessels and lymphatics concentrate the stored bile through absorption of water and inorganic salts. Bile in the gallbladder is much more concentrated than hepatic bile.[1] Bile is composed mostly of water (82 percent) and bile acids (12 percent). The remaining constituents include cholesterol, **bilirubin** (bile pigment), proteins, electrolytes, and mucus.[14]

SONOGRAPHIC APPEARANCE

Much of the biliary system is readily appreciated on sonography. It is especially common for the gallbladder, common hepatic duct, and common bile duct to be imaged. In the absence of disease, the other portions of the biliary system may prove to be difficult to appreciate if only because they are quite small.

Gallbladder

The sonographic appearance of the gallbladder is that of an anechoic or nearly anechoic pear-shaped structure in the right upper quadrant of the abdomen. (See Figure 6–10.) As mentioned, there is wide variation in shape and size of the gallbladder. The walls tend to be well defined, regular, and echodense, especially when the gallbladder is distended. In the "empty" gallbladder, the walls are thicker and may appear more irregular, with the central portion containing a few random echoes. (See Figure 6–11.) The wall thickness is usually 3 mm or less and may be difficult to measure when the gallbladder is in its partially distended, normal state.[5,9] Inadequate examination may lead to a false diagnosis of thickened walls and/or cholelithiasis. The nature of ultrasound tends to obscure one or both of the leading edges of the anterior (or proximal) wall of the gallbladder, making it difficult to determine where to place the measurement cursors.

The fundus may be difficult to visualize due to the close relationship of the gallbladder to the bowel. A shadow is often created by the bowel that partially obscures the fundus. Changing patient position or angling the transducer may be necessary to examine the entire gallbladder. Floating stones, **polyps** (protruding masses from the inner wall of the gallbladder), and other masses may be present in the fundus of the gallbladder and easily missed on casual examination.

Three landmarks may be helpful in locating the gallbladder on longitudinal imaging: the portal vein, the main lobar fissure, and the right kidney. The main lobar fissure may also be demonstrated just at the level of the gallbladder since it helps to form the "bed" in which the gallbladder lies. The main lobar fissure is considerably

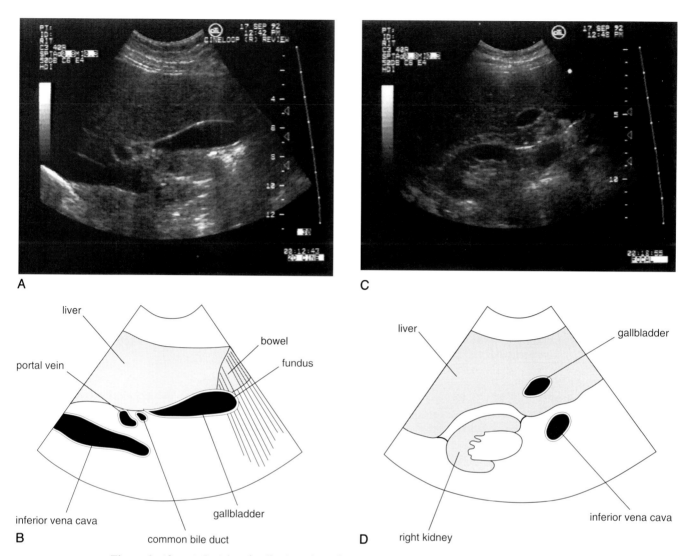

Figure 6–10. *A, B,* A longitudinal section of the gallbladder. Note that the fundus is partially obscured by bowel. *C, D,* A transverse section of the gallbladder.

Figure 6–11. Gallbladder wall thickness. The thickness of the gallbladder wall is usually less than 3 mm and should be noted on each study. Cholecystitis and carcinoma are just two examples of pathologic states which may alter the thickness and appearance of the gallbladder wall. Care must be taken not to falsely thicken the walls through too high gain and/or power settings.

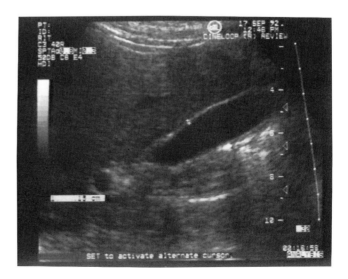

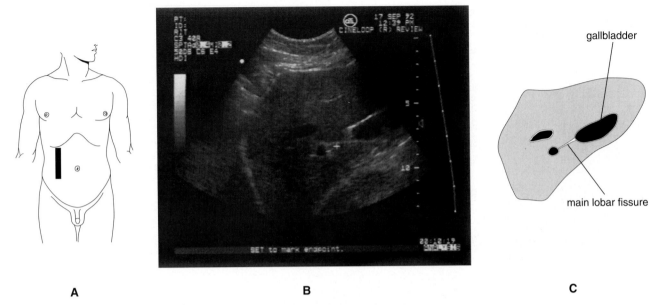

gallbladder

main lobar fissure

A   B   C

Figure 6–12. Relationship of the gallbladder to the main lobar fissure of the liver. *A,* Transducer position on patient. *B,* Longitudinal sonogram of main lobar fissure (cursor below "+") and gallbladder. *C,* Diagram of main lobar fissure and gallbladder.

more difficult to consistently appreciate than the portal vein, but is of value. Moreover, you will need to locate the portal vein in longitudinal sonogram to measure the common hepatic duct. (See Figure 6–12). Some sonographers locate the right kidney as an aid in locating the gallbladder. In most cases the gallbladder fundus is anterior to the superior pole of the right kidney.

An additional landmark for the gallbladder is the duodenum. In a transverse image taken at the level of the head of the pancreas, note that on a single plane drawn from midline to the right, the portal-splenic confluence,

the head of the pancreas, the duodenum, probably a portion of the liver, and then the gallbladder are seen. (Refer to Figure 6–2.) Remember this common relationship so that you can eliminate each anechoic structure as a possible gallbladder while scanning. Do not forget that the inferior vena cava is just posterior to the head of the pancreas and may be mistaken for an extremely posteriorly lying gallbladder. Remember also that the appearance of the duodenum changes depending on when and how much fluid the patient has ingested. Reference to all the landmarks will make locating the gallbladder easier.

At times, regardless of technique, the gallbladder simply will not be visualized. Nonvisualization may occur for a number of reasons. If the gallbladder fails to develop (agenesis) there will be nothing to image. This cause of nonvisualization is rare, however. A very small tube-like (vermiform or worm-like) gallbladder may appear as a bile duct and be missed on sonography. As has been noted, an empty gallbladder may be small and can be overlooked.

Shadows and other minor distortions related to the edge of the gallbladder walls and distal to the spiral valves of Heister are common. High-frequency sound produces a particularly striking shadow from these areas since it is more easily reflected than the lower frequencies. (See Figure 6–13.) Each shadow must be explored to determine whether it is natural or associated with disease. An acoustic shadow should be followed to its origin to learn whether it begins slightly more anteriorly and interrupts the representation of the wall. If it interrupts the wall, the shadow may indicate abnormal anatomy and deserves further study.

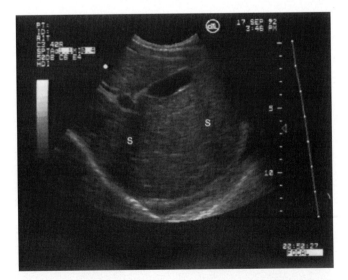

Figure 6–13. Normal wall shadowing from the gallbladder. It is common to find some shadowing from the walls of the gallbladder ("S") and from the area of the spiral valve of Heister with higher frequency transducers.

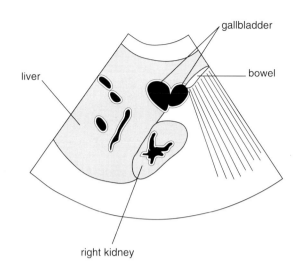

Figure 6–14. False appearance of a gallbladder variation. In this longitudinal section, it appears that a septation is present in the gallbladder. However, when the patient's position was changed, the gallbladder was seen to be folded onto itself. It is imperative that the patient be placed in at least two different positions during sonographic examination.

Ductal System

In the normal patient, bile ducts other than the common ducts are very small and usually not appreciated. Both the common hepatic duct and common bile ducts are larger in diameter and can be seen associated with the portal venous system. The common hepatic duct is usually located anterior to the right portal vein and on longitudinal sonogram may be noted as two echogenic short parallel lines separated by just 1 mm or so of anechoic space. (Refer to Figure 6–4.) The gallbladder is usually nearby, as is the main lobar fissure.

As noted, the common bile duct may be observed as part of Mickey's sign when traversed. It appears as a small round anechoic structure just anterior and slightly lateral on the right to the main portal vein, on scans taken at a transverse oblique angle. A perfectly round, anechoic duct structure will not be visualized consistently. Cutting the duct at an angle other than perfectly transverse may produce an oval structure. (Refer to Figure 6–5.)

SONOGRAPHIC APPLICATIONS

In most cases sonography is the method of choice for examining the biliary system. Some specific applications of sonographic examination of the biliary system follow:

Measuring the common hepatic duct
Measuring the common bile duct
Measuring the general volume of the gallbladder
Assessing the gallbladder and/or adjacent liver masses
Assessing possible obstruction of the biliary ductal system
Presence of stones in the gallbladder (cholelithiasis)

Presence of stones in the ductal system (choledocholithiasis)
Ruling out masses, including cysts, associated with the biliary system
Postsurgical follow-up (ie, cholecystectomy)

NORMAL VARIANTS

It may happen that the biliary system does not develop normally, and deviation occurs. Deviations are of special interest to the sonographer since they may challenge adequate examination. For example, what appears to be a septated gallbladder (a gallbladder with divisions or septations) may simply be one folded onto itself. If the patient's position is changed, the gallbladder may unfold to reveal no septation. (See Figure 6–14.) Other variations may be considered pathologic or may contribute to the development of disease. For instance, a gallbladder attached to the liver by a particularly long mesentery can mimic a "floating" gallbladder that is prone to torsion (twisting), as opposed to a gallbladder that is partially embedded in liver tissue.[15,16]

Gallbladder

Congenital abnormalities of the gallbladder are relatively common. In addition to the floating gallbladder, there may be hypoplasia (underdevelopment) or agenesis (complete failure of the gallbladder to develop). Both of these conditions are relatively rare, but must be ruled out as possible reasons for nonvisualization on sonography and other imaging modalities. At the opposite end of the scale is duplication of the gallbladder, with or without duplication of the cystic duct.[6]

More common are variations in gallbladder shape.[15] It may be bilobed (hourglass), septated, and/or folded into

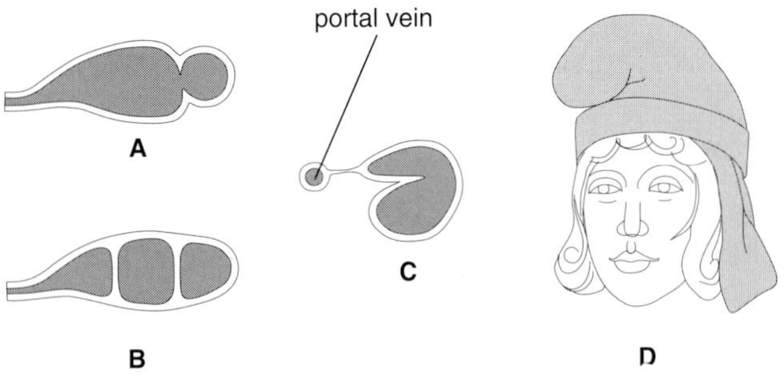

Figure 6-15. Typical gallbladder variations. Some possible shapes of the gallbladder: *A*, Bilobed gallbladder; *B*, True septated gallbladder; *C*, Gallbladder folded onto itself in what has been called the phrygian gallbladder; *D*, One possible shape of an early phrygian cap. This cap was worn by the early Roman freed slaves and later by French revolutionaries as a symbol of liberty.

any of several shapes. Septations tend to be associated with gallstone formation due to the stasis of gallbladder contents.[6] Septations may make it difficult to identify cholelithiasis. The most common variation in gallbladder shape is that of a phrygian cap.[15] In this case, the gallbladder is partially folded onto itself, so that it appears similar to the phrygian cap worn by the early Roman freed slaves and later by French revolutionaries as a symbol of liberty.[16-18] (See Figure 6-15.)

Biliary Ducts

Variations in the extrahepatic biliary ducts are common and may appear in almost any combination. As an example, the cystic duct may join the common hepatic duct at almost any point from the porta hepatis to the duodenum. With a very low juncture, the cystic duct may run parallel to the common hepatic duct for some distance. Accessory hepatic ducts are also fairly common and on sonographic examination may present as an "extra" tubular structure.[6] Such variations should not be an obstacle, though they may make it more difficult to identify every structure on the imaging screen.

A more easily recognized variation is the choledochal (or choledochus) cyst. Of the three types—congenital cystic dilation, intraduodenal (choledochocele), and congenital diverticulum—the first is the most common. A choledochal cyst is a localized dilatation of the common bile duct. When caused by a congenital diverticulum, it may appear as a separate or as a loosely connected structure to the common bile duct. The choledochocele (or intraduodenal) is formed by a section of the common bile duct that has entered the duodenum and enlarged. This is similar to the process involved in the formation of a ureterocele.[10]

Biliary atresia (congenital closure) may be diffuse or focal in the extrahepatic ducts, or intrahepatic. Diffuse extrahepatic biliary atresia is the most common.[6,10,15]

REFERENCE CHARTS

Associated Physicians

Surgeon: Involved in the diagnosis of biliary disease as well as surgical intervention.

Internist: Involved in the diagnosis and medical treatment of biliary disease.

Radiologist: Performs and interprets the various imaging tests used to diagnose biliary disease.

Common Diagnostic Tests

Oral Cholecystogram (OCG): A contrast material (dye) is ingested by the patient the night before the test. Information on structure and function of the gallbladder is obtained. This test is performed by a radiologist assisted by a radiologic technologist, and is interpreted by the radiologist.

Nuclear Medicine (HIDA Scan): A minute amount of a radiopharmaceutical is injected. It passes through the bloodstream to the liver, then to the biliary system and eventually into the duodenum. Functional information is the primary focus of this test, and some structural information is also obtained. This test is performed by a nuclear medicine technologist and interpreted by the radiologist.

Computed Axial Tomography (CT Scan): A radiologic examination in which cross-sectional x-ray images of the biliary system and other abdominal structures are obtained. A contrast medium may be administered to differentiate between disease and normal anatomy Structural information is the primary focus of this test, but some functional information may be obtained. It is performed by a radiologic technologist and is interpreted by the radiologist.

Cholangiography: A contrast material is injected into the biliary system either by catheter (ie, T-tube cholangiogram) or by needle (transhepatic cholangiogram) under radiographic guidance. This yields structural information about the entire biliary system, especially about obstruction. It may be performed before, during, or after surgery. Surgeons, surgical assistants, radiologists, and radiologic technologists are involved in the procedure, and it is interpreted by the radiologist.

Endoscopic Retrograde Cholangiopancreatography (ERCP): In this endoscopic, radiographically guided examination, the ampulla of Vater is cannulized through a tube inserted into the patient's upper gastrointestinal tract. Contrast material is then injected to fill and delineate the pancreatic and bile ducts. Information on obstructive processes is the objective. This type of endoscopy is usually performed by the gastroenterologist assisted by the radiologist. The gastroenterologist interprets the endoscopic results and the radiologist interpretes the radiologic findings.

Laboratory Values

Serum bilirubin: Adult: direct (conjugated): < 0.5 mg/dl
indirect (unconjugated): ≤ 1.1 mg/dl
urine: negative
Infant: total: 1 to 12 mg/dl

Urobilinogen: Fecal: 50 to 300 mg/24 hours
Urine: Men: 0.3 to 2.1 Ehrlich units/ 2 hours
Women: 0.1 to 1.1 Ehrlich units/ 2 hours[19]

Normal Measurements

Gallbladder (note that the shape of the gallbladder may be more important):
Length: 8 to 9 cm as measured from the neck to the fundus of a completely bile-filled gallbladder.
Diameter: about 3 cm

Common hepatic duct:
Length: highly variable
Diameter: 1 to 4 mm, in some normal persons up to 7 mm

Cystic duct:
Length: 1 to 3.5 cm
Diameter: up to 3 mm

Common bile duct:
Length: variable
Diameter: 1 to 7 mm, up to 10 mm post-cholecystectomy

Vasculature

Nonapplicable.

Affecting Chemicals

Nonapplicable.

References

1. Price S, Wilson LM: Pathophysiology, 3rd ed. New York, McGraw-Hill, 1986, 299.
2. Romanes GJ: Cunningham's Textbook of Anatomy, 11th ed. London, Oxford University Press, 1972, 61, 459–460.
3. Cohen L, Atwood R, Newelt M: Ultrasound of the normal fetal chest, abdomen, and pelvis. Obstet Gynecol 1(1):240, 1991.
4. Hagen-Ansert S: Textbook of Diagnostic Ultrasonography, 3rd ed. St. Louis, CV Mosby, 1989, 229.
5. Cosgrove DO, McCready VR: Ultrasound Imaging: Liver–Spleen–Pancreas. New York, Wiley, 1982, 226–227.
6. Netter F: Digestive system. The CIBA Collection of Medical Illustrations. Summit, NJ, CIBA Pharmaceutical, CIBA-Geigy, 3(III):22–23, 123, 1975.
7. Schwartz SI: Gallbladder and extrahepatic biliary system. Principles of Surgery, 5th Ed. New York, McGraw-Hill, 1989, 1381–1382.
8. Gray H: Anatomy, Descriptive and Surgical, 1901 ed. Philadelphia, Running Press, 1974, 942.
9. Mittelstaedt C: Abdominal Ultrasound. New York, Churchill Livingstone, 1989, 86–87.
10. Bisset RAL, Khan AN: Differential Diagnosis in Abdominal Ultrasound. London, Bailliere Tindall, 1990, 58, 63, 65–66.
11. Dorland WA: Dorland's Illustrated Medical Dictionary, 27th ed. Philadelphia, WB Saunders, 1988, 732.
12. Kawamura DM: Diagnostic Medical Sonography. Philadelphia, JB Lippincott, 1992, vol III.
13. Wilson SA, Gosnick BB, vanSonnenberg E: Unchanged size of dilated common bile duct after a fatty meal: results and significance. Radiology 160:29–31, 1986.
14. McPhee MS, Greenberger NJ: Diseases of the gallbladder and bile ducts. In Harrison TR (ed.). Principles of Internal Medicine. New York, McGraw-Hill, 1987, 1358–1359.
15. Schoenfield LJ: Gallstones and other biliary diseases. Clinical Symposia. CIBA, 1982:(34,4); 32.
16. Picken M: The Fashion Dictionary. New York, Funk and Wagnalls, 1957, 49–50.
17. Harrison M: The History of the Hat. London, William Clowes, 1960, 22.
18. Wilcox RT: The Mode in Hats and Headdress. New York, Scribner's, 1945, 6–15.
19. Ford RD (ed.): Diagnostic Tests Handbook. Springhouse, PA, Springhouse, 1987, 61, 217–219, 673.

Chapter 7

THE PANCREAS

MICHAEL C. FOSS
REVA ARNEZ CURRY
BETTY BATES TEMPKIN

Objectives:

Describe the gross anatomy of the pancreas.

Describe the function of the pancreas.

Describe the epigastric vessels which surround the pancreas.

Describe the blood supply to the pancreas.

Describe the sonographic appearance of the pancreas in the transverse view, using vascular landmarks.

Describe the sonographic appearance of the pancreas in the sagittal view, using vascular landmarks.

Describe other imaging modalities that may be used to examine the pancreas.

Define the key words.

Key Words:

Acini cells
Alpha cells
Ampulla of Vater
Beta cells
Caudal pancreatic artery
C-loop of the duodenum
Common bile duct
Delta cells

Dorsal pancreatic artery
Duct of Santorini
Duct of Wirsung
Endocrine
Exocrine
Gastroduodenal artery
Glucagon
Insulin
Isles of Langerhans
Pancreatic arcades
Pancreatic body
Pancreatic duodenal arteries
Pancreatic head
Pancreatic juice
Pancreatic magna arteria
Pancreatic neck
Pancreatic section
Pancreatic tail
Portal-splenic confluence
Prehilar section
Prepancreatic section
Somatostatin
Splenic artery
Splenic vein
Superior mesenteric artery
Superior mesenteric vein
Suprapancreatic section
Uncinate process

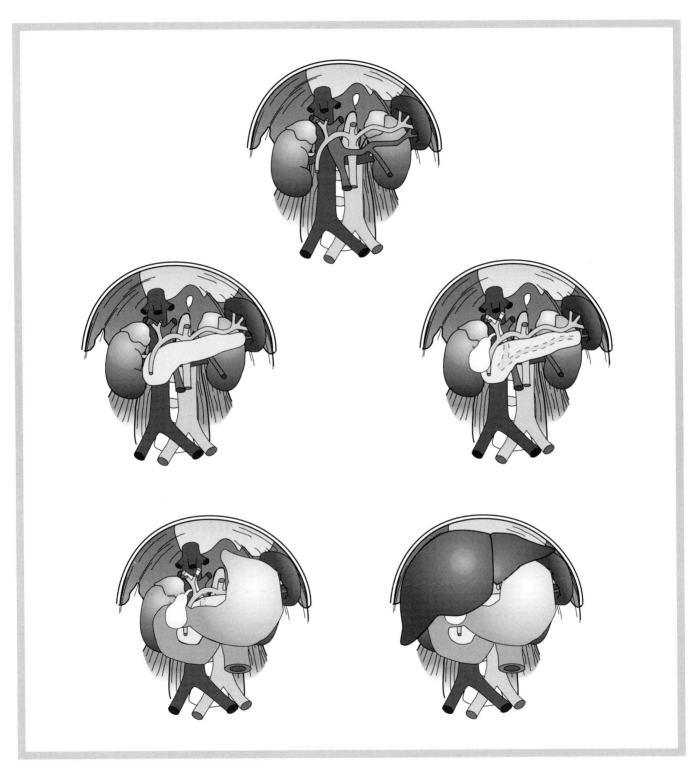

The pancreas and surrounding anatomic layers. See Figure 4-3 E, F, G, H, I, pp. 44-47, for more details.

INTRODUCTION

The pancreas has been and continues to be a most interesting challenge to image by sonography. Its close relationship to the stomach, duodenum and proximal jejunum of the small intestine, and the transverse colon of the large intestine may obscure much of the pancreatic structure. This is especially true in the case of the poorly prepped patient. In spite of these obstacles, sonography is very useful in the evaluation of the pancreas.

The pancreas and biliary tree are closely related. The pancreatic duct usually joins the common bile duct before both vessels enter the duodenum. (See Figure 7–1.) (The reader is advised to review the description of the biliary tree in Chapter 6 before proceeding.)

PRENATAL DEVELOPMENT

The pancreas is formed from ventral and dorsal diverticula of the primitive foregut. The diverticula rotate and fuse, with the ventral portion forming most of the head of the pancreas.

LOCATION

The pancreas is located in the epigastrium and left hypochondrium. It lies horizontally across the aorta and is shaped like an upside down "U"—the ends of the "U" appearing to have been pulled outward. (The shape of the pancreas has also been described as dumbbell.) Most of the pancreas is retroperitoneal; however, a portion of the head is surrounded by peritoneum. Behind the pancreas are connective prevertebral tissue, the inferior vena cava, aorta, and diaphragm.[1,2] Anterior to the pancreas are the stomach and transverse colon.

Understanding surrounding vessel anatomy is essential to locating the pancreas. In describing pancreatic anatomy, we move from right to left, beginning with the head of the pancreas and ending with the tail.

The **head** of the pancreas is cradled in the **C-loop of the duodenum** and is anterior to the inferior vena cava. The **neck** is anterior to the superior mesenteric vein and portal/splenic confluence.[3–6] The **portal/splenic confluence** is the area where the splenic vein meets the superior mesenteric vein. (See Figure 7–2.) Together, these veins form the portal vein. The inferior mesenteric vein also drains into the splenic vein before the latter receives the superior mesenteric vein.[1,7,8]

The **body** of the pancreas is anterior to the **superior mesenteric artery** of the aorta. It is usually the smallest part of the organ. The **splenic vein** lies just posterior to the body and tail, closely following the shape of the gland. (See Figure 7–2.) The **tail** of the pancreas can be seen near the hilum of the spleen.[1,7,8]

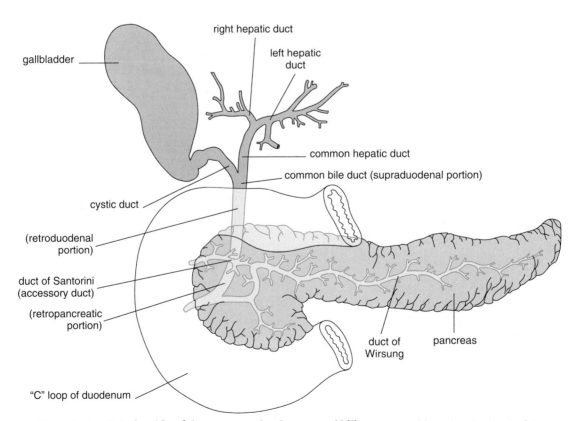

Figure 7–1. Relationship of the pancreas, duodenum, and biliary system. Note that the head of the pancreas is partially surrounded by the C-loop of the duodenum. The union of the main pancreatic duct and distal common bile duct is shown.

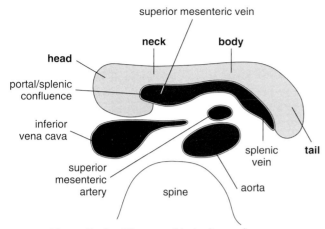

Figure 7–2. The portal/splenic confluence.

SIZE

The total length of the pancreas ranges between 12 and 18 cm.[1,2,4,7-9] It is approximately 2.5 cm thick, 3 to 5 cm wide, and weighs between 60 and 80 g.[1,4,9,10] It is important to note the overall contour of the gland along with its size. Is the contour smooth, well-defined, and without localized enlargement which appears to be out of place compared with the rest of the gland? This is important because a portion of the gland may be enlarged, yet fall within normal limits. Therefore, an assessment of glandular contour is essential when evaluating size.

Anterior posterior measurements of the head, body, and tail vary widely.[1,7,8,11] The head ranges between 2 and 3 cm in its anterior posterior dimension, though a size as high as 4 cm has been noted.[1,7,8,11] (We question whether the uncinate process, a medial extension of the head, may be contributing to these wide ranges.) Additional measurements include those of the neck, between 1.5 and 2.5 cm; the body, between 2 and 3 cm; and the tail, between 1 and 2 cm.[7,8,11] According to one reference, the "top normal" measurements for the adult pancreas were 3 cm for the head, 1 cm for the neck, 2.2. cm for the body, and 2.8 cm for the tail.[1] Readers are advised to consult the scanning protocols at their institutions to determine the acceptable range.

The vessels surrounding the pancreas are important in assessing pancreatic size. Slightly lateral and to the right

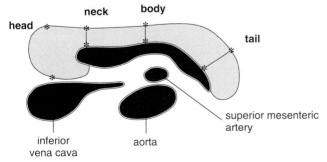

Figure 7–3. Caliber placement for measuring the head, neck, body, and tail of the pancreas.

of the portal/splenic confluence, the head can be measured. Directly anterior to the confluence is the neck. Medial to the neck is the body, anterior to the superior mesenteric artery and splenic vein. The splenic vein should be seen in its entirety in order to measure the tail, which can be identified close to the hilum of the spleen. Figure 7–3 shows caliber placement to measure parts of the pancreas. Note the use of the epigastric vessels as landmarks.

GROSS ANATOMY

As mentioned earlier, the pancreas consists of four parts: head, neck, body, and tail. The **head** lies to the right of the portal/splenic confluence and medial to the C-loop of the duodenum. (Formation of the confluence was explained earlier.) One part of the confluence, the **splenic vein**, carries blood from the spleen, while the second part of the confluence, the **superior mesenteric vein**, drains the small bowel and proximal colon. Both veins meet at the confluence to form the **portal vein**.[2-4]

Two vessels can be seen in the head: the **common bile duct** in the posterior portion, and the more anterior **gastroduodenal artery**. The common bile duct courses behind the first part of the duodenum and part of the head of the pancreas. It then enters the head on its way to the duodenum. (See Figure 7–1.)[4,5,12] The gastroduodenal artery is a branch of the common hepatic artery of the celiac axis. It supplies blood to the head of the pancreas and the duodenum. (See Figure 7–4.)[3,4]

The **uncinate process** is a posteromedial projection of pancreatic tissue which extends from the head. One way to visualize this area is to draw an imaginary line from the middle of the portal/splenic confluence to the middle

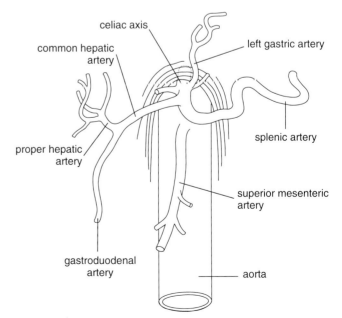

Figure 7–4. Celiac axis and branches. Note the gastroduodenal artery.

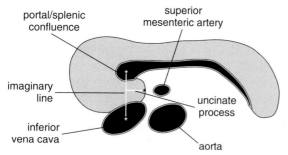

Figure 7–5. Transverse view showing imaginary line drawn from the middle of the portal/splenic confluence to the middle of the inferior vena cava to show the uncinate process.

of the inferior vena cava on a transverse scan (longitudinal view) of the pancreas. The tissue located to the left of the imaginary line is most likely the uncinate process. (See Figure 7–5.)

The **neck** of the pancreas is found immediately anterior to the portal/splenic confluence or superior mesenteric vein. Structurally, it is located between the pancreatic head and body. (Some sonographers may not consider the neck to be an individual structure, but include it as part of either the head or the body.)

The **body** of the pancreas is anterior to the aorta and superior mesenteric artery. The body and tail can be seen immediately anterior to the splenic vein. This vein follows the shape of the gland, coursing posteriorly from the spleen to help form the main portal vein.

The portion of the pancreas to the left of the aorta (and the body of the pancreas) is the **tail**. The tail extends from the left side of the abdomen to or in close proximity to the hilum of the spleen, and anterior to the superior pole of the left kidney.

The arterial supply of the pancreas includes blood from **pancreaticoduodenal arteries** and branches of the **splenic artery**. The anterior and inferior pancreaticoduodenal arteries supply the head and part of the duodenum. These arteries comprise part of the **pancreatic arcades**—the vascular connections between the hepatic, splenic, and superior mesenteric arteries which supply the head of the pancreas.[1]

The **splenic artery** supplies the body and tail of the pancreas and consists of four sections: **suprapancreatic** (the first 3 cm of the artery as it arises from the celiac axis), **pancreatic**, **prepancreatic** (before it leaves the pancreas), and **prehilar** (before it enters the spleen). The **dorsal pancreatic artery** arises from the suprapancreatic section; the **pancreatica magna**, or great, **artery** from the pancreatic section; and the **caudal pancreatic artery** from the prepancreatic or prehilar sections. (See Figure 7–6.)[1,10]

PHYSIOLOGY

The pancreas is a digestive (**exocrine**) and hormonal (**endocrine**) gland. The gland is mostly exocrine: only 2 percent of the gland's weight is endocrine tissue.[9] The exocrine function is carried out by the **acini cells** of the pancreas, which can produce up to 2 liters of pancreatic juice per day.[4] Acini resemble grape clusters with small areas of endocrine tissue interspersed between.

Pancreatic juice is composed of enzymes which help digest fats, proteins, carbohydrates, and nucleic acids. Pancreatic enzymes which aid in digestion include amylase, which digests carbohydrates; lipase, fat; trypsin, chymotrypsin, and carboxypepidase, proteins; and nucleases, nucleic acids.[2–4,9,12] The largest component of

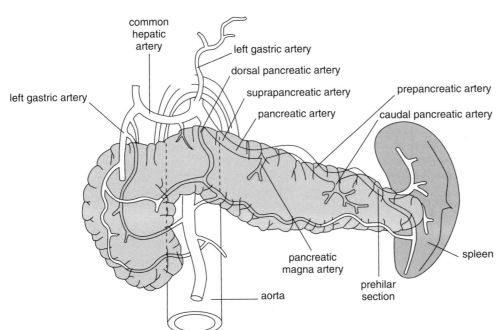

Figure 7–6. The suprapancreatic, pancreatic, prepancreatic, and prehilar sections of the splenic artery are shown. Note the origin of the dorsal pancreatic, pancreatic magna, and caudal pancreatic arteries from the splenic artery.

TABLE 7–1. Components of Pancreatic Juice

ENZYME	ACTS ON
Amylase	Carbohydrates
Lipase	Fats
Trypsin, Chymotrypsin, Carboxypeptidase	Proteins
Nucleases	Nucleic Acids
Socium Bicarbonate	Hydrochloric Acid

pancreatic juice is sodium bicarbonate, a substance needed to neutralize hydrochloric acid produced in the stomach. Bicarbonate is produced by cells lining the pancreatic duct. (See Table 7–1.)[10]

Chyme (partially digested food) in the duodenum stimulates the release of hormones which act on pancreatic juice formation. These hormones are cholecystokinin, gastrin, acetylcholine, and secretin.[4,10] The first three stimulate acini cells to produce digestive enzymes; the last-named, secretin, stimulates production of sodium bicarbonate.

Pancreatic juice moves into the duodenum through the main pancreatic duct, the **duct of Wirsung**, a vessel approximately 2 mm in diameter. In about 77 percent of cadavers, the duct of Wirsung meets the common bile duct before both enter the duodenum through the **ampulla of Vater**.[4] An accessory duct, the **duct of Santorini**, is a normal variant which enters the duodenum approximately 2 cm superior to the main duct. (See Figure 7–1.)[3,4] The sphincter of Oddi, a muscle surrounding the ampulla, relaxes to allow pancreatic juice (and, if the gallbladder has been stimulated, bile) to flow into the duodenum.[4]

The endocrine portion of the pancreas is located in the alpha, beta, and delta cells, in the **isles of Langerhans**.[3,4,6,10] **Beta cells** comprise 60 percent to 70 percent of the endocrine cells and produce **insulin**, a hormone which causes glycogen formation from glucose in the liver.[3,4,10] It also enables cells with insulin receptors to take up glucose. Hence, blood sugar decreases. **Alpha cells** comprise 15 percent to 20 percent of endocrine tissue and produce **glucagon**, a hormone which causes the opposite effect—cells release glucose in order to meet the immediate energy needs of the body. Glucagon also stimulates the liver to convert glycogen to glucose, thus increasing blood sugar levels. **Delta cells** comprise an even smaller percentage of endocrine tissue and produce a substance called **somatostatin**. This hormone inhibits the production of both insulin and glucagon.[4,10] The pancreatic hormones are released in minute quantities directly into the bloodstream. (See Table 7–2.)

TABLE 7–2. Pancreatic Hormones

HORMONE	TYPE OF CELL	ACTION
Insulin	Beta	Glucose → Glycogen
Glucagon	Alpha	Glycogen → Glucose
Somatostatin	Delta	Alpha/Beta Inhibitor

SONOGRAPHIC APPEARANCE

Echogenicity of the pancreas varies, but it is generally expected to have a slightly more echodense appearance than the typical liver, although the texture is not as homogeneous. The borders of the pancreas are usually well defined with a smooth, curvilinear contour. The main pancreatic duct can be seen as two short, highly reflective lines, about 2 mm apart, within the body of the pancreas. These reflective lines may be observed in other parts of the pancreas. *Note*: The pylorus of the stomach lies anterior to the pancreas. The collapsed walls of the pylorus (from an empty stomach) may lie across the pancreas and resemble the pancreatic duct. Having the patient drink water will fill the stomach, allow the stomach wall to be differentiated, and avoid confusion.

On transverse views, the long axis of the pancreas is shown, surrounded by epigastric vessels. The head contains two small, circular, anechoic structures: the posterior common bile duct and the anterior gastroduodenal artery. (See Figures 7–7 through 7–9.) Anterior to the portal/splenic confluence is the pancreatic neck. The gland is thinner at this point and merges into the body, located directly anterior to the superior mesenteric artery and the larger aorta. Both vessels will appear anechoic and circular, with highly reflective borders. (See Figures 7–10 through 7–13.) The splenic vein marks the tail and body of the pancreas and can be seen coursing from the hilum of the spleen. It is anechoic, curvilinear, and follows along the posterior border of the pancreas. (See Figures 7–14 and 7–15.) The splenic vein enlarges at the confluence, marking the entrance of the superior mesenteric vein.

Sagittal views of the pancreas will show the gland in transverse sections. The first transverse section is the head. It can be seen posteroinferior to the homogeneous liver, and anterior to the elongated, anechoic inferior vena cava. (See Figure 7–16.) A more medial section shows a transverse view of the neck. A smaller amount of tissue may be noted in this section; an enlongated vessel at the posterior border denotes the superior mesenteric vein. (See Figure 7–17.) A more medial view shows the body of the pancreas anterior to the elongated, anechoic superior mesenteric artery and the similar, but larger, aorta. (See Figures 7–18 and 7–19.) Another section to the left of the body will show the tail. It can be seen anterior to the circular, anechoic splenic vein. (See Figures 7–20 and 7–21.) This vein can also be seen posterior to the pancreatic body.

NOTE: Look for changes in the contours of the veins and arteries between transverse and sagittal views. Recognizing the appearance of the epigastric vessels on both views will help the sonographer identify surrounding structures.

ACKNOWLEDGMENTS: Special thanks to the sonographers of Jeanes Hospital and Nazareth Hospital, Philadelphia, PA, for providing sonograms of the pancreas.

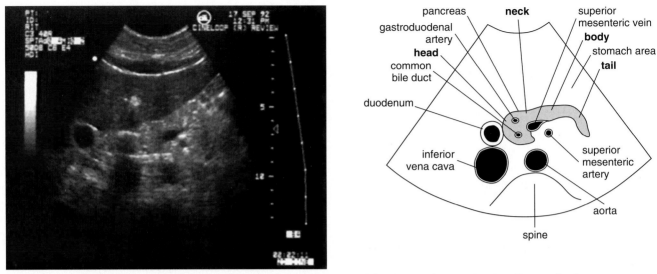

Figure 7–7. A transverse image showing the common bile duct and gastroduodenal artery in the head of the pancreas.

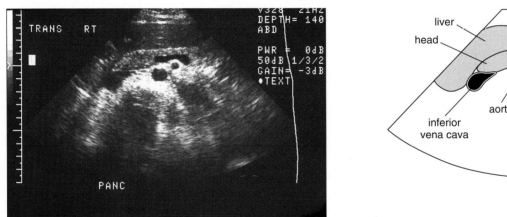
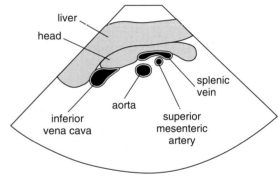

Figure 7–8. Transverse image showing the head of the pancreas (remember that transverse views show the long axis of the pancras). (Image provided by Carol Prives, RDMS, Nazareth Hospital, Philadelphia, PA.)

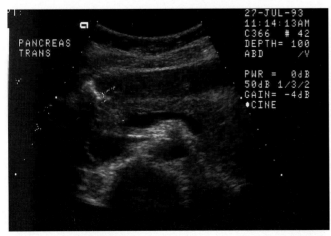
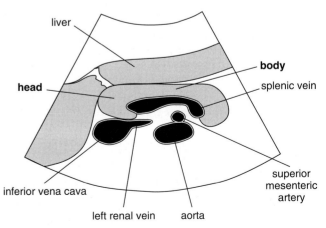

Figure 7–9. Transverse image showing the head of the pancreas. Note the portal/splenic confluence and left renal vein. (Image provided by Jeanes Hospital, Philadelphia, PA.)

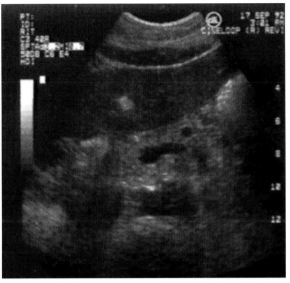
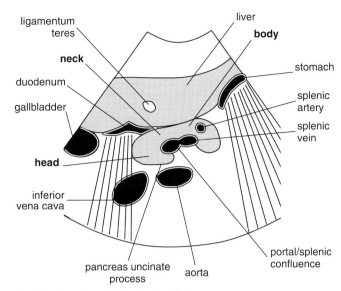

Figure 7–10. Transverse image showing a longitudinal section of the body of the pancreas.

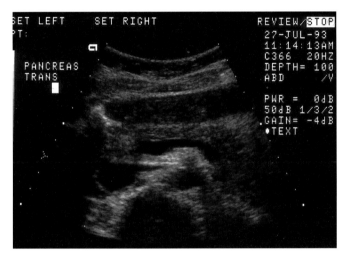
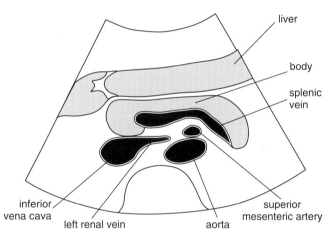

Figure 7–11. Transverse image of the body of the pancreas. (Image provided by Jeanes Hospital, Philadelphia, PA.)

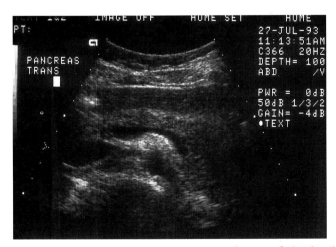
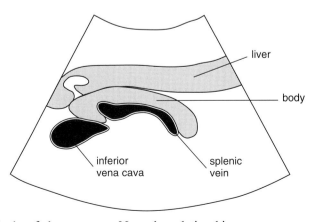

Figure 7–12. Transverse image of the head and body of the pancreas. Note the relationship between the inferior vena cava and head. (Image provided by Jeanes Hospital, Philadelphia, PA.)

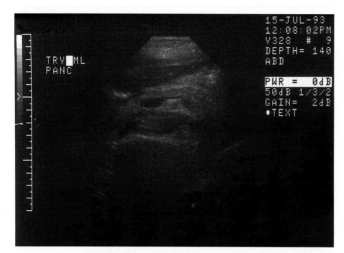 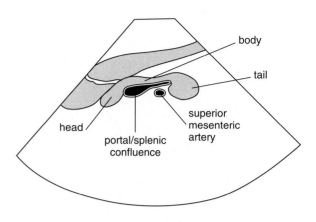

Figure 7–13. Transverse image showing the body of the pancreas. Note its small size compared with that of the head and tail. (Image provided by Rose Merna-Weston, RDMS, Nazareth Hospital, Philadelphia, PA.)

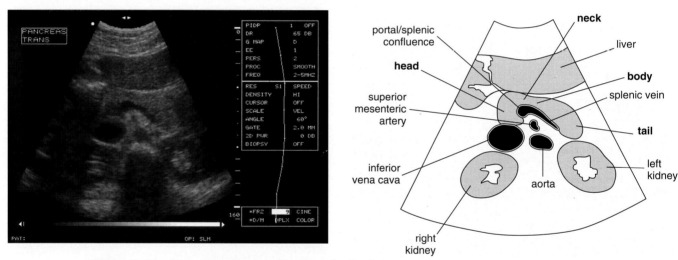

Figure 7–14. Transverse image of body and tail of the pancreas. (Image provided by Jeanes Hospital, Philadelphia, PA.)

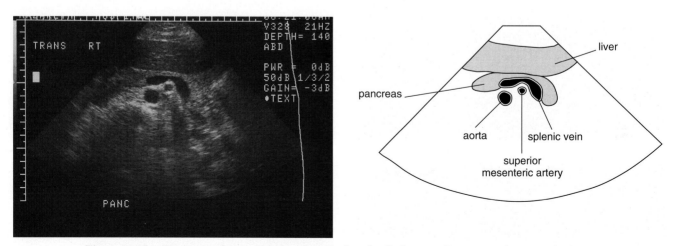

Figure 7–15. Transverse image showing the splenic vein. Only a small amount of pancreatic tissue can be seen. (Image provided by Carol Prives, RDMS, Nazareth Hospital, Philadelphia, PA.)

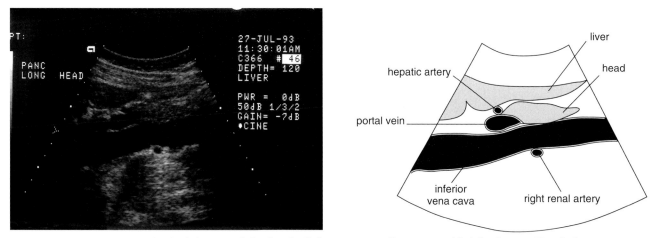

Figure 7–16. Sagittal image of the head of the pancreas. (Image provided by Jeanes Hospital, Philadelphia, PA.)

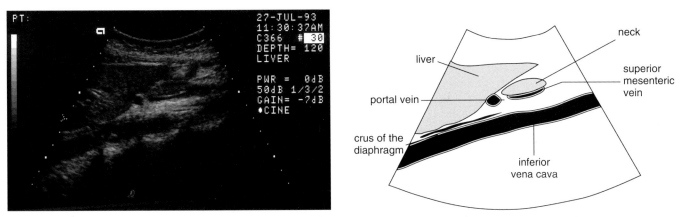

Figure 7–17. Sagittal image of the neck of the pancreas. (Image provided by Jeanes Hospital, Philadelphia, PA.)

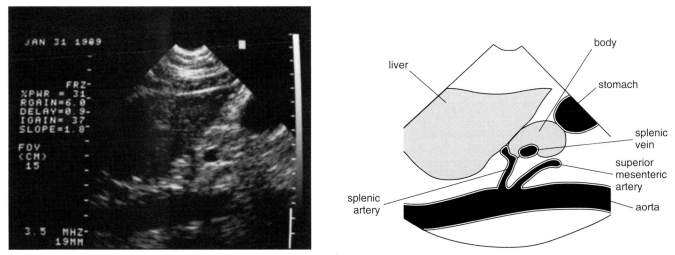

Figure 7–18. Sagittal image of the body of the pancreas between the celiac axis and superior mesenteric artery.

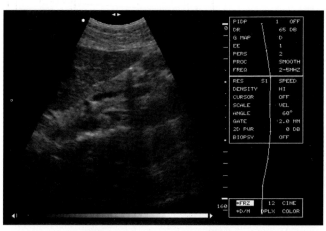
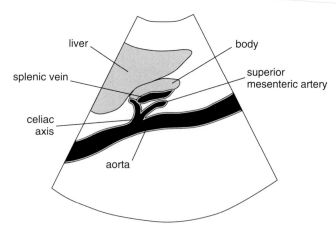

Figure 7–19. Sagittal image of the body of the pancreas. (Image provided by Jeanes Hospital, Philadelphia, PA.)

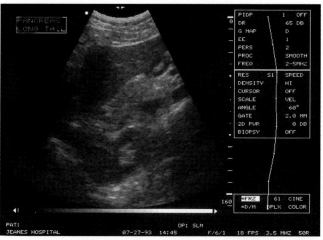
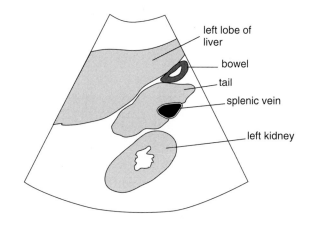

Figure 7–20. Sagittal image of the tail of the pancreas. Note that the tail lies between the bowel and the left kidney. (Image provided by Jeanes Hospital, Philadelphia, PA.)

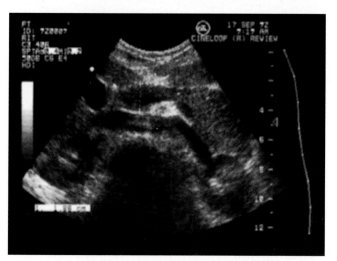
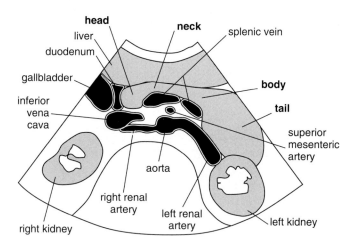

Figure 7–21. Transverse image showing an enlarged tail. This patient has a congenital malformation in which the tail of the pancreas is partially duplicated.

SONOGRAPHIC APPLICATIONS

Some uses of pancreatic sonography include the following:

Structural measurements
Distal biliary tree measurements
Identification of pancreatic masses
Identification of epigastric masses
Main pancreatic duct measurements
Adjacent associated biliary masses
Biliary obstruction
Diagnosis and follow-up of acute and chronic pancreatitis
Diagnosis and follow-up of pancreatic pseudocysts

NORMAL VARIANTS

Annular pancreas is a condition in which a ring of pancreatic tissue surrounds the second portion (C-loop) of the duodenum.

Ectopic (heterotopic, aberrant) pancreas is tissue that has no vascular or structural connection to the body of the pancreas. Since ectopic tissues may be as small as 1 cm in size, the condition is extremely difficult to detect on sonography.

Partial duplication of the tail of the pancreas is very rare. On transverse images, the tail may appear to be grossly enlarged. (See Figure 7–21.)

REFERENCE CHARTS

Associated Physicians

Surgeon: Involved in surgery of the pancreas.

Internal Medicine: Involved in diagnosing and treating pancreatic disease.

Radiologist: Performs and interprets most of the tests used to diagnose pancreatic and related diseases.

Common Diagnostic Tests

General Radiography: Except for the appearance of calcifications, plain radiography is not very revealing for pancreatic disease. An upper gastrointestinal (UGI) series, a study in which the patient swallows barium to outline the stomach and duodenum, detects pancreatic masses or enlargement through displacement of the C-loop of the duodenum by the mass. The UGI series is performed by a radiologist assisted by a radiologic technologist. The radiologist interprets the examination.

Endoscopic Retrograde Cholangiopancreaticoduoden-ography (ERCP): A tube is placed into the duodenum via the esophagus and stomach. Within the tube are fiberoptics to allow visualization of the anatomy and a means for inserting a catheter. The catheter tip is placed in the end of the common bile duct (or the pancreatic duct, depending on the anatomical configuration). A contrast medium is injected into the biliary system, which visualizes structures retrogradely (in the reverse direction). This examination is usually performed and interpreted by a gastroenterologist and a radiologist. Radiologic technologists may assist physicians in performing this procedure.

Computed Axial Tomography (CT Scan): A contrast material may or may not be administered. An x-ray beam passes through the patient to be detected by a series of devices that provide an electrical signal to a computer. The computer then arranges the data into a sectional image of the body. Structural and some functional information may be obtained. This examination is performed by a radiologic technologist and is interpreted by a radiologist.

Magnetic Resonance Imaging (MRI): Images are similar in format to those of a CT scan; however, the images are generated using a strong magnetic field instead of radiation as in CT. A magnetic resonance imaging technologist or a radiologic technologist performs the examination and a radiologist interprets the study.

Angiography: A contrast material is injected into an epigastric vessel to visualize the vascularity of the pancreas of a suspected lesion. This examination is performed by a radiologist assisted by a radiologic technologist. The radiologist interprets the study.

Laboratory Values[13]

Serum Tests:

Amylase: 60–80 units

Lipase: < 1.5 U/mL

Glucose (fasting): 65–110 mg/dL

(all sugars): 80–120 mg/dL

Urine Tests:

Amylase (2 hr): 35–260 units/hr

Alkaline Phosphatase: < 3.5 U/8 hr

Normal Measurements

Total length: 12.5–15 cm

Approximate anterior posterior measurements:

Head:	2.00–3 cm	**Body:**	1.20–2.8 cm
Neck:	1.00–2 cm	**Tail:**	2.00–2.8 cm

Vasculature

Arterial Supply to the Head and Neck of The Pancreas:

Gastroduodenal Artery—Pancreaticoduodenal Arteries—Pancreatic Arcades

Arterial Supply to the Body and Tail of the Pancreas:

Splenic Artery—Suprapancreatic Artery—Pancreatic Artery—Prepancreatic Artery—Prehilar Artery

Affecting Chemicals

Prolonged alcohol ingestion over a period of years (alcoholism) is toxic to the pancreas.

References

1. Friedman AC, Birns MT: Embryology, anatomy, histology, and physiology. In Friedman AC (ed.). Radiology of the Liver, Biliary Tract, Pancreas and Spleen. Baltimore, Williams & Wilkins, 1987, 619–641.
2. van DeGraaff KM: Concepts of Human Anatomy and Physiology, 2nd ed. Dubuque, Wm C. Brown, 1989, 882–884.
3. O'Rahilly R: Anatomy: A Regional Study of Human Structure, 5th ed. Philadelphia, WB Saunders, 1986, Chapter 36.
4. Frick H, Leonhardt H, Starck D: Human Anatomy 2: Special Anatomy: Viscera and Nervous System, Classification of Muscles and Vessels, Organization of Lymphatics and Nerves. New York, Thieme Medical, 1991, 139–141.
5. Schmidt RF, Thews G (eds.): Human Physiology. New York, Springer-Verlag, 1989, Chapter 29.
6. Guyton AC: Textbook of Medical Physiology. Philadelphia, WB Saunders, 1991, 718–719.
7. Balthazar EJ: CT diagnosis and staging of acute pancreatitis. Radiol Clin North Am 1989;27(1):19–24.
8. Federle MP, Burke VD: Pancreatitis and its complications: Computed tomography and sonography. Seminars Ultrasound CT MR 5:414–418, 1984.
9. Anthony CP, Thibodeau GA: Textbook of Anatomy and Physiology. St. Louis, CV Mosby, 1983, Chapters 19 and 20.
10. Rubin E, Farber JL: Pathology. Philadelphia, JB Lippincott, 1988, Chapter 15.
11. Craig M: Pocket Guide to Ultrasound Measurements. Philadelphia, JB Lippincott, 1988, 30.
12. Hole JW: Essentials of Human Anatomy and Physiology, 3rd ed. Dubuque, Wm C. Brown, 1989, Chapter 11.
13. Byrne CJ, Saxton DF, Pelikan PK, Nugent PM: Laboratory Tests: Implications for Nursing Care. Reading, Addison-Wesley, 1986, Appendix C.

Chapter 8

THE URINARY SYSTEM

REVA ARNEZ CURRY
BETTY BATES TEMPKIN
G. WILLIAM SHEPHERD

Objectives:

Describe the function of the urinary system.

Describe the location of the kidneys, ureters, urinary bladder, and urethra.

Describe the size of the kidneys, ureters, urinary bladder, and urethra.

Describe the sonographic appearance of the urinary system.

Describe associated physicians, diagnostic tests, and laboratory values.

Define the key words.

Homeostasis	medulla
Major calyces	pelvis
Minor calyces	sinus
Morrison's pouch	tubule
Nephron	Renin
Renal capsule	specific gravity
corpuscle	Ureters
cortex	Urethra
hilum	Urinary bladder

Key Words:

Afferent arteriole	Column of Bertin
Aldosterone	Cr
Antidiuretic hormone	Efferent arteriole
Arcuate arteries	Erythropoietin
Bowman's capsule	Gerota's fascia
BUN	Glomerulus

INTRODUCTION

The urinary system include two kidneys, a ureter for each kidney, a urinary bladder, and a urethra. The kidneys are excretory organs which maintain the body's chemical equilibrium through the excretion of urine, a waste product. Each kidney has a ureter that carries the urine to the urinary bladder for temporary storage. Urine

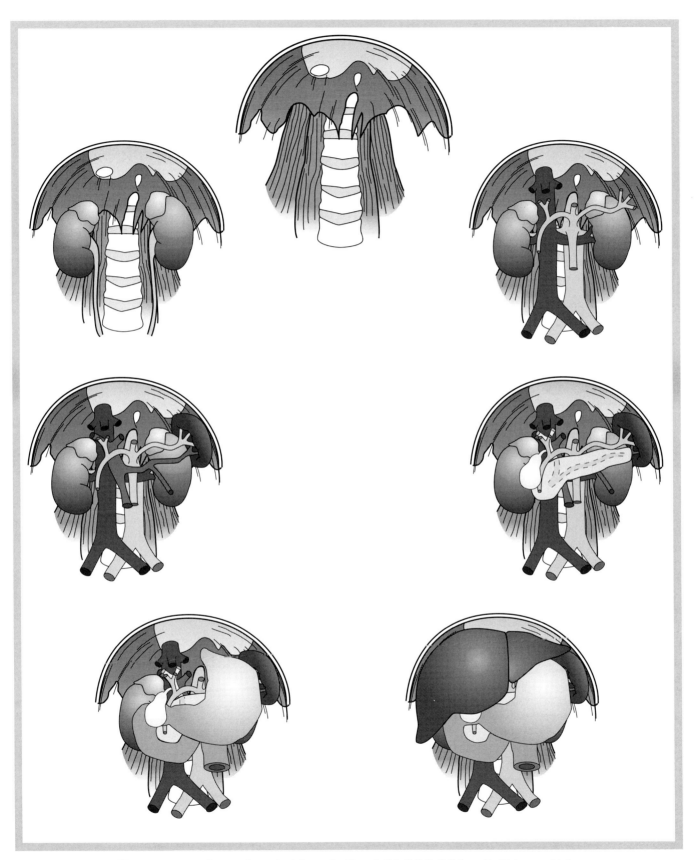

The urinary system and surrounding anatomic layers. See Figure 4–3 A, B, D, E, G, H, I, pp. 44–47, for more details.

is excreted from the bladder to outside of the body through the urethra, a membranous canal. Detoxification, blood pressure regulation, and the maintenance of the correct balance of pH, minerals, iron, and salt levels in the blood are functions of the urinary system.

PRENATAL DEVELOPMENT

The kidneys pass embryonically through three developmental stages. The pronephros and mesonephros appear in the fourth to fifth week of gestation and are precursors to the metanephros.[1,2] The embryonic kidneys are drained by the mesonephric (wolffian) ducts.[3] The paramesonephric ducts are located alongside the mesonephric ducts (para = next to). It is from this site that the reproductive organs will develop.[3] The permanent kidney—the metanephros—appears toward the end of the fifth week of gestation. It is derived from the mesodermal tissue of the embryo and is not functional until the end of the eighth week.[1] The kidneys initially lie in the pelvic cavity. As the embryo grows, the kidneys move up into the abdomen.[2,4]

Congenital defects in renal development include ectopic kidney (located away from the normal position), renal agenesis (unilateral or bilateral absence of the kidney[s]), horseshoe kidney (both kidneys joined together at their superior or inferior poles).[2] Variants in the renal vasculature and ureters may also occur. For example, multiple renal arteries occur in 25 percent of the United States population.[5] Variations of the ureter occur much less frequently, in 2 percent of that population.[6] Seventy-five percent of these variations consist of partial bifurcation of the ureter, with the remaining 25 percent, total duplication of the ureter along its entire length.[6]

LOCATION

The kidneys are bean-shaped, retroperitoneal organs that lie one on each side of the spine between the peritoneum and the back muscles. The kidney has a lateral convex and a medial concave border.[7] The liver displaces the right kidney inferiorly, hence it is located lower than the left kidney and has a slightly shorter ureter.[7] The kidneys and ureters comprise the upper urinary tract, while the urinary bladder and urethra form the lower urinary tract.[7] The kidneys lie in the lower thoracic and lumbar area, between the twelfth thoracic and fourth lumbar vertebrae.[1,8] Deep inspiration causes the kidneys to descend.[6,7] (See Figure 8–1.)

Anterior to the right kidney are the right adrenal gland, right lobe of the liver, second part of the duodenum, hepatic flexure of the colon, and jejunum or ileum of the small bowel.[7,9,10] (See Figure 8–2.) Refer to Table 8–1, which describes portions of the right kidney covered by these structures.

Anterior to the left kidney are the tail of the pancreas, the left adrenal gland, spleen, jejunum, stomach, and the splenic flexure of the colon.[7,9,10] See Figure 8–2, and refer to Table 8–2, which describes portions of the left kidney covered by these structures.

Posterior to both kidneys are the diaphragm, the psoas muscle, the transversus muscle, and the quadratus lumborum muscle.[6,7] See Figure 8–3 and refer to Table 8–3, which lists structures posterior to the kidneys.

The **ureters** are tubular, retroperitoneal structures which begin as an expanded area, the **renal pelvis,** in the hilum of each kidney. The ureters extend inferiorly along the psoas muscle. They travel from the renal hilum into the abdominopelvic cavity, and finally enter the urinary bladder posteriorly.[6,8] (See Figure 8–1C.)

The right ureter is posterior to the duodenum, terminal ileum, and right colic, ileocolic, and gonadal vessels. The left ureter is posterior to the colon, and the left colic and left gonadal (testicular or ovarian) vessels.[6,9,10]

The abdominal portion of both ureters passes anteriorly to the psoas muscle and the bifurcation of the common iliac arteries. The pelvic portions of the ureters pass posteriorly to the ductus deferens in the male and uterine artery in the female.[6,9]

Both ureters empty posteriorly into the **urinary bladder,** a hollow, muscular, retroperitoneal organ that is posterior to the symphysis pubis.[6,9] The male urinary bladder is anterior to the seminal vesicles and the rectum, and superior to the prostate gland. The ductus deferens, on its superior, slightly lateral course from the scrotum, crosses the ureter anteriorly, before descending into the prostate gland.[3] (See Figure 8–4.) The female urinary bladder is anterior to the vagina, posterior cul-de-sac, and rectum.[6,7,9] (See Figure 8–5.)

The **urethra** is a membranous canal which conveys urine out of the urinary bladder. It exits inferiorly via the neck of the urinary bladder.[1,6,9] The male urethra is much longer than the female urethra, and also functions as a pathway for seminal fluid.[7]

SIZE

The normal adult kidney is approximately 9 to 12 cm in length, 2.5 to 4 cm in depth, and 4 to 6 cm in diameter.[1-3] The kidney may shrink due to atrophic changes associated with age, circulatory insufficiency, or renal disease.[7] If only one kidney is present (ie, congenital absence of a kidney), it may be larger than normal, due to hypertrophy necessary to accommodate the increased workload.[11]

The neonatal kidney measures 3.3 to 5.0 cm in length, 1.5 to 2.5 cm in depth, and 2 to 3 cm in diameter.[12,13] The pediatric kidney is proportionately larger than the adult and may extern inferiorly to the iliac crest.[3]

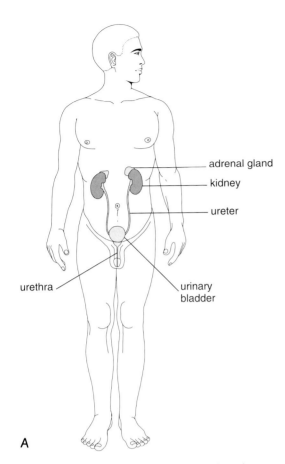

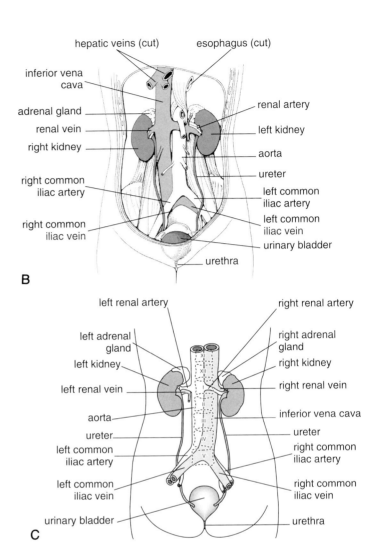

Figure 8–1. The urinary tract. *A,* Adrenal glands, kidneys, ureters, urinary bladder, and urethra. *B,* Frontal view of the urinary system shows how the ureters cross the iliac vessels anteriorly. *C,* Posterior view shows the urinary tract from behind. Note frontal placement of the ureters.

TABLE 8–1. Anterior Structures Which Cover the Right Kidney

STRUCTURE	PORTION OF KIDNEY COVERED
Right adrenal	Superior–medial
Right lobe of liver	Lateral
Second part of duodenum	Medial
Hepatic flexure of colon and jejunum or ileum of small bowel	Inferior

TABLE 8–2. Anterior Structures Which Cover the Left Kidney

STRUCTURE	PORTION OF KIDNEY COVERED
Tail of pancreas	Medial
Left adrenal gland	Superior–medial
Spleen	Superior–lateral
Jejunum	Inferior
Stomach	Superior
Splenic flexure of colon	Lateral

TABLE 8–3. Structures Posterior to Kidneys

STRUCTURE	PORTION OF KIDNEY COVERED
Diaphragm	Superior
Psoas muscle	Medial
Transversus muscle	Lateral
Quadratus lumborum muscle	Between lateral and medial portions

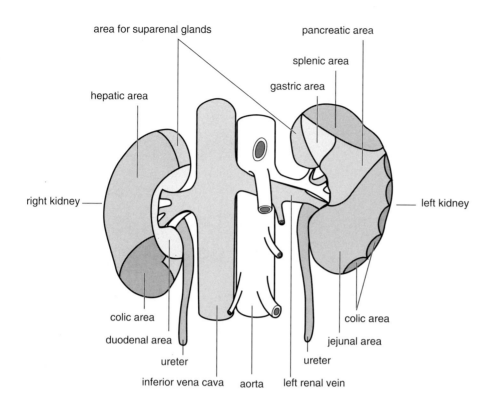

area for suparenal glands

pancreatic area

hepatic area

splenic area

gastric area

right kidney

left kidney

colic area

colic area

duodenal area

jejunal area

ureter

ureter

inferior vena cava

aorta

left renal vein

Figure 8-2. Frontal view of the kidneys showing the overlying structures (adrenals, liver, duodenum, hepatic flexure, jejunum, stomach, splenic flexure, spleen, and pancreatic tail). See Tables 8-1 and 8-2 for correlation.

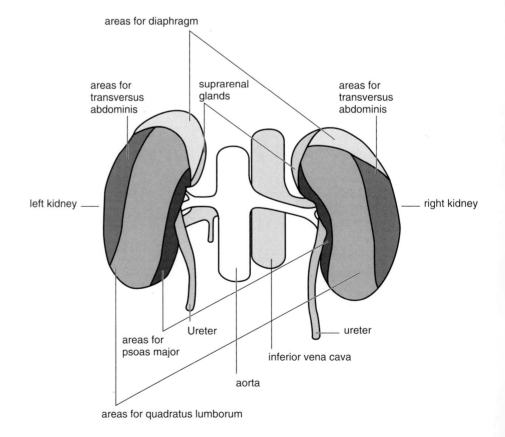

areas for diaphragm

areas for transversus abdominis

suprarenal glands

areas for transversus abdominis

left kidney

right kidney

Figure 8-3. Posterior view of the kidneys showing the structures covering the kidneys from behind (diaphragm, psoas and quadratus lumborum, and transversus muscles). See Table 8-3 for correlation.

areas for psoas major

Ureter

ureter

inferior vena cava

aorta

areas for quadratus lumborum

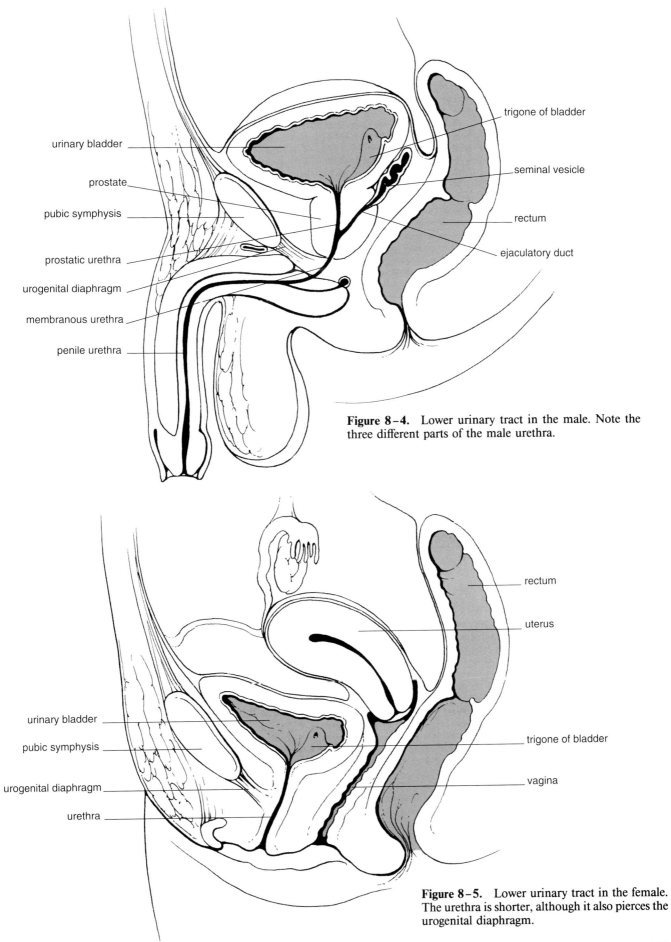

urinary bladder

prostate

pubic symphysis

prostatic urethra

urogenital diaphragm

membranous urethra

penile urethra

trigone of bladder

seminal vesicle

rectum

ejaculatory duct

Figure 8–4. Lower urinary tract in the male. Note the three different parts of the male urethra.

urinary bladder

pubic symphysis

urogenital diaphragm

urethra

rectum

uterus

trigone of bladder

vagina

Figure 8–5. Lower urinary tract in the female. The urethra is shorter, although it also pierces the urogenital diaphragm.

The ureters are hollow narrow tubes ranging from 25 to 30 cm in length.[1,14] The diameter ranges between 4 and 7 mm.[6] In a cadaver, the diameter is a uniform 5 mm throughout the length.[14] The ureters transport urine to the bladder through peristaltic action.[6,10,15]

The urinary bladder is a symmetrical hollow organ, whose size depends on the quantity of contained urine. The wall of a distended bladder will normally measure 3 to 6 mm depending on the degree of bladder distension.[16,17] The male urethra is 20 cm in length, while the female is considerably shorter, approximately 3.5 cm in length.[3]

GROSS ANATOMY

Upper Urinary Tract

The kidney consists of an upper, a middle, and a lower pole. It has several protective coverings which cushion and protect the entire organ. (See Figure 8–6.) First, it is covered with a tough, fibrous capsule. Second, a layer of perirenal fat surrounds the encapsulated kidney and is continuous with the fat in the renal sinus.[7] The third layer, the renal fascia, surrounds the kidney and perirenal fat.[1,18] Another term for the renal fascia is fascia of Gerota or **Gerota's fascia.**[14] Gerota's fascia is surrounded by yet another layer of fat, called pararenal fat.[1,18] This layer is especially thick posterior to Gerota's fascia.[7]

The renal fascia anchors the kidneys and limits any infection arising from them.[7,18] The double layer of renal fat (perirenal and pararenal) accommodates kidney movement during respiration.[7]

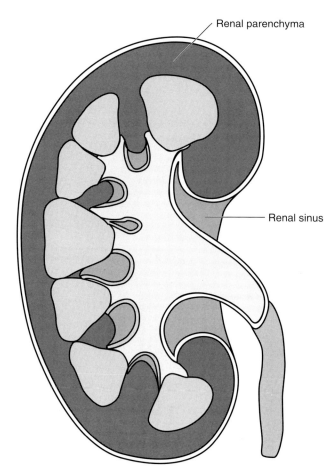

Figure 8–7. Simplified drawing of the kidney showing the renal parenchyma and sinus.

There has been some confusion regarding the various names given to the tissues which cover the kidneys. Some common alternative terms are listed in Table 8–4.

For the purposes of this text, two distinct areas—the renal sinus and the renal parenchyma—will be described. A dissected view of the kidney is shown in Figure 8–7.

The renal parenchyma consists of two areas. The outer portion of the parenchyma is the **cortex.** (See Figure 8–7.) It contains the renal corpuscle and the proximal and distal convoluted tubules of the nephron.[1,18] The inner portion of renal parenchyma is called the **medulla;** it contains the loop of Henle (also called renal loops). Thus, filtration takes place in the renal cortex and reabsorption occurs in the medulla.[6,15]

The medulla consists of eight to 18 medullary pyramids.[1,6,7,15] The pyramids are triangular structures with a narrow tip, called the apex, and a broad base. A renal

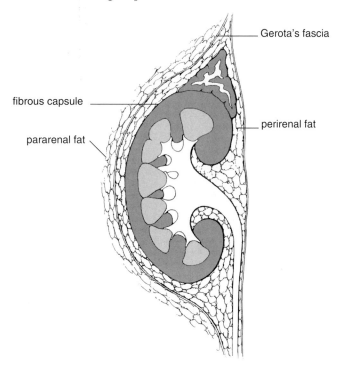

Figure 8–6. Four layers surrounding the kidney: fibrous capsule, perirenal fat, Gerota's fascia, and pararenal fat.

TABLE 8–4. Common Names for Tissues Covering Kidneys

Perinephric fat = adipose capsule		= packing fat of Zuckerkandl
Perirenal fascia = perinephric fascia	= fascia of Gerotas
Pararenal fat = pararenal body		

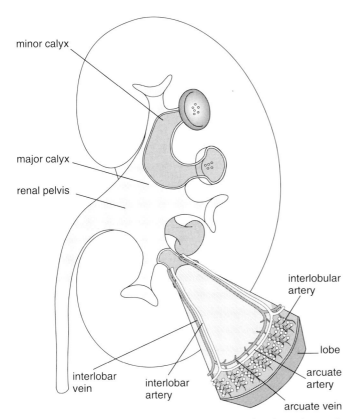

Figure 8-8. Renal lobe. Note that the lobe is triangular and bordered by the interlobar vasculature. The arcuate and interlobular vessels and the surrounding cortical tissue form the base of the lobe.

lobe consists of a pyramid, bordered on both sides with interlobar arteries and veins, with cortical tissue at its base.[3] (See Figure 8-8.)

The pyramids are separated by bands of cortical tissue called **columns of Bertin.**[7,8,18] The function of the renal pyramids is to convey urine to the minor calyces.[6,7,18] Thus, the number of renal pyramids will equal the number of minor calyces. The minor calyces also form the border of the area of the renal sinus. (See Figure 8-7.)

The **renal sinus** is the central portion of the kidney. It includes the minor calyces, the major calyces, the renal pelvis, renal artery and vein, fat, nerves, and lymphatics.[1,7,8,18] There are usually two to three major calyces which receive urine from the **minor calyces.** (See Figure 8-7.) The **major calyces** convey urine to the upper, expanded end of the ureter, the **renal pelvis.**[7,8] The **hilum** is the area where the renal artery enters the kidney and the renal vein and ureter exit.[1,6,18] (See Figure 8-7.)

NOTE: Students studying the kidney for the first time often mistakenly assume that the renal sinus and the renal pelvis are identical structures. This probably occurs because both the sinus and pelvis are in close proximity. It may be helpful to note that the renal pelvis is contained *within* the renal sinus and is its largest component. Other major parts of the sinus include fat (an extension of the perirenal fat), and the renal artery and vein.

The **ureters** begin in the kidney as the renal pelvis. They are composed of three layers of tissue, an inner mucosal layer, a medial layer of longitudinal and circular smooth muscle, and an outer fibrous layer.[1,6,9,15] Ureteral peristalsis transports urine to the urinary bladder.[6,9,14] The ureters enter the bladder posteriorly at the trigone area.[9,18] Urine is carried into the urinary bladder between intervals of several seconds and several minutes depending on the state of hydration.[1,7] Blood is supplied to the ureters by branches from the renal, internal spermatic, hypogastric, and inferior vesical arteries.[21]

Lower Urinary Tract

The **urinary bladder** consists of four layers of tissues—an inner mucosa, a submucosa layer, the muscularis, and the outer serosa.[1,9] The mucosa folds when the bladder is empty, and distends and becomes smooth when the bladder is full.[1] The muscularis layer is comprised of three layers of smooth muscle, called the detrusor muscle.[1] The outermost layer, the serosa, is located at the superior portion of the bladder. It is an extension of pelvic peritoneum.[1] (See Figure 8-9.)

The inferior portion of the urinary bladder is comprised of a posterior base (the trigone area) and the neck, which communicates with the urethra.[1,7] The inferior-lateral surfaces of the bladder meet anteriorly, and are in

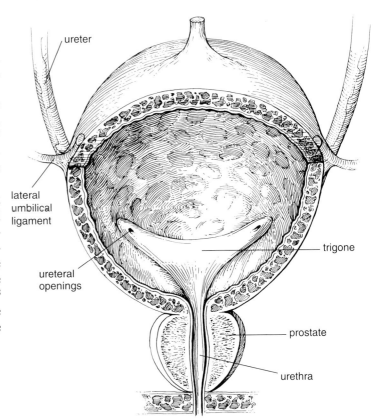

Figure 8-9. Urinary bladder. Note the triangular area, the trigone where the ureters enter. Also shown is the lateral umbilical ligament.

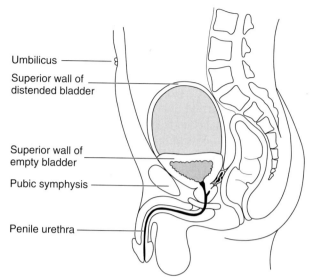

Figure 8–10. Difference between an empty and a distended urinary bladder. Note how the superior portion of the distended bladder moves toward the umbilicus.

contact with the pelvic floor muscles.[7] (See Figure 8–9.)

The anterior portion of the urinary bladder lies behind the pubic bone and the symphysis pubis.[7] Only the superior portion of the urinary bladder is covered by an extension of peritoneum. The location of the superior portion is variable, depending on the amount of urine in the bladder. (See Figure 8–10.)

The urinary bladder is anchored to the pelvis by ligaments.[5,7] Ligaments extending anteriorly from the bladder neck attach to the pubic bones. These ligaments are called pubovesical in the female, and puboprostatic in the male.[7] Laterally, ligaments extend to fuse with the tendinous arch of the obturator internus muscles. These attachments are called lateral ligaments.[7] Blood is supplied to the urinary bladder by the superior, middle, and inferior vesicles, derived from the anterior trunk of the hypogastric. The obturator and inferior gluteal arteries also supply small visceral branches to the bladder and in the female additional branches are derived from the uterine and vaginal arteries.[21]

The **urethra** consists of a membranous, hollow canal which conveys urine from the bladder to the outside. The male urethra is approximately 20 cm in length, compared with the female urethra, which is approximately 3.5 cm in length.[8,10,15] The male urethra is composed of three parts.[5,8,10,18] The first portion, the prostatic urethra, receives secretions from the prostate gland. The second part is the short membranous urethra, which pierces the urogenital diaphragm. The third portion is the longest. It is the penile urethra and extends the entire length of the penis. The female urethra is composed of the membranous urethra, which also pierces the urogenital diaphragm.[7,8] Male and female urethras are shown in Figures 8–4 and 8–5.

PHYSIOLOGY

As the primary excretory organs (see Chapter 3), the principal function of the kidneys is urine production and **homeostasis** (maintenance of normal body physiology).[1,5,8,15] The kidneys excrete metabolic waste products and maintain blood volume, and function independently. A unilateral condition (complete obstruction, congenital absence of a kidney, trauma or removal of a kidney) will not affect the remaining kidney's function; the healthy kidney will accommodate the increased workload. Failure of both kidneys however, will lead to uremia, a toxic and fatal condition if untreated.[8,18]

The kidneys filter approximately 1200 ml of blood per minute and produce on average 150 ml of urine daily.[1,4,6,7] The excreted urine is 95 percent water and 5 percent nitrogenous waste and inorganic salts.[8] Nitrogeneous waste consists of the byproducts of metabolism. The amount of nitrogenous waste is measured by **blood urea nitrogen (BUN)** and **creatinine (Cr)** laboratory tests,[8] which measure the kidneys' ability to get rid of waste. Normal ranges for BUN and Cr are 26 mg per dl and 1.1 mg per dl respectively.[19] Another laboratory test which can assess the kidneys' ability to concentrate urine is specific gravity.[8] **Specific gravity** is a measure of how much dissolved material is present in the urine. The higher the quantity of dissolved solutes, the higher the specific gravity. For example, specific gravity is higher when the kidneys must preserve water (eg, during exercise), to compensate for water lost in sweat.[8] The volume of urine therefore is decreased. The normal range of specific gravity is 1.101 to 1.025 (the specific gravity of distilled water, which has no solutes, is 1.000).[8]

The functional unit of the kidney is the **nephron.** There are over a million microscopic nephrons in each kidney.[1,4,6,7] The nephron functions by moving metabolic products from areas of high concentration to areas of low concentration.[1,6] This is accomplished through osmosis, the passive transport of cellular material. Another method is active transport, which uses cellular energy to move material from one area to another.[1,14]

There are two types of nephrons, named for their location in the kidney and the length of their loops (the loop of Henle is discussed later in this chapter).[1,7,8,18] Juxtamedullary nephrons originate in the inner third of the renal cortex and have longer loops of Henle than cortical nephrons located in the outer two thirds of the renal cortex. (See Figure 8–11.)

The nephron consists of a **renal corpuscle,** which includes Bowman's capsule and the glomerulus; and a **renal tubule,** which includes the proximal convoluted tubule, loop of Henle (with descending and ascending branches), distal convoluted tubule, and a collecting duct.[1,7,8,18] (See Figure 8–12.) The medulla contains the loop of Henle and collecting duct. The renal cortex contains the renal corpuscle and the proximal and distal convoluted tubules.

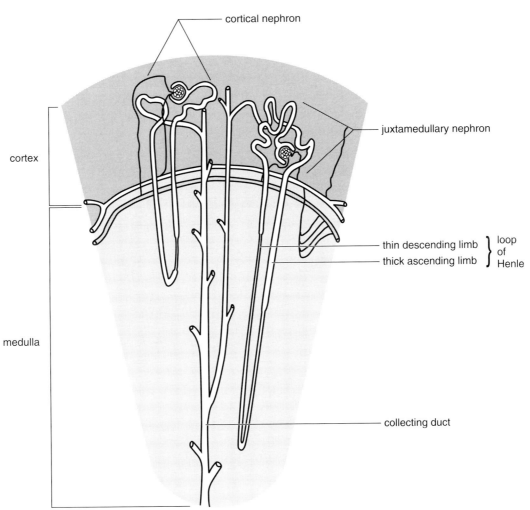

Figure 8–11. Cortical and juxtamedullary nephrons. The loop of Henle is longer in the juxtamedullary nephron.

Blood reaches the nephron in the following manner: Blood enters the kidney through the renal artery, a branch of the aorta. The renal artery forms interlobar arteries, which travel between the renal pyramids. The interlobar arteries branch into **arcuate arteries,** located at the base of the renal pyramids. From the arcuate arteries, the interlobular arteries travel into the renal cortex.[1,18] The interlobular arteries branch into **afferent arterioles,** which carry blood into the glomerulus of the nephron.

How the Nephron Works

The filtration which takes place in the **glomerulus** is the first step in urine formation.[1,7,8,18] As blood enters the glomerulus, afferent arterioles carrying the blood branch into capillaries. As the vessels narrow, the blood pressure in the vessels increases. Most capillaries have a blood pressure of approximately 25 mm Hg (mercury). However, in the glomerulus, the pressure is 60 to 90 mm Hg. This higher blood pressure forces a plasma-like fluid from the blood to filter into Bowman's capsule.[20] This

"nephric filtrate" contains water, salts, glucose, urea, and amino acids. Proteins and cells, which are too large to pass through the semipermeable walls of the glomerular capillaries, remain in the blood.[20]

Osmotic pressure forces water to return to the blood. This pressure is created by the difference in protein content of the fluid in the proximal convoluted tubule and the plasma in the glomerular capsule.[1] The protein concentration in the proximal convoluted tubule is 2 to 5 mg per 100 ml compared with the capsule concentration of 6 to 8 mg per 100 ml. This concentration gradient creates osmotic pressure, which returns water from the proximal convoluted tubule back to the plasma in the glomerular capsule, where it is returned into the blood.

The fluid which enters the glomerulus is called ultrafiltrate. The volume of filtrate produced per minute is 115 ml for women and 125 for males.[1] This means that the body's entire blood volume is filtered approximately every 40 minutes.[1] Ninety-nine percent of the blood volume is returned, and 1 percent is excreted.[1,18]

Tubular reabsorption is the process by which sub-

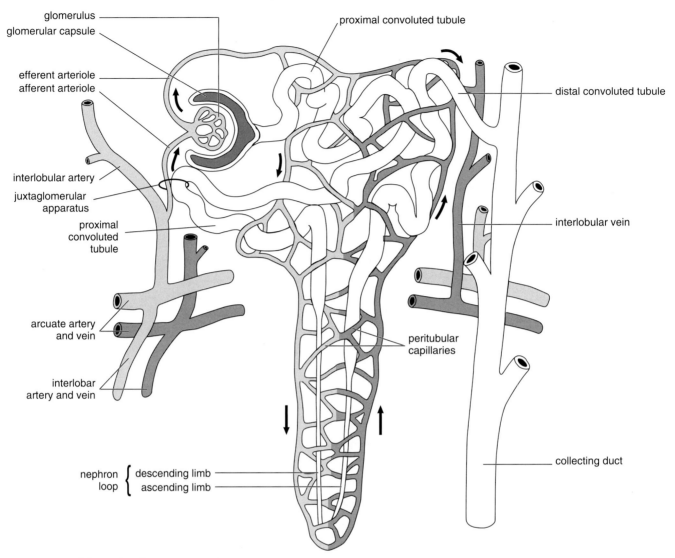

Figure 8–12. Enlarged view of nephron. Glomerulus, proximal and distal convoluted tubules, loop of Henle, and collecting duct are shown. Note juxtaglomerular apparatus.

stances in the plasma solute that are useful to the body are reabsorbed into the bloodstream.[1-3,6] These substances include water, glucose, vitamins, amino acids, bicarbonate ions, and chloride salts of magnesium, sodium, calcium, and potassium. Reabsorption takes place in the proximal convoluted tubule and the descending and ascending **loop of Henle.** Sixty-five percent of the salt and water in the ultrafiltrate is reabsorbed from the proximal convoluted tubule, and 20 percent is reabsorbed from the loop of Henle.[1] The amount of reabsorption of the remaining ultrafiltrate is dependent on hormonal influence and takes place in the distal convoluted tubule.[1,7] Tubular resorption takes place through active transport and expends a large amount of energy. It has been estimated that 6 percent of total calories consumed by the body at rest (no physical activity) may be required for tubular resorption.[1]

Blood from the **efferent arteriole** supplies the peritu-

bular capillaries, which in turn supply the proximal and distal convoluted tubules, and the vasa recta.[1,18] (See Figure 8–12.) The vasa recta are a series of intertwining capillary loops which surround the juxtamedullary nephron.[1] (See Figure 8–11.) Through osmotic pressure, the vasa recta trap salt and urea in the medulla and move water back into the blood. This mechanism is called the countercurrent multiplier system and helps the kidneys maintain homeostasis.[1,18]

Blood from the peritubular capillaries drains into the interlobular veins which, in turn, drain into arcuate veins. The arcuate veins drain into the interlobar veins, which convey blood back to the renal vein. The renal veins carry blood to the inferior vena cava.[1,14,18]

Tubular secretion is the process whereby waste substances, including ammonia, drugs, hydrogen, and potassium, are secreted into the distal convoluted tubule. The secretion process is controlled through active trans-

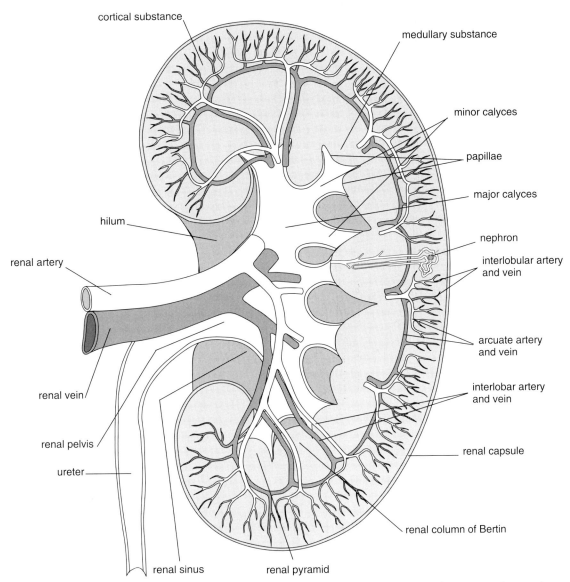

Figure 8-13. Dissected view of the kidney. The renal cortex, medulla, calyces, capsule, renal pelvis, and ureter are shown. Note the column of Bertin.

port.[1,7,9,18] Urine exits the distal convoluted tubule into the collecting tubule of duct. The collecting ducts convey urine to the renal pyramids. The apex of the pyramid lies within the minor calyx, which is part of the collecting system for urine. Several **minor calyces** empty urine into each major calyx; several **major calyces** empty urine into the renal pelvis. (See Figure 8-13.) The urine is emptied from the renal pelvis into the ureter, and by peristalsis is carried to the urinary bladder.[1,18]

Protective Mechanisms that Preserve Nephron Function

The kidneys are sensitive to changes in blood volume and have the capacity to alter blood volume to maintain homeostasis.[7] This is necessary because the kidneys need a large volume of blood for urine production and to nourish the cells lining the nephron. The latter are especially sensitive to anoxia (lack of O_2), and prolonged decrease in blood oxygen may result in irreversible cellular death.[7] Thus, there are several protective mechanisms that enable the kidneys to regulate blood volume and guard against anoxia.

A decrease in blood volume stimulates receptors in the left atrium of the heart and the lungs.[7] This activates the release of **antidiuretic hormone (ADH)** from the posterior pituitary gland. ADH increases the quantity of water returned from the distal collecting tubule to the bloodstream.[7] As a result, urine volume decreases and blood volume increases. Another hormone which affects blood volume is **aldosterone,** which is produced by the adrenal cortex and acts on the distal convoluted tubule.[7,8,18] A decrease in blood volume stimulates the release of aldosterone. Aldosterone causes salt and water to be reab-

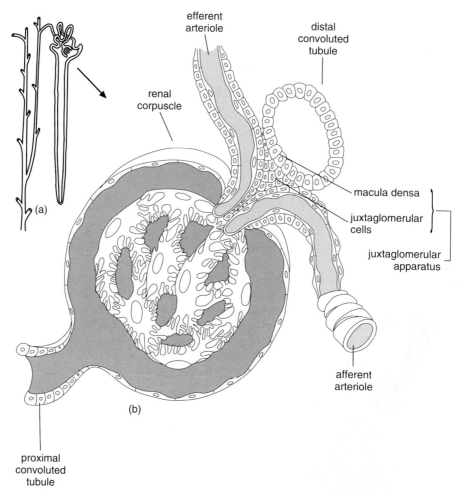

Figure 8–14. Juxtaglomerular apparatus. Note granular cells in the afferent and efferent arterioles. The macula densa are located in the distal convoluted tubule.

sorbed from the nephron into the bloodstream, which increases blood volume.

A third mechanism affecting blood volume is the juxtaglomerular apparatus. This system is located at the point where the afferent and efferent arterioles and distal convoluted tubule come into contact. (See Figure 8–14.) A decrease in blood volume is detected by granular cells in the afferent arteriole. The granular cells release **renin**, which acts on angiotensinogen in the blood to increase systemic pressure.[7] Cells in the distal convoluted tubule in contact with the afferent and efferent arterioles are called macula densa. (See Figure 8–14.) It is believed that the macula densa can inhibit renin secretion when the blood volume returns to normal.[1]

The kidneys produce another hormone which affects blood volume. **Erythropoietin** is released in response to a decrease in oxygen (eg, due to hemorrhage).[7] Erythropoietin acts on bone marrow, causing red blood cells to be produced. It also causes mature red blood cells stored in the bone marrow to be released into the bloodstream. This mechanism increases the number of red cells in the blood, thus enhancing the ability of the blood to carry oxygen.[7]

Another protective mechanism takes place during prolonged anoxia. Blood is shunted from the outer cortex to the inner cortex to maintain renal function.[7] The kidneys are also able to decrease resistance in the renal

TABLE 8–5. Protective Mechanisms

SOURCE	FUNCTIONS	EFFECT
Kidney	1. Decreases renal capillary bed resistance	Increases blood supply to kidneys
	2. Moves blood from outer cortex to inner cortex	Preserves renal function in severe blood loss
	3. Makes erythropoietin	Increases amount of red blood cells to carry oxygen
Juxtaglomerular apparatus of kidney	Makes renin	Increases systemic pressure
Adrenal cortex	Secretes aldosterone	Increases blood volume
Posterior pituitary gland	Secretes antidiuretic hormone	Increases blood volume

capillary bed (increasing the blood supply to the kidneys), when systemic pressure drops.

Refer to Table 8–5 which summarizes the kidneys' protective mechanisms.

SONOGRAPHIC APPEARANCE

In a longitudinal section the adult kidney appears as a smooth, contoured, elliptical structure. (See Figure 8–15.) In transverse section the kidney appears rounded and broken medially by the hilum. The renal vein and artery can be seen in the hilar region. (See Figure 8–16.)

Kidneys

A detailed description of the sonographic pattern of different parts of the kidney follows. Refer to Figures 8–15 and 8–16 to identify the parts described. The

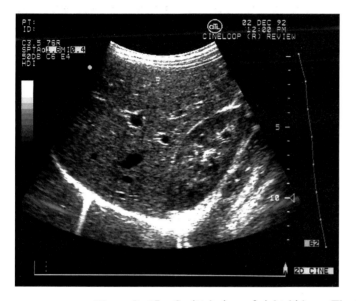
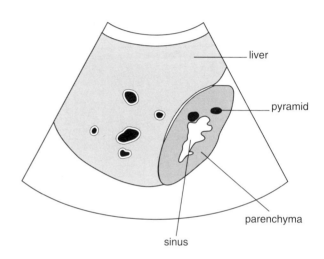

Figure 8–15. Sagittal view of right kidney. The liver is superior to the kidney. The curvilinear, echogenic line between the liver and right kidney is Morrison's pouch, a peritoneal space. Note the anechoic areas in the renal parenchyma representing the renal pyramids. Areas of high level echoes in the center of the kidney represent the renal sinus.

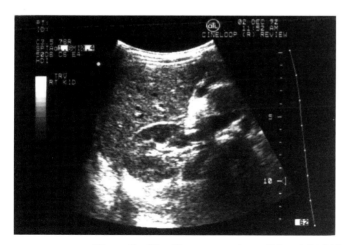
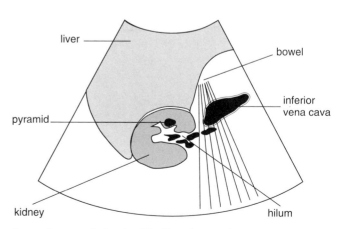

Figure 8–16. Transverse view of the right kidney shows the rounded pole. The liver is anterior. Note the hilar area, where the renal artery and vein are located.

description begins "outer edge" first (the renal capsule), and ends with the center of the kidney, the renal sinus.

The **true capsule** appears echogenic and surrounds the cortex.[22]

The **parenchymal cortex** appears as mid-gray or medium to low-level homogeneous echoes that are less than or equal to the echogenicity of the normal liver or spleen.[5,22]

The **arcuate vessels** appear as echogenic dots that may be seen at the corticomedullary junction.

The **medullae** (medulla, sing.) of the parenchyma appear as triangular, round, or blunted hypoechoic areas to the more urine-filled anechoic areas. The pyramids depict the medullary portion of the kidney.

The **sinus** appears as the echogenic center of the kidney.[5] The sinus is echogenic due to surrounding fat. The renal pelvis and infundibulum are not seen if collapsed; otherwise they appear anechoic.

Figures 8–17 through 8–20 show sagittal views of the right and left kidneys. Transverse views of both kidneys are shown in Figures 8–21 through 8–24.

Renal vasculature (arteries and veins) from both kidneys can be seen on a transverse view. (See Figure 8–25.)

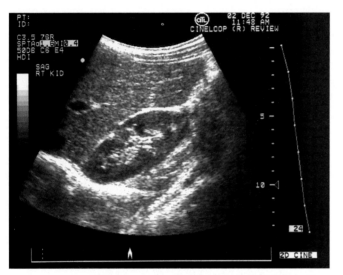
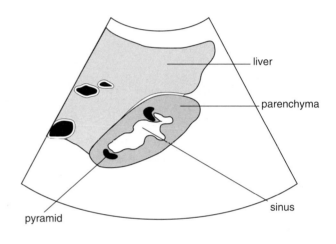

Figure 8–17. Sagittal view of the right kidney better shows the echogenic renal sinus.

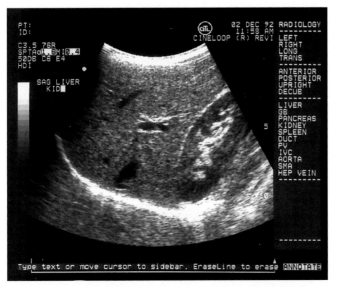
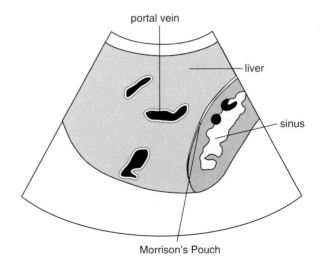

Figure 8–18. Sagittal view of the right kidney again shows the echogenic renal sinus. Morrison's pouch is also visualized.

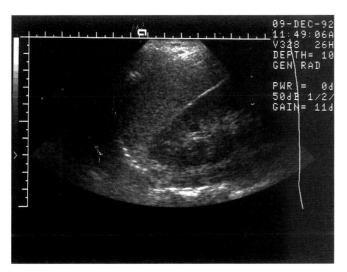
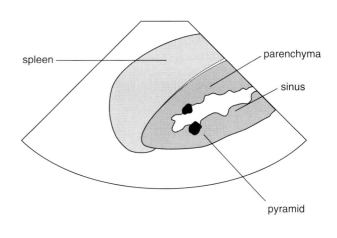

Figure 8–19. Coronal view of the spleen and left kidney. The lower pole is not seen, but several renal pyramids and the renal sinus are visualized.

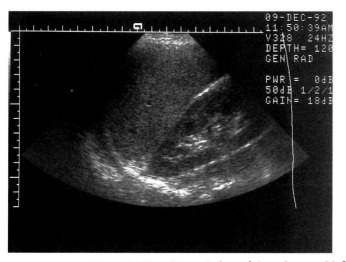
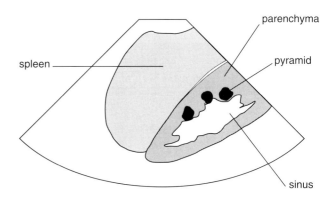

Figure 8–20. Coronal view of the spleen and left kidney. Both are better visualized, especially the renal sinus. Several pyramids are also visualized.

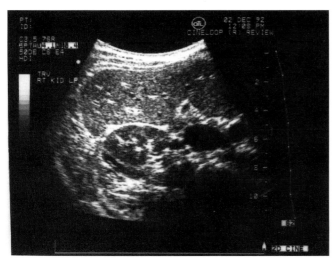
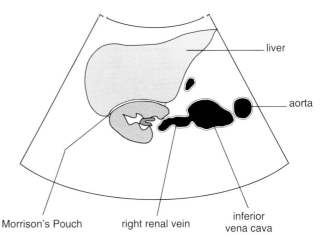

Figure 8–21. Transverse view of liver and right kidney. Morrison's pouch is more clearly visualized here than in the sagittal view. Also shown is a portion of the right renal vein entering the IVC. The aorta is adjacent to the IVC.

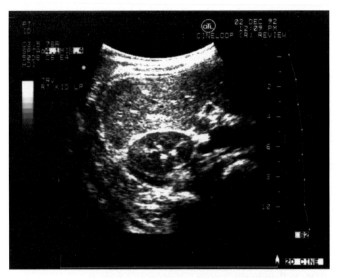
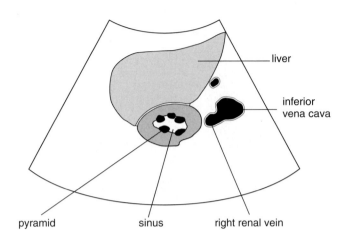

Figure 8–22. Transverse view of the liver and the right kidney. Renal pyramids are more clearly visualized. A portion of the right kidney and IVC is also shown.

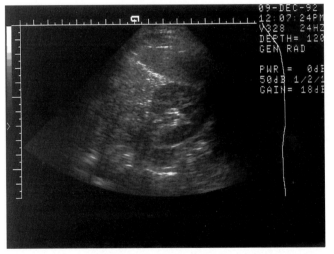
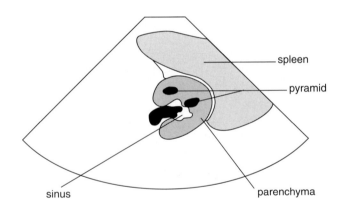

Figure 8–23. Transverse view of spleen and left kidney. The renal pyramids and hilum are clearly visualized.

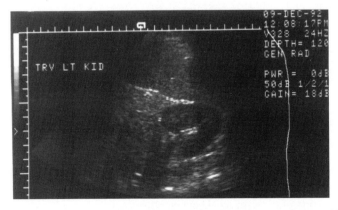
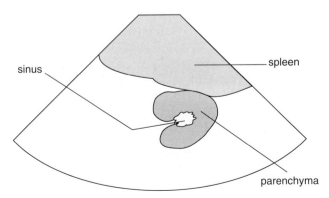

Figure 8–24. Transverse spleen and left kidney. The renal sinus can be seen.

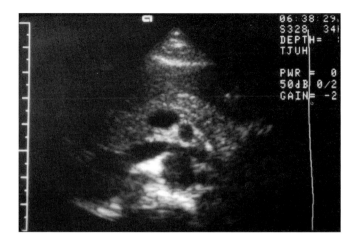

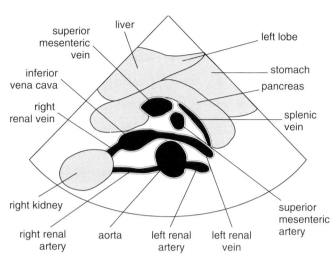

Figure 8–25. Transverse view of the epigastric region: Left lobe of the liver, and pancreas, are shown. Posterior to the pancreatic neck is the superior mesenteric vein. The left and right renal veins and arteries are seen. Also visualized is the superior mesenteric artery and part of the splenic vein.

Ureters

The ureters are not normally visible. However, the effect of ureters' ejecting urine into the bladder, called "ureteral jets," can be observed on real-time examination.

Urinary Bladder

In transverse section the bladder appears somewhat squared by the laterally laying psoas muscles. Anteriorly, the sides appear rounded. (See Figure 8–26.) In longitudinal section the posterior surface of the bladder may be somewhat indented by an anteverted uterus or an enlarged prostate. (See Figure 8–27.) It is important to note that the size and shape of the bladder vary due to the quantity of urine stored. Nevertheless, the distended bladder should appear symmetrical.

The bladder lumen is not visible if it is collapsed; otherwise it appears anechoic. The distended bladder wall appears as a smooth, thin echogenic line.

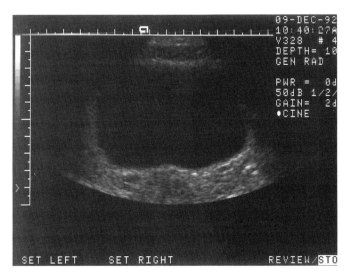

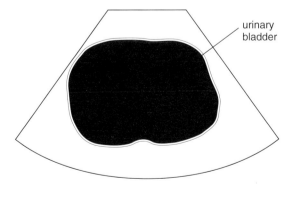

Figure 8–26. Distended urinary bladder.

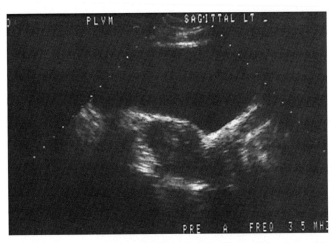
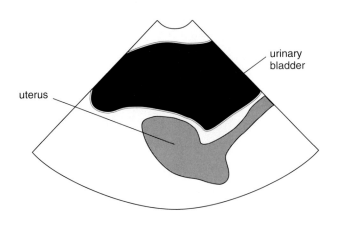

Figure 8-27. Overly distended urinary bladder. Note the uterus posterior to the bladder.

Urethra

The urethra when visualized appears echogenic.

NOTE: Renal Doppler may be used to assess arterial and venous blood flow in kidneys. It is also used in assessing blood flow in renal transplantation patients. However, research has shown that renal Doppler alone cannot effectively evaluate transplant patients for signs of acute rejection.[23,24] Renal Doppler has also been used to detect vascularity in renal tumors and atriovenous malformations.[25,26]

The Adrenal Glands

The adrenal glands are only briefly discussed in this section, because in the adult they are difficult to visualize sonographically.[17] The glands are much more readily detected in fetuses and young children. This has been attributed to adrenal size. The infant adrenal is proportionately larger than the adult adrenal. At birth, the adrenal is one third the size of the kidney, whereas in the adult, it is one thirteenth the size of the kidney.[27]

This section will take a brief look at the anatomy and physiology of the adrenal gland.

The adrenals are paired endocrine organs located at the superior and medial border of the kidneys.[7] They are approximately 2 inches in length, 1.1 inch in diameter, and 0.4 inch in depth.[1,28] The glands are enclosed with the kidneys in Gerota's fascia and are surrounded by fat.[7] Each gland consists of an outer cortex and an inner medulla. (See Figure 8-28.) The cortex and medulla function independently; thus the adrenal is actually two hormonal glands in one.

The cortex contains three areas called zones. Each zone produces steroid hormones, commonly called corticoids.[1,7] The zone at the outermost portion of the cortex is called the zona glomerulosa. It produces mineralocorticoids, of which the most important is aldosterone; aldosterone regulates sodium and potassium levels. The next zone is called the zona fasciculata. It produces glucocorticoids. Cortisol is its primary substance; it regulates glucose metabolism. The innermost zone is called the zona reticularis. It supplements the sex hormones produced by the reproductive organs—ovaries and testes.

The adrenal medulla is composed of chromaffin cells.[1] They secrete epinephrine and norepinephrine. The adrenals produce four times as much epinephrine as norepinephrine. These hormones are responsible for the "flight or fight" response. Their effects include an increase in heart and respiratory rates and dilatation of the coronary blood vessels.

SONOGRAPHIC APPLICATIONS

Sonography is used to evaluate several aspects of the urinary system. Common considerations include the following:

Renal size
Detection and composition of renal masses and cysts
Urinary system obstruction
Renal abscess
Renal hematoma
Enlarged ureters
Urinary bladder masses
Renal transplantation
Doppler evaluation of renal blood flow abnormalities
Sonographically guided biopsies of renal parenchyma or
   masses
Sonographically guided fluid aspirations

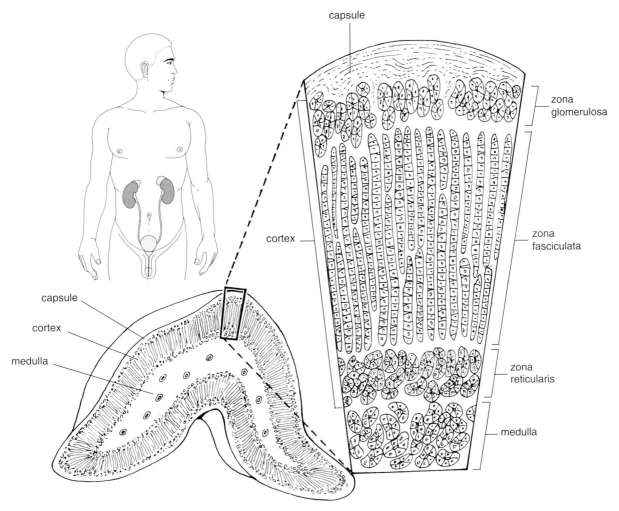

Figure 8–28. Zones of the adrenal cortex, zona glomerulosa, zona fasciculata, and zona reticularis. Also depicted is the adrenal medulla.

NORMAL VARIANTS

The following normal variants can be observed on ultrasound. (See Figure 8–29.)

Dromedary Hump

A dromedary hump is a localized bulge(s) on the lateral border of the kidney. It has the same sonographic appearance as a normal renal cortex. (See Figure 8–29A.)

Hypertrophied Column of Bertin

A hypertrophied column of Bertin occurs in varying degrees of size and may indent the renal sinus of the kidney. It has the same sonographic appearance as normal renal cortex. (See Figure 8–29B.)

Double Collecting System

A double collecting system occurs when the renal sinus is divided. (See Figure 8–29C.) Each sinus has a renal pelvis. A bifid (double) ureter may also be present.

Horseshoe Kidneys

A horseshoe kidney occurs when the kidneys are connected, usually at the lower poles. (See Figure 8–29D.) It has the same sonographic appearance as normal renal tissue. However, the junction between the two kidneys can be visualized on sonography.

Renal Ectopia

Renal ectopia occurs when one or both kidneys occur outside the normal renal fossa. Locations include the lower abdominal and pelvic region. Other ectopic locations (eg, intrathoracic) are rare.

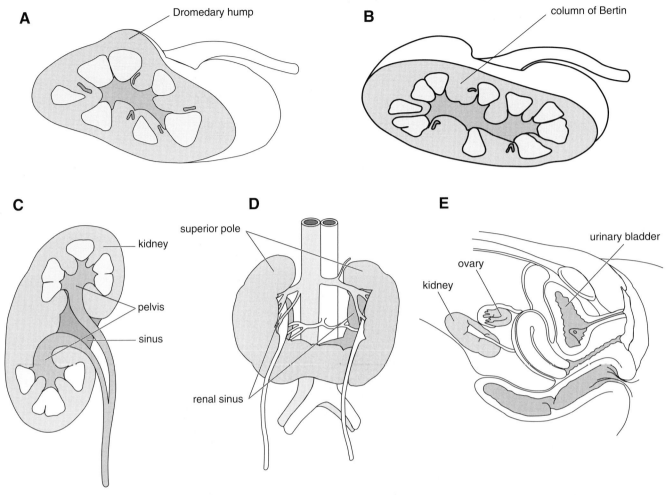

Figure 8–29. *A,* Dromedary hump; *B,* Column of Bertin; *C,* Double collecting system with double renal pelvis and partially bifid ureter; *D,* Horseshoe kidney connected at the lower poles; *E,* Sagittal adnexal view of the pelvis demonstrating an ovary and pelvic kidney.

REFERENCE CHARTS

Associated Physicians

Urologist: Specializes in surgical diseases of the urinary system in the female and genitourinary track in the male.

Nephrologist: Specializes in diseases of the kidney.

Radiologist: Specializes in the diagnostic interpretation of imaging modalities that assess renal disease.

This test is performed by a radiologic technologist and radiologist. The examination is interpreted by the radiologist.

Computed Axial Tomography (CT scan): A radiologic examination in which cross-sectional x-ray images are obtained of the kidneys and other urinary system structures to assess anatomy. A contrast medium may be administered to differentiate between pathology and normal anatomy. This test is performed by a radiologic technologist and radiologist. The examination is interpreted by the radiologist.

Common Diagnostic Tests

Intravenous Pyelogram (IVP): A radiologic examination in which a contrast medium ("dye") is injected into a vein and x-ray films are taken at specific intervals to observe kidney function and urinary system anatomy.

Laboratory Values

Blood Urea Nitrogen (BUN): Used to assess renal function. Normal BUN is 26 mg per dl. Elevation of this value may indicate renal disease.

Creatinine (Cr): Used to assess renal function. Normal Cr is 1.1 mg per dl. Elevation of this value may indicate renal disease.

Normal Measurements

Adult Kidney: 9 to 12 cm in length; 4 to 6 cm in diameter; 2.5 to 4 cm in depth.

Neonatal Kidney: 3.5 to 5.0 cm in length; 2 to 3 cm in diameter; 1.5 to 2.5 cm in depth.

Ureters: 28 to 34 cm in length; 6 mm in diameter.

Distended Urinary Bladder Wall: 3 to 6 mm in depth.

Female urethra: 4 cm in length.

Male Urethra: 20 cm in length.

Vasculature

Aorta—Renal Artery—Interlobar Artery—Arcuate Artery—Interlobular Artery—Afferent Arterioles—Glomerulus—Efferent Arteriole—Peritubular Capillaries—Interlobular Vein—Arcuate Vein—Interlobar Vein—Renal Vein—Inferior Vena Cava.

Affecting Chemicals

Aldosterone: A hormone which increases salt and water reabsorption by the kidneys.

Renin: A hormone which helps the kidneys maintain blood pressure.

Antidiuretic Hormone (ADH): A hormone which increases water reabsorption.

References

1. VanDeGraaff KM, Fox SI: Concepts of Human Anatomy and Physiology, 3rd ed., Chap 25. Dubuque, Wm C. Brown, 1992.
2. Moore K: Before We Are Born: Basic Embryology and Birth Defects, 3rd ed. Chaps 1, 14. Philadelphia, WB Saunders, 1989.
3. Langebartel DA: The Anatomical Primer: An Embryological Explanation of Human Gross Morphology. Baltimore, University Park Press, 1977.
4. Craig TS, Madsen KM: Anatomy of the kidney, Chap 1. In Brenner BM, Rector FC (eds.). The Kidney, 3rd ed. Philadelphia, Ardmore Publishers, 1986.
5. Wolfman NT, Bechtold RE, Watson NE: Chap 4. In Resnick L, Rifkin M (eds.). Ultrasonography of the Urinary Tract. Baltimore, Williams and Wilkins, 1991.
6. Frick H, Leonhardt H, Starck D: Human Anatomy Two, Chap 14. New York, Thieme, 1991.
7. Rogers AW: Textbook of Anatomy. New York, Churchill Livingstone, 1992.
8. Scanlon V, Sanders T: Essentials of Anatomy and Physiology, Chap 18. Philadelphia, FA Davis, 1991.
9. Snell RS: Clinical Anatomy for Medical Students, 2nd ed. Boston, Little, Brown, 1981.
10. Clements CD: Anatomy—A Regional Atlas of the Human Body, 2nd ed. Baltimore, Urban & Schwarzenberg, 1981.
11. Spitz L, Wurnig, P, Angerpointer TA eds.: Surgery in solitary kidney and corrections of urinary transport disturbances. Prog Pediatr Surg, Vol. 23, 1989.
12. McInnis AN, Felman AH, Laude JV, et al: Renal ultrasound in the neonatal period. Pediatr Radiol 12:15, 1982.
13. Scott JES, et al: Ultrasound measurement of renal size in newborn infants. Arch Dis Child 65:361–364, 1990.
14. Gosling A, Dixon S, Humpherson JR: Functional Anatomy of the Urinary Tract, Chap 1. Baltimore, University Park Press, 1982.
15. Jacob W, Francone CA: Elements of Anatomy and Physiology, 2nd ed., Chap 13. Philadelphia, WB Saunders, 1989.
16. Friedland GW, Cunningham J: The elusive ectopic ureterocele. Am J Radiol 116:792–811, 1972.
17. Abu-Yousef MM, Narayana AS, Brown RC, et al: Urinary bladder tumors studied by cystosonography, Part II: Staging. Radiology 153:227–231, 1984.
18. Martini F: Fundamentals of Anatomy and Physiology, 2nd ed., Chap 26. Englewood Cliffs, Prentice Hall, 1992.
19. Guyton, AC: Textbook of Medical Physiology, 8th ed., Chap 3. Philadelphia, WB Saunders, 1991.
20. Fong E, et al: Body structures and functions, 6th ed. Unit 31. New York, Delmar, 1984.
21. Gray H, Goss M: Anatomy of the Human Body, 27th ed. Philadelphia, Lea & Febiger, 1965, 1337–1345.
22. Coleman B: Genitourinary Ultrasound, Chap 1. New York, Igaku-Shoin, 1988.
23. Perrella RR, et al: Evaluation of renal transplant dysfunction by duplex Doppler sonography: A prospective study and review of the literature. Am Kidney Dis 20(6):544–550, 1990.
24. Drake DG, et al: Doppler evaluation of renal transplants in children: a prospective analysis with histopathologic correlation. Am J Radiol 154:785–787, 1990.
25. Kier R, et al: Renal masses: characterization with Doppler ultrasound. Radiology 176:703–707, 1990.
26. Takebayashi S, Aida N, Matsul K: Arteriovenous malformations of the kidneys: diagnosis and follow-up with color Doppler sonography in six patients. Am J Radiol 157:991–995, 1991.
27. Mittelstaedt C: Abdominal Ultrasound. New York, Churchill Livingstone, 1987.
28. Anthony CP, Thibodeau G: Textbook of Anatomy and Physiology, 14th ed. St. Louis, CV Mosby, 1983, 374–378.

Bibliography

Bo WJ, Wolfman NT, Krueger WA, et al: Basic Atlas of Sectional Anatomy with Correlated Imaging. 2nd ed. Philadelphia, WB Saunders, 1990.

Marsh DJ: Renal Physiology. New York, Raven Press, 1981.

Vander AJ: Renal Physiology, 2nd ed. New York, McGraw-Hill, 1980.

Walsh C, Gittes RF, Perlmutter AD, Stamey A: Campbell's Urology, 5th ed. Philadelphia, WB Saunders, 1986.

Weill FS, Rohmer P, Zeltner F: Renal Sonography, 2nd ed. New York, Springer-Verlag, 1987.

Chapter 9

THE SPLEEN

FELICIA M. JONES

Objectives:

Describe the function of the spleen.

Describe the location of the spleen.

Define size relationships of the normal spleen.

Describe the sonographic appearance of the normal spleen.

Describe the associated physicians, diagnostic tests, and laboratory values relevant to the normal spleen.

Define key words.

Key Words:

Culling	Mesoderm
Erythrocyte	Mesogastrium
Gastrolienal ligament	Omentum bursa
Hematopoietic	Phagocytosis
Hemoglobin	Pitting
Hemosiderin	Red pulp
Hypochondrium	Reticuloendothelial
Intraperitoneal	Splenic artery
Lienorenal ligament	Splenic cords
Lymph	Splenic hilum
Malpighian corpuscles	Splenic vein
Mesenchyme	White pulp

INTRODUCTION

The spleen is an **intraperitoneal** organ which lies in the left upper quadrant of the abdominal cavity. It is part of the **reticuloendothelial** system and is composed primarily of **lymph** tissue. Although the spleen is a component of the body's defense system, it is not essential to life and can be removed without adverse effects. (See Figure 9–1.)

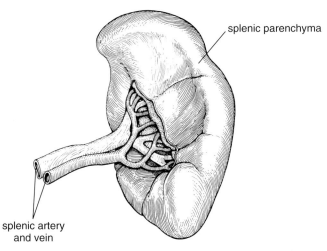

Figure 9–1. Normal splenic anatomy.

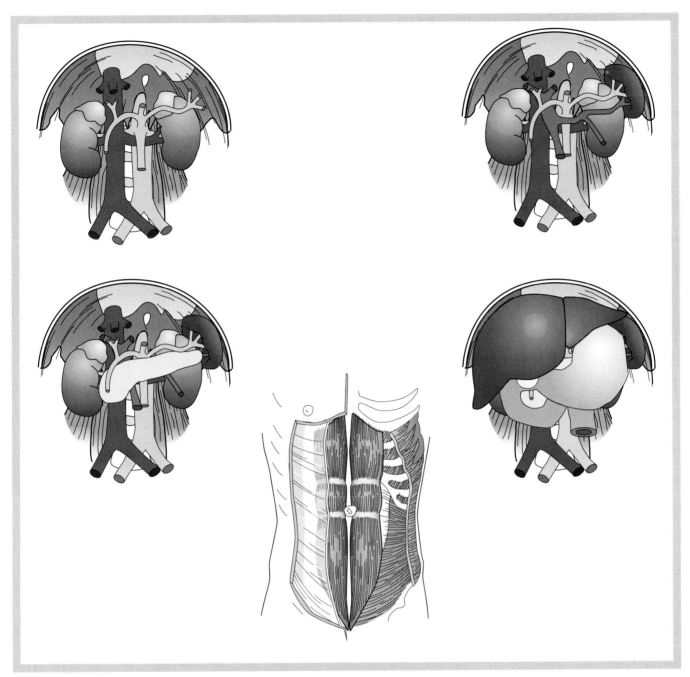

The spleen and surrounding anatomic layers. See Figure 4–3 D, E, F, I, J, pp. 44–47, for more details.

PRENATAL DEVELOPMENT

Development of the spleen begins at about the fifth week of gestation, arising from **mesodermal** cells. It begins as a thickening in the **mesenchyme** on the left side of the **mesogastrium** or the **omentum bursa**. These mesenchymal cells differentiate into two types of cells— reticular cells, and primitive free cells which resemble adult lymphocytes. The spleen is separated from the stomach by the **gastrolienal ligament** and from the left kidney by the **lienorenal ligament**. The fetal spleen is normally quite lobulated. (See Figure 9–2.)

The spleen begins to perform its **hematopoietic** or blood-cell producing functions by approximately the eleventh week of gestation. This activity is a result of tissue-myeloid functions. These functions generally end shortly after birth, but may reactivate in certain pathological conditions. In adult life the spleen will continue to produce lymphocytes.

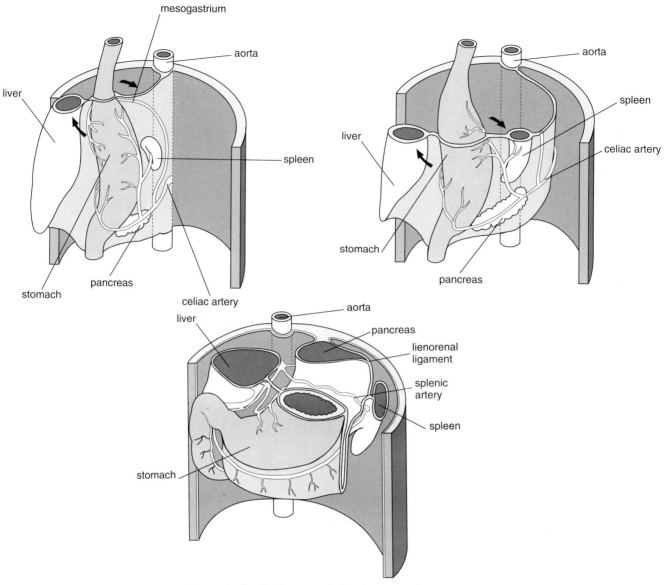

Figure 9–2. Early prenatal development of the spleen.

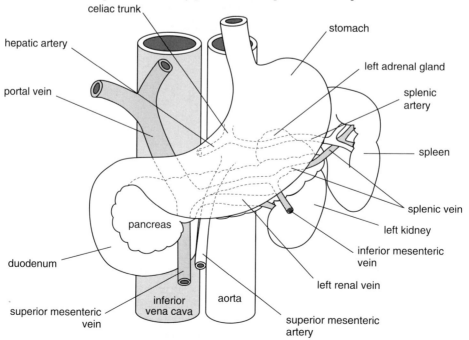

Figure 9–3. Surrounding splenic anatomic relationships.

By the fifth or sixth month of gestation, the spleen begins to assume its smooth ovoid adult shape and its adult functions. Its **white pulp**, which contains **malpighian corpuscles,** performs the **lymphocytic** functions. This distinct portion of the spleen begins to form late in fetal development.

The **red pulp** carries out various functions. The splenic cords house reticular cells, which are responsible for the reticuloendothelial functions of the spleen. This portion does not develop until after birth, when primary fetal blood cell formation ceases. The purpose of the red pulp is to destroy the degenerating red blood cells. It is called **phagocytosis.**

LOCATION

The spleen lies in the left hypochondrium, with its longest axis along the tenth rib. It lies posterolateral to the body and fundus of the stomach, posterolateral to the tail of the pancreas, and posterior to the left colic flexure. The left kidney is located posteroinferior to the medial portion of the spleen. Posterior to the spleen are the diaphragm; the lung; and the ninth, tenth, and eleventh ribs. The spleen is covered by peritoneum, with the exception of the hilum. This portion of the spleen, located medially, is where the vasculature enters and exits. (See Figure 9–3.)

SIZE

The size of the spleen may vary, but generally the longest dimension superior to inferior should be no greater than 12 or 13 cm. The largest transverse dimension (anterior to posterior) should be no larger than 7 or 8 cm.

The spleen is generally smooth in contour, with a convex superior surface and a concave inferior surface.

GROSS ANATOMY

The spleen is a highly vascular mass of lymphoid tissues located in the left upper quadrant of the abdomen. It is ovoid with a convex superior surface and a concave inferior surface. The spleen is entirely covered by the peritoneum except at the hilum, where all vessels enter and leave. The splenic vein exits the hilum and courses along the gastrolienal ligament to its confluence with the superior mesenteric vein to form the portal vein. The splenic artery, which originates at the celiac trunk of the aorta, often branches into two or more smaller arteries before entering the hilum.

The spleen's posterior location gives it the protection of the ribs. Consequently, the spleen is usually not palpable unless it is pathologically enlarged.

As described earlier, the spleen is composed of red pulp and white pulp. The white pulp consists of lymphatic tissue which surrounds and follows the smaller splenic arteries. The red pulp is looser and more vascular. It occupies all of the space not filled by white pulp or splenic cords.

PHYSIOLOGY

The spleen is composed of two components, red pulp and white pulp. The red pulp consists of the splenic sinuses and splenic cords. The sinuses are long, slender channels lined with epithelial cells. This portion of the spleen is a filter which aids in phagocytosis of degenerating red blood cells. The hemoglobin from these cells is further broken down into pigments. The most abundant pigment thus released is **hemosiderin.** Epithelial cells carry out the spleen's reticuloendothelial functions.

The white pulp is composed of lymphoid tissues. The primary components of this portion of the spleen are the malpighian corpuscles. This portion continues to produce lymphocytes in adult life. The white pulp also has a role in pigment and lipid metabolism.

Splenic functions can be divided into those related to the reticuloendothelial system and its functions as an organ. The reticuloendothelial system produces lymphocytes and plasma cells, as well as antibodies, and stores iron and metabolites.

As an organ, the spleen has the following functions: **erythrocyte** or red blood cell surface maturation; a reservoir; culling; pitting; disposal of degenerating or senescent erythrocytes; and regulation of platelet and leukocyte life span.

The ability of the spleen to store blood cells is due to its high smooth muscle content. Contraction of the smooth muscle causes the stored blood cells to be released when necessary. However, if the number of cells stored becomes excessive, splenomegaly will develop.

In its pitting function, the spleen removes senescent or abnormal red blood cells; in culling, it removes nuclei from the red blood cells as they pass through.

SONOGRAPHIC APPEARANCE

The spleen appears to be homogeneous in texture. It is very smooth and medium gray in color. It should be the same or less echogenic than the liver. Echogenic reflections may be seen that represent calcifications of small arterial walls or calcified granulomatous inclusions. The significance of the latter varies according to patient history. The organ may be difficult to visualize due to gas in the adjacent bowel and to the overlying ribs. It is often easiest to scan the spleen intercostally from a coronal approach. It is more readily visualized ultrasonically when pathologically enlarged. (See Figure 9–4.)

SONOGRAPHIC APPLICATIONS

The most common use of sonography in imaging the spleen is to detect its enlargement.

Previously, when articulated arm B scanning was in wide use, the rule of thumb was that if the spleen was visualized anterior to the aorta, it was pathologically enlarged. Today, with real time scanning, the determination of splenomegaly has become basically a subjective judgment. The more experience the sonographer and interpreting physician have, the more accurate their judgment will be.

Ultrasound can help assess splenic masses. Primary splenic masses are quite rare. Ultrasound is also useful in assessing splenic damage from blunt trauma, such as rupture or hemorrhage.

NORMAL VARIANTS

Accessory Spleen

Accessory spleen is found in up to 10 percent of the general population. These islands of tissue are usually less than 1 cm in diameter. More than one accessory spleen may be present, most often near the splenic hilum or attached to the tail of the pancreas.

Asplenia

This rare congenital abnormality may be associated with a congenital heart defect. If solitary, there are no complications. The liver may be visualized more distinctly to the left of the midline than usual.

Splenomegaly

This pathological finding is included because it is the most common splenic abnormality. It is most often due to complications of other organic disease. Splenomegaly is noted as a mass in the left upper quadrant. It may be due to recent trauma, portal venous congestion, systemic infection, or a blood disorder such as anemia.

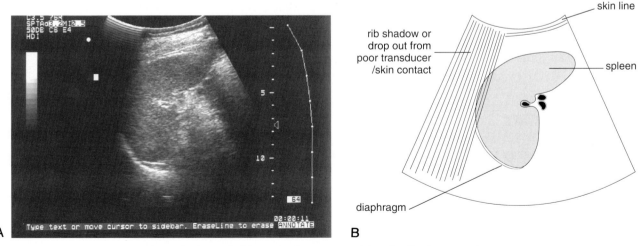

Figure 9–4. *A,B,* Normal spleen, coronal longitudinal approach.

Illustration continues on the opposite page.

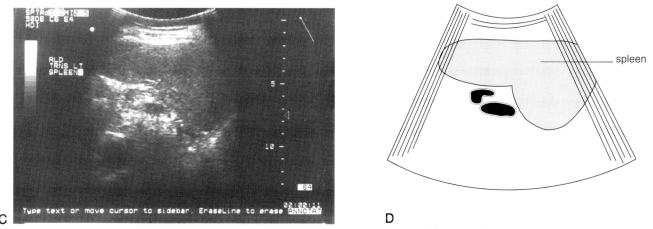

Figure 9–4. *C,D,* Normal spleen, a transverse left approach.

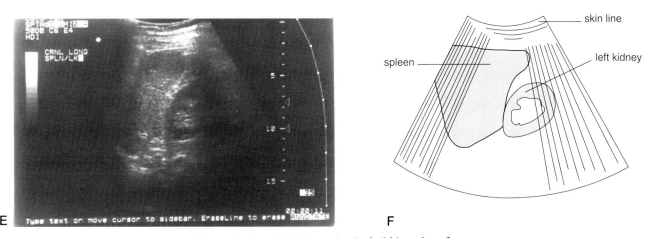

Figure 9–4. *E,F,* Normal splenic/kidney interface.

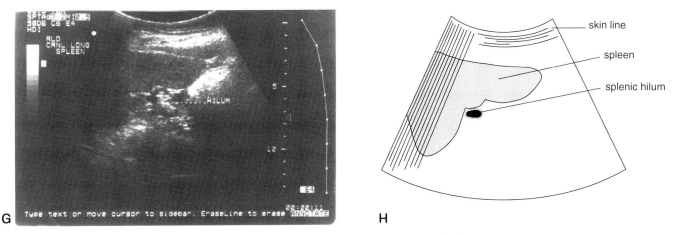

Figure 9–4. *G,H,* Normal spleen, showing splenic hilum.

REFERENCE CHARTS

Associated Physicians

Family Physician: Often serves as referring physician, coordinating patient care. In this capacity, the physician recommends referral to specialists when necessary.

Internist: Specializes in the diagnosis and treatment of internal disorders.

Surgeon: Specializes in performing surgical procedures.

Radiologist: Specializes in interpreting diagnostic imaging procedures.

Hematologist: Specializes in treating diseases of blood.

Common Diagnostic Tests

X-Ray: In this test, ionized electromagnetic waves create photographic images, which are then "read" and interpreted. It is performed by a radiologic technologist and interpreted by a radiologist.

Ultrasound: Nonionized sound waves generate diagnostic images in this test. The sound waves do not penetrate bone or air. The test is performed by a sonographer and interpreted by a radiologist.

Nuclear Medicine: This test involves intravenous injection of radionuclides to create diagnostic images. The radionuclides "tag" specific cells, so that the resulting image is specific to the area of interest. This test is performed by a nuclear medicine technologist and interpreted by a radiologist.

Computed Axial Tomography (CT Scan): The ionized waves create a cross-sectional x-ray image of the body. This test is performed by a radiologic technologist who is certified for "CT" or "CAT scan," and is interpreted by a radiologist.

Laboratory Values

Hematocrit: The hematocrit reading indicates the percentage of red blood cells per volume of blood. Normal values for men are 40 to 54 percent, for women, 37 to 47 percent. An abnormally low hematocrit points to internal bleeding.

Bacteremia: The presence of bacteria within the blood system, also known as sepsis. Symptoms include chills, fever, and possibly the presence of abscesses.

Leukocytosis: An increase in the number of circulating leukocytes (above 10,000 per cu mm). This finding is indicative of an infection of the blood. It may occur in hemorrhage, following surgery, in malignancies, during pregnancy, in toxemia, and may be due to leukemia.

Leukopenia: An abnormally low number of leukocytes in the blood (below 5000 per cu mm). This may develop due to certain drugs, or to a bone marrow disorder.

Thrombocytopenia: An abnormal decrease in the number of circulating platelets. The normal range is 150,000 to 350,000 per cu mm. The decrease may be due to internal hemorrhage.

Normal Measurements

The adult spleen is normally 12 or 13 cm in the superior to inferior axis; 6 or 7 cm in the medial to lateral axis; and 5 or 6 cm in the anterior to posterior plane.

Vasculature

The splenic venous sinuses unite to form venules which in turn merge to become the large splenic vein. The vein exits the hilum medially, coursing along the posterior border of the body and tail of the pancreas.

The spleen receives most of its blood supply through the splenic artery. This artery originates at the celiac axis from the aorta and courses laterally, serving as the superior border of the tail and body of the pancreas. The artery enters the splenic hilum medially, then branches into smaller arteries.

The smaller splenic arteries terminate in tiny capillaries which anastomose with the venous sinuses. The capillaries are permeable, which means that red blood cells can pass through them. This provides for the filtering functions of the spleen. (See Figure 9–5.)

Affecting Chemicals

Anticoagulants: Thin the blood in patients whose blood tends to clot abnormally, or patients who are at high risk for developing thromboemboli. Patients receiving such treatment are more likely to experience internal hemorrhage or bleeding from small cuts that does not clot in a normal manner. The patient's hematocrit should be monitored.

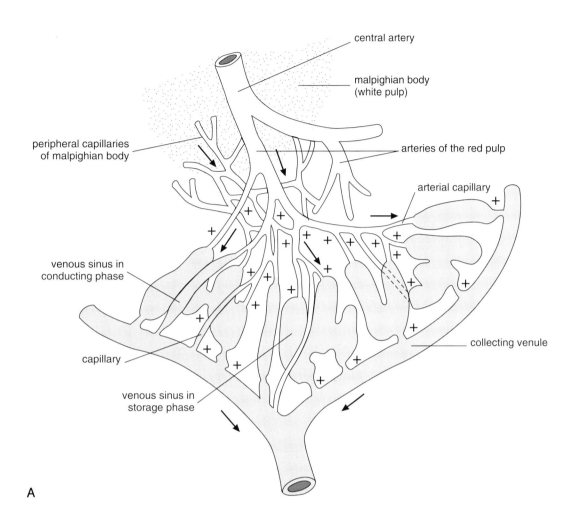

central artery

malpighian body
(white pulp)

peripheral capillaries
of malpighian body

arteries of the red pulp

arterial capillary

venous sinus in
conducting phase

collecting venule

capillary

venous sinus in
storage phase

A

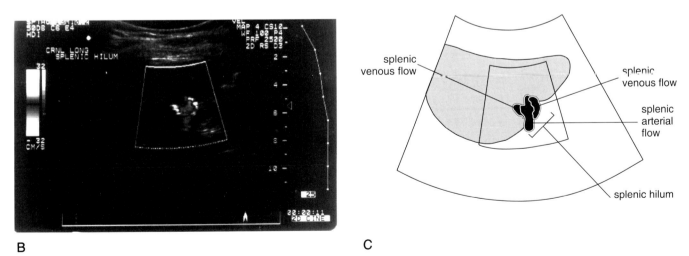

splenic
venous flow

splenic
venous flow

splenic
arterial
flow

splenic hilum

B

C

Figure 9–5. *A,* Vascular anatomy of the spleen. *B,C,* Normal splenic hilum with flow outlined by color Doppler image. (*A,* From Copenhaver WM: Bailey's Textbook of Histology, 16th ed. Baltimore, Williams & Wilkins, 1971, p. 361.)

Chapter 10

THE GASTROINTESTINAL SYSTEM

MARILYN DICKERSON

Objectives:

Differentiate the structures of the gastrointestinal tract.

Describe the functions of the gastrointestinal tract components.

Identify the five principal layers of bowel.

Know the vasculature of the gastrointestinal tract.

Describe the size of the gastrointestinal tract structures.

Describe the location of the gastrointestinal tract components.

Recognize the sonographic appearance of the gastrointestinal tract.

Describe the associated physicians, diagnostic tests, and laboratory values related to the gastrointestinal tract.

Define the key words.

Key Words:

Alimentary canal
Brunner's glands
Cardiac orifice
Cholecystokinin
Duodenal bulb

Foregut
Gastrin
Gastrohepatic ligament
Gastrophrenic ligament
Gastrosplenic ligament
Greater omentum
Gut signature
Haustra
Hepatic flexure
Hindgut
Lesser omentum
Lienorenal ligament
Ligament of Treitz
Meckel's diverticulum
Mediastinum
Mesentery
Mesogastrium
Mesothelium
Midgut
Mucosa
Muscularis
Omental bursa
Rectouterine pouch
Secretin
Serosa
Splenic flexure
Submucosa
Valves of Kerckring (valvulae conniventes)

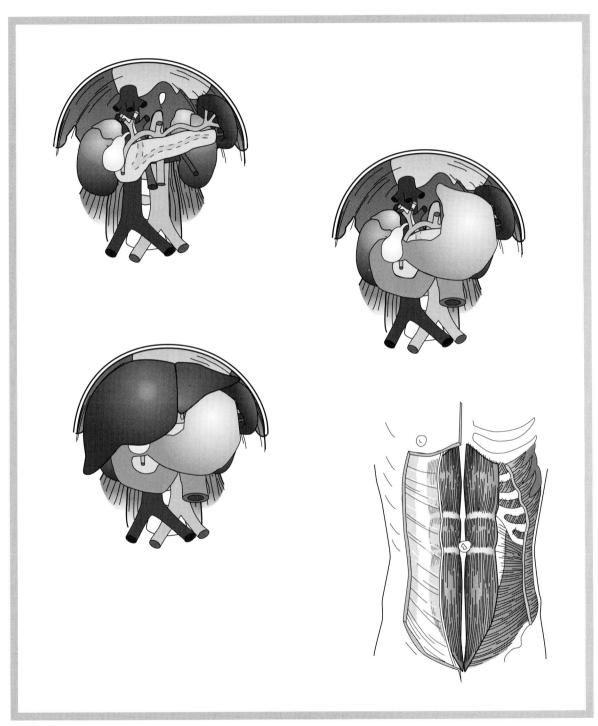

The gastrointestinal tract and surrounding anatomic layers. See Figure 4–3 G, H, I, J, pp. 46–47, for more details.

INTRODUCTION

The gastrointestinal (GI) tract includes the mouth, pharynx, esophagus, stomach, and small and large intestines. It is also known as the **alimentary canal**. (See Figure 10–1.)

The GI tract comprises a major portion of the digestive system. Food is ingested through the mouth and

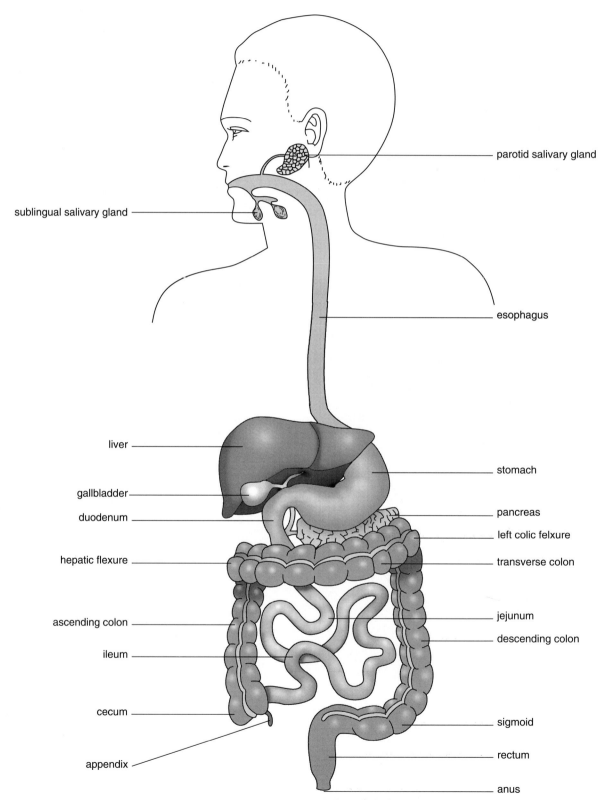

Figure 10–1. The gastrointestinal tract.

chewed. The salivary glands in the mouth release enzymes which initiate the breakdown of the food particles into small digestible molecules. The particles are then conveyed through the pharynx and esophagus to the stomach. In the stomach, food is mixed and the principal chemical changes occur; here food is reduced and converted to solution, stored, and then propelled into the small bowel.

Most of the digestive processes take place in the small bowel. Carbohydrates, proteins, fats, vitamins, and some fluids including water and electrolytes are digested and absorbed in the small bowel. The large bowel absorbs much of the remaining fluid and finally eliminates the undigested products.

PRENATAL DEVELOPMENT

The primitive gut develops from the posterior portion of the yolk sac during the fourth week of embryonic development.[1,2] It is divided into four parts: the foregut, the midgut, the hindgut, and the tailgut.[3]

A portion of the mouth, all of the pharynx, esophagus, stomach, and proximal duodenum originate from the **foregut** and are supplied with blood from the celiac axis artery. The remainder of the duodenum, the small bowel, and the colon as far as the middle and left thirds of the transverse colon originate from the **midgut**. Blood supply to the midgut is from the superior mesenteric artery. The **hindgut** gives rise to the remainder of the colon, supplied with blood from the inferior mesenteric artery. In the adult, these regions retain the same blood supply.[3] The tailgut is resorbed.

The mouth and pharynx develop from the cranial part of the foregut. The tracheoesophageal septum divides the cranial portion of the foregut into the laryngotracheal tube and the esophagus.[2]

The stomach originates as a fusiform dilatation of the caudal portion of the foregut.[2,3] It is suspended from the dorsal wall of the abdominal cavity by the dorsal mesentery and attaches, along with the duodenum, to the developing liver and the ventral abdominal wall by the ventral mesentery.[2] The liver, growing into the ventral mesentery, divides the mesentery into the falciform ligament and the lesser (gastrohepatic) omentum.[3] The dorsal mesentery bulges ventrally as the greater omentum; the spleen appears in its craniolateral portion.[3]

The final position of the stomach is the result of two rotations. The first rotation is 90 degrees around a vertical axis, moving the dorsal **mesogastrium** to the left and creating the **omental bursa** (lesser peritoneal cavity). The second rotation is around an anteroposterior axis, moving the pylorus to the right and superiorly and the proximal portion of the stomach to the left, resulting in the gastric cavity running from superior left to inferior right.[4]

During embryogenesis, the midgut herniates out of and then back into the abdominal cavity. (See Figure 10–2.) While outside, the midgut rotates 270 degrees counterclockwise and then returns to the abdomen. Thus the root of the mesentery becomes fixed, with one end at the ligament of Treitz and the other in the right iliac fossa. The colon returns next; distal bowel first and cecum, last. The colon wraps around the central small bowel and becomes fixed around the edge of the abdomen. This yields a "picture frame" for the small bowel.[5]

The duodenum develops from both the caudal portion of the foregut and the cranial portion of the midgut, forming a c-shaped loop that projects ventrally.[2] The lumen of the duodenum becomes reduced and may be obliterated by epithelial cells.[2] Normally the duodenum recanalizes and the lumen is restored.[3]

The embryonic duodenum is the site of origin of the liver and pancreas, and thus, the excretory ducts of these two organs discharge into the developed structure.[4]

The intestines project into the umbilical cord during

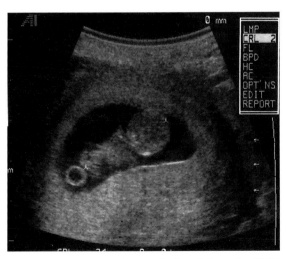
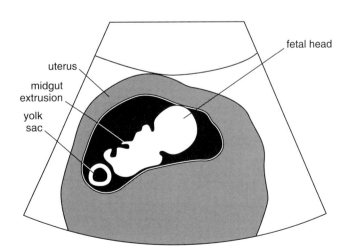

Figure 10–2. A 9-week-old fetus with normal midgut herniation into the cord.

the fifth week of embryonic development and return to the abdomen, coiling, during the tenth week, when the abdominal cavity has enlarged.[1] Peristalsis occurs by the eleventh week, swallowing begins at week 12, and the intestines begin to fill with meconium. By the twentieth week the gastrointestinal tract has reached its normal configuration and relative size.[1]

The anal canal opens during week 7, when a membrane that separates the rectum from the exterior ruptures.[1]

LOCATION

The mouth is placed at the origin of the alimentary canal, bound ventrally by the lips, laterally by the cheeks, anteriorly by the hard and soft palate, and posteriorly by the tongue. It communicates posteroinferiorly with the pharynx.[6]

The pharynx is placed behind the nose, mouth, and larynx. It extends from the undersurface of the skull to the level of the cricoid cartilage in front and to the intervertebral disk between C5 and C6 behind.[6]

Superiorly, the pharynx contacts the body of the sphenoid and basilar process of the occipital bone; inferiorly, it is continuous with the esophagus. Posteriorly, the pharynx is connected with the cervical portion of the vertebral column and the longus colli muscles. Anteriorly, it forms attachments to the lower jaw, the tongue, the hyoid bone, and the thyroid and cricoid cartilages. Laterally, the pharynx is in contact with the common and internal carotid arteries and the internal jugular veins.[6]

The esophagus begins at the level of the cricoid cartilage of the neck, which is the level of the sixth cervical vertebra.[7] The esophagus is a continuation of the pharynx and ends at the stomach, after passing through the left dome of the diaphragm at the T10 level. It courses posterior to the trachea from the C7-T4 vertebral bodies.[8]

As the esophagus continues through the thorax, it courses through the posterior portion of the middle **mediastinum** and is in contact with the aorta and its branches, the tracheobronchial tree, the heart, the lungs, and the interbronchial lymph nodes. Descending below the bifurcation of the trachea, it is in contact with the left atrium (base) of the heart.[8]

The esophagus lies anterior to vertebral bodies C7 through T8. It courses inferiorly to the right of and slightly anterior to the descending aorta to enter the left diaphragmatic dome at T10.

The terminal part of the esophagus lies in a groove on the posterior aspect of the left lobe of the liver.[8] It connects with the cardiac region of the stomach. The entrance of the esophagus into the stomach occurs at the **cardiac or esophageal orifice.** This orifice marks the juncture of the greater and lesser curvatures of the stomach.[9] The orifice is anterior to and slightly to the left of the abdominal aorta.[6] (See Figure 10–3.)

Above and to the left of the esophageal (cardiac) orifice, the fundus of the stomach curves superiorly to the left undersurface of the diaphragm.[6,8]

The stomach lies in the left upper quadrant, within the left hypochondrium and epigastric regions.[6,8,9] Its lower aspect lies on the transpyloric plane as it crosses the midline to reach its terminal point at the duodenum of the small intestine.[8]

The left hemidiaphragm separates the stomach from the pleura of the left lung and the apex of the heart.[8]

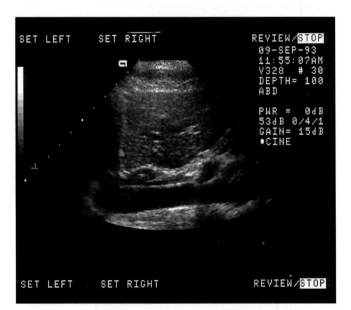

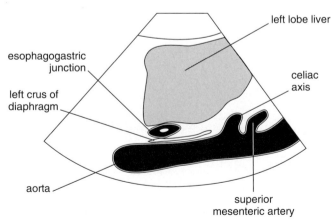

Figure 10–3. Longitudinal section just to the left of the midline, demonstrating the esophagogastric junction posterior to the left lobe of the liver.

The anterior surface of the stomach is in contact with the diaphragm, the thoracic wall formed on the left by the seventh, eighth, and ninth ribs, the left lobe of the liver, and the anterior abdominal wall.[6]

The stomach is suspended within the peritoneal cavity.[9]

The posterior surface of the stomach is related to the diaphragm, the gastric surface of the spleen, the left adrenal gland, the superior portion of the left kidney, the anterior surface of the pancreas, the splenic flexure of the colon, and the ascending layer of the transverse mesocolon. These structures form a shallow bed on which the stomach rests.[5] A small portion of the stomach, proximal to the cardiac orifice and in contact with the diaphragm and left adrenal gland, is not covered by peritoneum.[6]

Posteroinferior to the stomach are the lesser sac, the pancreas, the left adrenal gland, the transverse colon, and the spleen.[8]

The lesser curvature of the stomach marks the right border of the organ, extending between the esophageal (cardiac) and pyloric orifices.[6]

The greater curvature marks the left border, descending in front of the left crus of the diaphragm along the left side of the eleventh and twelfth thoracic vertebrae. This curvature crosses the first lumbar vertebra as it courses to the right and ascends to the pylorus.[6]

The body of the stomach is in contact on the left with the left costal margin and the anterior abdominal wall. Inferiorly, it descends to the midlumbar vertebral level.[8]

The antrum of the pylorus is near the midline and begins as a slight dilatation at the angular incisure in the lesser curvature.[8,9] The antrum ascends, blending into the pyloric canal, which lies on the transpyloric plane between L1 and L2 vertebral bodies.[8]

The pyloric orifice communicates with the duodenum. With the stomach empty, the pylorus is just to the right of the midline at the L1 vertebral level. (See Figure 10–4.) A fully distended stomach may cause the pylorus to become situated 5 to 8 cm to the right of midline.[6]

The small bowel is divided into three portions: duodenum, jejunum, and ileum, is related anteriorly to the greater omentum and the abdominal wall, and is connected to the spine by a fold of peritoneum, the **mesentery**.[6] The small bowel is contained in the central and lower part of the abdominal cavity, and is surrounded superiorly and laterally by the large intestine, partly extending below the pelvic brim anterior to the rectum.[6]

The first portion of the duodenum begins at the pylorus and ends at the neck of the gallbladder,[6] posterior to the left lobe of the liver and medial to the gallbladder.

The **duodenal bulb** (first or superior portion) is peritoneal, supported by the hepatoduodenal ligament, and passes anterior to the common bile duct and the gastroduodenal artery, the common hepatic artery, the hepatic portal vein, and the head of the pancreas.[6,9] (See Figure 10–5.)

The descending duodenum is retroperitoneal and runs posteriorly, parallel and to the right of the spine.[5,6] It extends from the gallbladder neck, at the level of the first lumbar vertebra, to the body of the fourth lumbar vertebra.[6]

The transverse colon crosses anterior to the middle third of the descending duodenum and is connected by a small amount of connective tissue.[6] The head of the pancreas is medial to this portion; lateral to it is the hepatic flexure of the colon.[6] This portion receives the common bile duct via the ampulla of Vater and secondary pancreatic duct (Santorini's duct) if that is present.[6,9]

The transverse (third) portion of the duodenum begins at the right of the fourth lumbar vertebra and passes from right to left, anterior to the great vessels and dia-

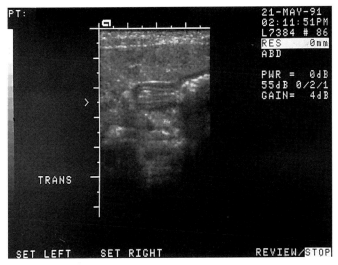

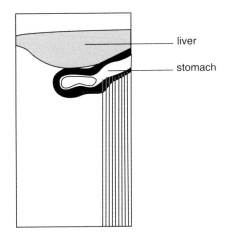

Figure 10–4. Transverse section demonstrating the long axis of the pylorus.

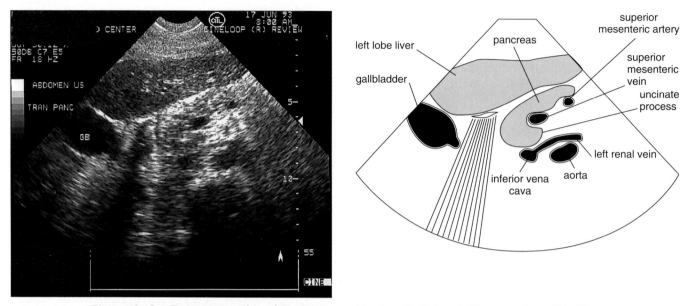

Figure 10-5. Transverse section of the duodenum/duodenal bulb located between the gallbladder and the head of the pancreas.

phragmatic crura, ending in the fourth portion just to the left of the aorta.[6]

The superior mesenteric vessels course anteriorly to the transverse (third) portion of the inferior duodenum.[8,9]

The gallbladder, the right lobe of the liver, and the medial portion of the left lobe of the liver are anterior to the c-shaped duodenum.[8]

The fourth portion ascends superiorly on the left side of the spine and aorta as far as the level of the upper border of the second lumbar vertebra, where it bends ventrally and downward to join the proximal jejunum at the duodenojejunal flexure.[4,6] The ascending portion lies on the left crus of the diaphragm.[4]

The ascending (fourth) portion is held in place by the **suspensory ligament (ligament of Treitz)**, a fibromuscu-

lar band which courses from the left toward the right crus of the diaphragm.[4,9] The bowel leaves its retroperitoneal position and becomes intraperitoneal at the level of the suspensory ligament.[4]

At the duodenojejunal flexure, the jejunum is contained within the peritoneum.[9] The jejunum occupies the umbilical and left iliac regions, while the ileum occupies the umbilical, hypogastric, right iliac, and pelvic regions and terminates in the right iliac fossa by opening into the inner side of the origin of the large intestine.

The large intestine begins in the right inguinal region.[6] The cecum is situated below the iliocecal opening as a blind cul-de-sac.[8] The vermiform appendix opens into the cecum approximately 2 to 3 cm below the opening. (See Figure 10-6.) The ascending colon arises from the right iliac fossa, across the iliac crest, to the visceral

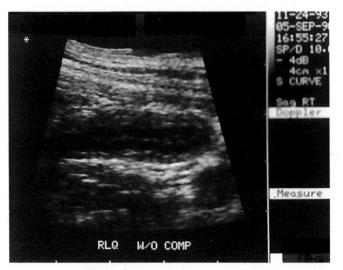

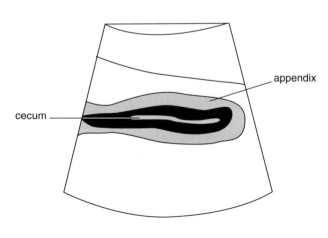

Figure 10-6. Section of normal appendix. The appendix is not usually identified; this was a false positive.

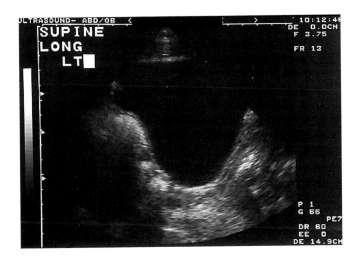

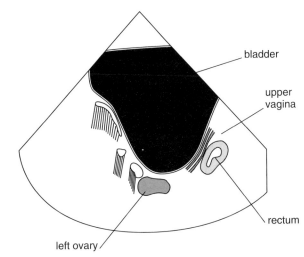

Figure 10–7. Longitudinal section of the rectum in the pelvis.

surface of the right lobe of the liver. It bends at this point (**hepatic or right flexure**) and becomes the transverse colon, which crosses the abdomen anterior to the duodenum and just below the transpyloric plane.[8]

The pancreas is posterosuperior to the transverse colon.[5]

Inferior to the spleen, the colon bends (**splenic flexure**) to descend on the left side of the abdomen into the left iliac fossa and over the pelvic brim, where it becomes the sigmoid colon.[8] The pelvic sigmoid colon reaches the midline anterior to the sacrum, where it becomes the rectum, which then descends into the pelvic cavity to the level of the pelvic floor (diaphragm).[8] (See Figure 10–7.) The rectum penetrates the levator ani muscle to become the anal canal.[10]

At this point the anal canal crosses the pelvic floor and the gastrointestinal tract terminates through the opening of the anus.

SIZE

The pharynx is just under 10 cm in length and is broader in the transverse than in the anteroposterior diameter. The largest portion is opposite the cornua of the hyoid bone; its narrowest portion is at the termination in the esophagus.[6]

The esophagus is a muscular tube approximately 23 cm in length.[6] It is the narrowest part of the alimentary canal, and is most contracted at the origin and at the point where it passes through the diaphragm.[6]

The size of the stomach varies considerably.[6] In the adult male its capacity is 2 to 4 liters. The greatest length of the stomach is from 25 to 30 cm, from the top of the fundus to the bottom of the greater curvature; its widest diameter is 10 to 12 cm. The distance between the two openings ranges from 7 to 15 cm.[6]

The pyloric canal is 2 to 3 cm in length.[9]

The small intestine is approximately 6 m in length and 4 cm in diameter. It decreases in size from the origin to the termination.[6]

The duodenum is the smallest, widest, and most fixed portion of the small intestine, measuring some 25 cm in length.[6,9] It is subdivided into four parts. The superior duodenum (duodenal bulb) is 3 to 5 cm in length, the descending duodenum is approximately 10 cm in length, and the transverse and ascending portions are each 2.5 to 5 cm in length.[9]

The jejunum comprises the upper two fifths of the remaining small intestine or some 2.3 m. Its width is approximately 4 cm.[6] The ileum contains the lower three fifths (3.5 m) of the small bowel and is some 3 cm in diameter.[6]

The large intestine is nearly 2 m in length, largest at the cecum and gradually diminishing in size to the rectum.[6]

GROSS ANATOMY

The gut is a long, hollow tube composed of multiple layers contained within the abdominopelvic cavity and attached by mesentery.[8]

The esophagus is the most muscular structure of the GI tract.[9] Its outer muscular layer is composed of longitudinal fibers; its inner muscle layer has a circular axis.[4]

The arteries which supply the esophagus derive from the inferior thyroid branch of the subclavian artery, the descending thoracic aorta, the gastric branch of the celiac axis, and the left inferior phrenic artery of the abdominal aorta.

The stomach consists of smooth muscle cells arranged in three layers: an outer longitudinal layer, an inner oblique layer, and a circular middle layer. The two outer layers increase in thickness toward the small bowel.[8]

The stomach has three parts: the fundus superiorly, the body (corpus), which is the major portion of the stomach, and the pylorus. The pylorus is subdivided into three regions: the antrum, the pyloric canal, and the pyloric sphincter.[9]

Five ligamentous structures of the mesentery support the stomach. The **greater omentum**, the **gastrophrenic ligament**, the **gastrosplenic ligament**, and the **lienorenal ligament** support the surface of the greater curvature. The lesser curvature is supported by the **gastrohepatic ligament** of the **lesser omentum**.[9]

Arterial flow to the stomach is supplied by the right gastric branch, the pyloric and right gastroepiploic branches of the hepatic artery, the left gastroepiploic branch and vasa brevia from the splenic artery, and the left gastric artery.[6,9]

Veins of the stomach are generally parallel to the arterial vessels and drain into the portal system.[9]

The small intestine, like the esophagus and the large intestine, has a two-layered muscular structure, with the outer layer of cells arranged longitudinally and the inner layer of cells following a circular axis.

The duodenum, the jejunum, and the ileum are the parts of the small intestine.

The duodenum is the c-shaped, most proximal portion of the small bowel and contains four segments: superior, descending, transverse, and ascending.[4]

The first portion of the duodenum is not fixed, whereas the remaining portions of the small bowel are bound to the neighboring viscera and the posterior abdominal wall by the extensive peritoneal fold, the mesentery, which allows for freest motion.[4,6] The fan-shaped mesentery contains blood vessels, nerves, lymphatic glands, and fat between its two layers.[6]

The jejunum is distinguishable from the ileum by the presence of greater vascularity, the presence of **Brunner's (duodenal) glands**, which are similar to the pyloric glands of the stomach, large and thickly set valvulae conniventes, and larger villi.[6] The valvulae conniventes (**valves of Kerckring**) are large folds of mucous membrane which project into the lumen of the bowel and serve to retard the passage of food and provide a greater absorbing area.[11] They begin to appear about 3 to 5 cm beyond the pylorus and almost entirely disappear in the lower part of the ileum.[6] The ileum connects to the large intestine at the ileocecal orifice.[8]

The large intestine is both shorter and larger than the small gut. This large gut contains the vermiform appendix; the cecum; the ascending, transverse, descending, and sigmoid colons; the right and left colic flexures; the rectum; the anal canal; and the anus.[8]

The colon is divided into segments called **haustra**.[8]

The celiac, superior, and inferior mesenteric arteries supply the small and large intestines. The celiac artery, arising off the anterior abdominal aorta, supplies the duodenum from its right gastric, gastroduodenal, and superior pancreaticoduodenal branches.[9] (See Figure 10–8.)

The superior mesenteric artery (SMA) arises from the anterior surface of the abdominal aorta, passes between the head and neck of the pancreas, and supplies branches to the intestines. The SMA branches to the small bowel include the inferior pancreaticoduodenal, the jejunal, and the ileal arteries.[8] (See Figure 10–9.)

The SMA branches to the large intestine include the ileocolic, the right colic, and the middle colic arteries.[8]

The inferior mesenteric artery (IMA) supplies the large intestine from the left border of the transverse colon to the rectum, arising from the anterior surface of the abdominal aorta at the level of the third lumbar vertebra and descending retroperitoneally.[8]

Branches of the IMA include the left colic, the sigmoid, and the superior rectal arteries.[8]

Venous return from the small and large intestines

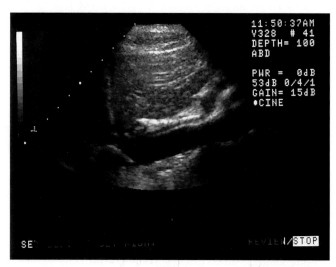
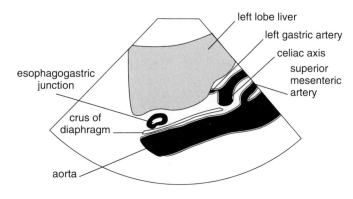

Figure 10–8. Longitudinal section demonstrating the left gastric artery.

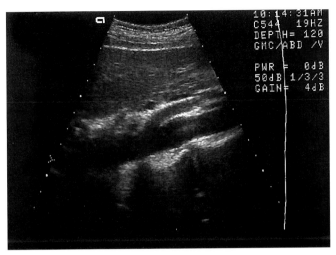
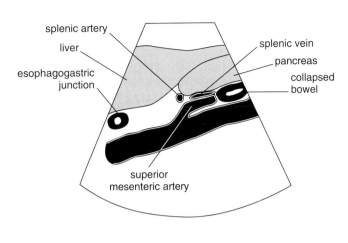

splenic artery
liver
esophagogastric junction
superior mesenteric artery
splenic vein
pancreas
collapsed bowel

Figure 10-9. Longitudinal section of the superior mesenteric artery.

empties into the portal system via vessels that parallel the SMA branches. These channels may drain directly into the portal vein, the splenic vein, and the inferior mesenteric vein or the superior mesenteric vein.[4]

The superior mesenteric vein courses to the right of the SMA and joins the splenic vein to form the portal vein, which enters the liver as its major blood supply.

PHYSIOLOGY

The primary functions of the GI tract are the digestion and absorption of nutrients.

The GI tract is the largest endocrine organ in the body.[12] When food is eaten, nervous activity, distention, and chemical stimulation of the GI tract result in the release of hormones from endocrine cells scattered throughout the mucosa from the stomach to the colon.[12] These hormones influence intestinal absorption and act on the secretion of enzymes, water, and electrolytes. The absorption of water, electrolytes, and nutrients influences the motility and growth of the GI tract.[12]

Several GI hormones are well known. **Gastrin** is an endocrine hormone released from the stomach which stimulates the secretion of gastric acid.[12] **Cholecystokinin** is released by the presence of fat in the intestine and serves to regulate gallbladder contraction and gastric emptying.[12] **Secretin** is released from the small bowel and as "nature's antacid" it stimulates the secretion of bicarbonate, naturally decreasing the acid content of the intestine.[12]

The digestive system breaks down food products—carbohydrates, fats, and proteins—into small, absorbable nutrients.

The GI tract plays a major role in digestion. Food products are reduced to small, absorbable molecules by chemical actions. These actions are initiated by the enzymes present in the juices of the tract.

Food transport and digestion begin in the mouth. The oral cavity, pharynx, and esophagus are coordinated to prepare the food for transport and to transport it to the stomach.[13] The esophagus has two major functions: transport of the food from the mouth to the stomach, and prevention of reflux of the gastrointestinal contents.[14]

The esophagus transports swallowed material from the pharynx to the stomach, using muscular contractions. The lower esophagus acts as a sphincter, controlling the passage of material entering the stomach.[13] Reflux is prevented by closure of the upper and lower esophageal sphincters between swallows.[14]

The stomach performs important functions related to the storage and digestion of food. It holds a large volume of ingested material, thus providing a storage function.

Digestion involves the breakdown, or hydrolysis, of nutrients to smaller molecules so that they can be absorbed or transported across the intestinal cell.[14] Muscles of the stomach contract and mix the material ingested with gastric juice, thereby facilitating the digestive function of the stomach.[15] The stomach contents are then propelled into the duodenum of the small bowel.

The digestion and absorption of all major food products takes place in the small bowel.[16] After the products mix with digestive secretions and enzymes, carbohydrates are reduced to monosaccharides and disaccharides, proteins to peptides and amino acids, and fats to monoglycerides and fatty acids.[14] These nutrients are then absorbed through the intestinal mucosa into the bloodstream. They enter the general circulation via the capillaries into the portal system, or via the lacteals into the intestinal lymphatics.[14] The remaining contents are moved to the large bowel for elimination.

In the large bowel, intestinal material is transformed from a liquid to a semisolid state by the time it reaches the descending and sigmoid colons, as water and electrolytes are absorbed.[17] Most of the absorption process occurs in the cecum.[14] In the sigmoid and rectum, the material is stored and then eliminated.

SONOGRAPHIC APPEARANCE

Visualization of the bowel is impeded by the presence of air or gas within the lumen, which will reflect the sound and thus prevent transmission of the beam. (See Figure 10–10.) The sonographic appearance of bowel is dependent on the presence or absence of air, gas, feces, or fluid within the lumen, and on the recognition of anatomic landmarks.

The layers of the bowel wall create a characteristic appearance on sonography called a **gut signature**, wherein up to five layers can be visualized.[18,19] The first, third, and fifth layers are echogenic, while the second and fourth layers are hypoechoic, with an average total thickness of 3 mm if distended and 5 mm if undistended.[18,19]

Investigators differ as to the histologic structure of the wall layers visible on sonography.[18-22] Pozniac describes the five principal layers as follows: **mucosa** directly contacts the intraluminal contents and is lined with epithelium having many folds, which increase the absorptive surface and give the mucosal layer its high echogenicity. The **submucosa** beneath it contains blood vessels and lymph channels in connective tissue. The third layer, **muscularis**, contains the circular and longitudinal bands of fiber. The **serosa** is a thin, loose layer of connective tissue, surrounded by the outermost single cell layer of **mesothelium** covering the intraperitoneal bowel loops.[20]

The esophagus is normally recognized at the esophagogastric (EG) junction on a longitudinal scan of the aorta, just to the left of the midline. (See Figure 10–11.) It appears as a target lesion, surrounded by the crura of the diaphragm and anterior to the aorta along the posterior aspect of the left lobe of the liver. The normal esophageal wall measures 5 mm.[7] In the neck, it may be seen

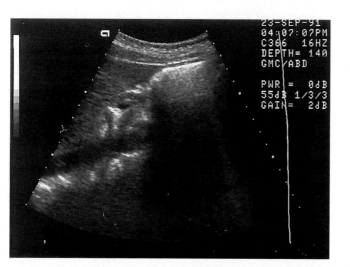
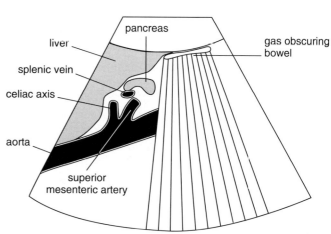

Figure 10–10. Longitudinal section of the abdominal aorta obscured by overlying gas-filled bowel.

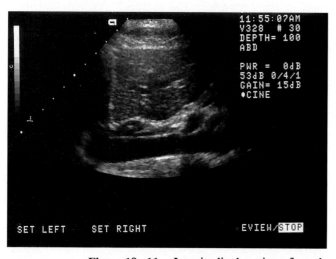
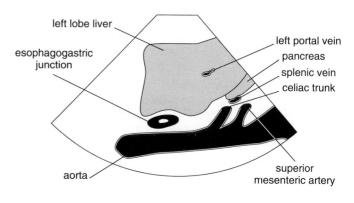

Figure 10–11. Longitudinal section of esophagogastric junction anterior to the abdominal aorta.

posterior to the thyroid gland on the left and is usually recognized by its bull's-eye appearance.[23] (See Figure 10–12.)

Empty loops of bowel also demonstrate the target (bull's-eye) pattern: a thin, hypoechoic sonolucent periphery with an echogenic center of varying size.[24]

The stomach can usually be identified by its characteristic location between the free edge of the left lobe of the liver and the anterior surface of the spleen.[24]

Separation of the fundus of the stomach and the left hemidiaphragm suggests a pathologic process in the subphrenic space, such as an abscess.[5]

The collapsed antrum of the stomach lies anterior to the pancreas.[25] (See Figure 10–13.)

A large mass in the pancreas will displace the stomach anteriorly and perhaps superiorly.[5] Posterior displacement of the stomach is most probably caused by an enlarged left lobe of the liver, since this lobe is the only

structure anterior to the stomach. Splenic enlargement tends to displace the stomach medially.[5]

A fluid-filled stomach may simulate a cystic mass such as a pseudocyst in the left upper quadrant.[24] (See Figure 10–14.) Sonographic visualization of peristalsis helps to identify bowel and thus differentiate it from cystic masses.

The duodenal bulb is related to the gallbladder and the transverse colon near the hepatic flexure. It is lateral to the head of the pancreas. The duodenum, the gallbladder, and the proper vascular landmarks form a triad that helps to localize the head of the pancreas.[25] Gas in the duodenum, however, may mimic mass lesions or pseudomasses in the pancreas, or a stone-filled gallbladder.[25] (See Figure 10–15.)

A distended gallbladder will indent the superolateral aspect of the duodenal bulb and the descending duodenum.[5]

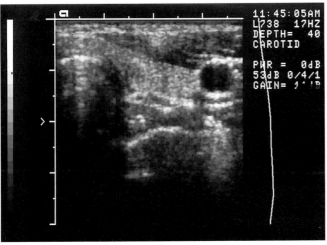
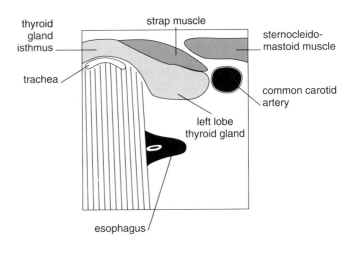

Figure 10–12. Transverse section of the esophagus posterior to the left lobe of the thyroid gland.

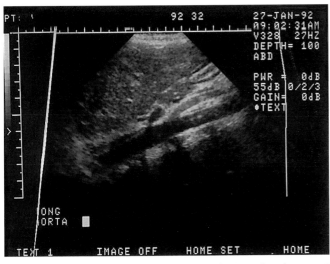
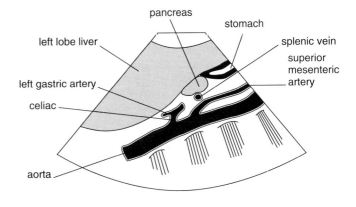

Figure 10–13. Longitudinal section just to the left of the midline, demonstrating the collapsed stomach antrum anteroinferior to the pancreas.

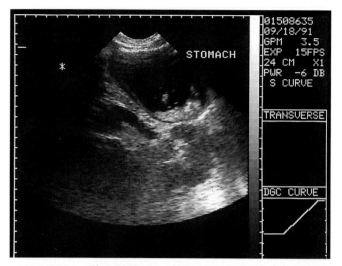
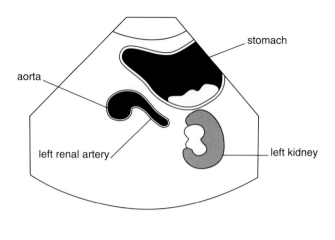

Figure 10-14. Transverse section of a fluid-filled stomach visualized anterior to the left kidney.

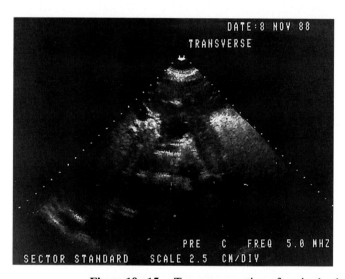
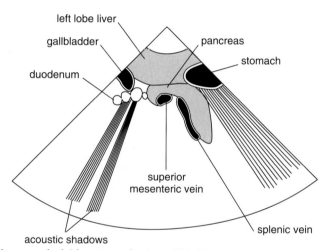

Figure 10-15. Transverse section of gas in the duodenum mimicking stones in the gallbladder or a pseudomass in the head of the pancreas.

The proximal portion of the jejunum is inferior to the body and tail of the pancreas and anterior to the left kidney. (See Figure 10-16.)

The cecum is medial to the anterior superior iliac spine, and anterior to the iliopsoas muscle.

The vermiform appendix is usually posterior to the cecum, though it may project over the pelvic brim.[26]

The ascending colon is anterolateral to the lower pole of the right kidney. It ascends along the right paracolic gutter to the liver, where it passes anteriorly to the kidney and the descending duodenum as it courses left to form the hepatic flexure.[27]

The collapsed transverse colon may be seen, on longitudinal scans, inferior to the plane of the pancreas and stomach.[23] (See Figure 10-17.) It lies beneath the anterior abdominal wall, throughout its course, and passes anterior to the left kidney as it courses caudally to form the splenic flexure.[27]

The right colic flexure is inferior to the right lobe of the liver and at a lower level than the left colic flexure, which is inferior to the spleen.[25] The right colic (hepatic) flexure may produce artifacts simulating gallbladder disease if it is gas filled, while the left colic (splenic) flexure may mimic the left kidney.[23]

The descending colon is posterior and extends from the splenic flexure to the sigmoid, adjacent to the left flank.[27]

The sigmoid colon is anterior to the external iliac vessels and the sacrum. In females, it is posterior to the posterior surface of the uterus and the upper part of the vagina, and in males, posterior to the urinary bladder.[9] (See Figure 10-18.)

The rectum is posterior to the lower uterine segment and the vagina in the female, with the peritoneum over its anterior surface extending to the uterine surface. This forms the **rectouterine pouch**, the pouch of Douglas (pos-

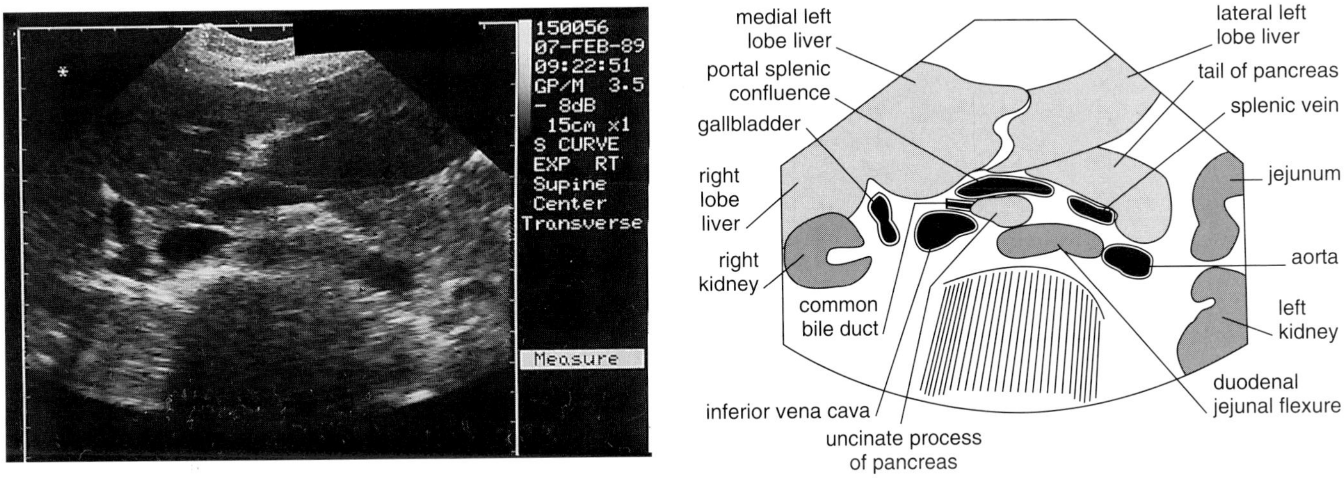

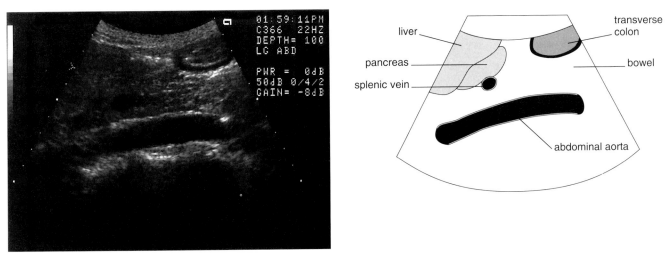

Figure 10–16. Transverse section demonstrating the region of the duodenojejunal flexure posterior to the uncinate process of the pancreas. The jejunum is that portion of small bowel located anterior to the left kidney.

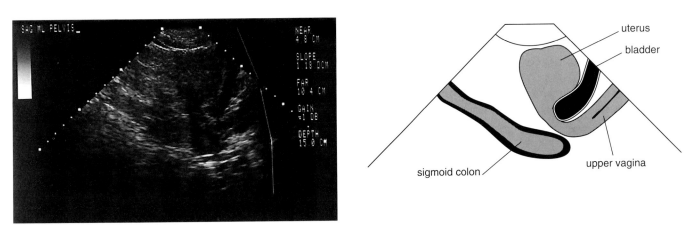

Figure 10–17. Compressed transverse colon noted on a longitudinal section. The transverse colon is seen inferior to the plane of the pancreas and stomach and anterior to the abdominal aorta.

Figure 10–18. Sigmoid colon, superior and posterior to the uterus and the upper vagina.

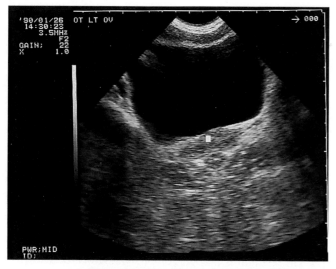 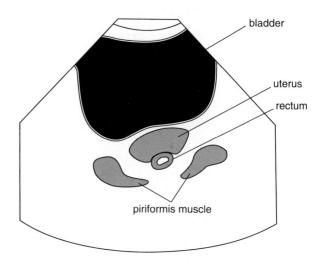

Figure 10–19. Transverse section of rectum posterior to the uterus and anterior to the piriformis muscle.

terior cul-de-sac).[10] It is posterior to the prostate gland, the seminal vesicles, and the bladder in the male, and anterior to the levator ani muscles in both the male and female pelvis. (See Figure 10–19.)

SONOGRAPHIC APPLICATIONS

Ultrasound helps to narrow the differential diagnosis of bowel disorders by visualization of the bowel wall and its layers.[20]

Thickening of the bowel wall occurs with infiltration, inflammation, edema, or neoplastic invasion,[18–20,24] thus allowing for sonographic recognition of the pathologic process. Causes of wall thickening include pyloric stenosis, hematoma, intussusception, tumor, appendicitis, and edema.[5,18–20,24]

Inflammation causes ulceration of bowel. Deep or submucosal inflammation such as that found in Crohn's disease causes thickening of the bowel wall.[5]

With serosal inflammation, the inflammatory mass may indent or displace the bowel. Appendicitis is an inflammatory process which exerts such an effect on the cecum.[5]

Normal bowel loops demonstrate peristalsis and are compressible; an inflamed appendix does not exhibit peristalsis and is not compressed.[28] The normal appendix is rarely visualized, except occasionally in a thin

patient or when it is surrounded by ascites.[29] Appendicoliths and periappendiceal abscesses can also be visualized.[29]

Bowel becomes dilated when it is obstructed and when ileus occurs. Ileus causes paralysis of bowel loops. Peristalsis is absent in the affected loop or loops of bowel, which results in gas accumulating in the paralyzed loop. Localized ileus commonly occurs near an inflammatory process.[5]

If bowel becomes obstructed, gas does not pass through the GI tract, and builds up proximal to the obstructed loop. The portion of bowel distal to the obstruction becomes decompressed.[5]

Doppler imaging can be used to assess malrotation of the bowel, which is frequently associated with malposition of the superior mesenteric artery and vein, and the detection of varices as well as the determination of directional flow within them.[30]

Endosonography is useful in evaluating the esophagus, the stomach, and the rectum.

The normal thickness of the esophageal wall is approximately 3 mm as five identifiable layers.[21] (See Figures 10–20 and 10–21.)

Esophageal and gastric lesions assessed with endosonography include varices, typically located in the EG junction, intramural tumors, and peptic ulcers, which typically demonstrate thickening of all the gut wall layers.[19]

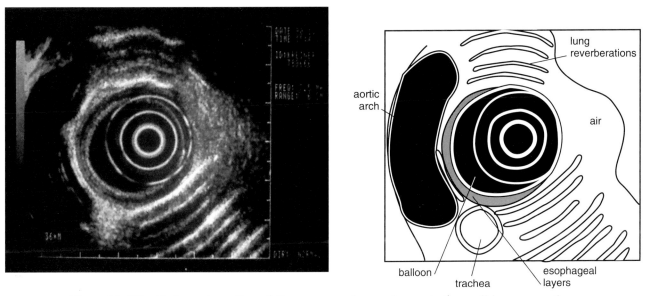

Figure 10–20. Endoscopic section of the upper esophagus, demonstrating wall layer separation. (Photo courtesy of Wui Chong, M.D., Vanderbilt Medical Center.)

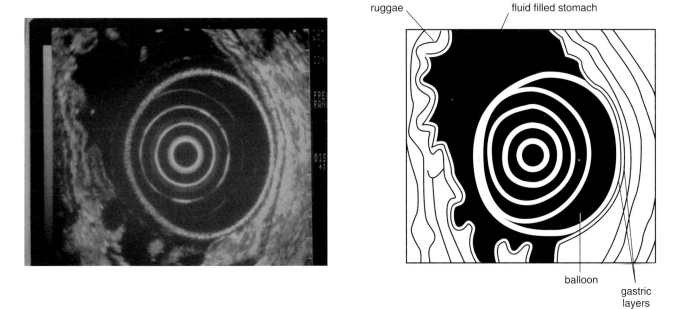

Figure 10–21. Endoscopic section of stomach demonstrating five identifiable wall layers. (Photo courtesy of Wui Chong, M.D., Vanderbilt Medical Center.)

Endoscopic sonography can also depict direct extension of gastrointestinal malignancies into adjacent soft tissues, and perivisceral adenopathy.[29]

Transrectal endosonography is typically used to identify and stage previously detected cancer.[19] Endorectal ultrasound is considered at least as accurate as CT for the preoperative staging of rectal carcinoma.[29]

NORMAL VARIANTS

Two to three percent of the population have **Meckel's diverticulum**—the remains of the prenatal yolk stalk (vitelline duct), projecting from the side of the ileum.[9,27] The diverticulum measures between 5 and 25 cm in length and is attached by a peritoneal fold.[27]

REFERENCE CHARTS

Associated Physicians

Gastroenterologist: Specializes in treating diseases of the gastrointestinal tract, including the stomach, small and large bowel, the gallbladder, and bile ducts.

Internist: Specializes in studying the physiology and pathology of internal organs and diagnosing and treating disorders of those organs.

Oncologist: Specializes in the study and treatment of tumors and malignancies.

Pediatrician: Specializes in guiding the development of children. They are concerned with the prevention and treatment of childhood diseases.

Surgeon: Utilizes operative procedures to treat diseases, trauma, and organ deformity.

Proctologist: Treats disorders of the colon, rectum, and anus.

Otolaryngologist: Specializes in the diagnosis and treatment of diseases and injuries of the ears, nose, and throat.

Radiologist: Specializes in performing and interpreting radiologic diagnostic studies of the gasrointestinal tract.

Common Diagnostic Tests

Examination	Use
ABDOMINAL PLAIN FILM	Bowel gas
	Intestinal obstruction
	Carcinoma
	Appendicolith
	Volvulus

This radiograph is used to evaluate bones and soft tissue densities of the intra-abdominal contents. Fluid-filled loops of bowel may be seen as tubular densities. Bowel gas patterns are evaluated and compared with normal gas patterns. Identification of the air-filled stomach, portions of the small intestine, and portions of the colon is possible. The examination is performed by a radiologic technologist and interpreted by a radiologist.

Examination	Use
UPPER GI SERIES	Hernia
	Strictures
	Obstruction
	Inflammation
	Carcinoma
	Lesions
	Reflux
	Diverticula
	Ulcer disease
	Neoplasms
	Gastritis
	Focal dilatation
	Edema
	Wall thickening

The upper GI series is a set of fluoroscopic and radiographic examinations used to evaluate the GI tract from the esophagus to the small bowel. Fluoroscopy permits observation of real time motion of the tract. Contrast media are used to increase the density of the GI tract so that the anatomy and mucosal detail are visualized. Barium sulfate is most commonly used for these procedures. An iodinated contrast medium is another preparation used to opacify the tract for optimum visualization. Compression and palpation are techniques used by radiologists who perform and interpret the fluoroscopic examinations. Radiologic technologists assist the physician by adjusting the equipment controls, maintaining adequate film supplies, preparing media, and providing patient care and positioning.

These examinations include the following: barium swallow and small-bowel follow-through.

Examination	Use
UPPER GI ENDOSCOPY	Biopsy
	Localized bleeding
	Dye injection
	Polyp removal
	Stent placement
	Ulcer follow-up
	Obstruction
	Hemorrhage control

Upper GI endoscopy is used for diagnostic and therapeutic indications. Following appropriate patient preparation, the endoscope is placed in the throat of the sedated patient. It must be swallowed. The scope is guided through the esophagus and into the stomach and duodenum and provides direct visualization of the upper GI tract. Photography, cytology, and biopsy sampling supplement the procedure, which is usually performed and interpreted by a gastroenterologist.

Examination	Use
BARIUM ENEMA	Obstruction
	Tumors
	Inflammation

Similar to the upper GI series, this examination involves the study of the colon. Single or double contrast media are used in the fluoroscopic procedure. Barium sulfate is infused into the cleaned rectum and x-ray studies are performed. The procedure is also used therapeutically in children with nonstrangulated intussusception. A radiologist performs and interprets the examination. A radiologic technologist assists the physician.

Examination	Use
COLONOSCOPY	Polyp removal
SIGMOIDOSCOPY	Bleeding
ANOSCOPY	Lesion evaluation
	Inflammatory bowel

These procedures are done to further evaluate an abnormality previously identified by barium enema. For the colonoscopy, the sedated patient is given a rectal examination, followed by insertion of the colonoscope. Air is infused into the anus and the instrument is moved through the colon to the cecum and terminal ileum. The diagnostic evaluation involves structure visualization, photography, and biopsy or lesion removal. The procedures are similar in sigmoidoscopy, in which the sigmoid colon and rectum are examined, and anoscopy, in which the perianal region and the distal rectum are examined, utilizing smaller probes. The procedures are performed and interpreted by gastroenterologists.

Laboratory Values

WB	—	Whole blood
P	—	Plasma
S	—	Serum
U	—	Urine
A	—	Arterial
V	—	Venous

Test	Normal	Increase	Decrease
CO_2	A:19–24 mM		Severe diarrhea
	V:22–26 mM		
Carcinoembryonic antigen (CEA) (P)	0–25 mg/ml	Inflammatory bowel disease	
Cholesterol (S)			
Total	150–250 mg/dl		Cancer, fat malabsorption
HDL cholesterol (P)	29–77 mg/dl		
LDL cholesterol (P)	62–185 mg/dl		
VLDL cholesterol (P)	0–40 mg/dl		
Lipids (S)			
Total	400–800 mg/dl		Fat malabsorption
Cholesterol	150–250 mg/dl		
Triglycerides	10–190 mg/dl		
Phospholipids	150–380 mg/dl		
Fatty acids	9.0–15.0 mM/l		
Chloride (CL^-)(U)	110–254 mEq/24 hr		Polyoric obstruction, diarrhea
Potassium (K^+)(U)	25–100 mEq/l		Diarrhea, malabsorption
Sodium (NA^+)(U)	75–200 mg/24 hr		Diarrhea

Normal Measurements

Nonapplicable.

Vasculature

ARTERIAL SYSTEM

Vessel	Branch of	Supplies
Esophageal artery	Descending thoracic aorta	Esophagus
Inferior thyroid esophageal branch	Subclavian artery	Esophagus
Left inferior phrenic esophageal branch	Abdominal aorta	Esophagus
Left gastric artery	Celiac artery	Stomach
Esophagus		
Right gastric artery	Hepatic artery	Stomach, duodenum
Short gastric arteries (vasa brevia)	Splenic artery	Stomach
Gastroduodenal artery	Hepatic artery	Stomach, duodenum
Supraduodenal artery	Gastroduodenal artery	Duodenum
Right gastroepiploic artery	Gastroduodenal artery	Stomach, greater omentum
Left gastroepiploic artery	Splenic artery	Stomach, omentum
Superior pancreaticoduodenal artery	Gastroduodenal artery	Pancreas, duodenum
Inferior pancreaticoduodenal artery	Superior mesenteric artery	Pancreas, duodenum
Superior mesenteric artery	Abdominal aorta	Midgut
Inferior mesenteric artery	Abdominal aorta	Hindgut
Right colic artery	Superior mesenteric	Large intestine
Middle colic artery	Superior mesenteric	Transverse colon
Ileocolic artery	Superior mesenteric	Cecum, ASCD., Colon, ileum Appendix
Left colic artery	Inferior mesenteric	DESC. Colon
Sigmoid artery	Inferior mesenteric	Sigmoid colon
Hemorrhoidal artery	Inferior mesenteric	Rectum, anal canal, anus
Superior rectal artery	Inferior mesenteric	Rectum

VENOUS SYSTEM

Vessel	Tributary to	Drains
Esophageal vein	Azygos	Esophagus
Left gastric vein	Splenic vein	Stomach, esophagus
Right gastric vein	Portal vein	Stomach
Superior mesenteric vein	Portal vein	Midgut
Inferior mesenteric vein	Splenic vein	Hindgut
Portal vein	Liver	GI tract
Left gastroepiploic vein	Splenic vein	Stomach, omentum
Right gastroepiploic vein	Superior mesenteric vein	Stomach, pancreas
Pancreaticoduodenal vein	Splenic vein	Pancreas, duodenum
Ileocolic vein	Superior mesenteric vein	Intestine
Right colic vein	Superior mesenteric vein	Colon
Middle colic vein	Superior mesenteric vein	Colon
Left colic vein	Inferior mesenteric vein	Sigmoid
Superior hemorrhoidal veins	Inferior mesenteric vein	Rectum, anal canal, anus
Superior rectal veins	Inferior mesenteric vein	Rectum

Affecting Chemicals

Nonapplicable.

References

1. Guyton AC: Textbook of Medical Physiology, 8th ed. Philadelphia, WB Saunders, 1991.
2. Moore KL: The Developing Human: Clinically Oriented Embryology, 4th ed. Philadelphia, WB Saunders, 1988.
3. Monie I: Embryology. In Margulis AR, Burhenne HJ (eds.). Alimentary Tract Radiology, vol. 1. St. Louis, CV Mosby, 1989, 215–230.
4. Linder HH: Clinical Anatomy. Norwalk, CT, Appleton & Lange, 1989.
5. Jones B, Braver JM: Essentials of Gastrointestinal Radiology. Philadelphia, WB Saunders, 1982.
6. Gray H: Anatomy, Descriptive and Surgical, 15th ed. New York, Crown Publishers, 1977.
7. Torres WE: Radiology of the Esophagus. In Gedgaudas-McClees (ed.). Handbook of Gastrointestinal Imaging. New York, Churchill Livingstone, 1987.
8. Basmajian JV, Slonecker CE: Grant's method of Anatomy, 11th ed. Baltimore, Williams & Wilkins, 1989.
9. April EW: Anatomy. Media, PA, Harwall, 1984.
10. Applegate EJ: The Sectional Anatomy Learning System: Concepts. Philadelphia, WB Saunders, 1991.
11. Thomas CL: Taber's Cyclopedic Medical Dictionary, 13th ed. Philadelphia, FA Davis, 1977.
12. Johnson LR: Gastrointestinal Hormones. In Johnson LR (ed.). Gastrointestinal Physiology. St. Louis, CV Mosby, 1977, 1–11.
13. Weisbrodt NW: Esophageal Motility. In Johnson LR (ed.). Gastrointestinal Physiology. St. Louis, CV Mosby, 1977, 12–19.
14. Greenberger NJ, Isselbacher KJ: Disorders of Absorption. In Braunwald E, Isselbacher KJ, et al. (eds.). Harrison's Principles of Internal Medicine. New York, McGraw-Hill, 1987, 1260–1276.
15. Weisbrodt NW: Gastric Motility. In Johnson, LR (ed.). Gastrointestinal Physiology. St. Louis, CV Mosby, 1977, 20–27.
16. Castro GA: Principles of Digestion and Absorption. In Johnson LR (ed.). Gastrointestinal Physiology. St. Louis, CV Mosby, 1977, 95–108.
17. Weisbrodt NW: Motility of the Large Intestine. In Johnson LR (ed.). Gastrointestinal Physiology. St. Louis, CV Mosby, 1977, 35–41.
18. Wilson SR: The Gastrointestinal Tract. In Rumack CM, Wilson SR, Charboneau JW (eds.). Diagnostic Ultrasound, vol 2. St. Louis, Mosby Year Book, 1991, 181–207.
19. Wilson SR: Ultrasonography of the gastrointestinal tract. In Rifkin MD (ed.). Syllabus: Special Course Ultrasound 1991. Oak Brook, IL, Radiological Society of North America, Inc., 1991, 307–318.
20. Pozniac MA, Scanlon K, Yandow, D: Ultrasound in the evaluation of bowel disorders. Semin Ultrasound, CT, MR 8:366–384, 1987.
21. Botet JF, Lightdale C: Endoscopic sonography of the upper gastrointestinal tract. Am J Radiol 156:63–68, 1991.
22. Rifkin MD: Endorectal ultrasound of the rectal wall. Semin Ultrasound, CT, MR 8:424–431, 1987.
23. Ngo C, Sarti DA: Simulation of the normal esophagus by a parathyroid adenoma. J Clin Ultrasound 15:421–424, 1987.
24. Gooding GAW, Filly RA, Laing FC: Ultrasound of the Alimentary Tube. In Margulis AR, Burhenne HJ (eds.). Alimentary Tract Radiology, vol. 1. St. Louis, CV Mosby, 1989, 197–214.
25. Sarti DA: Diagnostic Ultrasound Text and Cases, 2nd ed. Chicago, Year Book, 1987.
26. Agur AMR: Grant's Atlas of Anatomy, 9th ed. Baltimore, Williams & Wilkins, 1991.
27. Janower ML: The Colon: Anatomy and Examination Techniques. In Tavares JM, Ferruchi JT (eds.). Radiology: Diagnosis-Imaging-Intervention, vol. 4. Philadelphia, JB Lippincott, 1988, 1–7.
28. Laing FC: Ultrasonography of the acute abdomen. Radiol Clin North Am 30:389–404, 1992.
29. Carroll BA: Ultrasonography of the gastrointestinal tract. Radiology 172:605–608, 1989.
30. Fernbach SK, Feinstein KA: Selected topics in pediatric ultrasonography–1992. Radiol Clin North Am 30:1011–1031, 1992.

Chapter 11

THE ABDOMINAL AORTA

JERRY PEARSON

Objectives:

Discuss the embryologic development of the aorta and its major branches.

Describe the normal location, course, and size of the aorta.

Describe the layers (gross anatomy) of an artery.

Describe the location of the aortic branches and the organs supplied by those branches.

Discuss the function of the aorta.

Describe the sonographic appearance of the aorta and its branches.

Describe the associated laboratory values and diagnostic tests

Define the key words.

Key Words:

Aorta	Common iliac
Celiac artery	arteries
Common hepatic artery	Gastroduodenal artery

Gonadal arteries	Splenic artery
Inferior mesenteric artery	Superior mesenteric artery
Left gastric artery	Suprarenal artery
Proper hepatic artery	Tunica media
Renal artery	

INTRODUCTION

Although all body vessels are important, the **aorta** is especially vital because the blood flowing to the abdominal organs and lower extremities must pass through at least some part of this vessel in order to reach its destination. Thus, because of the large volume of blood which it transports, the aorta is considered one of the two great vessels of the abdomen.

PRENATAL DEVELOPMENT

The cardiovascular system is the first system to begin to function in the embryo.[1,2] This is necessary to provide

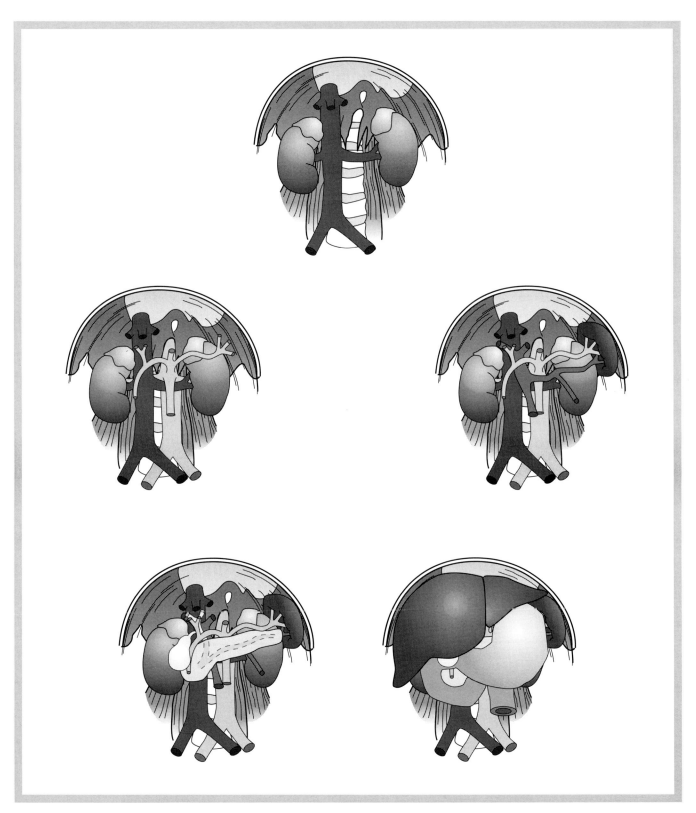

The abdominal aorta and surrounding anatomic layers. See Figure 4–3 C, D, E, G, I, pp. 44–47, for more details.

an adequate supply of nutrients and oxygen to the other body systems as they develop. The vascular portion of the cardiovascular system develops from mesodermal cells, the angioblasts, during the third week. At this time, all vessels are composed of endothelium; thus, the location of vessels in relation to the heart determines which vessels are arteries and which vessels are veins. During the third week, there are two dorsal aortas which are extensions of the two endocardial heart tubes. (See Figure 11–1.) The aortas quickly fuse into a single vessel after this period.[1,2]

The single aorta has several branches. Numerous intersegmental arteries branch posteriorly and feed the embryo. Eventually many of these arteries become the lumbar arteries. (See Figure 11–1.) In addition, the common iliac arteries and the median sacral artery develop from intersegmental arteries. The vitelline artery complex branches anteriorly from the aorta and extends into the yolk sac. The celiac artery, superior mesenteric artery, and inferior mesenteric artery develop from this complex.[1] The umbilical arteries branch off the inferior aspect of the anterior aorta and return the deoxygenated blood to the placenta. The umbilical arteries eventually give rise to the internal iliac arteries and superior vesical artery.[1] The majority of the remaining vessels develop from the primitive vascular network by forming chan-nels connecting the organ systems to existing capillaries and vessels.

LOCATION

The aorta is a retroperitoneal structure coursing in a superior-to-inferior direction along the left side of the spine. This tubular structure originates from the heart at the left ventricular outflow tract and follows a candy-cane-shaped loop down into the thoracic cavity. This portion, considered the thoracic aorta, is not visualized when an abdominal sonogram is performed. After the aorta passes posteriorly to the diaphragm at the aortic hiatus on the posterior superior portion of the diaphragm, it is termed the abdominal aorta. It continues to course inferiorly giving off several branches, many of which can be visualized by sonography. The abdominal aorta bifurcates into the **common iliac arteries** slightly to the left of the umbilicus. (See Figure 11–2.) The aorta is lateral and to the left of the spinal column. It is posterior to the left lobe of the liver, body of the pancreas, pylorus of the stomach, splenic artery, splenic vein, and left renal vein. It is anterior to the musculature of the back.

The abdominal aorta (AO) has many branches. (See Figures 11–3 and 11–4.) There is considerable variation

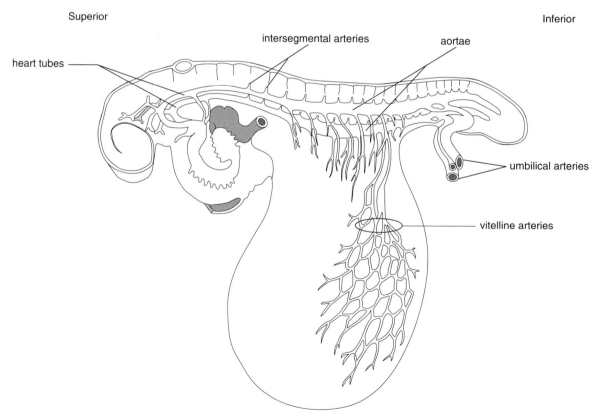

Figure 11–1. Representation of aortic development at approximately the third embryologic week.

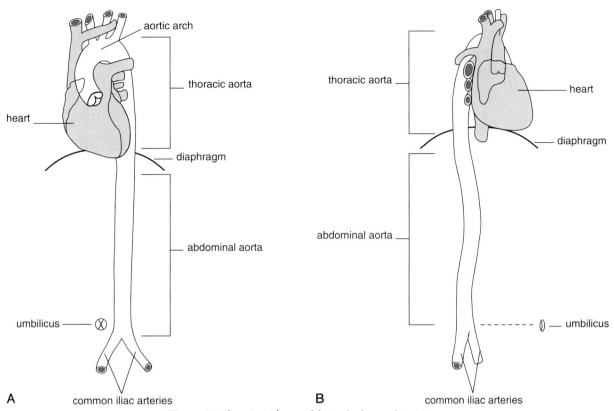

Figure 11-2. Anterior and lateral views of the aorta.

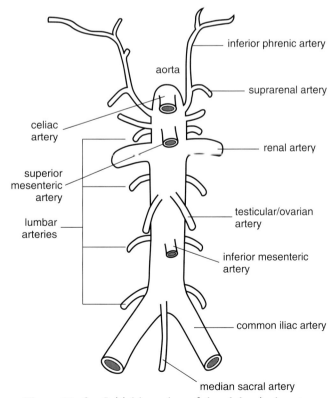

Figure 11-3. Initial branches of the abdominal aorta.

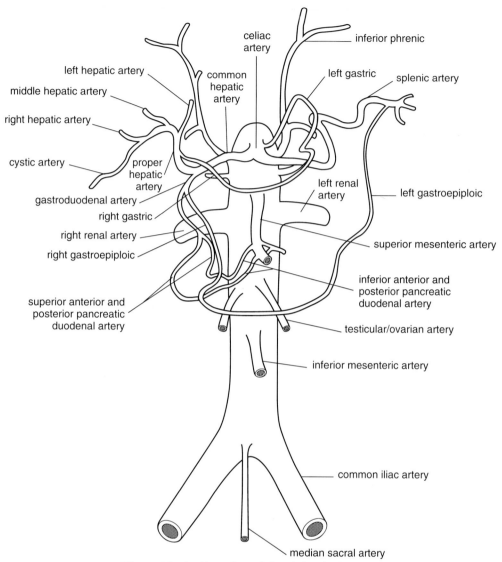

Figure 11–4. Branches of the abdominal aorta.

in the origin and course of these vessels; therefore, only the most common configurations will be discussed.

Directly after the aorta passes posteriorly to the diaphragm, the inferior phrenic arteries branch off the anterior-lateral aspect of the aorta and course superiorly to supply the underside of the diaphragm. At approximately the same level, the celiac trunk (also known as the **celiac artery** or celiac axis) branches anteriorly from the aorta. The celiac artery (CA), often measuring less than 1 cm, further branches into the left gastric (LGA), splenic (SPA), and common hepatic arteries (CHA). The **left gastric artery** courses superiorly and to the left. It doubles back to supply the left side of the lesser curvature of the stomach and eventually anastomoses with the right gastric artery. The **splenic artery** supplies the spleen, pancreas, and left side of the greater curvature of

the stomach as it courses horizontally to the left with a slight inferior-to-superior angulation. The pancreas is supplied primarily via the main, dorsal, caudal, and great pancreatic arteries, which branch from the splenic artery. The left side of the greater curvature of the stomach is supplied by the left gastroepiploic artery, which branches from the distal end of the splenic artery. The **common hepatic artery** pursues a horizontal course to the right and branches into the gastroduodenal (GDA) and proper hepatic artery (PHA). The **gastroduodenal artery** courses inferiorly, supplying the right side of the greater curvature of the stomach via the right gastroepiploic artery and the pancreatic duodenal area via the superior-anterior and superior-posterior pancreatic duodenal arteries. The **proper hepatic artery** courses superiorly, supplying the liver via the right, middle, and left hepatic arteries.

The cystic artery feeds the gallbladder after it branches from the right hepatic artery. The right gastric artery, which supplies the right side of the lesser curvature of the stomach, commonly originates from either the gastro-duodenal, common hepatic, or proper hepatic artery. One can easily realize the celiac axis and its branches are of extreme importance in supplying the majority of the abdominal organs, the stomach, and the duodeum.

The origin of the next most inferiorly located branch of the aorta varies. The **suprarenal arteries** commonly originate from the level of the celiac axis to the level of the superior mesenteric artery, which is located a few centimeters inferior to the celiac axis. The suprarenal arteries, also termed the adrenal arteries, originate bilaterally from the lateral aspect of the aorta and course horizontally to the adrenal glands.

Moving inferiorly, the **superior mesenteric artery** (SMA) branches from the anterior aspect of the aorta within centimeters of the celiac axis. The SMA continues an anterior-inferior course and divides into several arteries which supply the largest portion of the small intestine as well as the ascending colon and part of the transverse colon. In addition, the inferior-anterior pancreatic duodenal artery and the inferior-posterior pancreatic duodenal artery originate from the SMA and feed the pancreatic head and duodenal area. Within a few centimeters of the origin of the SMA, the **right and left renal arteries** branch from the lateral aspect of the aorta. Both arteries course horizontally and supply the kidneys; however, the right renal artery (RRA) has a longer course than the left renal artery (LRA) because the aorta sits on the left side which forces the RRA to travel a greater distance. In addition, it should be noted that the RRA normally courses posteriorly to the inferior vena cava (IVC) to reach the right kidney.

Inferior to the superior mesenteric artery and renal arteries, the **gonadal arteries** originate from the anterior aspect of the aorta and course inferiorly to their respective organs. The left artery often originates slightly superiorly to the right artery. The male gonadal arteries are termed the testicular arteries, and the female gonadal arteries are termed the ovarian arteries.

The **inferior mesenteric artery** (IMA) is the next major artery that branches from the aorta. It originates from the anterior aspect of the aorta and pursues the anterior-inferior course dividing into several other smaller arteries supplying the transverse colon, descending colon, and rectum.

The median sacral artery supplies the sacrum and is the most inferior branch of the aorta; however, the aorta does bifurcate at this point into the **common iliac arteries**, which, along with their branches, supply the pelvis and lower extremities. One should also note that lumbar arteries originate bilaterally from the lateral aspect of the aorta throughout the entire length of the aorta.

SIZE

Although the size of the vessel varies depending upon body habitus, it is accepted that the average anterior-posterior diameter of the normal aorta is 2cm at the most superior portion of the abdomen.[3] Coursing inferiorly, it decreases in size with an average measurement of 1.5cm at its bifurcation into the iliac arteries.[3,4] This vessel should not exceed 3cm at any level. It has been suggested that the best method to decrease observer variation when measuring the aorta is to take the anterior-posterior measurement in the longitudinal plane.[5] One should always be consistent in the technique used to measure this vessel, to ensure consistent results.

GROSS ANATOMY

The aorta, like other vessels, has three layers (tunica intima, tunica media, and tunica adventitia. (See Figure 11–5.)[6,7] Their thickness varies. Arteries often have a thicker **tunica media** to allow for greater elasticity.

PHYSIOLOGY

The primary function of the aorta and its branches is to channel blood to organs and tissues to ensure oxygen-

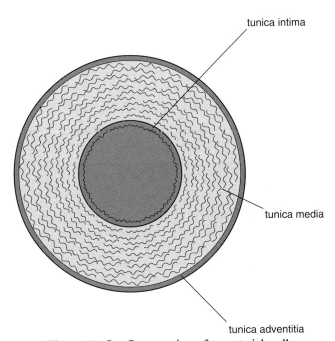

Figure 11–5. Cross-section of an arterial wall.

ation and metabolism. The arterial system also serves other functions.

Although the arteriole-capillary system is primarily responsible for the other functions such as blood pressure maintenance and assisting in the control of bleeding, the aorta does participate in these functions. The venous system is capable of maintaining blood pressure through its valves; however, valves are not present in the arterial system. Thus, the aorta and large arteries use a different mechanism to maintain blood flow during diastole. As the ventricles contract during systole, blood is quickly sent into the aorta, forcing the expansion of the vessel wall. As a result, potential energy is stored in the vessel wall.[7,8] As the aortic valve in the heart closes and diastole ensues, the arterial wall recoils to release the stored potential energy. The wall recoil forces blood to continue its forward movement; thus, the blood pressure is maintained. In addition, multiple nerve and chemical receptors are present throughout the arterial system which respond to various stimuli. The many local and systemic chemical and neurologic events can cause vasoconstriction or vasodilatation. For instance, renin is released from the kidney in the event of bleeding. Renin acts on angiotensin II, which initiates vasoconstriction; thus, blood pressure is maintained through vasoconstriction. In addition, chemical-humoral reactions allow for vasoconstriction of certain arterial segments, which can result in increased organ perfusion or heat dissipation. As is evident, the aorta and its branches play a critical role in homeostasis.

SONOGRAPHIC APPEARANCE

Arterial vasculature should normally display an anechoic center with echogenic walls that clearly delineate it from adjacent structures. Larger vessels will often display significant pulsatility, which will assist in proper identification. In the longitudinal plane, the aorta is a tubular, highly pulsatile structure slightly anterior and to the left of the spine.[3-5] The proximal portion of the aorta is often seen as a curvilinear structure as it courses from posterior to anterior after piercing the diaphragm. The aorta continues to course anteriorly until it bifurcates; however, this slight degree of posterior-to-anterior angulation results in the mid and distal aorta displaying more of a linear configuration than the proximal portion. (See Figure 11–6.) Note that the aorta is often tortuous; thus, identification of a significant portion in the longitudinal plane can be difficult. Although it is not always possible, one should attempt to identify the layers of the vessel to assist in excluding pathology. The tunica intima often appears as a bright echogenic line on the innermost portion of the vessel wall. The tunica media is felt to be represented by the echo-free area between the echogenic tunica intima and tunica adventitia. The tunica adventitia is the fibrous outermost section of the vessel which appears as a moderately echogenic line separating the vessel from other structures.

Although the aorta has many branches, the branches that are demonstrated with reasonable consistency are the celiac axis, superior mesenteric artery, renal arteries, and common iliac arteries. The celiac axis is most easily seen in transverse plane slightly superior to the pancreas. The vessel is recognizable as it branches anteriorly from the aorta by displaying the characteristic shape of a seagull. (See Figure 11–7.) The splenic artery and the common hepatic artery represent the wings of the bird. The CA will appear as a short tubular structure branching anteriorly from the aorta. (See Figure 11–8.)

The SMA can also be identified in the longitudinal plane as a linear structure branching anteriorly from the

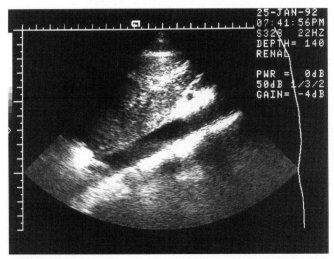

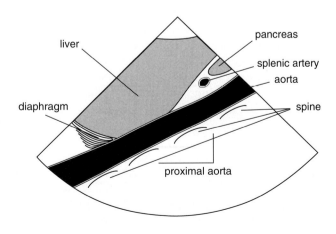

Figure 11–6. Longitudinal section of the proximal aorta.

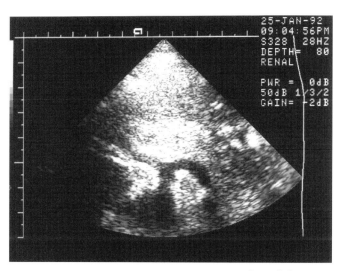

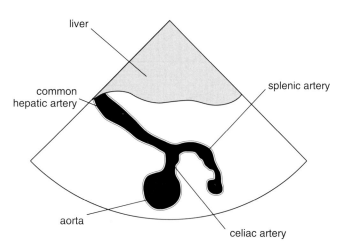

Figure 11-7. Transverse section of the aorta, celiac artery, common hepatic artery, and splenic artery.

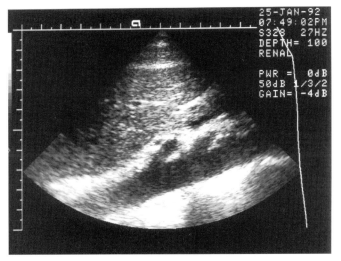

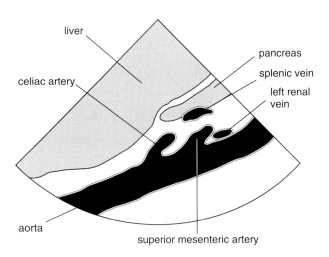

Figure 11-8. Longitudinal section of the midaorta showing branches of the celiac artery and superior mesenteric artery.

aorta slightly inferior to the CA. (See Figure 11-8.) The SMA courses posteriorly to the pancreas and can usually be identified more easily in the transverse plane as a circular, anechoic structure surrounded by echogenic parapancreatic fat directly posterior to the splenic vein. (See Figure 11-9.)

The renal arteries are usually most easily seen in the transverse plane as small-diameter curvilinear structures branching laterally from the aorta. (See Figure 11-10.) Although the left renal artery is very difficult to identify in the longitudinal plane, the right renal artery can usu-

ally be identified in the longitudinal plane directly posterior to the inferior vena cava. (See Figure 11-11.) The inferior mesenteric artery is the next most inferiorly located vessel; however, it is not consistently demonstrated.

As was discussed, the aorta bifurcates into the common iliac arteries at the level of the umbilicus. This bifurcation is most easily demonstrated in the transverse plane. One will see the single aorta divided into two separate vessels as the transducer is angled or moved inferiorly. (See Figures 11-12 to 11-14.)

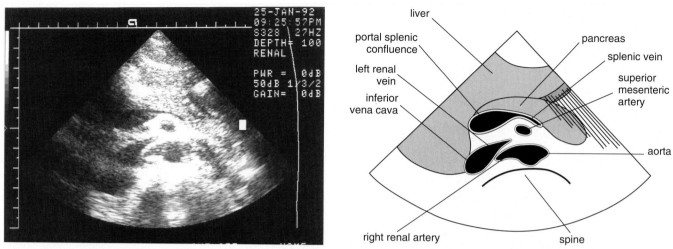

Figure 11–9. Transverse section of the midaorta displaying the superior mesenteric artery branch.

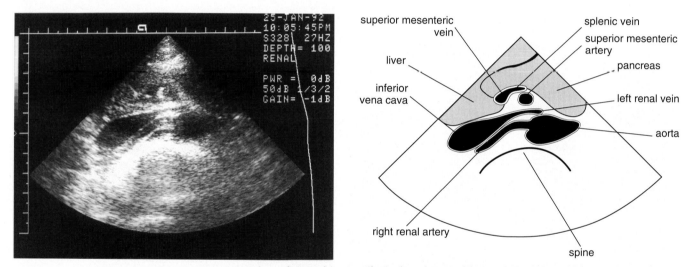

Figure 11–10. Transverse section of the midaorta displaying the curvilinear right renal artery.

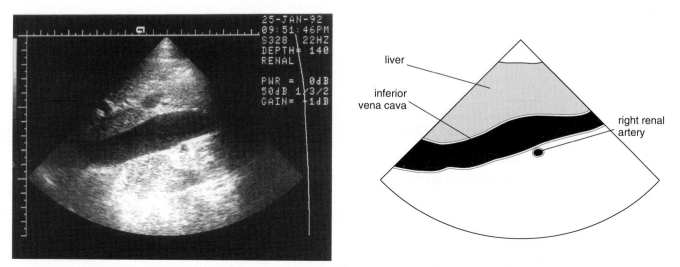

Figure 11–11. Longitudinal section of the inferior vena cava delineating the right renal artery.

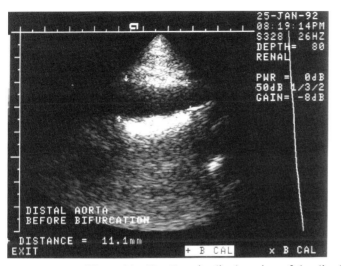
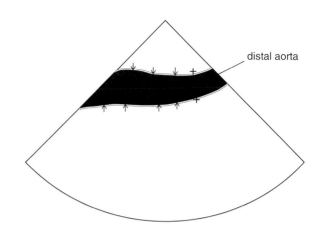

Figure 11–12. Longitudinal section of the distal aorta (arrows). Note decrease in aortic diameter preceding bifurcation (calibers).

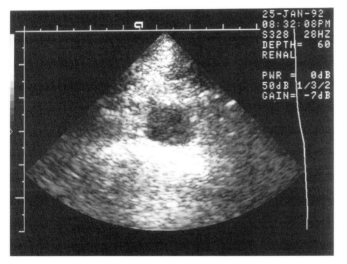
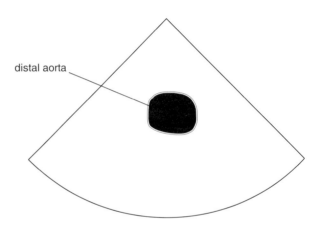

Figure 11–13. Transverse section of the distal aorta just prior to bifurcation into the common iliac arteries.

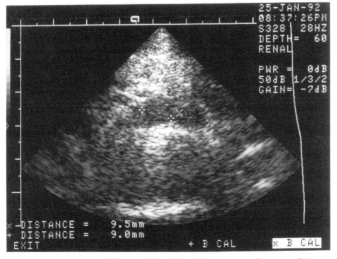
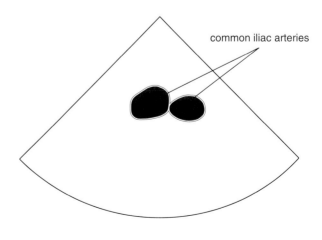

Figure 11–14. Transverse image of the common iliac arteries distal to the bifurcation.

SONOGRAPHIC APPLICATIONS

The aorta and its branches are primarily evaluated to detect aneurysms and stenosis. Fusiform, saccular, and dissecting aneurysms can be readily identified. Stenosis of the celiac artery, superior mesenteric artery, renal artery, and iliac artery can also be identified with the aid of Doppler sonography. Stenosis is often the causative factor in other disease states such as bowel ischemia due to SMA stenosis, or renovascular hypertension due to renal artery stenosis. In addition, grafts can be evaluated for patency and complications using Doppler sonography.

NORMAL VARIANTS

Nonapplicable.

REFERENCE CHARTS

Associated Physicians

Many physicians may be involved in care of the patient with a disorder of the aorta or its branches, depending on the organ affected. The vascular surgeon, who specializes in the surgical treatment of the vasculature, is the primary physician who treats the arterial system.

Common Diagnostic Tests

Diagnostic tests to evaluate the arterial system include duplex Doppler sonography, color-flow Doppler, plethysmography, segmental blood pressures, arteriography, computerized tomography, and magnetic resonance imaging.

Duplex Doppler Sonography: Duplex Doppler sonography can indicate flow patterns within the vasculature, and these abnormalities indicate certain disease states such as stenosis and aneurysms. (This chapter includes only a limited discussion of Doppler sonography as an aid in evaluating the aorta and its branches.) The normal Doppler waveform may be a low resistance waveform, a high resistance waveform, or a combination waveform. A low resistance waveform occurs when there is no reverse flow and significant diastolic flow is present throughout the cardiac cycle. This is generally seen when the diastolic flow is approximately one third of the normal peak systolic flow. A low resistance waveform should be present in arteries which feed low resistance beds such as the brain, kidneys, and abdominal organs. (See Figure 11–15.) A normally high resistance waveform will exhibit a sharp systolic upstroke along with reduced diastolic flow, and it may display reverse flow. High resistance waveforms will be seen in the external carotid artery, extremities, and the preprandial SMA. (See Figure 11–16.) A combination waveform will show attributes of both low and high resistance waveforms. This type of waveform is seen in the common carotid artery and abdominal aorta. (See Figures 11–17 and 11–18.) In addition, most waveforms should not exhibit spectral broadening. Spectral broadening can be detected as excessive echoes within the window of the waveform. Various abnormalities within these waveforms such as increased peak systolic velocities, increased diastolic velocities, significant spectral broadening, flow reversal, and other findings assist one in ascertaining the presence of pathology in the vessel or the organ supplied by the vessel. (It should be noted that this discussion does not explain Doppler sonography sufficiently to allow one to interpret Doppler waveforms.) A sonographer or vascular technologist performs this examination and often presents a preliminary impression. A physician, usually a radiologist or vascular surgeon, interprets the sonogram.

Color Flow Doppler: Color flow Doppler or color imaging often gives similar results to duplex sonography; however, its main use is to facilitate in locating vessels for duplex sonography or to ascertain the presence and location of flow in a structure. (See Figures 11–19 and 11–20.) Recent improvements in equipment may shortly allow for color imaging to be used much like duplex sonography. Personnel responsible for performing and interpreting duplex sonography have similar functions in this examination.

Plethysmography and Segmental Blood Pressure: Although plethysmography and segmental blood pressures are primarily used to evaluate vascular disease of the extremities, they can assist in determining the presence and extent of occlusive aortic disease. There are several types of plethysmographs; the function of each is to measure volume changes within an area.[6] Thus, one can ascertain the volume of blood and extent of arterial disease within that particular area. In addition, segmental blood pressures can be used in conjunction with plethysmography or separately to ascertain blood flow to an area. When compared to normal values, the pressure information can also indicate the presence or severity of disease. A sonographer or vascular technologist performs this examination and often provides a preliminary impression. A vascular surgeon usually interprets the examination.

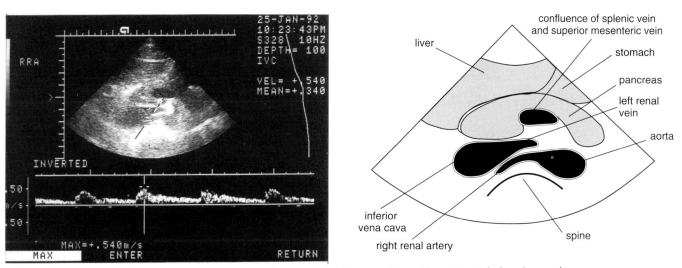

Figure 11-15. Normal right renal artery Doppler waveform. Note that this is a low resistance waveform (the diastolic flow is approximately one third of the peak systolic flow, indicating a low resistance vascular bed).

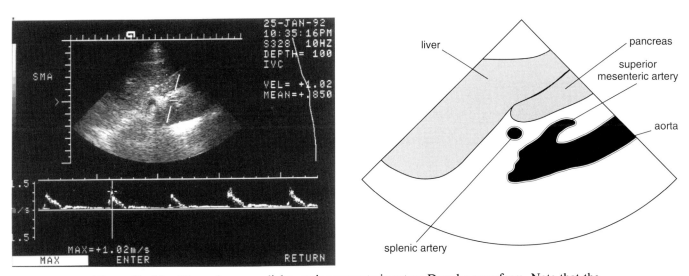

Figure 11-16. Normal preprandial superior mesenteric artery Doppler waveform. Note that the diastolic flow, as compared to the low resistance renal artery waveform, is much less in relation to the peak systolic flow. The preprandial superior mesenteric artery waveform is considered a high resistance waveform.

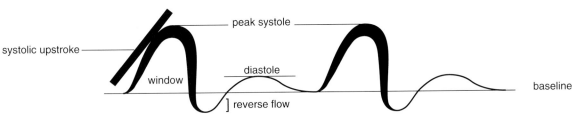

Figure 11-17. Doppler waveform throughout two cardiac cycles.

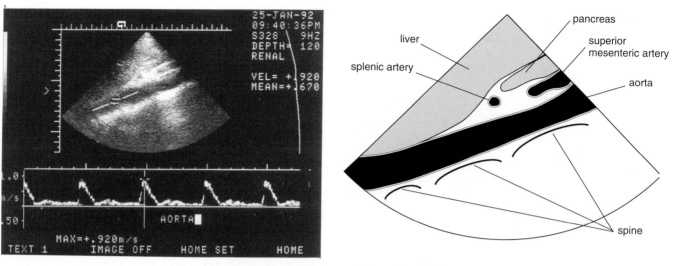

Figure 11–18. Normal aortic Doppler waveform.

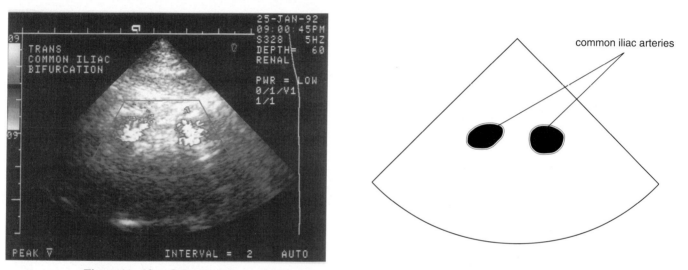

Figure 11–19. Color Doppler sonogram demonstrating the common iliac arteries. (See Color Plate 4 at the back of this book.)

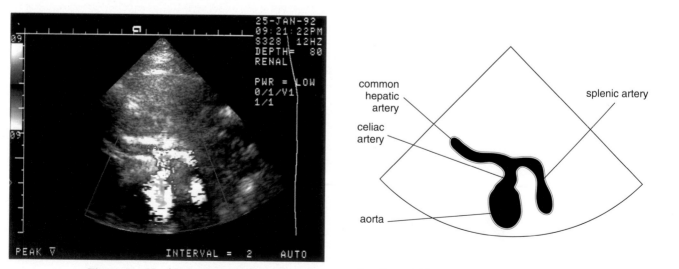

Figure 11–20. Color Doppler sonogram demonstrating flow within the aorta, celiac artery, splenic artery, and common hepatic artery. (See Color Plate 5 at the back of this book.)

Arteriography: Arteriography is most often considered the gold standard when evaluating the aorta and its branches. In the arteriogram, dye is injected into the vessel supplying the target area and several radiographs are then taken. A radiologist assisted by a radiologic technologist performs this examination. The radiologist interprets this examination.

Computed Axial Tomography (CT scan): CT is often utilized to evaluate the aorta. This examination consists of a series of sequential radiographs taken over the target area. The images are computer reconstructed in two or three dimensions, enabling excellent identification and differentiation of structures. Structures can be evaluated with or without the aid of contrast material. A radiologic technologist performs this examination and a radiologist interprets it.

Magnetic Resonance Imaging (MRI): MRI is rapidly increasing in applications, which now include the vascular area. The images are similar in format to those of CT. The resolution is often superior, however, the image being created by magnetic field, not by radiation. A magnetic resonance imaging technologist or radiologic technologist performs this procedure, and a radiologist interprets the examination.

Laboratory Values

Many laboratory values are based on the arterial system, most of which indicate the functioning of other organs. Hematocrit (the percentage of red blood cells to whole blood) is used to measure possible bleeding from the arterial system; measurement of red blood cells aids in this determination. An abnormal decrease in red blood cells may also point to bleeding. Levels of cholesterol and lipids may indicate the potential for pathology or suggest the current arterial disease state; however, they cannot directly measure either. The arterial vascular system is complex. One should be well acquainted with its anatomy, physiology, sonographic appearance, and associated tests to ensure that the patient receives the highest quality of care.

Normal Measurements

The diameter of the normal aorta measures 2cm at its most superior aspect in the abdomen, diminishing to approximately 1.5cm as it courses inferiorly. The normal aorta should not exceed 3cm at any point.

Vasculature

Aorta-inferior phrenic
Aorta-celiac axis—left gastric
  —splenic—left gastroepiploic
  —common hepatic—proper hepatic—left hepatic
                      —right hepatic
    —gastroduodenal—left gastroepiploic
          —superior, anterior and posterior pancreatic duodenal artery
          —inferior anterior and posterior pancreatic duodenal artery
Aorta—superior mesenteric
Aorta—gonadals
Aorta—inferior mesenteric
Aorta—common iliacs

Affecting Chemicals

Nonapplicable.

References

1. Moore KL: The Developing Human; Clinically Oriented Embryology, 4th ed. Philadelphia, WB Saunders, 1988.
2. Netter FH: The CIBA Collection of Medical Illustrations, vol 5, Heart. Summit, N.J., CIBA Division of CIBA-Geigy, 1978.
3. Mittelstaedt CM: Abdominal Ultrasound. New York, Churchill Livingstone, 1987.
4. Anderhub B: Manual of Abdominal Sonography. Baltimore, University Park Press, 1983.
5. Yucel KE et al: Sonograhic measurement of abdominal aortic diameter: intraobserver variability. Ultrasound Med 10:681–683, 1991.
6. Zweibel WJ (ed): Introduction to Vascular Ultrasonography, 2nd ed. Philadelphia, WB Saunders, 1986.
7. Gay W-R, Rothenburger A: Color Atlas of Physiology, 4th ed. (Trans. Joy Wieser). New York, Thieme, 1991.
8. Ganong WF: Review of Medical Physiology, 12th ed. Los Altos, Lange Medical Publications, 1985.

Chapter 12

THE INFERIOR VENA CAVA

JERRY PEARSON

Objectives:

Discuss the prenatal development of the inferior vena cava (IVC).

Discuss the normal location and course of the IVC.

Discuss the major tributaries which feed into the IVC along with the organs that are emptied by the tributaries.

Discuss the function of the IVC.

Describe the sonographic appearance of the IVC and commonly visualized tributaries.

Describe associated diagnostic tests related to the IVC.

Define the key words.

Key Words:

Cardinal venous system	Lumbar veins
Common iliac veins	Renal veins
Hepatic veins	Vitelline vein
Inferior vena cava	

INTRODUCTION

The **inferior vena cava** (IVC) is one of the two great abdominal vessels. Like all other veins, the IVC transports blood toward the heart. Thus, the sonographer must have a full understanding of this vasculature to adequately evaluate the abdomen during a sonographic examination.

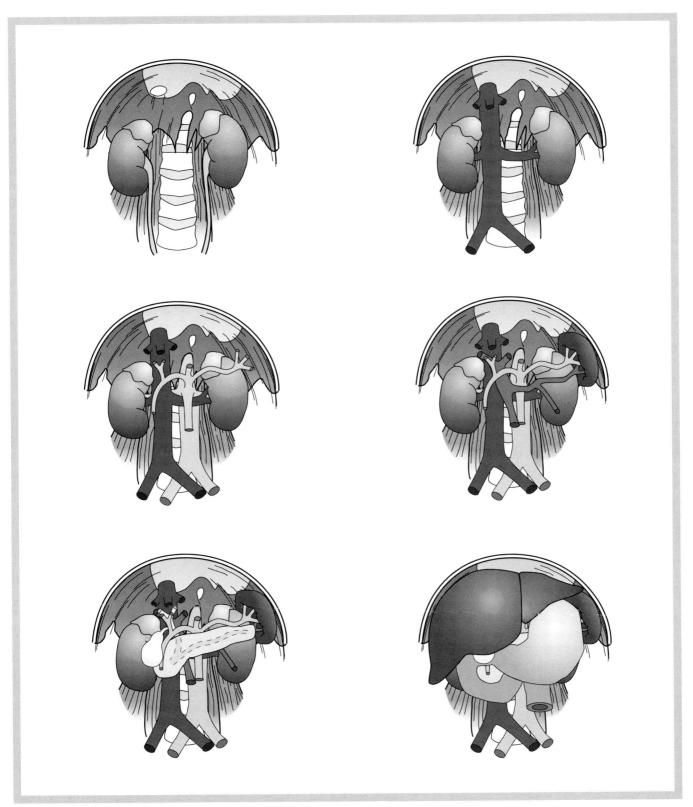

The inferior vena cava and surrounding anatomic layers. *See* Figure 4–3 B, C, D, E, G, I, pp. 44–47, for more details.

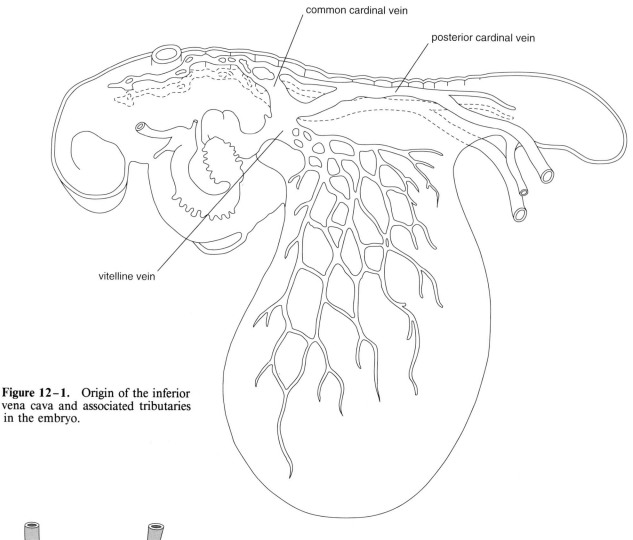

common cardinal vein

posterior cardinal vein

vitelline vein

Figure 12–1. Origin of the inferior vena cava and associated tributaries in the embryo.

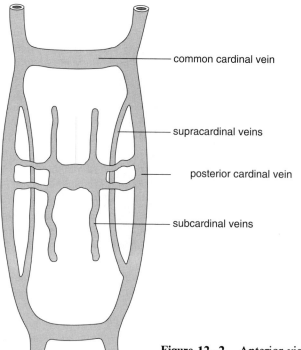

common cardinal vein

supracardinal veins

posterior cardinal vein

subcardinal veins

Figure 12–2. Anterior view of the cardinal venous system.

PRENATAL DEVELOPMENT

The development of the IVC is very complex which predisposes it to multiple anatomic variations. The IVC and its tributaries are formed from a portion of the **vitelline vein** and portions of the **cardinal venous system** within the embryo.[1–3] (See Figures 12–1 and 12–2.) The posterior cardinal veins (PCVs), subcardinal veins, and supracardinal veins are formed during the sixth, seventh, and eighth weeks of embryonic development, respectively. The PCVs regress during this time period and do not evolve into a portion of the IVC; however, they do serve as a base for the development of the subcardinal and supracardinal veins. Enormous anastomoses and regressions of these veins give rise to the IVC and its tributaries.

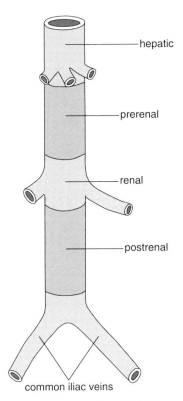

Figure 12-3. Sections of the inferior vena cava.

zant that the IVC can have many possible congenital variations including double IVC, IVC located on the left, absence of certain portions of the IVC, or a combination of these.[1-3] This is due to its complex development, as previously discussed. Many tributaries, including the lumbar veins, right gonadal vein, renal veins, and hepatic veins, will empty into the IVC as it continues its superior course and pierces the diaphragm at the caval hiatus to enter the right atrium of the heart. The IVC is located posterior to the intestines and the body of the liver. It is medial to the right kidney. The IVC is located more posteriorly as it courses superiorly.

The IVC has many tributaries; however, several contain multiple configurations or are not suitable for sonographic evaluation. Thus, only major tributaries will be discussed. (See Figure 12-4.) As previously mentioned, the IVC is formed from the convergence of the common iliac veins, which empty the lower extremities and pelvis at approximately the level of the umbilicus. The **lumbar veins**, which empty into the lateral aspect of the IVC, are the next most superior branch. These horizontally coursing veins empty the posterior abdominal wall and are located bilaterally. In addition, there is usually more than one pair that continue emptying into the IVC to the level of the renal veins. Moving superiorly, the right gonadal vein, which courses parallel to the IVC, empties

The IVC is considered to have four sections. (See Figure 12-3.) Beginning superiorly, the first area encountered is the hepatic section, located directly posterior to the liver where the hepatic veins empty into the IVC. The hepatic section of the IVC and hepatic veins develop from the proximal vitelline vein. The next section is termed the prerenal section. It extends from just inferior to the hepatic veins to slightly superior to the renal veins and is derived from a subcardinal vein. The renal section is the next most inferiorly located area of the IVC. The renal veins and multiple tributaries are located within this section, which terminates almost immediately after the branching of the renal veins. The subcardinal and supracardinal veins undergo multiple anastomoses to form this level. The final section is the postrenal section, which is formed from a supracardinal vein. The postrenal section of the IVC extends from just inferior to the renal veins until the common iliac veins converge into the IVC.

LOCATION

The IVC is formed by the convergence of the **common iliac veins**, which empty the lower extremities and pelvis. The IVC continues to course superiorly through the retroperitoneum along the anterior lateral aspect of the spine and to the right of the aorta. One should be cogni-

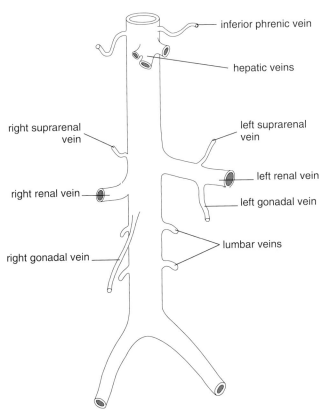

Figure 12-4. The inferior vena cava and its major tributaries.

into the anterior lateral aspect of the IVC. Within a few centimeters superiorly, the **renal veins** empty into the IVC. Although the right renal vein generally empties only the right kidney or sometimes the right adrenal gland via the right suprarenal vein, the left renal vein has additional tributaries which it assists in draining. The left gonadal vein courses parallel and lateral to the IVC and empties into the left renal vein. In addition, the left suprarenal vein follows a course similar to that of the left renal vein into which it eventually empties. Many smaller tributaries may also drain into the left renal vein. Note that the normal right renal vein is much shorter than the left renal vein. The left renal vein passes anteriorly to the aorta and posteriorly to the superior mesenteric artery as it courses from the left kidney. The right suprarenal vein often empties into the IVC slightly superior to the right renal vein. The next major tributaries are the hepatic veins. There are most commonly three **hepatic veins**, which course from the inferior aspect, deep within the liver, to the superior aspect of the liver where they empty into the IVC. Generally, the right hepatic vein empties the right lobe of the liver, the middle hepatic vein empties the caudate lobe, and the left hepatic vein empties the left lobe of the liver. The most superior branches of the IVC are the inferior phrenic veins, which course in a superior-to-inferior direction draining the diaphragm and emptying into the lateral aspect of the IVC. One should note that several vein locations parallel the locations of their sister arteries.

SIZE

The diameter of the IVC will increase during a Valsalva maneuver or inspiration and commonly decrease during expiration. Although the diameter of the IVC varies, it is considered dilated if it exceeds 3.7 cm.[3]

GROSS ANATOMY

In general, venous walls are thinner because their tunica media is thin in comparison to that of the arterial system. This is because a highly tensile vessel is not needed, as the venous network is a low pressure system.

PHYSIOLOGY

The IVC and its associated tributaries have the primary function of returning deoxygenated blood to the heart. Because the pressure on the venous side of the circulatory system is low in comparison to the arterial side, the venous circulation contains valves, which prevent backflow of blood during diastole.

The momentum of the blood during systole forces the valves open. Once the momentum decreases and the blood is not pushed forward, the valve closes and prevents retrograde flow. In various diseases, the valves may not function and this will cause retrograde blood flow. Blood is also moved forward by a decrease in thoracic pressure which pulls the blood into the right atrium. In this case the IVC simply acts as a transportation vehicle.

SONOGRAPHIC APPEARANCE

Venous vasculature should normally display an anechoic center with thin, hyperechoic walls. During real-time examination, one will note that the IVC displays

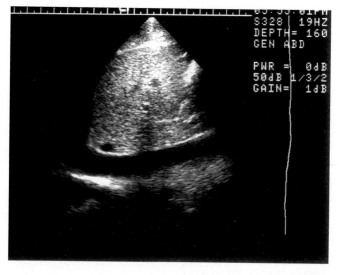

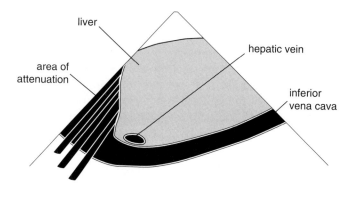

Figure 12–5. Longitudinal image of the inferior vena cava.

significant variation in diameter as compared to the arterial vasculature. In addition, small moving echoes are often noticed within the lumen of the IVC. The reason for these echoes is debated; however, it is agreed that they are related to the flow of blood within the vessel.

As the transducer is longitudinally placed in the epigastric area, the hepatic section of the IVC can be seen as a tubular, elastic structure located directly posterior to the liver. (See Figure 12–5.) In some instances, the IVC may appear to be coursing through the liver parenchyma, especially in the most superior section of the liver. The hepatic veins can often be seen at this level as linear structures originating in the liver and emptying into the IVC. (See Figure 12–6.) It is evident that the hepatic veins increase in diameter as they approach the IVC. In the transverse plane, the hepatic veins can once

again be seen as anechoic linear structures, whose walls are not obvious, emptying into the IVC. (See Figure 12–7.) One often notices a characteristic "bunny ear" pattern with this image. The renal veins are the next most inferiorly located venous structures which are consistently recognized. The left renal vein is seen as a curvilinear structure emptying into the lateral aspect of the IVC as it courses anterior to the aorta and posterior to the superior mesenteric artery from its origin in the left kidney. (See Figure 12–8.) The right renal vein is also seen as a curvilinear structure emptying into the lateral aspect of the IVC at this level. The gonadal vein and lumbar veins are not consistently imaged. However, the common iliac veins are most easily visualized in the transverse plane at approximately the umbilicus immediately before they converge to form the IVC.

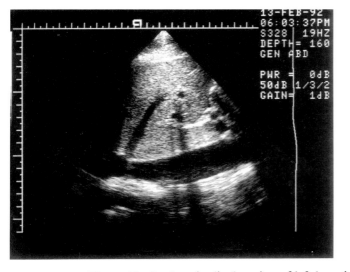 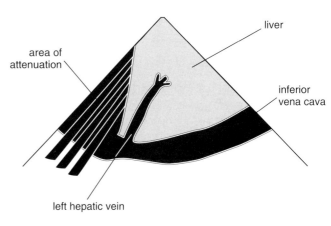

Figure 12–6. Longitudinal section of left hepatic vein emptying into the inferior vena cava.

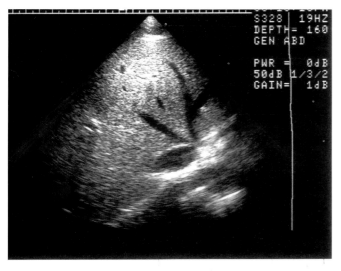 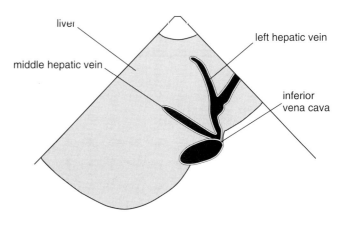

Figure 12–7. Transverse section of the liver showing the middle hepatic vein and left hepatic vein emptying into the inferior vena cava.

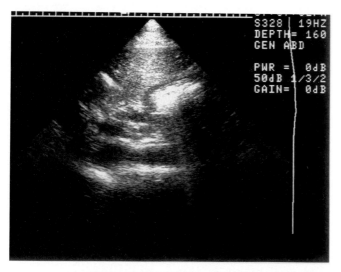

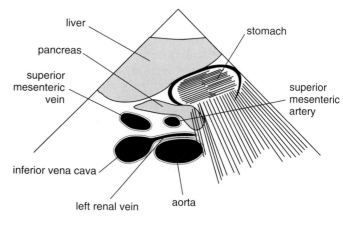

Figure 12–8. Transverse section of the abdominal vasculature demonstrating the circular inferior vena cava aorta, and superior mesenteric artery along with the curvilinear left renal vein coursing posterior to the superior mesenteric artery and anterior to the aorta.

SONOGRAPHIC APPLICATIONS

The IVC and its visible branches are primarily evaluated to detect intraluminal thrombosis and tumor invasion. The thrombosis may be due to numerous causes. Tumor invasion most commonly occurs in the renal veins and often extends into the IVC. The venous system can be evaluated by many diagnostic modalities. However, sonography is continually increasing in diagnostic accuracy and acceptance by medical professionals. Thus, sonographers must have a complete understanding of this system to ensure that each patient receives the best care possible.

NORMAL VARIANTS

Variations of the IVC can occur because of its complex formation. There may be a double IVC or a left positioned IVC, or a portion of the vessel may be absent. However, these are not common.

REFERENCE CHARTS

Associated Physicians

Generally, vascular surgeons treat the patient whose disorder involves the venous system. However, other physicians are often involved depending on the other organs or organ systems involved. In addition, internists—internal medicine practitioners—often render care to patients who do not require surgery.

Common Diagnostic Tests

The following diagnostic tests are commonly used to evaluate the venous system: duplex Doppler sonography, color Doppler, continuous wave Doppler sonography, impedance flow plethysmography, venography, computerized tomography, and magnetic resonance imaging.

Duplex Doppler Sonography: Although veins of the extremities can be evaluated with B-Mode imaging and compression, one also needs to assess the flow dynamics of the area. Thus, duplex Doppler is necessary to ensure an adequate examination. A normal venous flow pattern should be spontaneous and phasic (change with respiration). Proximal compression and distal augmentation are also used to assess venous flow. Abnormalities often suggest disease. The abdominal venous system displays characteristic Doppler waveforms. (See Figure 12–9.) A sonographer, vascular technologist, or nurse performs this examination and often provides a preliminary impression. A physician, usually a radiologist or a vascular surgeon, interprets the findings.

Color Flow Doppler: Color Doppler can often assist in determining flow characteristics in the abdomen and extremities by quickly identifying flow and turbulence. Continuous wave Doppler is also helpful in determining the status of extremity veins. The Doppler signal is amplified by a loudspeaker, which allows the examiner to hear an audible signal. Abnormalities in this signal indicate disease. The same personnel who perform and interpret duplex sonography also perform and interpret this examination.

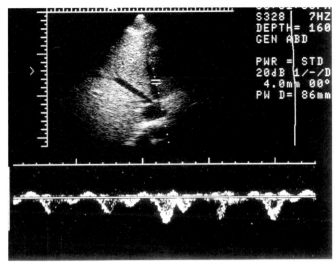 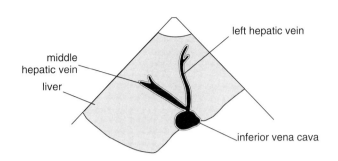

Figure 12-9. Transverse section of the liver demonstrating a normal spontaneous and phasic Doppler pattern from the left hepatic vein.

Impedance Flow Plethysmography: Impedance flow plethysmography is the technique of measuring the blood volume change of an area.[4] Strain gauge plethysmography is generally used when evaluating veins. Bilateral inflatable cuffs are placed on the proximal portion of the extremities along with gauges that measure change in extremity size. As the cuffs are inflated, the flow of blood toward the heart is stopped and blood accumulates distal to the cuff, causing the extremity to increase in size. Next, the cuffs are deflated, allowing the blood to rush from the extremity back toward the heart. The strain gauge presents a readout of this rate of volume change. The results between extremities are compared as well as to established normals. If the flow of blood toward the heart is abnormally slow, some type of blockage should be considered; this test should be done in conjunction with B-mode imaging, continuous wave sonography, and/or duplex sonography to ensure accuracy. The same personnel who perform and interpret duplex and color sonography also perform and interpret this examination.

Venography: Venography is considered by many the gold standard when detecting venous disease. Dye (contrast material) is injected into the target vein and serial radiographs are taken. Defects in filling indicate the presence of disease. This is a highly invasive test, and reactions to the injected dye are of great concern. This procedure is performed by a radiologist assisted by a radiologic technologist. The radiologist interprets this examination.

Computerized Axial Tomography (CT Scan): CT is sometimes done to evaluate the abdominal venous system; however, it is rarely used to determine the disease state of extremities. This examination consists of a series of sequential radiographs, which are computer reconstructed to identify various structures. A radiologic technologist performs this examination and a radiologist interprets the findings.

Magnetic Resonance Imaging (MRI): MRI is infrequently called upon to evaluate the venous system. Furthermore, it is not utilized to assess the extremity veins. The images are similar in format to those of CT; however, the images are generated using a strong magnetic field instead of radiation as in CT. A magnetic resonance imaging technologist or radiologic technologist performs this exami-nation and a radiologist interprets the examination.

Laboratory Values

Almost all blood laboratory values are taken from the venous system; however, the majority of examinations indicate the status of other organs or body systems. As with the arterial system, the percentage of red blood cells to whole blood (hematocrit) indicates possible bleeding from the venous system.

Normal Measurements

The IVC will vary with respiration; however, it should not exceed 3.7cm.

Vasculature

IVC—inferior phrenic veins
IVC—hepatic veins
IVC—renal veins
IVC—gonadal veins
IVC—lumbar veins
IVC—iliac veins

Affecting Chemicals

Nonapplicable.

References

1. Netter, FH.: The CIBA Collection of Medical Illustrations, vol. 5, Heart. Summit, N.J., CIBA Division of CIBA-Geigy, 1978.
2. Moore, KL.: The Developing Human; Clinically Oriented Embryology, 4th ed. Philadelphia, WB Saunders, 1988.
3. Mittelstaedt, CM.: Abdominal Ultrasound. New York, Churchill Livingstone, 1987.
4. Zwiebel, WJ (ed).: Introduction to Vascular Ultrasonography, 2nd ed. Philadelphia, WB Saunders, 1986.

Chapter 13

THE PORTAL VENOUS SYSTEM

JERRY PEARSON

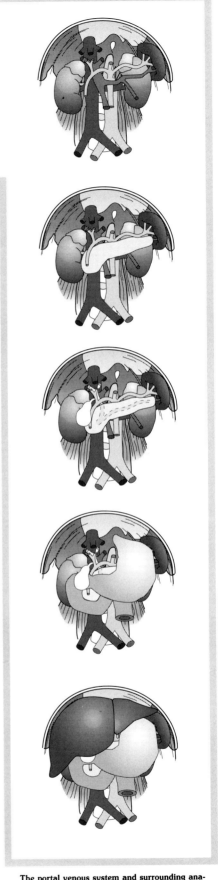

The portal venous system and surrounding anatomic layers. See Figure 4–3 D, E, F, G, H, I, pp. 44–47, for more details.

Objectives:

Discuss the embryologic development of the portal vein.

Discuss the normal location, course, and size of the portal vein.

Discuss the normal location of the portal vein tributaries.

Describe the function of the portal venous system.

Describe the sonographic appearance of the portal vein and its tributaries.

Discuss associated diagnostic tests.

Define the key words.

Key Words:

Inferior mesenteric vein
Left portal vein
Main portal vein
Portal triad
Right portal vein
Splenic vein
Superior mesenteric vein

INTRODUCTION

The portal venous system is unique because it is the system that supplies blood to the liver for metabolic processes. This blood originates from organs within the gastrointestinal tract which include the stomach, small intestine, large intestine, and spleen. Disruption to the flow can cause multiple adverse effects. Therefore, it is imperative that the sonographer understand the many factors associated with the portal system.

PRENATAL DEVELOPMENT

The portal vein develops during approximately the eighth embryologic week.[1] The vitelline veins undergo several anastomoses, forming a vascular network that gives rise to the main portal vein.[1,2] (See Figure 13–1.) The venous tributaries are also formed from the primitive vascular network, and they join the main portal vein at its inferior aspect.

LOCATION

The portal vein is an intra-abdominal structure normally measuring less than 13mm.[2,3] It is formed by the confluence of the splenic vein and the superior mesenteric vein directly posterior to the head of the pancreas. (See Figure 13–2.) The **splenic vein** drains the spleen and courses from lateral to medial directly posterior to the pancreas. The **superior mesenteric vein** courses from inferior to superior and drains the small intestine and portions of the large intestine via several smaller branches. The **inferior mesenteric vein** also courses from inferior to superior as it drains the large intestine via several smaller branches. This vessel most often empties blood into the splenic vein; however, there is considerable variance regarding where the inferior mesenteric vein joins the portal system. There are several other tributaries which empty into the portal vein including the left and right gastric veins, pancreaticoduodenal veins, and gastroepiploic veins. There is significant variability regarding where these vessels enter the system.

After the main portal vein forms, it continues to course superiorly approximately 5 to 6 cm.[2] At this point it divides into right and left branches. The left branch continues to course horizontally and branches into medial and lateral subdivisions. The left lateral subdivision feeds the left lobe of the liver. The right branch of the portal vein continues to course to the right and branches into anterior and posterior subdivisions. It should be noted that both right and left portal veins give off multi-

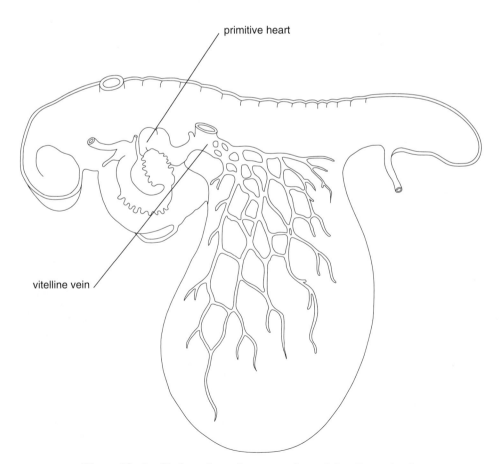

Figure 13–1. Early embryo demonstrating origin of portal vein.

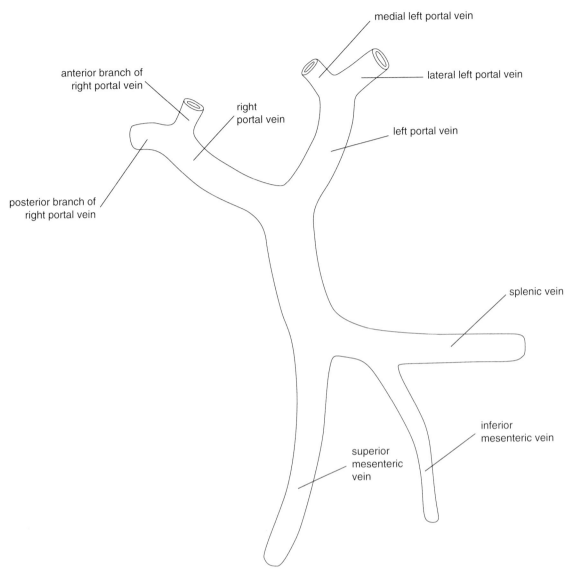

Figure 13-2. Portal venous system.

ple subdivisions, and variations in location are commonplace.

SIZE

The portal vein is an abdominal structure normally measuring less than 13 mm.

GROSS ANATOMY

Refer to location.

PHYSIOLOGY

The function of the portal vein and its tributaries is to deliver blood from the spleen and gastrointestinal tract (esophagus, stomach, and small and large intestines) to the liver for metabolism and detoxification. This system is much different from the arterial supply to the liver or the systemic venous supply, which empties the liver after the arterial and portal venous blood has been delivered to the organ. As has been noted, this is a vital and unique function.

SONOGRAPHIC APPEARANCE

The portal veins are one portion of the **portal triad** (made up of the hepatic arteries, bile ducts, and portal veins) located throughout the liver. However, the portal veins can generally be distinguished from other structures, especially hepatic veins, by their highly echogenic walls. This echogenicity is a result of the high collagen content in the walls of the portal veins. (See Figure 13-3.)

In transverse section, one visualizes the beginning of the **main portal vein** as an oval, anechoic structure,

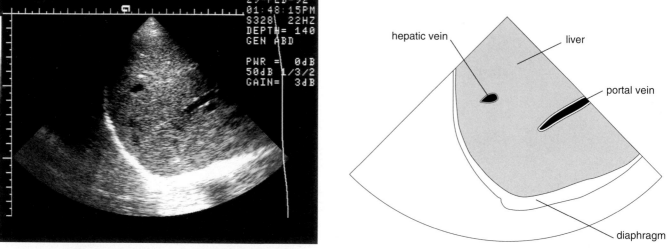

Figure 13–3. Longitudinal section, right lobe of the liver, showing a hepatic vein without echogenic walls and a portal vein with echogenic walls.

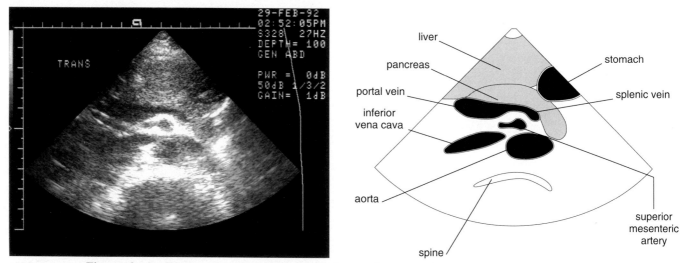

Figure 13–4. Transverse section of the epigastric area demonstrating the linear anechoic splenic vein joining the portal vein.

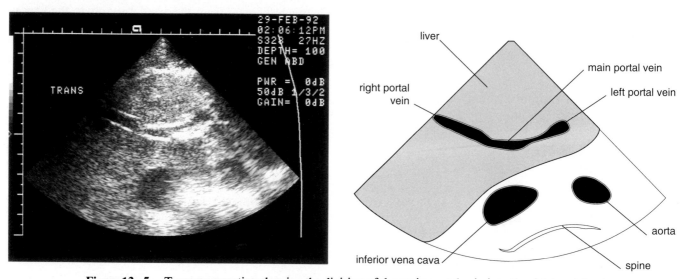

Figure 13–5. Transverse section showing the division of the main portal vein into the right portal vein and left portal vein.

where the splenic vein and superior mesenteric vein join directly posterior to the neck of the pancreas. (See Figure 13–4.) Superiorly to this location, the main portal vein can be seen as it branches into right and left portal veins. (See Figure 13–5.) The **left portal vein** can often be followed further to the left and be seen branching into its medial and lateral subdivisions. (See Figure 13–6.) The left lateral branch is more commonly visualized than the medial branch, and the lateral branch feeds the traditional left lobe of the liver.[4] The **right portal vein** can be seen in the transverse plane as a linear horizontal structure coursing to the right. It shortly bifurcates into its anterior and posterior branches. (See Figure 13–7.)

In a longitudinal plane, the main portal vein can be seen as a linear anechoic structure directly posterior to the pancreatic neck as it joins the superior mesenteric vein. (See Figure 13–8.) Moving laterally, the right portal vein can be imaged. The bile ducts are generally imaged as linear anechoic structures located anterior to the circular right portal vein. (See Figure 13–9.) One can often see smaller echogenic portal vein tributaries throughout the liver parenchyma which are routinely imaged in this section. In the left lobe of the liver, it is often more difficult to image the normal portal vein. However, it appears as small anechoic circular structures with echogenic walls when imaged. (See Figure 13–10.)

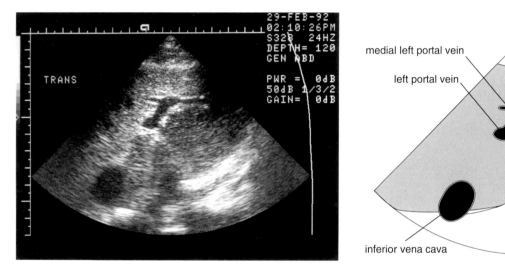

Figure 13–6. Transverse section of the left lobe of the liver demonstrating the left portal vein dividing into its medial and lateral subdivisions.

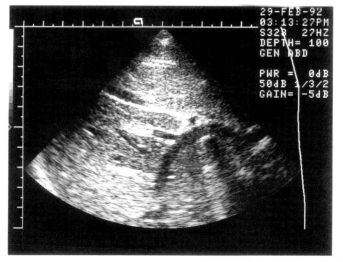
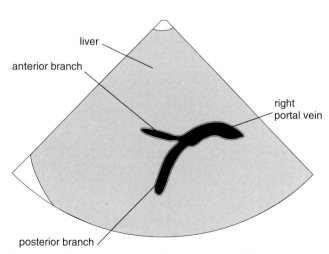

Figure 13–7. Transverse section of the right lobe of the liver demonstrating the division of the right portal vein into its anterior and posterior divisions.

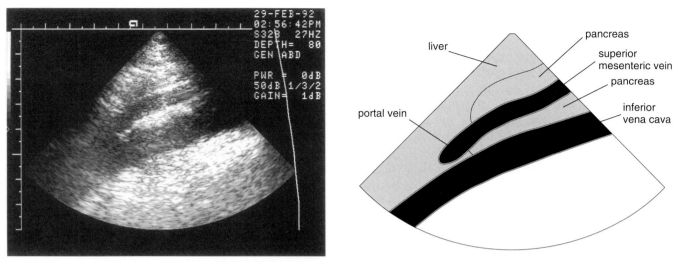

Figure 13–8. Longitudinal oblique section of the epigastric area demonstrating the joining of the superior mesenteric vein to the main portal vein. Note the pancreatic tissue visible anterior and posterior to the portal vein, superior mesenteric vein, and inferior vena cava.

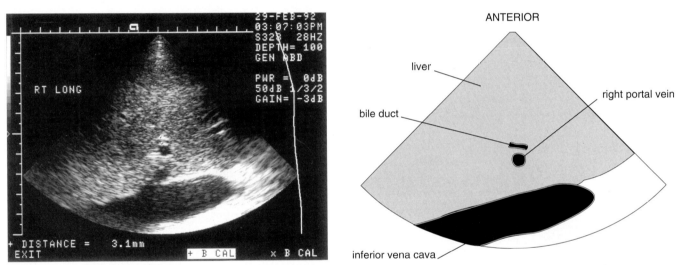

Figure 13–9. Longitudinal section demonstrating the circular anechoic section of a right portal vein with echogenic walls. A linear anechoic duct with hyperechoic walls is located directly anterior to the right portal vein.

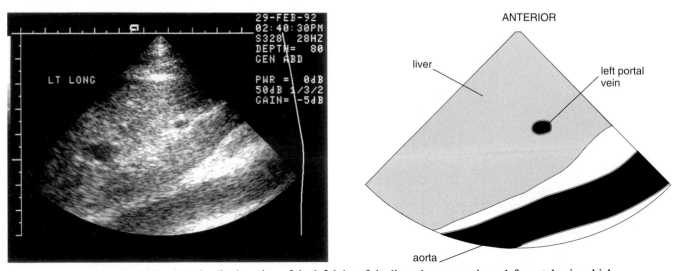

Figure 13–10. Longitudinal section of the left lobe of the liver demonstrating a left portal vein which appears as a circular anechoic structure with echogenic walls.

SONOGRAPHIC APPLICATIONS

Because the portal vein can be consistently imaged with sonography, it is often evaluated to detect tumor invasion and thrombosis. In addition, the most common reason for examination of the portal vein is to uncover portal vein hypertension. One should note, however, that this pathology involves more structures than the portal vein including the abdominal cavity, spleen, and liver. These organs are often more indicative of portal vein hypertension. Furthermore, evaluating the portal vein with color Doppler and duplex Doppler is far superior as a diagnostic tool than evaluating the structure with only B-mode imaging.

As stated earlier, the portal system is unique because it carries blood and nutrients from the bowel and abdominal organs to the liver for metabolism and detoxification. Thus, pathologies that affect other organs are often the reason for portal vein pathology. Therefore, one needs to have a good understanding of this system to ensure that the patient receives the highest quality sonographic examination possible.

NORMAL VARIANTS

Nonapplicable.

REFERENCE CHARTS

Associated Physicians

Various physicians may be involved in caring for the patient who has a disorder of the portal vein, depending on the problem. A physician who specializes in internal medicine may treat the patient whose portal vein hypertension is due to cirrhosis of the liver or one who is not a surgical candidate or does not require surgery. Various surgical specialists may treat the patient who requires surgery.

Common Diagnostic Tests

Diagnostic tests may include duplex Doppler sonography, color sonography, venography, computerized tomography, and magnetic resonance imaging.

Duplex Sonography: Duplex sonography can detect the direction and magnitude of flow within a portal vein. Flow should be toward the liver from the portal vein, and the protal venous system should display phasic flow in response to respiration. (See Figure 13–11.) This examination and the color flow examination provide extremely valuable information in a short time pe-

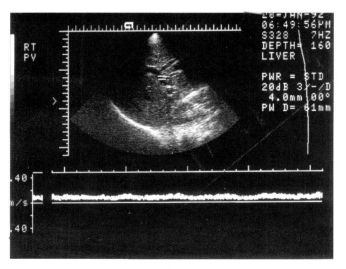
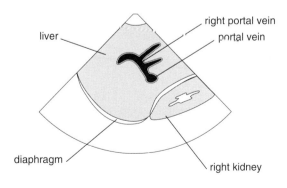

Figure 13–11. Longitudinal section of the right lobe of the liver demonstrating a normal Doppler waveform of the right portal vein. Note the phasic flow (variation) of the Doppler signal in response to respiration. In addition, note that the flow is above baseline. In this case, blood is flowing into the liver, which is normal.

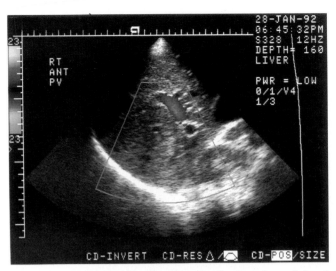

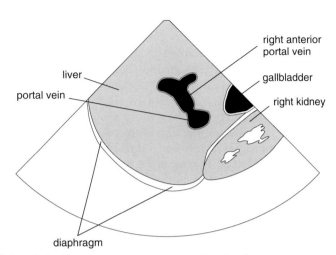

Figure 13–12. Longitudinal section of the right lobe of the liver demonstrating normal color flow Doppler. Note that flow toward the transducer is indicated in red. Thus, the flow is toward the transducer (into the liver) in this case. (See Color Plate 6 at the back of this book.)

riod and without the use of ionizing radiation. Thus, duplex sonography and color flow sonography are often utilized. A sonographer or vascular technologist usually performs this examination and often provides a preliminary impression. A radiologist interprets the findings.

Color Flow Sonography: Color flow sonography reveals information similar to that derived from duplex sonography. However, color flow imaging can often yield this information much faster. (See Figure 13–12.) The same personnel who perform and interpret duplex sonography also perform and interpret color flow sonography.

Direct Portal Venography: Although not usually done given today's technological environment, direct portal venography can be carried out by injecting contrast material (dye) into the splenic or portal vein and taking radiographs of the area as the contrast agent is transported throughout the system. This examination provides information related to portal vein anatomy and intraluminal contents. A radiologist assisted by a radiologic technologist performs this examination. The radiologist interprets it.

Computed Axial Tomography (CT Scan) and Magnetic Resonance Imaging (MRI): CT and MRI can also be done to evaluate the portal vein. In CT, a series of sequential radiographs are taken over the area of interest. The information is stored in a computer which converts the data into a two- or three-dimensional image. CT is not the best method, as it may be difficult to ascertain intraluminal contents. MRI, although not widely utilized, can often distinguish subtle differences in tissues within the portal system. In MRI, a magnetic field generates data, and a computer converts the information into a diagnostic image. Although MRI is non-ionizing, it has several limitations because of the matnetic field. A radiologic technologist performs the CT and MRI examinations. A radiologist interprets the findings.

Benefits of Sonography: Clinical data often suggest portal vein pathology. Sonography can easily verify the intraluminal contents and the direction of flow, in addition to indicating other pathological findings of the abdomen. Thus, sonography is often used as a diagnostic tool in evaluating the system.

Laboratory Values

Generally, laboratory values do not directly indicate portal vein pathology. However, a tumor, or cirrhosis of the liver, for example, will produce various laboratory and clinical data that could point to portal vein involvement in the disorder.

Normal Measurements

The main portal vein should measure less than 13 mm.

Vasculature

Left Portal Vein   Splenic Vein — Inferior
Mesenteric Vein

Main Portal Vein

Right Portal Vein   Superior Mesenteric Vein

Affecting Chemicals

Nonapplicable.

References

1. Moore, KL: The Developing Human: Clinically Oriented Embry-ology, 4th ed. Philadelphia, WB Saunders, 1988, 286.
2. Netter, FH: The CIBA Collection of Medical Illustrations, vol. 3, Digestive System, Part III: Liver, Biliary Tract and Pancreas). Summit, N.J.: CIBA, Division, CIBA-Geigy, 1978.
3. Weinreb J, et al: Portal vein measurements by real-time sonogra-phy. Am J Radiol 139:497, 1982.
4. Mittelstaedt, CM: Abdominal Ultrasound. New York, Churchill Livingstone, 1987.

SECTION IV

PELVIC SONOGRAPHY

Chapter 14

THE MALE PELVIS

MICHAEL J. KAMMERMEIER

Objectives:

Describe the location of the scrotum, testicles, epididymis, ductus (vas) deferens, seminal vesicles, and prostate.

Describe the size of the testicles and prostate.

Identify the gross anatomy of the scrotum, testicles, ducts, prostate, and penis.

Describe the sonographic appearances of the testicles, seminal vesicles, prostate, and penis.

Identify the associated physicians, related diagnostic tests, and laboratory values.

Define the key words.

Key Words:

Anterior fibromuscular stroma
Buck's fascia
Central zone
Convoluted seminiferous tubules
Corpus cavernosum
Corpus spongiosum
Cremaster muscle
Denonvillier's fascia
Ductus (vas) deferens
Ductus epididymis

Efferent ducts
Ejaculatory Ducts
Epididymis
Inguinal canal
Levator ani muscle
Median raphe
Mediastinum testis
Obturator internus muscle
Pampiniform plexus
Penis
Perineum
Peripheral zone
Periurethral glandular zone
Prostate
Rectum
Rete testis
Scrotum
Semen
Seminal vesicles
Spermatic cord
Spermatogenesis
Testicles/Testis
Transition zone
Tunica albuginea
Tunica dartos
Tunica vaginalis
Urethra
Verumontanum

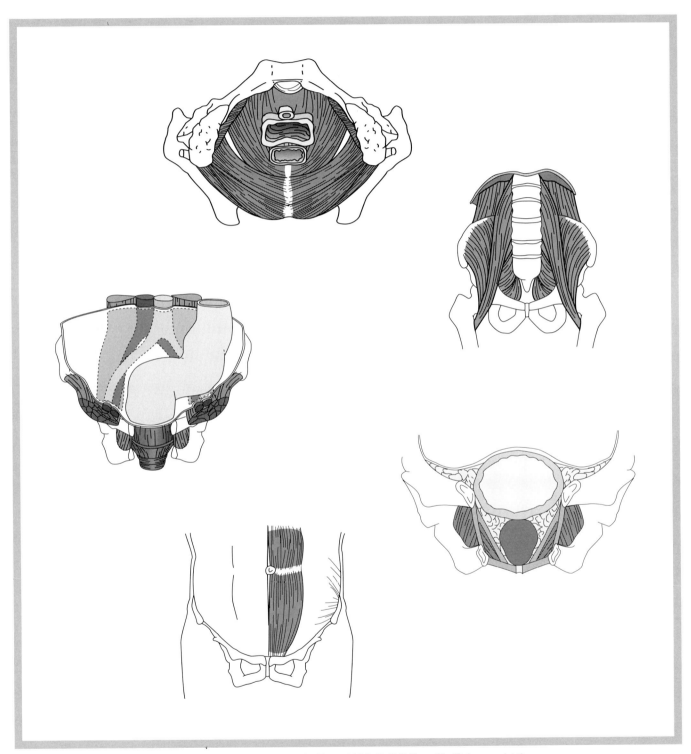

Anatomic layers of the male pelvis. See Figure 4–4 A, B, C, E, F, pp. 48–49, for more details.

INTRODUCTION

This chapter on the male pelvis/genitourinary system includes the scrotum, testicles, seminal vesicles, prostate, penis, and related structures. Other structures within the male pelvis, ie, the urinary bladder, ureters, muscles, and vasculature which are described elsewhere, are not included (see Figure 14–1).

PRENATAL DEVELOPMENT

Gender is initially determined by the presence (male) or absence (female) of the Y chromosome during conception. Until the seventh or eighth week of gestation, male and female embryos appear identical.[1]

The testicles arise in the fetal upper abdomen near the developing kidneys.[1,2] In the fourth month, the testes descend to the level of the urinary bladder, where they will remain until approximately the seventh month of gestation. The testes descend through the **inguinal canal** and into the scrotum after the seventh month. This descent is hormonally controlled and usually happens dur-

ing the last month of gestation but occasionally does not occur until the first weeks of neonatal life.[2]

The prostate develops during the third month of gestation.[1] The apex of the urinary bladder (already formed) narrows to form the prostatic urethra. Prostate buds develop as outgrowths of the urethra. These buds develop into tubules, which elongate and multiply to form the lobes of the new prostate gland.[1]

The external genitals of both male and female embryos remain undifferentiated until the eighth week of gestation.[1] Prior to the eighth week, all embryos have a region called the genital tubercle. The genital tubercle is an elevated area between the coccyx and the umbilical cord where the mesonephric and paramesonephric ducts empty.[1,2] In males, the genital tubercle elongates and develops into the penis.

LOCATION

The **scrotum** is a sac of cutaneous tissue that supports the testicles, or testes, the paired organs of reproduction. The **testes** are the male gonads and are classified as both

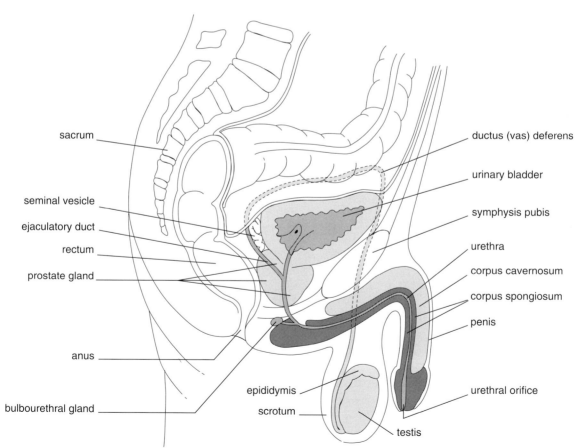

Figure 14–1. Male pelvis. Sagittal cross-section of the male pelvis illustrating the relationships of genital organs to surrounding structures.

endocrine and exocrine glands. The testes produce sperm, which are transported through a network of ducts (exocrine function) that store and transport the sperm. The accessory organs, the seminal vesicles and the prostate, add secretions, called **semen** to the sperm. The penis has two functions: it ejects sperm and semen from the body and excretes urine.

Scrotum and Contents

The scrotum is a pouch of skin that is continuous with the abdomen. It is suspended from the base of the male pelvis between the **perineum** and the penis. The scrotum contains the testicles, epididymis, and the proximal portion of the ductus deferens.

The **epididymis** is connected to the superior portion of the testis and runs along the posterior aspect to the base of the testis. The epididymis drains into the ductus deferens at the base of the testis. The **ductus deferens** courses superiorly and exits the scrotum through the **inguinal canal**. Once inside the abdominal cavity, each ductus deferens courses along the lateral aspect of the urinary bladder and turns medially and posteriorly to connect with the seminal vesicles.

Seminal Vesicles

The **seminal vesicles** are paired glands that lie posterior to the urinary bladder just superior to the prostate. Each seminal vesicle angles medially toward the apex of the bladder and lies medial to the ureters. Each seminal vesicle joins with its corresponding ductus deferens to form an **ejaculatory duct.** The two ejaculatory ducts course through the prostate gland and empty into the prostatic urethra.

Prostate

The **prostate** is a doughnut-like gland that lies inferior to the urinary bladder surrounding the proximal urethra. The prostate lies behind the symphysis pubis and is separated posteriorly from the **rectum** by the two layers of **Denonvillier's fascia.** Laterally, the prostate is supported by the **obturator internus** and **levator ani muscles.**[1] Prostatic secretions are conveyed through numerous prostatic ducts to the prostatic urethra, located at the central core of the prostate. The fluids are then carried outside the body through the penis via the distal urethra and finally exit through the external urethral orifice.

SIZE

Testis

The normal adult testicle measures approximately 3 to 5 cm (1.5 to 2 inches) in length, 2 to 3 cm (1 inch) in anterior to posterior dimension, and 2 to 3 cm (1 inch) in width.[2,3] Between the ages of 12 and 17 years, the testicle undergoes rapid growth. Prior to age 12, the average testicular volume is less than 5 mL. After maturity, the average testicular volume is approximately 25 mL with the testicle weighing between 10 and 15 g.[2] The testicle gradually decreases in size with advancing age.

Epididymis

The epididymis is actually a single, tightly wrapped tube—the ductus epididymis. When unwrapped, the ductus epididymis measures about 6 m (20 feet) in length and about 1 mm in diameter.[2] The epididymis (head, body, and tail combined), as seen grossly, measures only 3.8 cm (1.5 inches) in length.[2,3] The epididymis empties into the ductus deferens, which measures approximately 45 cm (18 inches) in length.[2]

Seminal Vesicles

The seminal vesicles are convoluted pouch-like structures emptying into the distal portion of the ductus deferens to form the ejaculatory ducts. Each seminal vesicle measures approximately 5 cm (2 inches) in length and less than 1 cm in diameter.[2,4]

Prostate

The prostate is a single gland weighing about 20 g.[1] It normally measures approximately 4 cm (less than 2 inches) transversely, 3 cm (1.5 inches) in anteroposterior dimension, and 3.8 cm (1.5 inches) in cephalocaudal dimension.[1] Unlike most other organs that atrophy with age, the prostate sometimes enlarges owing to benign changes in the gland, infection, presence of malignant tumors, or other causes.[1,4,5]

GROSS ANATOMY

Figure 14–2 illustrates the scrotum and its contents.

Scrotum

The skin and superficial fascia of the scrotum are continuous with those of the abdomen. Externally, the scrotum is divided into lateral portions by a median ridge called the **raphe.** Internally, the scrotum is divided into sacs by a septum consisting of the dartos, or **tunica dartos.** The dartos contains superficial fascia and contractile tissue, which is also continuous with the subcutaneous tissue of the abdominal wall and is abundantly supplied by small vessels. Just posterior to the dartos lies the external spermatic fascia, which is a continuation of the external oblique fascia of the abdominal wall. The

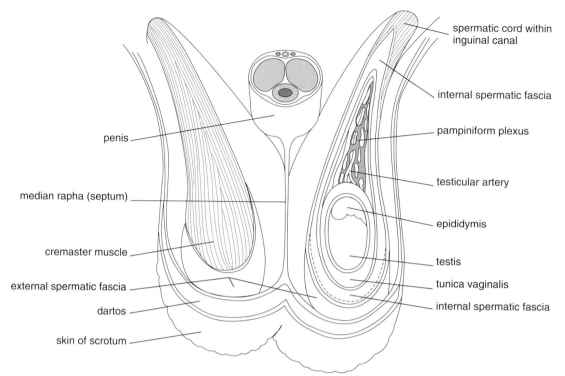

Figure 14–2. Dissected scrotum and its contents.

cremaster muscle surrounds each testicle and extends into the abdomen over the spermatic cord. The cremaster muscle is covered by the cremasteric fascia; this is continuous with the internal oblique fascia of the abdomen. Contraction of the cremaster muscle performs the important function of regulating the temperature of the testicles. Deep to the cremaster muscle is the innermost fascial layer of the scrotum, the internal spermatic fascia or infundibuliform fascia. This inner fascia surrounds the covering layers of the testicles, the **tunica vaginalis.** The tunica vaginalis consists of two layers derived from the perineum, an outer parietal layer that is closely attached to the internal spermatic fascia, and an inner visceral layer which is closely attached to the testicle.[2]

Testis

Figure 14–3 illustrates the testis, epididymis, and ductus (vas) deferens.

Each testis is covered by a dense, white fibrous tissue called **tunica albuginea** testis. The tunica albuginea extends into the posterior wall of the testicle and forms the **mediastinum testis** and interlobar septae. The septae of the mediastinum radiate into the testicle and separate into 200 to 300 lobules.[2,3] Each lobule contains one to three **convoluted seminiferous tubules,** which produce sperm through a process called **spermatogenesis.** The seminiferous tubules empty the spermatozoa into the straight tubules, which lead to a network of ducts called the **rete testis.** The rete testis is located within the medi-astinum testis and this network connects and exits the testis through the mediastinum testis as a series of coiled **efferent ducts.**[2,3]

The blood supply to the testicles is via the internal spermatic arteries, which arise from the midabdomen as branches of the aorta just inferior to the renal vessels.[2] The right testicular vein drains into the inferior cava at the level near the renal veins. The left testicular vein drains into the left renal vein.[5]

Epididymis

The **epididymis** is composed mostly of a single convoluted tube, the **ductus epididymis,** encapsulated by a serosal layer.[2] The ductus epididymis is lined by pseudostratified columnar epithelium, and its walls contain a thin layer of smooth muscle. The ductus epididymis is subdivided into a head (globus major), body, and tail (globus minor).[2,3] The head of the epididymis is the larger, superior portion consisting mostly of the efferent ducts that empty into the ductus epididymis. The body runs along the posterior aspect of the testis and contains the ductus epididymis. The tail is the smaller, inferior portion, where the ductus epididymis empties into the ductus deferens.

Ductus (vas) Deferens

The **ductus deferens** is a thicker, less convoluted continuation of the ductus epididymis. Three smooth mus-

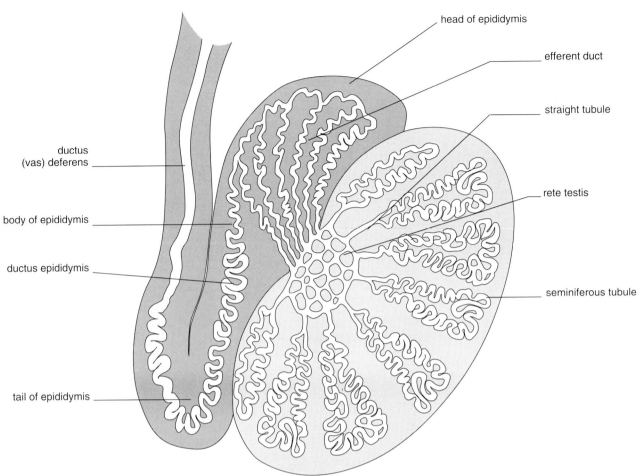

Figure 14-3. Enlarged longitudinal cross-section of testis, epididymis, and ductus (vas) deferens illustrating the complex network of ducts needed to transport sperm.

cle layers contribute to this duct's increased thickness. At its terminal portion near the seminal vesicles, the ductus deferens dilates; this area is referred to as the *ampulla of the deferens.*[2]

Spermatic Cord

The two spermatic cords extend from the scrotum through the inguinal canals and internal inguinal rings into the pelvis. Each **spermatic cord** contains the ductus deferens, testicular arteries, venous **pampiniform plexus** (veins which drain the testes and become the spermatic veins superiorly), lymphatics, autonomic nerves, and fibers of the cremaster muscle.[1-3]

Seminal Vesicles

The seminal vesicles are paired glands each encapsulated by connective tissue. Beneath the connective tissue is a thin layer of smooth muscle that surrounds the submucosa and mucous membrane. The seminal vesicles join with the ductus deferens to form the ejaculatory ducts, which course through the prostate and empty into the prostatic urethra.[1,2]

Prostate

The prostate is shaped like a cone with a central core, the prostatic urethra.[1,6] The tip of the cone, or apex, is the inferior margin of the prostate and provides an exit for the urethra. The base of the gland is the superior aspect, which is in contact with the urinary bladder. The prostate is perforated by the two ejaculatory ducts, which enter the prostate at its posterior margin and course obliquely and anteriorly to join the prostatic urethra near the verumontanum, an area close to the center of the prostate.[1,5,6]

The prostate consists of a small anterior fibromuscular region and a much larger posterior glandular region. The **fibromuscular stroma** is located anterior to the prostatic urethra and is generally of less clinical significance because most pathology occurs in the glandular areas. The posterior glandular portion of the prostate has been described as consisting of zones. Dividing the glandular

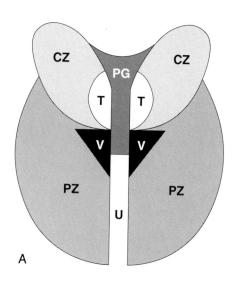

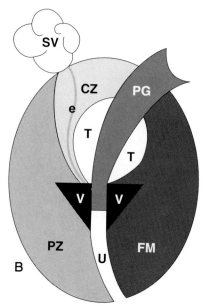

Figure 14-4. *A,* Zonal anatomy of the prostate in the coronal plane. PG = periurethral glandular tissue (or zone); CZ = central zone; T = transition zone; V = verumontanum; PZ = peripheral zone; U = prostatic urethra. *B,* Zonal anatomy of prostate in the sagittal plane. SV = seminal vesicles; CZ = central zone; E = ejaculatory duct; PG = periurethral glandular tissue (or zone); T = transitional zone; V = verumontanum; PZ = peripheral zone; FM = fibromuscular stroma; U = prostatic urethra.

prostate into zones is probably the most useful representation for imaging the prostate.[6] There are four zones within the glandular prostate: the peripheral zone, the central zone, the transition zone, and the periurethral glandular tissue or zone.[6]

The **peripheral zone** is the largest, making up approximately 70 percent of the glandular prostate. This zone occupies the area lateral and posterior to the distal prostatic urethra. The **central zone** forms about 20 percent of the glandular prostate and is located at the superior edge bordering the bladder and seminal vesicles. The ejaculatory ducts course through this zone. The **transition zone** comprises only about 5 percent of the glandular prostate and has two lobes situated on the lateral aspects of the proximal prostatic urethra superior to the verumontanum. The transition zone borders the central zone posteriorly and laterally and the fibromuscular tissue anteriorly. The tissue that lines the proximal prostatic urethra forms the **periurethral glandular zone.**[6] Figure 14-4A depicts the zonal anatomy of the prostate in the coronal plane; Figure 14-4B illustrates the prostatic anatomy in the sagittal plane. The prostate is surrounded by a thin capsule consisting of dense fibrous tissue and smooth muscle. This capsule connects with the muscle layers of the prostatic urethra. The prostatic urethra is divided by the **verumontanum** (area near the center of the prostate) into proximal and distal segments. These proximal and distal segments form an angle of approximately 35 degrees at the verumontanum.[1,6]

Penis

Figure 14-5A illustrates the gross anatomy of the penis in the coronal plane; Figure 14-5B depicts penile anatomy in the transverse plane.

The **penis** is composed of three cylindrical masses of tissue. There are two **corpora cavernosa** situated dorsolaterally and a single **corpus spongiosum** in the midventral region, which contains the spongy **urethra.** The three corpora are bound and separated by the fibrous tissue called the **tunica albuginea.** Superficial to the tunica albuginea is **Buck's fascia,** a thick fibrous envelope, and a loosely applied covering of skin.[2]

The three corpora are composed of smooth muscle and erectile tissue that enclose vascular cavities. The penis becomes enlarged and erect when engorged with venous blood.

The blood supply to the penis and urethra is via the paired internal pudendal arteries, branches of the internal iliac arteries. These arteries divide into a deep artery of the penis and the bulbourethral artery. The deep artery of the penis supplies the corpora cavernosa. Branches of the dorsal artery and bulbourethral artery supply the corpus spongiosum, glans penis, and urethra.[2]

The main veins of the penis are the superficial dorsal vein and the deep dorsal vein. The superficial dorsal vein is located outside Buck's fascia while the deep dorsal vein is beneath Buck's fascia. The superficial and deep dorsal veins connect with the pudendal venous plexus, which drains the penis via the internal pudendal vein.

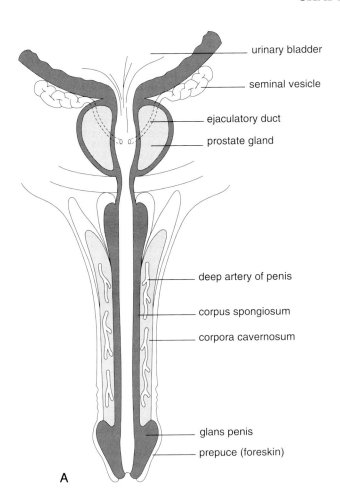

- urinary bladder
- seminal vesicle
- ejaculatory duct
- prostate gland
- deep artery of penis
- corpus spongiosum
- corpora cavernosum
- glans penis
- prepuce (foreskin)

A

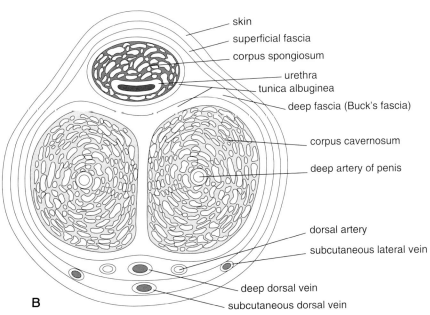

- skin
- superficial fascia
- corpus spongiosum
- urethra
- tunica albuginea
- deep fascia (Buck's fascia)
- corpus cavernosum
- deep artery of penis
- dorsal artery
- subcutaneous lateral vein
- deep dorsal vein
- subcutaneous dorsal vein

B

Figure 14–5. *A*, Gross anatomy of the penis in the coronal plane. *B*, Gross penile anatomy in the transverse plane.

PHYSIOLOGY

The process by which genetic information is passed from one generation of a species to the next is called *reproduction*. In human reproduction, 23 chromosomes are passed from the male gamete, or sperm cell, to the female gamete, or ovum, which also contains 23 chromosomes. Through the union of these gametes, a zygote is formed, containing a total of 46 chromosomes. Multiple divisions of the zygote develop into a new organism.

The male gametes, or spermatozoa, are produced in the testes by the process of meiosis. The seminiferous tubules within the testicle are lined with spermatogonia. These spermatogonia develop into mature spermatozoa through the process of **spermatogenesis.** The entire process takes approximately 2 to 3 weeks. Approximately 300 million spermatozoa mature every day.[2] The spermatozoa are transported out of the testes into the ductus epididymis, where the final maturation of the sperm occurs. The spermatozoa can remain viable in storage for up to 4 weeks, after which time they are reabsorbed. The function of the ductal system is to store and help propel the sperm during ejaculation.[2]

The production of sperm might be considered the most important function of the male reproductive system, but without the secretions of the accessory organs, the sperm could not survive to complete the process of reproduction. The **seminal vesicles** secrete an alkaline, viscous fluid rich in fructose, which contributes to sperm viability. This fluid constitutes about 60 percent of the volume of semen.[2,6]

The **prostate** also produces and secretes an alkaline fluid. Its secretions constitute between 13 and 33 percent of the volume of semen.[6] This alkaline fluid is believed to neutralize the acid environment of the vagina, uterus, and fallopian tubes, where fertilization of the ovum takes place.

The reproductive function of the penis is to eject semen into the vagina. Sexual stimulation increases the blood supply to the penis. The penile arteries dilate as the penis is engorged with blood. Expansion of these arteries and blood sinuses within the corpora cavernosa causes compression of the veins which drain the penis; thus most of the blood is retained, resulting in an erection. During ejaculation, increased pressure within the urethra causes the urinary bladder sphincter to close. This mechanism prevents urine from being expelled during ejaculation and semen from entering the bladder.[2]

SONOGRAPHIC APPEARANCE

Scrotal Contents

Sonographically, normal testicular parenchyma is homogeneous, containing medium-level echoes similar in ultrasound appearance to those of the thyroid gland.[7,8] (See Figures 14–6 and 14–7.) The highly echogenic line running along the long axis of the testis demonstrates the mediastinum testis. This is a normal finding and should not be mistaken for pathology. A few millimeters of anechoic fluid are also normally seen between the two layers of the tunica vaginalis. Excess fluid may indicate pathology (hydrocele).[7,8]

The head of the epididymis is seen superior and posterior to the testicle. The body and tail of the epididymis are not normally identified.[8] The echogenicity of the epididymis is equal to or slightly greater than that of the

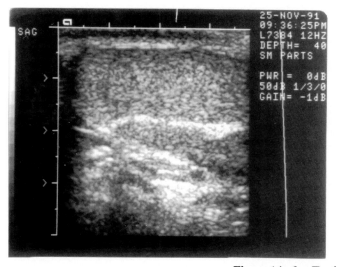
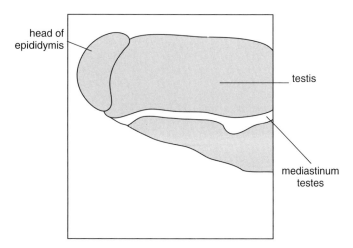

Figure 14–6. Testis in the sagittal plane.

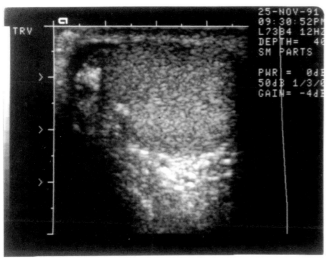

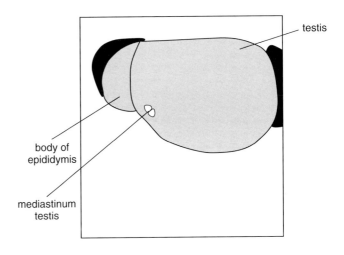

Figure 14–7. Scrotum in the transverse plane.

normal testicle.[7,8] However, the texture of the epididymis is generally more coarse in appearance.

The various layers of the scrotum are not normally differentiated on ultrasound. The combination of the scrotal wall layers typically appears as a single, highly echogenic stripe.[7]

The spermatic cord may be visualized at it courses through the inguinal canal. Color flow Doppler is useful in identifying the blood vessels within the cord; however, the ductus deferens is not normally seen.

Seminal Vesicles and Prostate

Ultrasound examination of the seminal vesicles and prostate may be performed by either the transabdominal method through a distended urinary bladder or by the transrectal approach. The transabdominal method is used only to assess the size of the glands, as most pathol-

ogy is not well demonstrated with this technique. The transrectal approach is superior for scanning the seminal vesicles and prostate because of the close proximity of the transducer to the area of interest.[1,6]

The transrectal ultrasound appearance of the seminal vesicles and prostate is described below.

Sonographically, the seminal vesicles are demonstrated as structures with low level echoes superior to the prostate.[6,9] In the transverse plane, the seminal vesicles are seen in their long axis. Figure 14–8 illustrates the seminal vesicles in the transverse plane. Normally they should be symmetrical in size, shape, and echogenicity. In the longitudinal or sagittal plane, the seminal vesicles are identified as ovoid structures with low level echoes superior to the prostate gland.[9] Figure 14–9 demonstrates the prostate and seminal vesicles in the longitudinal plane. The prostate is sonographically heterogeneous, with medium level echoes.[6] It contains glandular

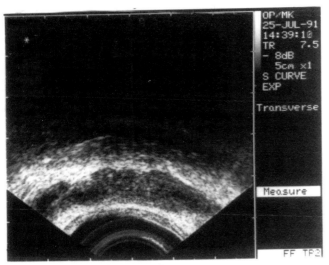

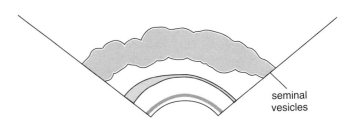

Figure 14–8. Seminal vesicles in the transverse plane.

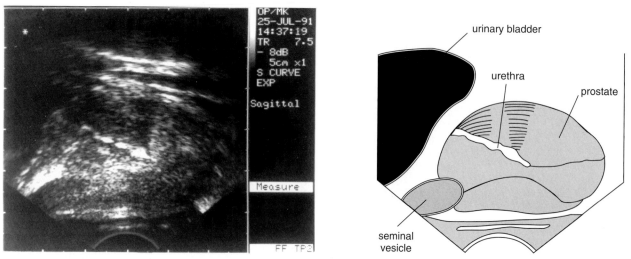

Figure 14-9. Normal sonographic relationship of the prostate and seminal vesicles in the longitudinal plane.

and fibromuscular tissue, which surrounds the prostatic urethra. The normal prostate should always appear symmetrical.[6,10,11] (See Figure 14-9).

Transrectally, in the transverse plane, the prostate will appear semilunar in shape near the base (superiorly) and will become more rounded near the apex (inferiorly). The normal prostate will appear hyperechoic to the normal seminal vesicles. An area of low level echoes situated anteriorly and in the midline represents the periurethral tissue and fibromuscular stroma. In the normal prostate, the central zone and transition zone cannot be individually distinguished, whereas the peripheral zone may appear more echogenic and homogeneous in comparison.[6,10] The peripheral zone occupies the posterior and lateral portions of the gland. (See Figure 14-10).

Longitudinally in the midline, the hypoechoic periurethral tissues will be visualized and may be difficult to differentiate from the anterior fibromuscular stroma, which can also appear hypoechoic.[6] The peripheral zone should normally be homogeneous and slightly more echogenic.[6,10,11]

Penis

The most extensive role of penile ultrasonography is in the evaluation of vasculogenic impotence. The advent of duplex ultrasound has made this diagnosis possible.[12] Another use of penile ultrasound is detection of pathologic abnormalities such as fibrosis, tumors, and periurethral diseases.

In the transverse plane, the corpus spongiosum will be seen in the midline, compressed by the transducer, and will appear elliptical in shape. Sonographically, the corpus spongiosum should be of homogeneous texture

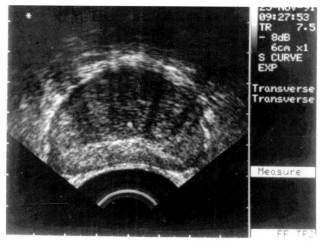

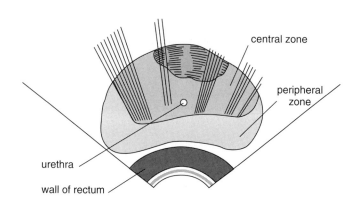

Figure 14-10. Normal prostate in the transverse plane.

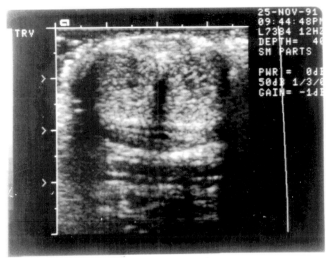

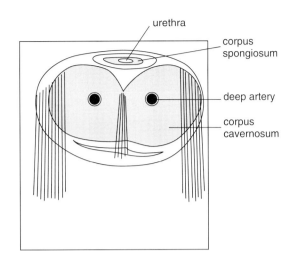

Figure 14–11. Penis in the transverse plane.

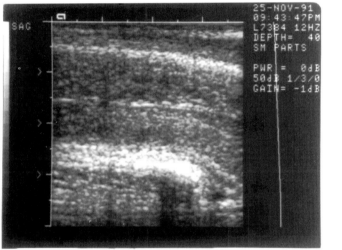

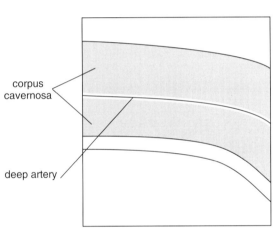

Figure 14–12. Penis in the longitudinal plane.

composed of medium level echoes.[12,13] The paired corpora cavernosa are posterior to the corpus spongiosum and appear symmetrically round or oval in shape also, with a medium level homogeneous echo texture.[12,13] The corpora cavernosa are covered by the highly echogenic tunica albuginea. The echogenic plane dividing the two appears symmetrically round or oval in shape also with a medium level homogeneous echo texture. The corpora cavernosa are covered by the highly echogenic tunica albuginea. The echogenic plane dividing the two corpora cavernosa is an extension of the tunica albuginea called the septum penis. Centrally located within the corpora cavernosa are cavernosal arteries, which can be identified by their echogenic walls and pulsations as seen in real time.[12,13] Figure 14–11 demonstrates the penis in the transverse plane.

In the longitudinal plane, each corpus cavernosum should remain homogeneous with highly echogenic tunica albuginea visualized above and below. The cavernosal arteries will be imaged in their long axis and appear as parallel echogenic lines, representing the walls of the artery, coursing through the middle of the corpora cavernosa.[13] Figure 14–12 illustrates the penis in the longitudinal plane.

SONOGRAPHIC APPLICATIONS

Scrotum

1. Testicular size
2. Inflammatory processes (epididymitis, orchitis)

3. Presence and composition of masses

4. Detection of peritesticular fluid collections (hydrocele)

5. Evaluation of scrotal trauma

6. Doppler evaluation to rule out testicular torsion

7. Evaluation of scrotal pain

8. Location of undescended testicles

Prostate

1. Prostatic size and echo texture

2. Evaluation of infection (prostatitis)

3. Detection of masses

4. Evaluation of benign prostatic hypertrophy (BPH)

5. Sonographic correlation of findings on a digital rectal examination

6. Sonographic correlation of evaluated serum prostatic specific antigen (PSA)

7. Evaluation of extracapsular spread of prostatic carcinoma

8. Evaluation of postoperative transurethral resection (TURP)

9. Ultrasound guided biopsies of prostatic lesions

Seminal Vesicles

1. Evaluate size, symmetry, and echo texture

2. Presence of cysts or calculi

3. Inflammatory processes

4. Congenital anomalies

Penis

1. Detection of fibrosis (Peyronie's disease)

2. Detection of scar tissue and plaques

3. Evaluation of tumors

4. Penile hematoma

5. Evaluation of periurethral disease

6. Doppler evaluation of vasculogenic impotence

NORMAL VARIANTS

Cryptorchidism is a failure of the testicles to descend into the scrotum. Common locations of undescended testes include the abdomen, inguinal canal, and at the external inguinal ring.

REFERENCE CHARTS

Associated Physicians

Urologist: Specializes in surgical diseases of the male genitourinary tract and female urinary system.

Common Diagnostic Tests

Magnetic Resonance Imaging (MRI): MRI is a noninvasive imaging modality, that is very useful in identifying soft tissue structures. It is performed by a radiologic technologist and interpreted by a radiologist.

Ultrasonography: Second to direct physical palpation by a urologist, it is the method of choice for evaluating the male genitourinary system. It is performed by a radiologic technologist and interpreted by a radiologist.

Laboratory Values

Serum Prostatic Specific Antigen (PSA): This is used to evaluate the function of the prostate. Normal serum PSA is less than 4.0. Elevated serum PSA may indicate disease but is not specific for carcinoma.

Normal Measurements

Normal adult testicle: 3 to 5 cm in length; 2 to 3 cm in width; 2 to 3 cm anteroposterior

Epididymis: 3.8 cm in length; uncoiled, 6 m

Ductus (vas) deferens: 45 cm

Seminal vesicles: 5 cm in length, less than 1 cm in diameter

Prostate: 4 cm transverse, 3 cm anteroposterior; 3.8 cm in length

Vasculature

Nonapplicable.

Affecting Chemicals

Nonapplicable.

References

1. Rifkin MD: Ultrasound of the Prostate. New York, Raven Press, 1988.
2. Tortora GJ, Anagnostakos NP: Principles of Anatomy and Physiology, 5th ed. New York, Harper and Row, 1987, 706–708, 713–718, 733–735.

3. Tanagho EA, McAninch JW: Smith's General Urology, 12th ed. Norwalk, CT, Appleton & Lange, 1988, 7–13.
4. DeVere White RW, Plamer JM: New Techniques in Urology. Mt. Kisco, NY, Futura, 1987, 235–240, 251–258.
5. Walsh PC, Gittes RF, Perlmutter AD, et al, eds: Campbell's Urology, 5th ed., vol. I. Philadelphia, WB Saunders, 1986, 47–69.
6. Kammermeier, MJ: Carcinoma of the prostate: What every sonographer should know. J Diagnostic Med Sonog 1991, 7:139–146.
7. Hoddic WK, Hricak H, Jeffrey RB: Scrotal sonography. Semin Urol III(2):146–147, 1985.
8. Krone KD, Carrol BA: Scrotal ultrasound. Radiol Clin N Am 23:121–129, 1985.
9. Asch MR, Toi A: Seminal vesicles: imaging and intervention using transrectal ultrasound. J Ultrasound Med 10:19–23, 1991.
10. Fornage BD: Normal ultrasound anatomy of the prostate. J Ultrasound Med Biol 12:1011–1021, 1986.
11. Dakin R, Bedigian K, Grube GL: Transrectal ultrasound of the prostate: technique and sonographic findings. J Diagnostic Med Sonog 1:1–5, 1989.
12. Hattery RR, King BF, Lewis RW, et al: Vasculogenic impotence: duplex and color Doppler imaging. Radiol Clin N Am 29:629–645, 1991.
13. Quam JP, King BF, James EM, et al: Duplex and color Doppler sonographic evaluation and vasculogenic impotence. Am J Radiol 153:1141–1147, 1989.

Bibliography

Benson BC, Vickers MA: Sexual impotence caused by vascular disease: Diagnosis with duplex sonography. Am J Radiol 153:1149–1153, 1989.
Coleman BG: Genitourinary Ultrasound; A Test/Atlas. New York, Igaku-Shoin, 1988, 375–380, 406–412.
Krysiewacz S, Mellinger BC: The role of imaging in the diagnostic evaluation of impotence. Am J Radiol 153:1133–1134, 1989.
Littrup PJ, Lee F, McLeary RD, et al: Transrectal ultrasound of seminal vesicles and ejaculatory ducts: clinical correlation. Radiology 168:625–628, 1988.
Resnick MI, Rifkin MD, eds: Ultrasonography of the Urinary Tract, 3rd ed. Baltimore, Williams & Wilkins, 1991, 300–309.
O'Reilly PH, George NJR, Weiss RM: Diagnostic Techniques in Radiology. Philadelphia, WB Saunders, 1990, 93–97.
Rifkin MD: Diagnostic Imaging of the Lower Genitourinary Tract. New York, Raven Press, 1985, 10–19, 21–26.
Rifkin MD, Kurtz AB, Pasto ME, Goldberg BB: Diagnostic capabilities of high-resolution scrotal ultrasonography: L perspective evaluation. J Ultrasound Med 4:13–19, 1985.
Schwartz AN, Lowe M, Berger RE, et al: Assessment of normal and abnormal erectile function: color Doppler flow sonography versus conventional techniques. Radiology 180:105–109, 1991.
Schwartz AN, Wang KY, Mack LA, et al: Evaluation of normal erectile function with color flow Doppler sonography. Am J Radiol 153:1155–1160, 1989.

Chapter 15

THE FEMALE PELVIS

DEBORAH D. WERNEBURG

Objectives:

Describe the anatomy, physiology, and function of the female reproductive organs of the pelvis.

Describe the sonographic appearance of the organs, muscles, and surrounding structures of the true pelvis.

Define physicians, diagnostic tests, laboratory values, and key words relevant to sonography of the female pelvis.

Define the key words.

Key Words:

Adnexa
Ampulla
Anteflexed uterus
Anterior cul de sac
Anteverted uterus
Bicornuate uterus
Broad ligaments
Cervix
Color flow Doppler

Cornu (cornua)
Corpus albicans
Corpus luteum
Cumulus oophorus
Dominant follicle
Endometrial canal (uterine cavity)
Endometrium
Estrogen
External os
False pelvis
Fimbria (fimbriae)
Follicle stimulating hormone (FSH)
Follicular antrum
Follicular phase
Germinal epithelium
Graafian follicle
Human chorionic gonadotropin (hCG)
Iliopsoas muscles
In vitro fertilization
Infundibulum of fallopian tube
Internal os
Interstitial segment of fallopian tube
Intrauterine contraceptive device (IUD, IUCD)
Isthmus of fallopian tube

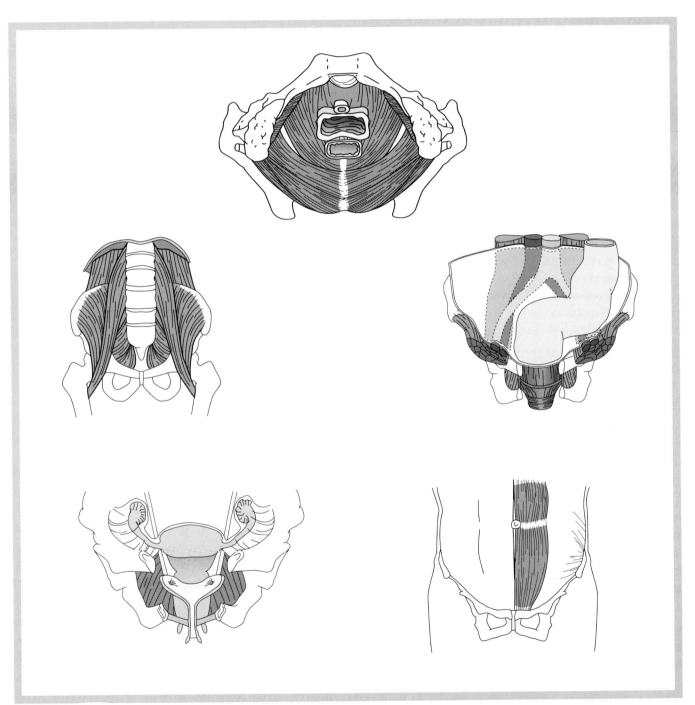

Anatomic layers of the female pelvis. See Figure 4–4 A, B, C, D, E, pp. 48–49, for more details.

Isthmus of uterus
Linea terminalis
Luteal phase of ovarian cycle
Luteinizing hormone (LH)
Menses
Müllerian ducts
Myometrium
Obturator internus muscles
Ovarian cortex
Ovarian hilum
Ovarian medulla
Ovulation
Pelvic diaphragm
Peritoneum
Posterior cul de sac
Progesterone
Proliferative phase of endometrium
Rectus abdominis muscles
Retroflexed uterus
Retroverted uterus
Round ligaments
Ruga (Rugae)
Secretory phase of endometrium
Spectral Doppler
True pelvis
Tunica albuginea
Uterine corpus
Uterine fundus
Vaginal fornix (fornices)

INTRODUCTION

The abdominopelvic cavity is a continuous space containing the major organs of the abdomen and pelvis. The pelvic cavity is the caudal portion of the abdominopelvic cavity, extending from the iliac crests superiorly to the pelvic diaphragm inferiorly.

The outer boundaries of the pelvic cavity are formed by the osseous pelvis. Deep to this bony framework lie the skeletal muscles lining the abdominopelvic cavity. The organs contained within the female pelvis include the urinary bladder, genital tract, ovaries, and pelvic colon.

The ovaries and the genital tract comprise the primary reproductive organs of the female. The ovaries are paired organs, responsible for the production of female gametes. The human ovum is fertilized within the fallopian tube. The fertilized ovum is transported to the uterus through the fallopian tube. The uterus provides a suitable environment for implantation of the fertilized egg and for fetal development. Together, the fallopian tubes, uterus, and vagina form the continuous muscular channel of the genital tract.

PRENATAL DEVELOPMENT

The reproductive organs develop with the urinary system from two urogenital folds in the early embryo. Each urogenital fold consists of a gonad and a mesonephros.

Differentiation of the gonads into ovaries or testes is dependent on the genetic make-up of the embryo. The gonads are initially located in a cephalad position and descend into the true pelvis during fetal development.

The mesonephros is the precursor of the metanephros,

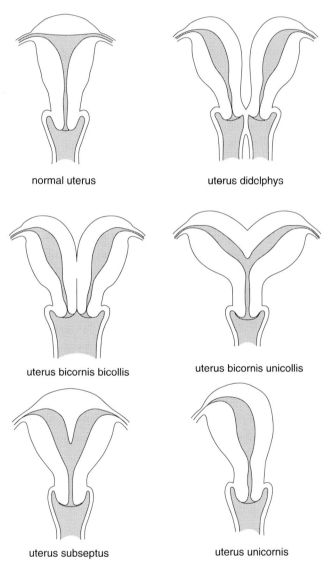

Figure 15-1. This figure illustrates some congenital uterine malformations, anatomical variations of the uterus, cervix, and vagina resulting from the incomplete fusion or agenesis of the Müllerian ducts. Complete duplication of the vagina, cervix, and uterine horns is seen in uterus didelphys. The bicornuate uterus has two uterine horns which are fused at one cervix (uterus bicornis unicollis) or at two cervices (uterus bicornis bicollis). Uterus subseptus is a milder anomaly marked by a midline myometrial septum within the endometrial canal. Occasionally only one Müllerian duct develops, forming a single uterine horn and a fallopian tube continuous with one cervix and vagina (uterus unicornis).

the urogenital sinus, the Wolffian (mesonephric) ducts, and the Müllerian (paramesonephric) ducts. The metanephros and the urogenital sinus form the urinary system. The Wolffian and Müllerian ducts form the male and female genital tracts, respectively. The Müllerian ducts of the female embryo fuse midline to form the vagina, uterus, and fallopian tubes. The Wolffian ducts degenerate in the female embryo, leaving only remnants along the broad ligaments and the vaginal walls.

Bicornuate uterus is the most common of numerous congenital malformations of the female genital tract. This abnormality is characterized by partial duplication of the uterus resulting from incomplete fusion of the müllerian ducts. (See Figure 15–1 for a depiction of various congenital malformations of the uterus.)

LOCATION

The uterus is located in the midregion of the true pelvis. This organ lies superoposterior to the urinary bladder and anterior to the sigmoid colon. The anterior and posterior walls of the uterus are lined by peritoneum.

The vagina extends from the uterus to the external genitalia. The vagina sits posterior to both the urinary bladder and the urethra. It is anterior to the rectum.

The fallopian tubes extend from the uterus to the ovaries, which are situated more laterally within the true pelvis. The tubes course within the peritoneal folds of the broad ligaments. They are lateral to the uterus, anteromedial to the ovaries, and posterior to the urinary bladder.

The ovaries lie within the peritoneal cavity, posterior to the broad ligaments. They are quite mobile and may be located anywhere within the adnexal regions. Most commonly, the ovaries are situated posterolateral to the uterus. They may lie posterior or superior to the uterus. While their anatomic position is variable, they cannot be located anterior to the uterus or broad ligaments.

The ureters and internal iliac vessels course posterior to the ovaries. The iliopsoas muscles border the ovaries laterally. The external iliac vessels lie anterolateral to each ovary.

SIZE

Uterus

The adult nulliparous uterus is approximately 8 cm in length, 3 cm anteroposteriorly, and 5.5 cm in width. The cervix is approximately 2 to 3 cm in length.

Age and parity are two important factors influencing uterine size and shape. The corpus and fundus of the uterus show considerably more variation in size than the more rigid cervix. In childhood, the uterus measures approximately 2.5 cm in length, 1 cm in thickness, and 2 cm in width. While the uterus is smaller in size, the cervix comprises a significantly greater proportion of the organ in the child than in the adult.

During puberty, the corpus and fundus enlarge and the uterus takes on its characteristic pear shape. The multiparous uterus may be significantly larger than the nulliparous uterus due to growth of the corpus and fundus. Following menopause, the corpus and fundus shrink, and the uterine size and shape are similar to those of childhood.

Ovaries

Normal ovarian size varies during the life span. The normal measurements during reproductive years range from 2.5 to 5 cm in length, 0.6 to 2.2 cm in thickness, and 1.5 to 3 cm in width. Prior to puberty and in the postmenopausal years, the ovaries are much smaller. Postmenopausal ovaries should not exceed 2 cm in length, 1 cm in thickness, and 2 cm in width.

Ovarian volume may also be used as a measure of normal size and is calculated as follows:

$$Volume = (length) \times (AP\ thickness) \times (width) \times (0.523)$$

In women between the ages of 15 and 55 years, normal ovarian volume ranges from 6 to 13 cc. These parameters may be exceeded when ovarian pathology exists or under normal conditions in the presence of a large follicle.

GROSS ANATOMY

Pelvic Skeleton

The pelvic skeleton consists of the sacrum, coccyx, and the innominate bones. The sacrum and coccyx constitute the distal segment of the vertebral spine, and form the posterior border of the pelvic cavity. The innominate bones encircle most of the pelvic cavity, forming its lateral and anterior margins. Each innominate bone is comprised of the ilium, ischium, and pubis. The innominate bones join posteriorly at the sacrum and coccyx and fuse anteriorly at the pubic symphysis. The iliac crests of the innominate bones define the most superior aspect of the pelvic cavity. The two iliac crests and the pubic symphysis are palpable external landmarks which aid in evaluating the pelvis. (See Figure 15–2.)

The **linea terminalis** is an imaginary line drawn along the internal circumference of the pelvic skeleton, from the pubic symphysis anteriorly along the arcuate lines of the innominate bones to the sacral promontory posteriorly. The linea terminalis serves as a boundary dividing the pelvic cavity into the false and true pelves. (See Figure 15–3.)

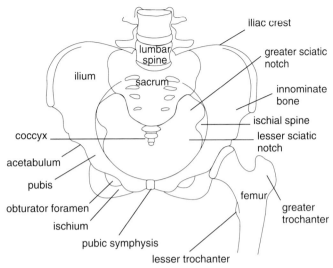

Figure 15-2. The pelvic skeleton.

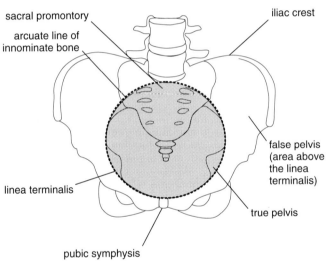

Figure 15-3. The linea terminalis extends from the sacral promontory, along the arcuate lines of the innominate bones, to the pubic symphysis. The true pelvis is the region deep to the linea terminalis. The false pelvis is the region of the abdomino-pelvic cavity which is superior to the linea terminalis and inferior to the iliac crests.

Figure 15-4. The true pelvis is a bowl-shaped cavity which tilts inferoposteriorly.

The **false pelvis** (major or greater pelvis) is defined as the more superior aspect of the pelvic cavity, extending from the iliac crests superiorly to the linea terminalis inferiorly. The remainder of the pelvic cavity extending from the linea terminalis to the pelvic diaphragm inferiorly is known as the **true pelvis** (minor or lesser pelvis). The true pelvis is a bowl-shaped cavity aligned posteriorly and inferiorly within the skeletal framework. The reproductive organs are contained within the true pelvis. (See Figure 15-4.)

Pelvic Musculature

Muscles of the False Pelvis

The major skeletal muscles of the false pelvis include the iliopsoas, rectus abdominis, and transverse abdominis muscles. The psoas major muscles are prominent paired muscles extending across the posterior wall of the abdominopelvic cavity. These muscles originate at the lateral aspects of the lower thoracic vertebrae and course anterolaterally in their descent to the iliac crests. The psoas muscles join the iliacus muscles at the level of the iliac crests to form the **iliopsoas muscles** of the false pelvis. Each iliopsoas muscle courses anteriorly along the linea terminalis and travels over the pelvic brim to insert into the lesser trochanter of the femur. (See Figure 15-5.)

Much of the anterior wall of the abdominopelvic cavity is formed by the **rectus abdominis muscles**, which extend from the sixth ribs and the xiphoid process down to the pubic symphysis. These paired muscles are intersected by transverse tendinous bands and are wrapped in a muscular sheath. The rectus sheath fuses midline at the linea alba. The transverse abdominis muscles form the anterolateral borders of the abdominopelvic cavity. This muscle group lies deep to the internal and external oblique muscles. (See Figure 15-6.)

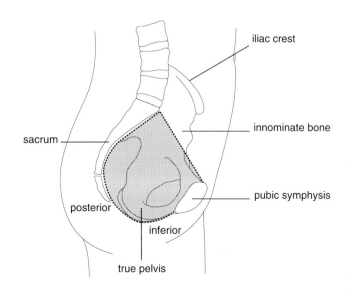

Figure 15–5. In the pelvic musculature, the psoas major muscles and the iliacus muscles join at the level of the iliac crests to form the iliopsoas muscles of the false pelvis. The iliopsoas muscle passes over the pelvic brim, exiting the false pelvis to reach the lesser trochanter of the femur.

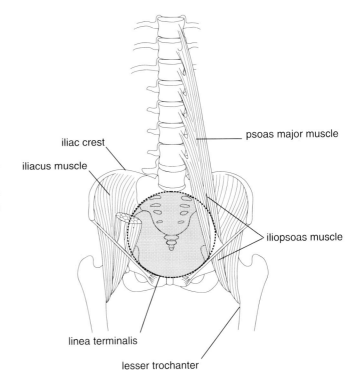

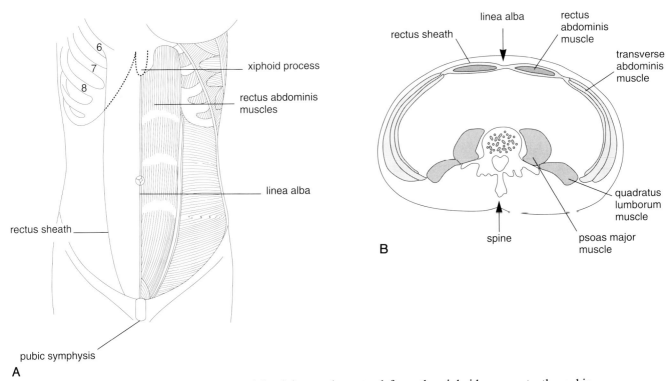

Figure 15–6. *A*, The rectus abdominis muscles extend from the xiphoid process to the pubic symphysis along the anterior abdominal wall. The muscular rectus sheath surrounding the rectus abdominis muscles fuses midline at the linea alba. *B*, Axial section through the midabdomen. The skeletal muscles lining the abdominopelvic cavity include the rectus abdominus muscles anteriorly, the transverse abdominis muscles laterally, and the psoas major and quadratus lumborum muscles posteriorly.

Muscles of the True Pelvis

The skeletal muscles of the true pelvis include the obturator internus muscles, the piriformis muscles, and the muscles of the pelvic diaphragm. The **obturator internus muscles** originate along the arcuate line of the innominate bones and course parallel to the lateral walls of the true pelvis. These triangular muscles narrow inferiorly to pass through the lesser sciatic notch. The obturator internus is secured to the medial aspect of the greater trochanter. The internal surface of this muscle is covered by a tough membranous layer called the obturator fascia.

The piriformis muscles originate in the most posterior aspect of the true pelvis, along the lower portion of the sacrum. These muscles travel anterolaterally, narrowing to pass through the greater sciatic notch. The piriformis muscles are attached to the superior aspect of each greater trochanter. (See Figure 15–7.)

The **pelvic diaphragm** is a group of skeletal muscles lining the floor of the true pelvis and supporting the pelvic organs. This muscular floor is composed of three paired muscles: the pubococcygeus, iliococcygeus, and coccygeus muscles. The pubococcygeus muscles are the

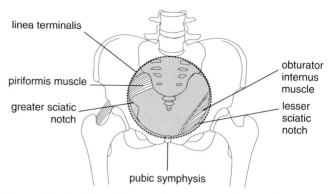

Figure 15–7. The obturator internus muscles line the lateral walls of the true pelvis. The piriformis muscles are situated in the posterior region of the true pelvis and course cross-grain to the obturator internus muscles.

most medial and anterior muscle pair of the pelvic diaphragm. These muscles extend from the pubic bones to the coccyx, encircling the urethra, vagina, and rectum.

The iliococcygeus muscles are located lateral to the pubococcygeus muscles. This pair extends from the obturator fascia and ischial spine anteriorly to the coccyx

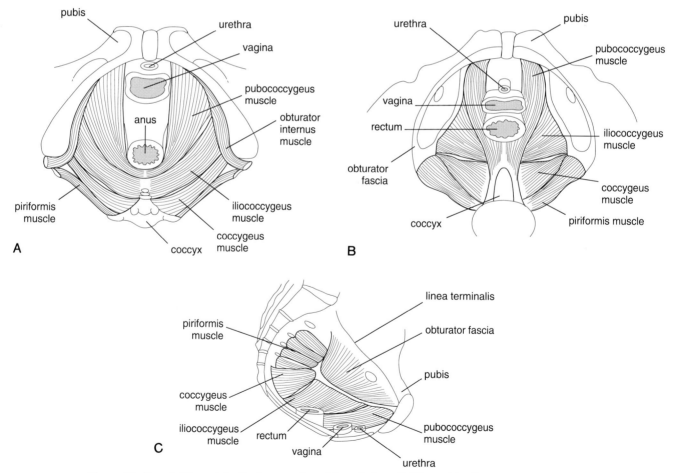

Figure 15–8. *A*, The pelvic diaphragm viewed from below. *B*, The pelvic diaphragm viewed from above. *C*, Lateral view of the pelvic diaphragm.

posteriorly. Together the pubococcygeus and iliococcygeus muscles form a hammock across the floor of the true pelvis and are termed the levator ani muscles. These muscles provide primary support to the pelvic viscera and aid in the contraction of the vagina and rectum. The coccygeus muscles are the most posterior muscle pair of the pelvic diaphragm. These muscles extend from the ischial spine to the sacrum and coccyx. (See Figure 15–8.)

Pelvic Organs

Urinary Bladder

The urinary bladder is a muscular sac which receives and stores urine produced by the kidneys. The bladder is posterior to the pubic symphysis and anterior to the uterus and vagina. The anterior surface of the bladder abuts the anterior abdominal wall. The space of Retzius contains extraperitoneal fat, which separates the anterior bladder wall from the pubic symphysis.

The superior and posterior walls of the bladder are lined by visceral peritoneum, which is continuous with the peritoneal lining of the abdominopelvic space. The peritoneum covering the bladder walls and extending over the uterine fundus creates a potential space between the bladder and the uterus, known as the **anterior cul de sac** (vesicouterine pouch). (See Figure 15–9.)

The ureters and the urethra communicate with the posteroinferior aspect of the bladder, at the trigone. The external urethral orifice is located between the labia minora of the external genitalia.

The bladder walls are primarily composed of a thick detrusor muscle. This muscle layer stretches thin when the bladder is greatly distended. The bladder walls are lined internally by a thin mucosa. A serosal lining covers the muscular walls of the bladder externally. (See Figure 15–10.)

Genital Tract

The vagina, uterus, and fallopian tubes all have the same basic structure: a narrow cavity enclosed by an inner mucosal lining, a smooth muscle wall, and an

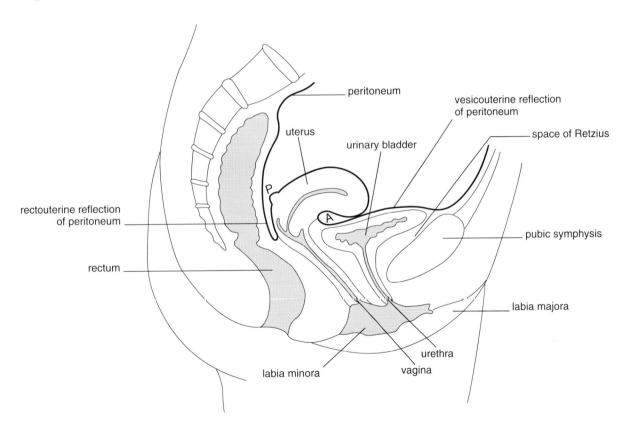

Figure 15–9. A midline sagittal plane through the female pelvis. The peritoneal lining of the abdominopelvic cavity is seen covering the superior aspect of the urinary bladder, the uterus, and the anterior region of the rectum. The anterior and posterior culs de sac are potential peritoneal spaces created by folds in the peritoneum.

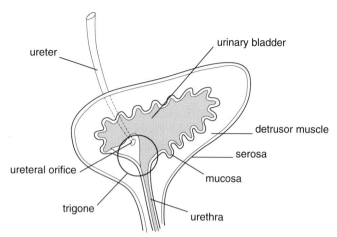

Figure 15-10. The urinary bladder wall is composed of an innermost mucosa; a thick, middle muscular layer; and an outer serosal lining. The trigone is the region of the urinary bladder where the ureters enter and the urethra exits this cavity.

outer layer of connective tissue. Variations in the mucosa and muscular walls of the genital tract are dictated by the location and function of each segment.

Vagina

The vagina extends from the uterine cervix to the external genitalia. The vagina receives the male penis during coitus and forms the distal portion of the birth canal. The vagina lies posterior to the urinary bladder and urethra and anterior to the rectum. The external orifice of the vagina is located posterior to the urethral orifice between the labia minora. The vaginal canal is a blunt-ended cavity approximately 9 cm in length. The uterine cervix protrudes through the anterior vaginal wall into the upper portion of the vaginal canal. The space within the vaginal canal encircling the cervix forms the anterior, posterior, and lateral **fornices** of the vagina. (See Figure 15–11.)

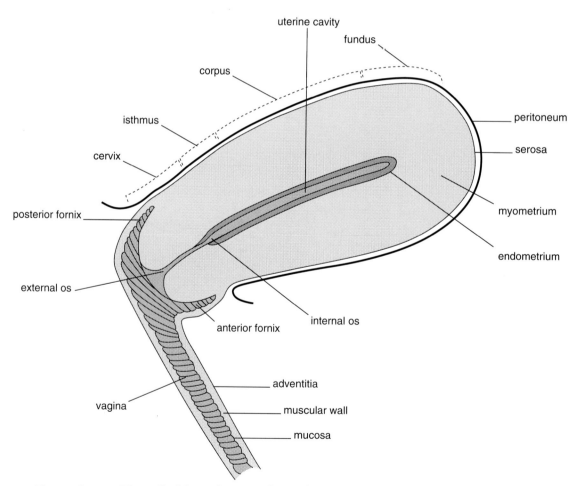

Figure 15–11. The wall of the vagina comprises an inner mucosa, a middle smooth muscle layer, and an outer adventitia. The anterior and posterior fornices of the vagina are seen as spaces between the vaginal walls and the portion of the cervix protruding into the vaginal canal. The uterine wall comprises an inner mucosa, called the endometrium; a thick, smooth muscle wall, called the myometrium; and an outer serosa. The regions of the uterus include the cervix, isthmus, corpus, and fundus. Note the narrow anteroposterior dimension of the uterine cavity.

The walls of the vagina conform to the general structure of the genital tract. The vagina has a mucosal lining of epithelial cells, a thin smooth muscle wall, and an outer adventitia. The vagina is highly elastic, permitting gross distention during parturition. In the relaxed state, the vaginal walls collapse together and the epithelial lining folds into transverse ridges, or **rugae**.

Uterus

The uterus is a pear-shaped organ resting on the dome of the bladder in the midpelvis. The uterus may be divided into four regions: the fundus, corpus, isthmus, and cervix. The **fundus** is the widest and uppermost segment of the uterus. It is continuous with the body of the uterus, called the **corpus**. The **isthmus** is a short, flexible region of the uterus between the corpus and cervix. The **cervix** is the most inferior region of the uterus which extends into the upper portion of the vaginal canal.

The fallopian tubes join the lateral aspects of the uterus, at the **cornua**. Passing through the thick muscular wall of the uterus, the fallopian tubes communicate with the **uterine cavity (endometrial canal)**.

The anteroposterior dimension of the endometrial canal is very thin. The width of this cavity is greatest near the uterine fundus and narrows toward the cervix. The cervical canal is continuous with the endometrial canal at the **internal os**. This canal communicates with the vaginal canal at the **external os**.

The uterine walls are composed of three tissue layers: the endometrium, myometrium, and serosa. The **endometrium** is the mucosal lining of the uterine cavity, consisting of ciliated epithelial cells and mucosal glands. During the menstrual cycle, the ovaries produce the hormones estrogen and progesterone, which stimulate cyclical changes in the endometrial lining of the uterus.

The **myometrium** forms the largest part of the uterine wall. This middle layer is composed of smooth muscle fibers, a rich vascular supply, and supporting connective tissue. During pregnancy, the myometrium enlarges dramatically through both cell growth and cell division. The myometrium is responsible for producing the radial muscle contractions necessary to expel the fetus at parturition. The serosa is a thin membranous layer surrounding the myometrium. (See Figure 15–12.)

The walls of the cervix are structurally unique compared with the rest of the uterus. The smooth muscle fibers are interlaced with collagen fibers, creating a more rigid framework. The cervical canal is lined by epithelial cells and mucus-secreting glands. The mucosal lining of the vaginal portion of the cervix is identical to the epithelial lining of the vagina.

The uterus normally tilts forward, resting on the dome of the bladder. The ligaments and peritoneal connections

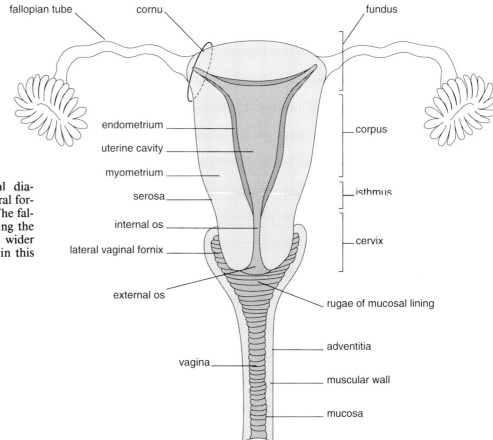

Figure 15–12. In this coronal diagram of the genital tract, the lateral fornices of the vagina are evident. The fallopian tubes can be seen adjoining the uterus at the cornua. Note the wider dimension of the uterine cavity in this plane.

of this organ allow considerable mobility within the true pelvis. This mobility affords subtle displacements of the uterus with filling of the urinary bladder or the rectum, as well as marked displacement of this organ during pregnancy.

The anterior and posterior walls of the uterus are covered by the peritoneal lining of the abdominopelvic cavity. The vesicouterine reflection of peritoneum expands over the urinary bladder and covers the anterior wall of the uterus. As previously noted, this reflection creates a shallow space within the peritoneal cavity, known as the **anterior cul de sac.** The rectouterine reflection of the peritoneum creates a larger potential space between the posterior wall of the uterus and the anterior wall of the rectum. The **posterior cul de sac** (pouch of Douglas or rectouterine pouch) is the most dependent space in the abdominopelvic cavity. Fluid collecting within the peritoneal cavity often drains into this space. (See Figure 15–9.)

The anterior and posterior peritoneal reflections covering the uterus extend anterolaterally to the walls of the true pelvis. These double folds of peritoneum extend from the uterine cornua to the lateral pelvic walls to form the **broad ligaments.** The broad ligaments are not true ligaments, and they provide minimal support for the uterus. The following structures are positioned between the two layers of each broad ligament: fallopian tube, round ligament, ovarian ligament, and vascular structures of the uterus and ovaries. These structures are surrounded by fat and cellular connective tissue, called the parametrium. The spaces within the peritoneal cavity located posterior to the broad ligaments are referred to as the adnexa. (See Figure 15–13.)

There are three paired ligaments which provide structural support to the uterus: the round ligaments, the cardinal ligaments, and the uterosacral ligaments. Each **round ligament** originates at the uterine cornu and courses within the broad ligament to the anterolateral

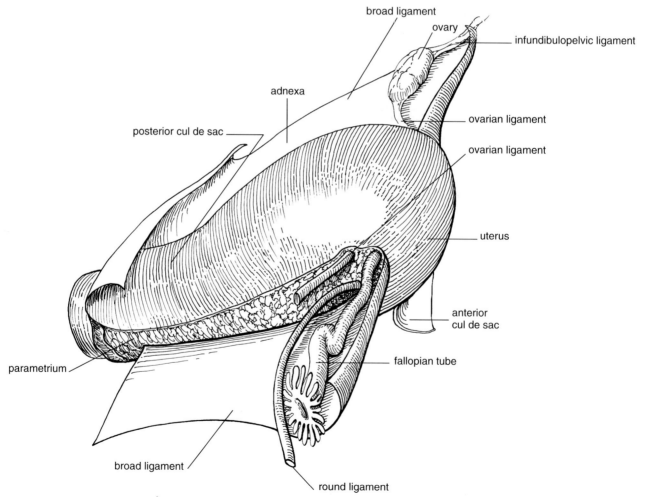

Figure 15–13. The broad ligaments are double folds of peritoneum extending from the lateral aspects of the uterus to the pelvic wall. The fallopian tubes, round ligaments, and ovarian ligaments are all located within the double folds of the broad ligaments. The ovaries are situated in the adnexa, the regions of the true pelvis posterior to the broad ligaments.

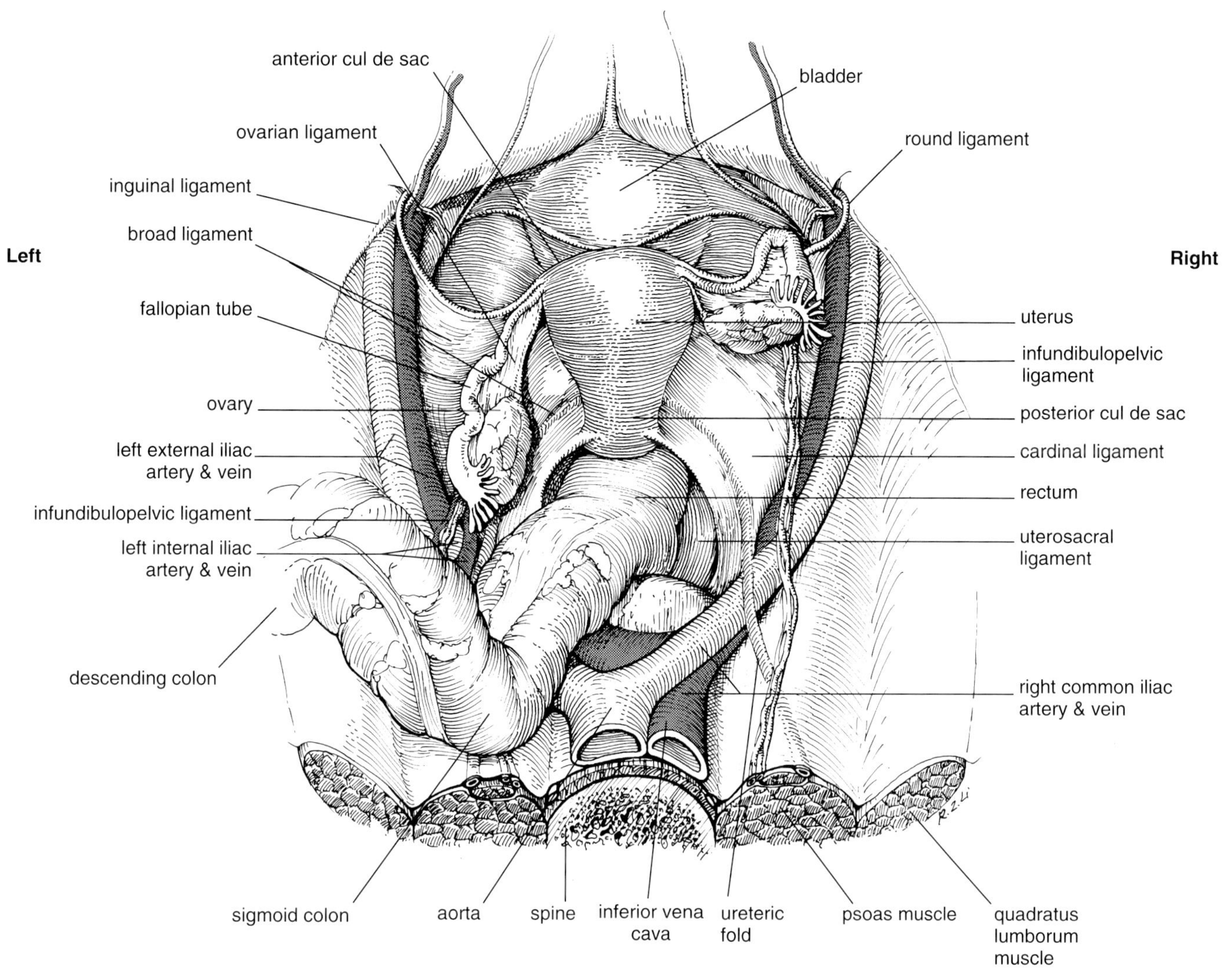

Figure 15–14. The cardinal ligaments and the uterosacral ligaments provide rigid support for the uterine cervix. The round ligaments extend from the cornua to the anterior wall of the pelvis. These ligaments pass through the inguinal canal and are secured to the external genitalia. The round ligaments maintain the anterior bend of the normal anteverted uterus.

pelvic wall. The round ligament passes over the pelvic brim and through the inguinal canal, and is secured at the labia majora. The round ligaments maintain the forward bend of the uterine fundus.

The cardinal and uterosacral ligaments provide more rigid support for the cervix. These ligaments maintain the normal axis of the cervix, roughly perpendicular to the vaginal canal. The cardinal ligaments extend from the upper cervix and isthmus to the obturator fascia at the lateral walls of the pelvis. The uterosacral ligaments extend from the posterior aspect of the cervix around the lateral walls of the rectum to the sacrum. (See Figure 15–14.)

The flexibility of the support structures of the uterus affords considerable variation in normal uterine position. The uterus is normally located in the midline of the true pelvis in an **anteverted** position. In this position, the uterine body is bent slightly forward at the isthmus so that the corpus and fundus rest on the dome of the bladder.

Anteflexion is defined by a marked anterior flexion of the uterus at the isthmus. A backward bend at the level of the isthmus defines the **retroflexed** position, in which the uterine fundus is angled back toward the posterior cul de sac.

Another common variation is **retroversion**. In this instance, the cervix is tilted posteriorly. This causes the uterine fundus to extend posteriorly toward the rectum. A retroverted and retroflexed uterus is angled posteriorly due to both the axis of the cervix and posterior flexion of the isthmus. These variations are demonstrated in Figure 15–15.

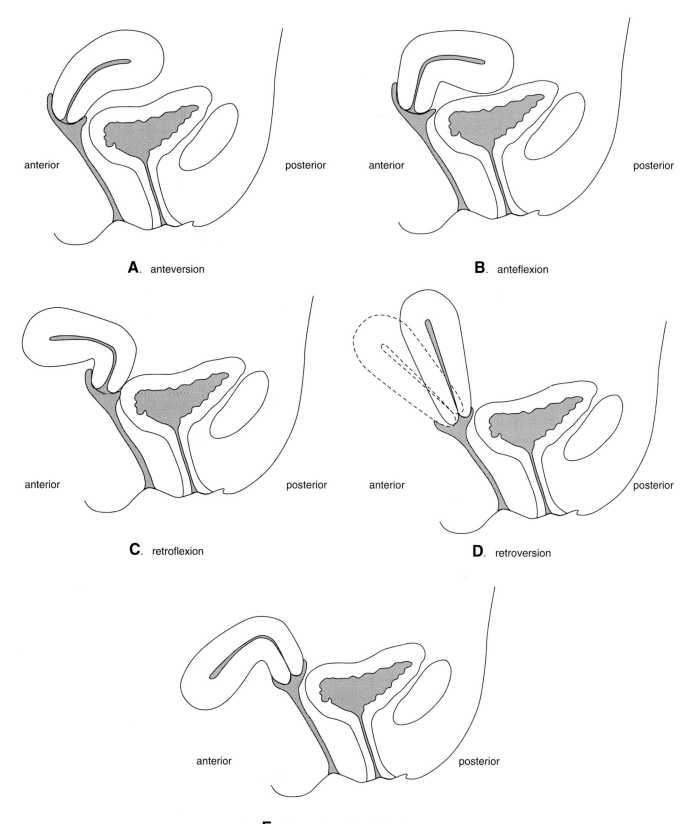

Figure 15-15. Variations in uterine position. *A*, Anteversion; *B*, Anteflexion; *C*, Retroflexion; *D*, Retroversion; *E*, Retroversion with retroflexion.

Fallopian Tubes

The fallopian tubes or oviducts are coiled, muscular tubes extending from the uterine cornua to the ovaries. The oviducts are approximately 10 cm in length and course within the parametrium of the broad ligaments. The connective tissue serosa of the fallopian tube is continuous with the outer tissue surrounding the oviduct. The fallopian tube conducts a mature ovum from the ovary to the uterus through gentle peristalsis of its smooth muscle walls. The mucosal lining of the tube consists of ciliated epithelial cells and secretory cells. The cilia propel a gentle current of fluid which aids in the transport of ova.

The fallopian tube may be divided into four segments: the interstitial segment, isthmus, ampulla, and infundibulum. The **interstitial** portion of the oviduct constitutes the first region of the tube which traverses the myometrium of the uterine cornu. Lateral to the interstitial portion is a short, straight segment of the tube, known as the **isthmus**.

The longest and most coiled portion of the fallopian tube is the **ampulla**. Fertilization most often occurs in the ampulla. The mucosal lining of the ampulla folds into complex matrices, filling much of the tubular lumen.

The **infundibulum** is the funnel-shaped portion of the oviduct which is closest to the ovary. The ovaries are located within the adnexal spaces. The infundibulum passes through the posterior aspect of the broad ligament to reach the ovary. The fallopian tube and the ovary are not intimately connected, thus the genital tract creates a channel between the outside and the peritoneal cavity. The **fimbriae** of the oviduct are fringe-like extensions of the infundibulum which overlie the ovary and direct the released ovum into the fallopian tube. (See Figure 15–16.)

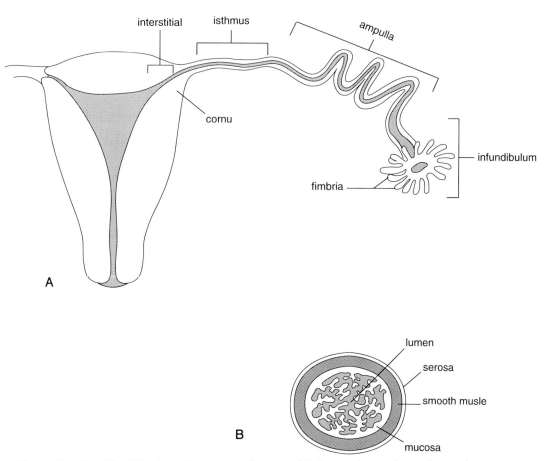

Figure 15–16. The fallopian tubes are continuous with the uterine cavity at the uterine cornua. The four regions of the oviduct include the interstitial segment, isthmus, ampulla, and infundibulum. *A*, The regions of the fallopian tube. *B*, Cross-section through the ampulla of the fallopian tube. This section demonstrates the intricate folds of the mucosal lining. The wall of the fallopian tube comprises the inner mucosa, a middle muscular layer, and the outer serosa.

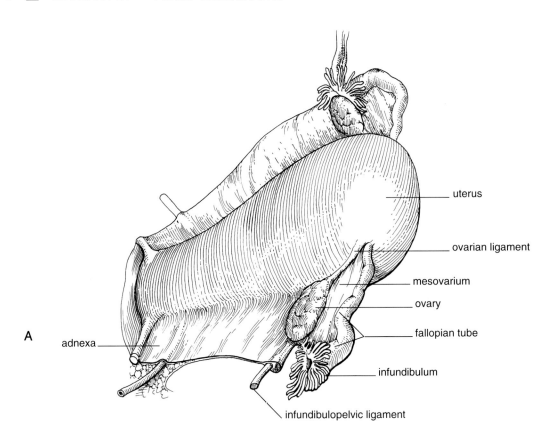

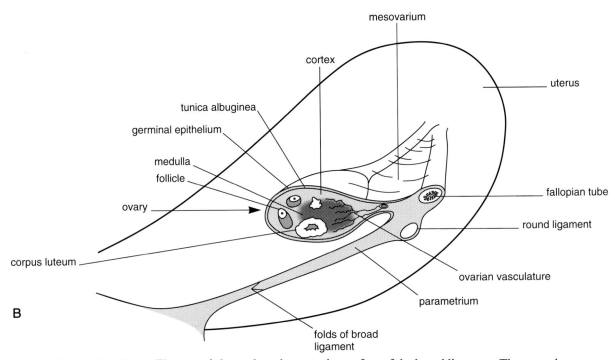

Figure 15–17. *A*, The ovary is located on the posterior surface of the broad ligament. The ovary is anchored in this position by the ovarian ligament, the infundibulopelvic ligament, and the mesovarium. The ovaries are the only organs located within the peritoneal cavity which are not covered by peritoneum. *B*, The innermost ovarian tissue is the medulla, composed of ovarian vessels, nerves, and connective tissue. Follicular development takes place in the cortex of the ovary. The cortex is surrounded by a fibrous capsule, called the tunica albuginea. The germinal epithelium is the outermost cellular layer.

Ovaries

The ovaries are almond-shaped organs lying on the posterior surface of the broad ligaments. They are the only organs within the abdominopelvic cavity not lined by visceral peritoneum. The **germinal epithelium** is a single layer of epithelial cells lining the outer surface of the ovary. (This name arose from the mistaken belief that the germ cells originated from this tissue layer.)

The **tunica albuginea** is a fibrous connective tissue capsule found beneath the epithelial layer. The ovarian stroma, or the body of the ovary, consists of the peripheral cortex and the central medulla. The cortex constitutes the bulk of ovarian tissue and is the site of oogenesis, the production of female gametes. The medulla contains the ovarian vasculature, lymphatics, and nerves supported by fibrous connective tissue. This highly vascular core communicates with the parametrium of the broad ligament at the **ovarian hilum**. The hilum is located along the superior and anterior aspect of the ovary.

There are two paired ligaments supporting the ovaries and maintaining their relative positions in the adnexal regions: The infundibulopelvic ligament extends from the infundibulum and the lateral aspect of the ovary to the lateral pelvic wall. The ovarian ligament supports the medial aspect of the ovary to the uterine cornu. This ligament lies within the peritoneal folds of the broad ligament. The mesovarium is a short double fold of peritoneum extending from the posterior aspect of the broad ligament to the ovarian hilum. (See Figure 15–17.)

Pelvic Colon

The portions of the large intestine contained within the true pelvis include the sigmoid colon and the rectum. The sigmoid colon is continuous with the descending colon in the left lower quadrant of the abdominopelvic cavity. (Refer to Figure 15–14.) The sigmoid colon is loosely secured to the posterior pelvic wall by the mesocolon. The sigmoid colon descends toward the rectum in the inferoposterior aspect of the pelvis minor. The rectum is largely retroperitoneal, and is situated posterior to the vagina.

When the bladder is empty, loops of small bowel rest in the anterior region of the abdominopelvic cavity. A distended urinary bladder pushes the small intestine superiorly, out of the true pelvis. The position of the small intestine relative to the pelvic organs becomes important in sonographic imaging.

Vasculature of the True Pelvis

The uterine artery is a branch of the internal iliac artery and supplies blood to the reproductive organs of the pelvis. The left and right uterine arteries divide into vaginal and uterine branches at the level of the cervix. The uterine branches course along the lateral aspect of the uterus toward the fundus. The arterial and venous uterine branches are located within the peritoneal folds of the broad ligament.

The uterine branches of each uterine artery give rise to the arcuate arteries. These arteries loop around the uterus and branch into the radial arteries. The radial arteries penetrate the myometrium and give rise to the straight arteries.

The straight arteries supply the first layer of endometrial tissue, with smaller branches, called the spiral arteries, perfusing the proliferating endometrium. Flow in the spiral arteries is responsive to hormonal changes of the menstrual cycle. The venous drainage of the uterus is analogous to its arterial supply.

The blood supply to the ovary is maintained by two separate vascular pathways. The uterine branches of the uterine artery and vein give rise to ovarian branches at the level of the cornu. The ovarian branches travel laterally within the broad ligament to reach the ovarian hilum.

The ovarian artery and vein provide an alternative vascular supply to this organ. The left and right ovarian arteries branch off the abdominal aorta inferior to the renal arteries. The ovarian arteries course anterior to the psoas and iliopsoas muscles within the retroperitoneum. They travel medially along the infundibulopelvic ligaments to reach the **ovarian hilum**. The ovarian veins follow a similar ascent to the inferior vena cava, with slight variation in that the left ovarian vein drains into the left renal vein. (See Figure 15–18.)

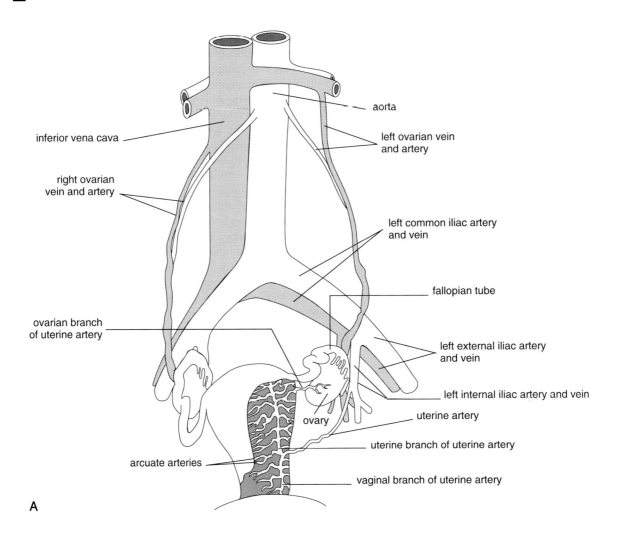

aorta

inferior vena cava

left ovarian vein and artery

right ovarian vein and artery

left common iliac artery and vein

fallopian tube

ovarian branch of uterine artery

left external iliac artery and vein

left internal iliac artery and vein

ovary

uterine artery

uterine branch of uterine artery

arcuate arteries

vaginal branch of uterine artery

A

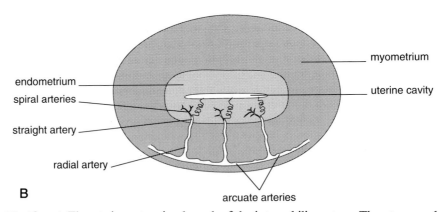

myometrium

endometrium

uterine cavity

spiral arteries

straight artery

radial artery

arcuate arteries

B

Figure 15–18. *A,* The uterine artery is a branch of the internal iliac artery. The uterus and vagina receive blood from branches of this artery. *B,* The arcuate arteries encircle the outer tissue of the uterus. The myometrium is penetrated by the radial arteries. The endometrium receives blood from the straight and spiral arteries. The spiral arteries become more dilated during the secretory phase of the menstrual cycle. During menses, the spiral arteries are shed along with much of the endometrial lining. The ovaries receive blood from branches of the uterine artery and from the ovarian arteries arising from the abdominal aorta.

PHYSIOLOGY

Between puberty and menopause, the female reproductive system normally undergoes monthly cyclical changes. The menstrual cycle usually follows a 28-day course, during which a single ovum reaches maturity and is released into the genital tract. Changes in the ovary and the endometrium throughout this cycle are controlled by hormones secreted by the anterior pituitary gland and by the ovary itself.

The Ovarian Cycle

At menarche the ovaries contain thousands of primordial follicles, each composed of a single primary oocyte and surrounding follicular cells. During the **follicular phase** of the ovarian cycle (days 1 to 14), 10 to 20 primordial follicles begin to mature. **Follicle stimulating hormone (FSH)** is a gonadotropin produced by the anterior pituitary gland which initiates follicular development. This initial maturation process results in the development of several follicles, each composed of multiple cellular layers.

The primary follicle contains the primary oocyte surrounded by a membranous protein layer, called the zona pellucida. This layer is encircled by proliferating follicular cells, collectively called the zona granulosa. Outer connective tissue layers of the primary follicle include the theca interna and the theca externa.

As each primary follicle grows, the oocyte reaches a mature size. The **follicular antrum** is a fluid-filled cavity which forms between the cellular layers of the zona granulosa. The developing oocyte rests along the wall of the follicular antrum and is surrounded by the **cumulus oophorus**, a layer of follicular cells continuous with the zona granulosa. At this stage of development, the oocyte and its surrounding structures are called the secondary follicle. The theca interna cells of multiple secondary follicles fulfill an endocrine function as they differentiate into estrogen-secreting cells. The hormone **estrogen** promotes proliferation of the endometrium.

While many follicles develop in the ovaries in response to FSH, only one follicle matures completely to be released at ovulation. Most of the follicles undergo follicular atresia beyond the stage of the secondary follicle. One secondary follicle continues to mature to become a **graafian follicle** prior to ovulation. The ovum continues to mature through meiotic division, forming the secondary oocyte. Now the oocyte floats freely within the enlarged follicular antrum of the graafian follicle. The follicular cells of the cumulus oophorus now completely surround the zona pellucida and the secondary oocyte, and are called the corona radiata. (See Figure 15–19.)

The theca interna cells of the graafian follicle continue to produce estrogen. The graafian follicle migrates to the surface of the ovary, while the remaining secondary folli-

cles undergo atresia. At approximately day 14 of the ovarian cycle, the mature ovum is expelled into the peritoneal cavity. The fimbria of the oviduct draw the released egg into the infundibulum.

At **ovulation**, 5 to 10 ml of follicular fluid are released into the peritoneal cavity, settling into the posterior cul de sac. The ruptured graafian follicle collapses, fills with blood, and is transformed into a temporary endocrine gland. This begins the **luteal phase** of the ovarian cycle (days 15 to 28). The remaining follicular structure is now called the **corpus luteum** and contains a central blood clot surrounded by granulosa luteal cells, theca luteal cells, and the theca externa.

The granulosa luteal cells enlarge and secrete **progesterone**, which promotes glandular secretions of the endometrium. The theca luteal cells continue the estrogen secretion of their precursors (theca interna), maintaining the proliferated endometrial lining of the uterus. The outer theca externa cells support the rich vascular network characteristic of an endocrine gland.

Luteinizing hormone (LH) is produced by the anterior pituitary gland throughout the ovarian cycle. This hormone promotes secretion of estrogen and progesterone by the ovary. Both estrogen and LH peak immediately prior to ovulation. While the corpus luteum is dependent on LH, progesterone negatively inhibits the production of LH. Consequently, the corpus luteum eventually regresses due to lack of LH stimulation, and only a fibrous tissue mass, called the **corpus albicans**, remains in the ovary. When the levels of estrogen and progesterone diminish, the thickened endometrial lining of the uterus is shed through menstruation. (See Figure 15–20.)

Pregnancy interrupts the normal menstrual cycle. Following implantation of the fertilized ovum, **human chorionic gonadotropin (hCG)** is secreted by the developing placenta. This hormone has an analogous function to LH, maintaining the corpus luteum. Thus, during pregnancy, the corpus luteum continues to secrete estrogen and progesterone throughout the first trimester. The placenta ultimately takes over this endocrine function and the corpus luteum regresses, forming the corpus albicans.

The Endometrial Cycle

The days of the menstrual cycle are numbered according to changes in the endometrial lining of the uterus. Days 1 through 5 generally correspond to **menses**, when the thickened endometrium is shed.

Proliferation is the second phase of the endometrial cycle, occurring between menses and ovulation. The endometrium thickens in response to estrogen, preparing the uterine cavity to receive the fertilized egg.

Ovulation usually occurs near the fourteenth day of the menstrual cycle, marking the beginning of the **secretory phase**. The production of estrogen and progesterone by the corpus luteum promotes continued proliferation

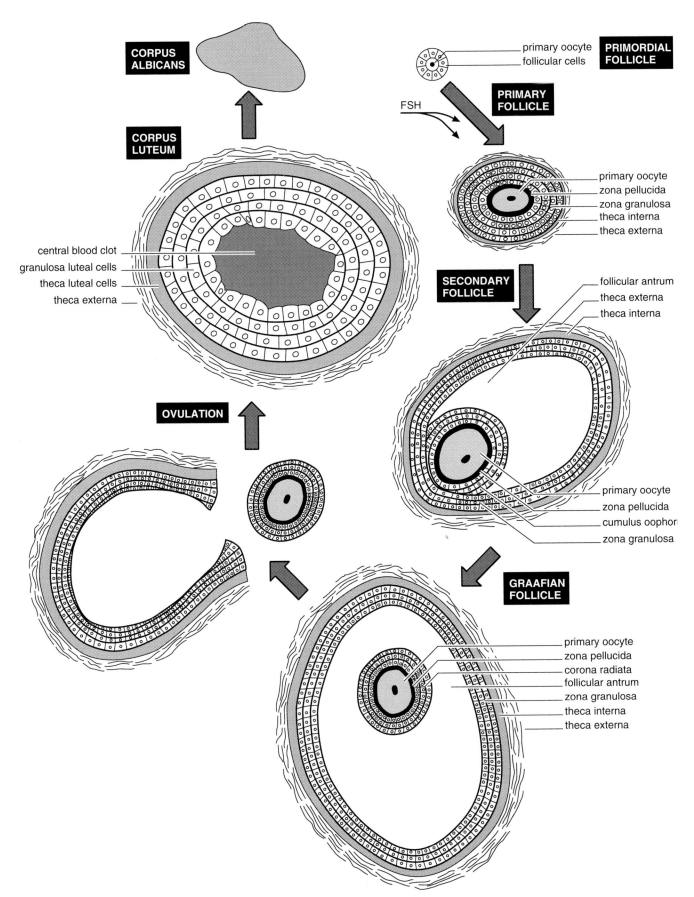

Figure 15–19. Growth and development of a follicle during the normal menstrual cycle.

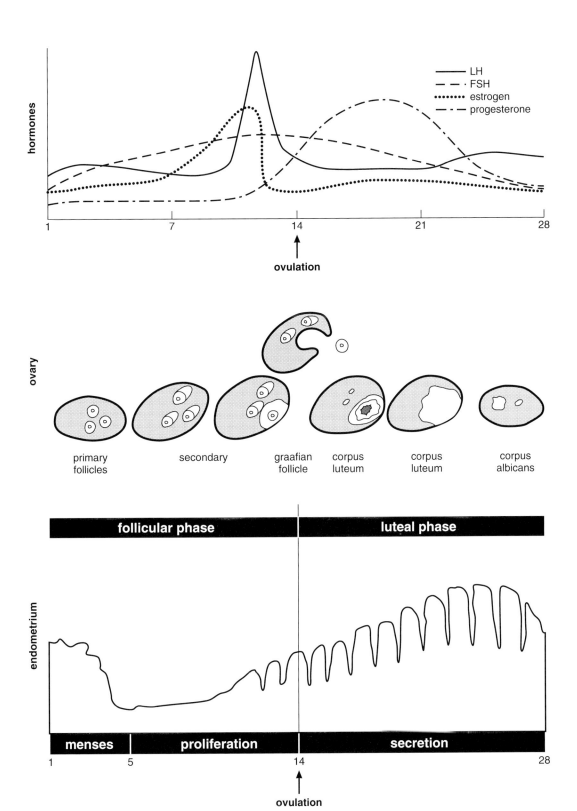

Figure 15–20. The menstrual cycle. The first day of bleeding corresponds to the first day of the female menstrual cycle. The thickened endometrial lining of the uterus is shed during menses. At this point, the production of follicle stimulating hormone promotes the follicular phase of the ovarian cycle. Developing follicles within the ovaries begin to produce estrogen, which in turn causes proliferation of the endometrial lining. At approximately day 14 of the menstrual cycle, luteinizing hormone peaks; at this point, ovulation occurs, and the graafian follicle releases a mature ovum. The latter half of the menstrual cycle corresponds to the luteal phase of the ovary, during which the corpus luteum produces estrogen and progesterone. These hormones promote the secretory phase of the endometrial cycle, during which the endometrium continues to thicken. Inhibited production of luteinizing hormone at the end of the menstrual cycle leads to a breakdown of the corpus luteum and the shedding of the endometrium with the onset of menses.

of the endometrium. Exocrine glands of the endometrial lining secrete a glycogen-rich mucus, preparing a suitable environment for implantation.

In the absence of fertilization, the production of LH, estrogen, and progesterone diminishes, and a new cycle begins on day 1 with menses. The timing of menses and proliferation in the endometrial cycle correspond to the follicular phase of the ovarian cycle (days 1 to 14). The secretory phase of the endometrial cycle corresponds to the luteal phase of the ovarian cycle (days 15 to 28).

SONOGRAPHIC APPEARANCE

Sonographic imaging of the female pelvis can be performed using transabdominal or transvaginal techniques. Transabdominal sonography requires a fully distended urinary bladder as an acoustic window through which to visualize the pelvic structures. Transvaginal sonography is performed using a high frequency transducer (5 to 7.5 MHz) which is inserted into the vagina in order to image the uterus, ovaries, and adnexa. This newer technique requires an empty bladder and is most often performed in conjunction with the traditional transabdominal method. Transvaginal sonography is limited in its field of view due to the lower penetration of higher frequency transducers. The primary advantage of this technique is its superior resolution.

The anterior approach of transabdominal pelvic sonography provides visualization of the true pelvis in sagittal and transverse planes. In transabdominal scanning, the most superficial anatomy is displayed at the apex of the monitor. The posterior region of the pelvis is displayed at the bottom of the screen, in the far field. In sagittal views, the left and right sides of the display screen correspond to cranial and caudal regions of the pelvis, respectively. In transverse views, the left and right sides of the screen correspond to the right and left sides of the pelvis, respectively. (See Figures 15–21 and 15–22.)

Understanding image orientation is more challenging in transvaginal sonography. Two types of transvaginal transducers are illustrated in Figure 15–23. The inferior approach of the transvaginal technique (through the vaginal canal) affords sagittal and coronal imaging planes of the true pelvis. In transvaginal scanning, the apex of the display screen corresponds to a caudal position, closest to the vagina in both the sagittal and coronal planes. The cranial region of the pelvis is displayed in the far field, at the bottom of the screen in both the sagittal and coronal planes. In sagittal views, the left and right sides of the display screen correspond to anterior and posterior regions of the pelvis, respectively. (See Figure 15–24.) In coronal views, the left and right sides of the screen correspond to the right and left sides of the pelvis, respectively. (See Figure 15–25.)

Image orientation in transvaginal sonography is de-

pendent on manipulation of the transducer and the steering angle of the ultrasound beam. Figure 15–26 illustrates a more anterior transvaginal approach and the corresponding orientation on the display monitor. In mastering this scanning technique, the sonographer must understand how changes in the position of the transvaginal probe affect image orientation.

Urinary Bladder

The fully distended urinary bladder appears as a large anechoic structure in the anterior region of the midpelvis. The inner mucosal lining of the bladder is a thin hyperechoic line along the circumference of the bladder. The mucosa is most readily visible where the transducer beam is perpendicular to the bladder wall. The middle muscular layer of the bladder wall stretches thin with bladder distention, and is not well seen. (See Figures 15–27 and 15–28.) When the bladder is only slightly distended, the relaxed detrusor muscle can be visualized as a hypoechoic layer surrounding the mucosa. (See Figure 15–29.) The detrusor muscle is more often appreciated in transvaginal scanning. (See Figure 15–30.)

The outer serosa of the bladder is indistinct sonographically. The urinary bladder is an extremely important landmark in sonographic imaging of the pelvis. Under normal conditions, neither the ureters nor the urethra are visualized in transabdominal or transvaginal pelvic sonography.

Musculature

The muscles most commonly visualized in transabdominal pelvic sonography include the iliopsoas muscles, the obturator internus muscles, and the muscles of the pelvic diaphragm. The skeletal muscles of the pelvis follow the characteristic sonographic pattern seen throughout the rest of the body. These muscles exhibit low level echoes with linear striations when imaged in a plane longitudinal to the muscle fibers. The skeletal muscles define the external borders of the abdominopelvic cavity.

In a transverse image of the pelvis, the iliopsoas muscles can be identified anteriorly as ovoid structures lateral to the urinary bladder. (See Figure 15–31.) They exhibit low level echoes with a distinct central echogenic focus due to the femoral nerve sheath. The iliopsoas muscles can also be identified in sagittal views along the lateral pelvic wall. (See Figure 15–32.)

The obturator internus muscles are best seen in transverse images of the true pelvis. These muscles appear as thin, linear low level echoes that are parallel to the lateral walls of the urinary bladder. (See Figure 15–33.)

The muscles of the pelvic diaphragm can be seen in transverse views of the cervix and vagina. The low level echoes of these muscles are seen in the far field of a

Text continued on page 241

DISPLAY MONITOR

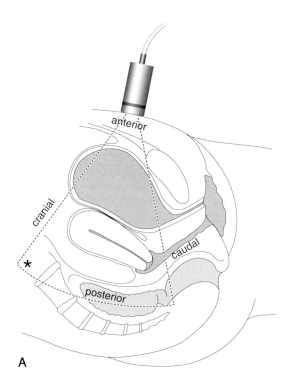

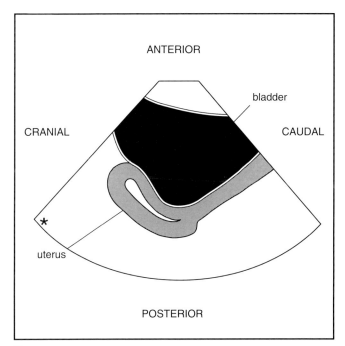

A

B

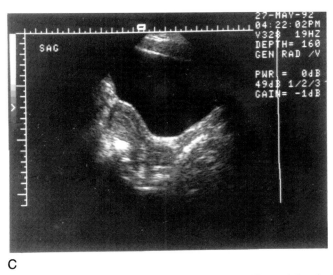

C

Figure 15–21. Transabdominal imaging in the sagittal plane. *A*, Transabdominal pelvic sonography is performed from an anterior approach using the fully distended urinary bladder as an acoustic window. In transabdominal pelvic sonography the anterior region of the pelvis is displayed in the near field, and the more posterior region of the pelvis is displayed in the far field of the image. *B*, In the sagittal plane, the left and right sides of the display monitor correspond to the superior and inferior regions of the pelvis, respectively. *C*, Corresponding sonogram of a midsagittal plane in transabdominal pelvic imaging. The fully distended urinary bladder is seen as an anechoic cavity in the near field of the image. The uterus is pushed posteriorly by the distended bladder, and is roughly perpendicular to the ultrasound beam.

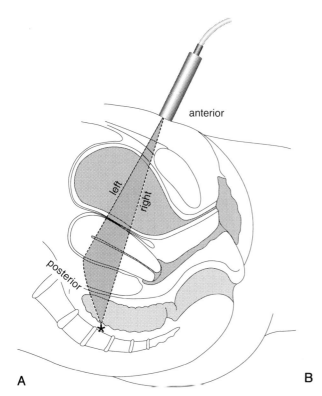

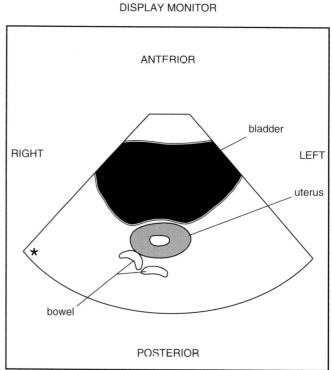

DISPLAY MONITOR

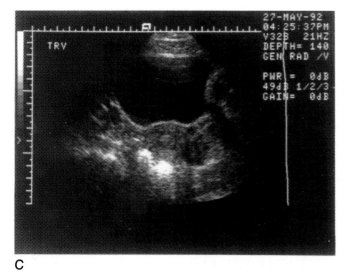

Figure 15–22. Transabdominal imaging in the transverse plane. *A,* Transducer position for transabdominal imaging of the pelvis in the transverse plane. The transducer has been rotated 90 degrees counterclockwise from the sagittal orientation. *B,* Image orientation of the transverse plane on the display monitor. The near and far fields of the transverse image correspond to the anterior and posterior regions of the pelvis, respectively. The left and right sides of the display monitor now correspond to the right and left sides of the pelvis, respectively. Transverse planes of the pelvis can be imaged at more superior or inferior levels of the pelvis by moving or angling the transducer cranially or caudally against the anterior abdominal wall. *C,* Corresponding sonogram for the transverse transabdominal approach. Note again that the distended urinary bladder is anechoic and seen in the near field of the image.

Figure 15–23. The transvaginal transducer is inserted vaginally so that the face of the transducer is against the cervix and vaginal fornices. The structures closest to the transducer are always displayed in the near field of the sonographic image. The transvaginal ultrasound beam is often transmitted from an angled transducer face, as illustrated by transducer A. Alternatively, the transvaginal transducer may emit sound waves directly from the end of the probe, as illustrated by transducer B. The transvaginal transducer has a small field of view due to the high frequency utilized in this technique. The sonographer must tilt the probe anteriorly, posteriorly, and laterally within the vagina in order to evaluate the entire pelvic region.

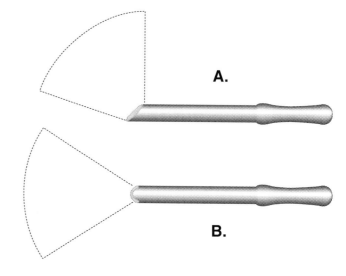

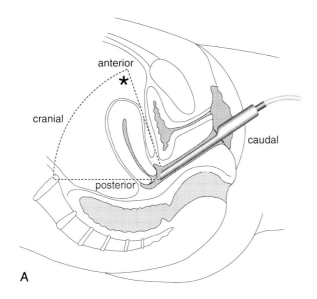

A

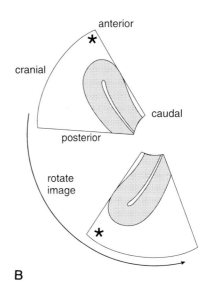

B

DISPLAY MONITOR

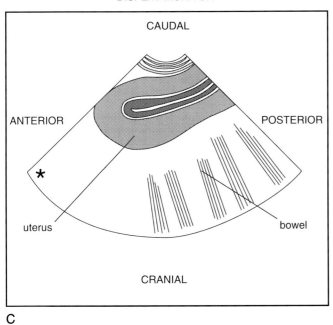

C

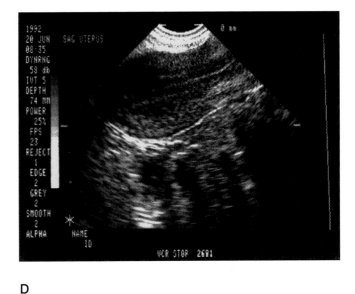

D

Figure 15-24. Transvaginal imaging in the sagittal plane. Transvaginal pelvic sonography is performed from an inferior approach, through the vaginal canal. The apex of the transvaginal image corresponds to anatomic structures which are closest to the face of the transducer. In the sagittal plane, the near field of the transvaginal image generally corresponds to the inferior region of the true pelvis. The far field of the transvaginal image, displayed at the bottom of the monitor, generally corresponds to the superior region of the true pelvis. The left and right sides of the display monitor correspond to anterior and posterior regions of the pelvis, respectively. *A*, *B*, and *C* illustrate the transvaginal approach and the rotation of the image on the display monitor. *D*, The corresponding sonogram of the midsagittal transvaginal plane.

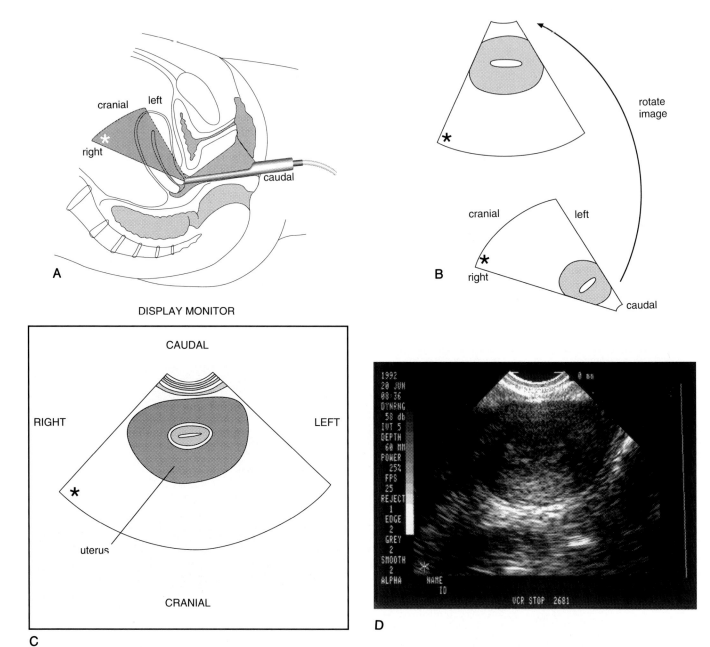

Figure 15–25. Transvaginal imaging in the coronal plane. By rotating the transvaginal transducer 90 degrees counterclockwise, the coronal plane of the pelvis is imaged. With an empty urinary bladder, the fundus of the anteverted uterus is tilted forward toward the anterior abdominal wall. Consequently, the coronal transvaginal imaging plane usually demonstrates a transverse section of the anteverted or anteflexed uterus. The near and far fields of the coronal transvaginal image correspond to inferior and superior regions of the pelvis. The left and right sides of the display monitor correspond to the right and left sides of the pelvis, respectively. *A, B,* and *C,* The coronal transvaginal scanning plane. Again, the image is rotated in order to display the apex of the sector image at the top of the display monitor. *D,* The corresponding sonogram, illustrating a transverse section of the uterus in the coronal plane of the pelvis.

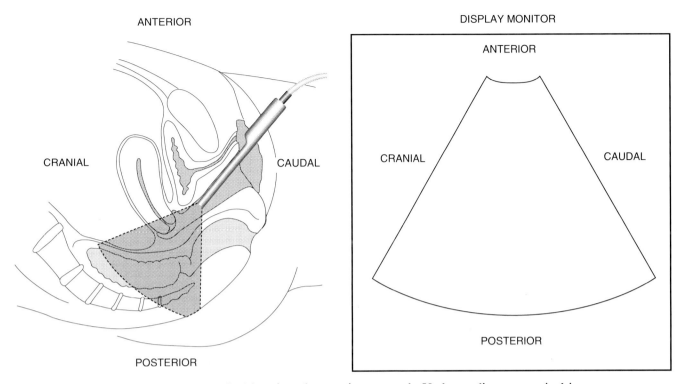

Figure 15–26. Transvaginal imaging: the anterior approach. Understanding transvaginal image orientation is likely to be the most difficult aspect of mastering this technique. The orientations of the sagittal and coronal planes illustrated in Figures 15–24 and 15–25 will be used consistently throughout this chapter. It is important to understand, however, that manipulation of the transvaginal transducer causes some variation from the standard image orientation described here. For example, when the transducer is lifted anteriorly (toward the pubic symphysis) the acoustic beam is directed more posteriorly. In this case, the near and far fields of the sagittal image correspond to anterior and posterior regions of the pelvis, respectively. Similarly, from a more anterior transvaginal approach, the left and right sides of the display monitor more closely correspond to superior and inferior regions of the pelvis. A posterior transvaginal approach would also cause significant variation in image orientation. Thus, image orientation for transvaginal sonography may vary between authors and ultrasound texts.

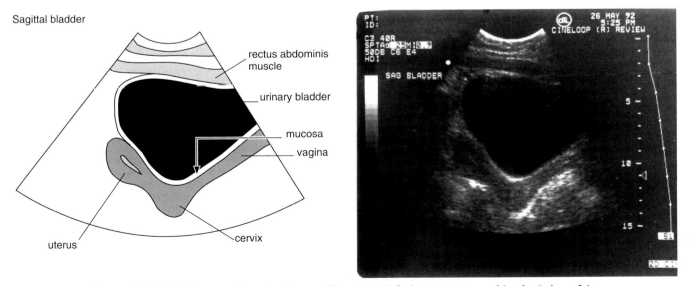

Figure 15–27. This transabdominal image of the true pelvis demonstrates a midsagittal view of the distended urinary bladder. The bladder mucosa is seen as a hyperechoic lining around the anechoic, fluid-filled cavity The muscular wall of the bladder is stretched thin due to distention; thus the detrusor muscle is not visible. The uterus is seen posterior to the urinary bladder.

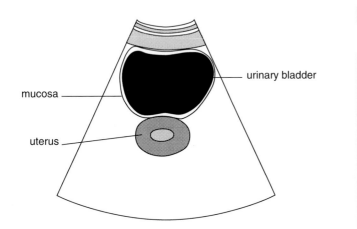

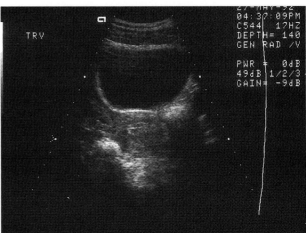

Figure 15–28. Transversely, the full urinary bladder is more square in shape in the transabdominal image. The hyperechoic mucosal lining is again seen along the circumference of the anechoic bladder. A transverse section of the uterus is seen posterior to the bladder.

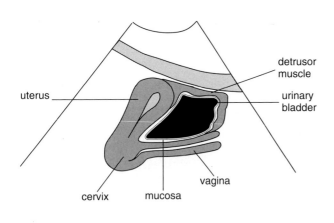

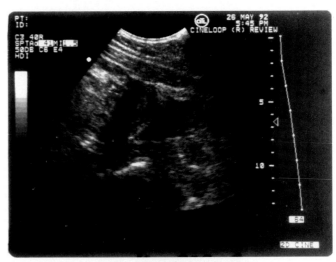

Figure 15–29. Sagittal transabdominal image of the midpelvis with an undistended urinary bladder. In this case the detrusor muscle is relaxed and is seen as a hypoechoic layer of the bladder wall. The hyperechoic inner mucosal layer is most visible where the transducer beam is angled perpendicular to the bladder wall. Note that the uterus is more difficult to visualize without the acoustic window of a full urinary bladder.

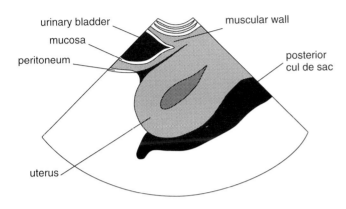
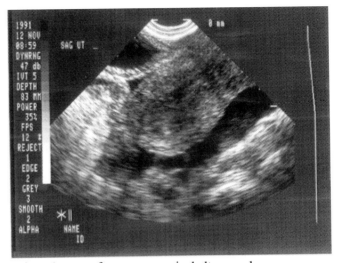

Figure 15–30. The urinary bladder should be empty in order to perform a transvaginal ultrasound examination. A small quantity of urine can be identified within the bladder transvaginally. The urinary bladder appears in the upper left corner of a sagittal transvaginal image. Remember that this region correlates to an anteroinferior anatomic location in transvaginal imaging. The inner mucosa of the bladder wall is less visible in this image, while the relaxed detrusor muscle and the peritoneal lining surrounding the bladder are clearly visualized. The uterus is seen posterior to the bladder, with a moderate quantity of anechoic fluid in the posterior cul de sac.

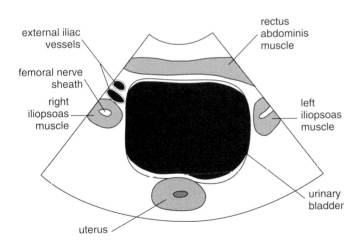
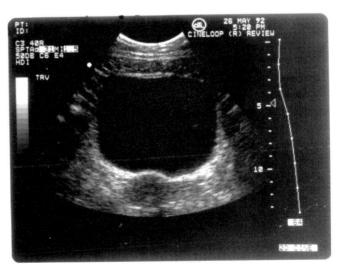

Figure 15–31. This transabdominal image illustrates the iliopsoas muscles in a transverse plane, seen lateral to the urinary bladder. These skeletal muscles have low level echoes with a central echogenic foci, corresponding to the femoral nerve sheath.

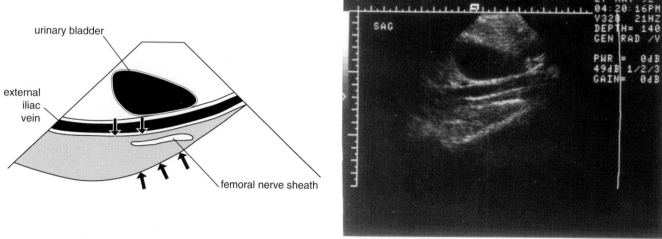

Figure 15–32. This transabdominal image illustrates a right parasagittal view of the pelvis, just lateral to the right ovary. This view demonstrates the low level echoes of the iliopsoas muscle (shown by arrows), with the central hyperechoic femoral nerve sheath. The external iliac vein is seen anterior to the muscle.

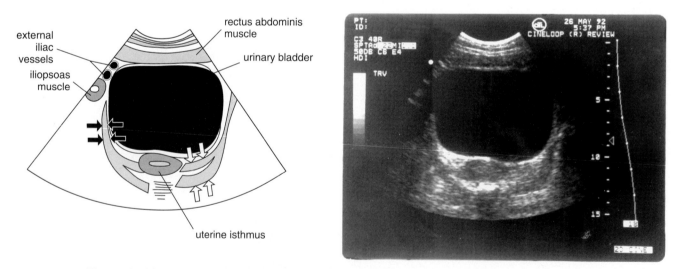

Figure 15–33. The obturator internus muscles can be seen transversely as thin structures with low level echoes, paralleling the lateral walls of the urinary bladder (shown by arrows). The levator ani muscles are seen hammocking across the pelvic floor, posterior to the uterus (shown by the open arrows). The right iliopsoas muscle is seen anterolaterally. The right external iliac artery and vein can be identified as circular anechoic structures anterior to the iliopsoas muscle. The rectus abdominis muscle is seen lining the anterior abdominal wall, anterior to the urinary bladder.

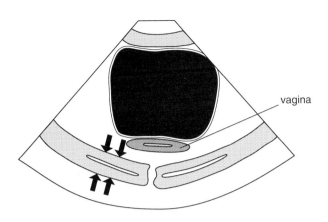

vagina

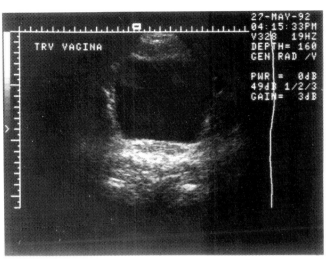

Figure 15–34. This transabdominal image of the transverse plane demonstrates the levator ani muscles posterior to the vagina (shown by arrows).

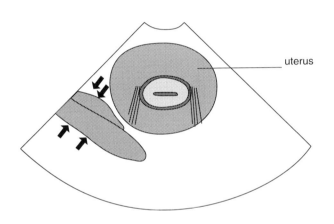

uterus

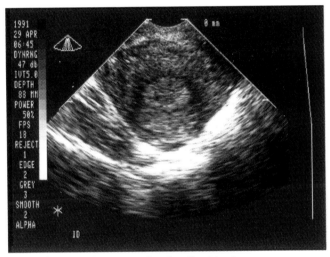

Figure 15–35. In this coronal, transvaginal image the pelvic musculature can be visualized in the right posterior region of the pelvis (shown by arrows). The muscles are obscured by overlying bowel gas in the left region of the pelvis.

transabdominal image. (See Figures 15–33 and 15–34.) The obturator internus muscles and the muscles of the pelvic diaphragm are more difficult to see in the sagittal plane. The skeletal muscles of the true pelvis can also be visualized in transvaginal sonography. However, overlying bowel gas and reduced penetration limit visualization of these deep structures. (See Figure 15–35.)

Vagina

The vagina can be identified posterior to the bladder neck in transabdominal imaging of the pelvis. Sagittally, the muscular walls of the vagina can be seen as parallel layers of medium to low level echoes separated by a thin, echogenic stripe of the vaginal mucosa. The vagina has a flattened, oval shape in a transverse plane. The muscle walls exhibit medium to low level echoes surrounding the central echogenic mucosal lining. The collapsed vaginal canal cannot normally be identified in transabdominal sonography. The rectum and the muscles of the pelvic diaphragm can be visualized posterior to the vagina. (See Figures 15–36 and 15–37.)

Uterus

The uterus is well visualized sonographically using either the transabdominal or the transvaginal approach. The uterine myometrium comprises the bulk of the uterine tissue and exhibits homogeneous, medium to low level echoes. The myometrium is isoechoic to the muscular walls of the vagina. The outer serosa of the uterus is not visualized sonographically. In sagittal views of the uterus, the endometrium is seen as a longitudinal, echogenic stripe lining the myometrium. (See Figure 15–38.)

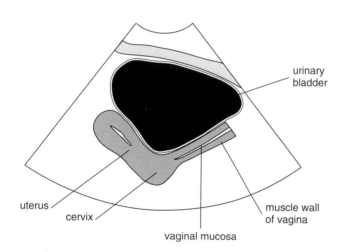

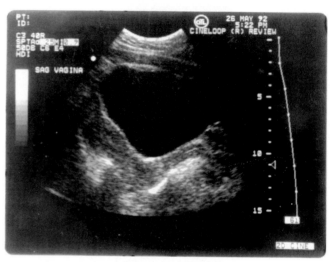

Figure 15-36. In the sagittal transabdominal image, the vagina is seen posterior and inferior to the distended urinary bladder. The muscular walls of the vagina reflect low to mid level echoes and surround the more hyperechoic central mucosal lining.

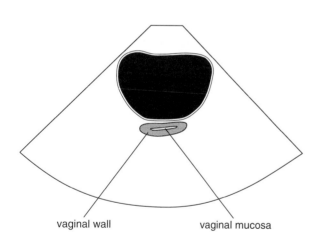

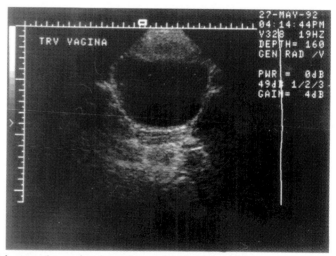

Figure 15-37. In the transverse transabdominal image, the vagina is again seen posterior to the urinary bladder. The vaginal mucosa is seen centrally and is hyperechoic compared with the muscular layer surrounding it.

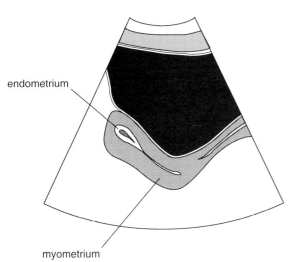

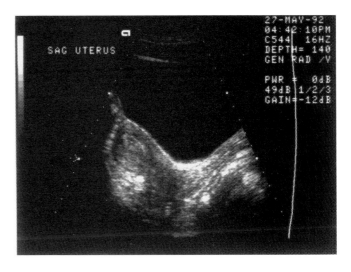

Figure 15-38. The uterus is demonstrated in a midsagittal transabdominal image. The uterine myometrium is made up of low to mid level echoes and is very similar in echotexture (isoechoic) to the muscular walls of the vagina. The endometrium is seen as a central more hyperechoic line within the uterus.

Transversely, the medium to low level echo texture of the uterine myometrium appears rounded and encircles the more echogenic endometrial lining. (See Figure 15-39.) Transvaginal images of the uterus are demonstrated in Figures 15-40 and 15-41. The width of the uterine cavity is greater than its anteroposterior dimension. Consequently, the endometrial stripe appears horizontal in transverse images of the uterus. The walls of the uterus are normally compressed together, collapsing the uterine cavity. Correct measurements of the uterus are illustrated in Figures 15-42 and 15-43.

The thickness and echopattern of the endometrium vary considerably throughout the menstrual cycle. Sonographic patterns have been described corresponding to the stages of the endometrial cycle.[1-3] During menses and early proliferation, the endometrium appears thin and

hyperechoic (Fig. 15-44). Prior to ovulation, the endometrium thickens and takes on a multilayered appearance. (See Figures 15-40, 15-41, and 15-45.) This sonographic appearance consists of a thin central echogenic lining surrounded by a thicker hypoechoic layer, which is separated from the myometrium by a thin, hyperechoic outer layer. This layered appearance continues during the early secretory phase. Prior to menses, the endometrium appears thick, hyperechoic, and homogenous. (See Figure 15-46.)

The thickness of the endometrium can be measured both transvaginally and transabdominally. This measurement is most accurately taken in the sagittal plane, as demonstrated in Figure 15-47. The high resolution of transvaginal imaging provides visualization of much of the uterine vasculature. Vessels coursing within the

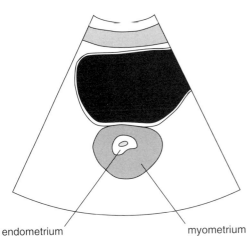

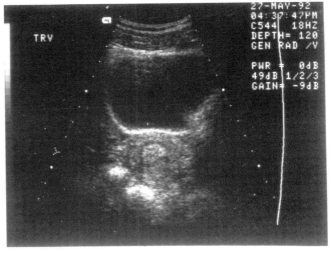

Figure 15-39. In the transverse transabdominal plane, the myometrium is seen encircling the more hyperechoic endometrium.

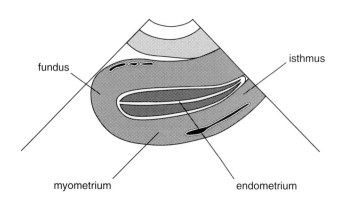

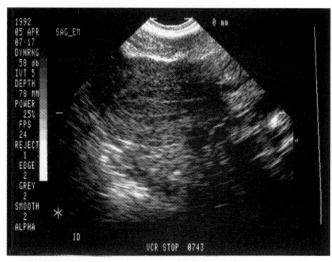

Figure 15–40. Transvaginally, the normal anteverted uterus is well visualized in the midsagittal plane. The bladder is empty and not visualized in this image. The uterine fundus is seen on the left side of the screen, corresponding to the anterior region of the true pelvis. The myometrium contains low to mid level homogeneous echoes. The endometrium is multilayered in appearance (preovulatory pattern).

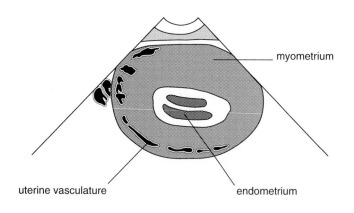

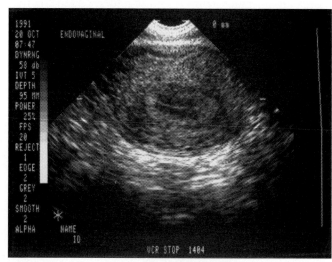

Figure 15–41. The transvaginal coronal plane demonstrates a transverse section through the anteverted uterus. Again, the myometrium contains low to mid level echoes, and the endometrium has a multilayered appearance (preovulatory pattern).

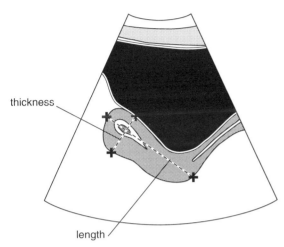

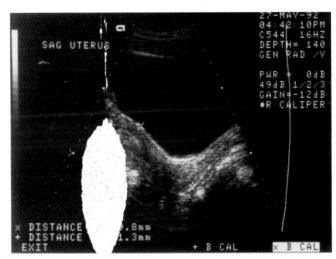

Figure 15–42. This transabdominal image demonstrates the longitudinal and anteroposterior measurements of the uterus, taken in the sagittal plane. The length of the uterus is measured from the fundus to the inferior cervical region. The anteroposterior thickness is measured perpendicular to the length at the widest region of the uterine corpus.

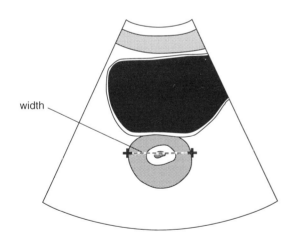

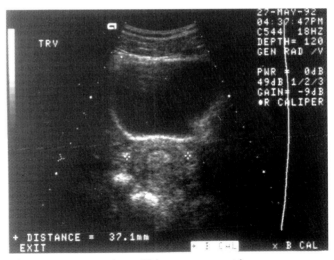

Figure 15–43. The width of the uterus is measured in the transverse plane. This measurement is taken at the widest region of the uterine corpus.

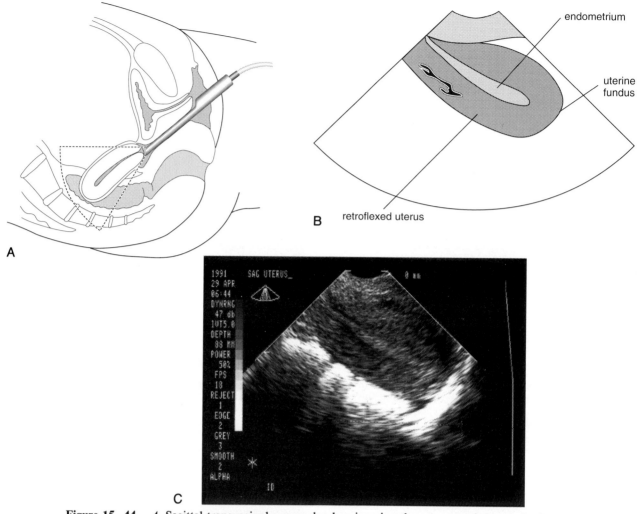

Figure 15-44. *A,* Sagittal transvaginal approach when imaging the retroverted uterus. *B, C,* The rotated sonographic image. Now the uterine fundus appears on the right of the screen, corresponding to the posterior region of the pelvis. The endometrium is thin and hyperechoic compared with the myometrial tissue. This sonographic pattern is consistent with early proliferation.

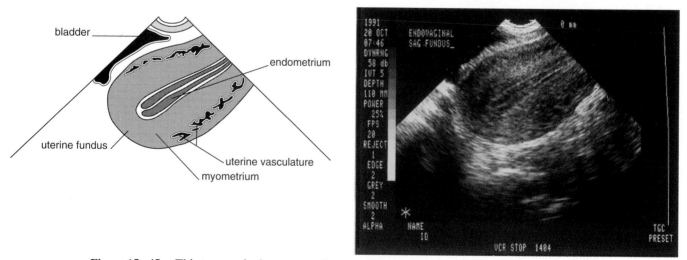

Figure 15-45. This transvaginal sonogram demonstrates an anteverted uterus prior to ovulation, in the sagittal scanning plane. Now the endometrium takes on a multilayered appearance. A central hyperechoic line can be identified surrounded by a thicker, hypoechoic layer, surrounded by a thin, hyperechoic border. A small quantity of urine is seen in the urinary bladder. The uterine vessels can be identified as anechoic areas along the periphery of the myometrium.

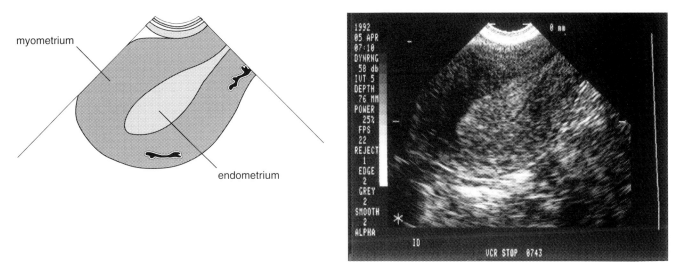

Figure 15-46. This sagittal transvaginal image demonstrates the thickened, more hyperechoic endometrium in the secretory phase.

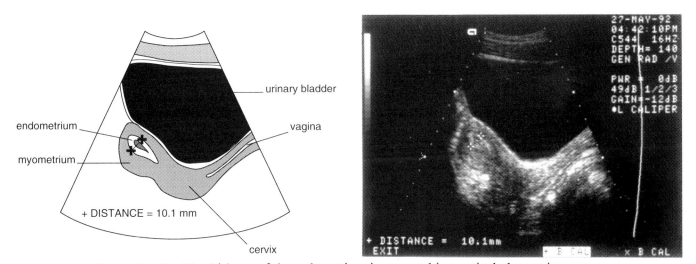

Figure 15-47. The thickness of the endometrium is measured in a sagittal plane at its greatest dimension.

peripheral myometrium appear as anechoic tubular structures.

The sonographic pattern of the cervix is similar to that of the rest of the uterus in a sagittal plane. (See Figure 15-48.) The muscular walls are homogeneous, medium to low level echoes, while the cervical mucosa is thin and echogenic. The cervix has a unique sonographic appearance in transverse or coronal images due to acoustic shadowing from the vaginal fornices. (See Figure 15-49.) Figures 15-50, 15-51, and 15-52 illustrate transvaginal images of the cervix.

Fallopian Tubes

The fallopian tubes are not routinely visualized in sonographic imaging. The region of the broad ligament and fallopian tube can be identified as a hypoechoic area extending laterally from the uterine cornu. (See Figure 15-53.) The small dimensions of the tube make it difficult to distinguish from the surrounding vasculature and tissue of the broad ligament. Advances in transvaginal imaging continue to improve visualization of these small structures.

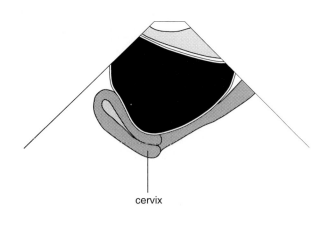
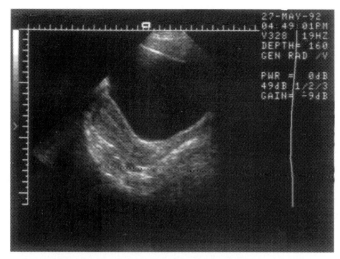

Figure 15–48. This sagittal transabdominal image demonstrates the cervix at the most inferior aspect of the uterus, closest to the vagina.

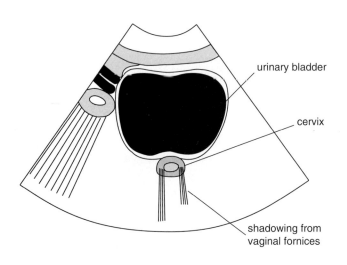
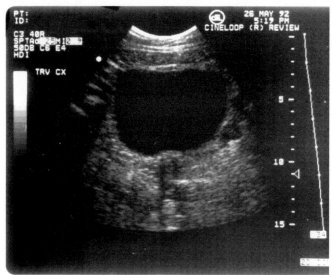

urinary bladder

cervix

shadowing from
vaginal fornices

Figure 15–49. In the transverse transabdominal image, shadowing from the vaginal fornices clearly denotes the level of the cervix.

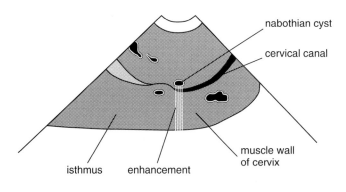
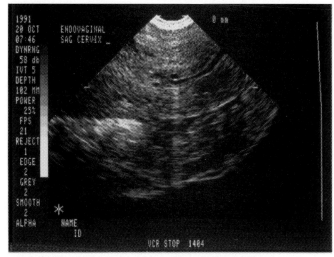

nabothian cyst

cervical canal

muscle wall
of cervix

isthmus   enhancement

Figure 15–50. The cervix is also well visualized transvaginally. This sagittal plane demonstrates a small quantity of anechoic fluid within the cervical canal. The uterus is in the normal anteverted position. A small nabothian cyst is seen within the wall of the cervix with posterior enhancement.

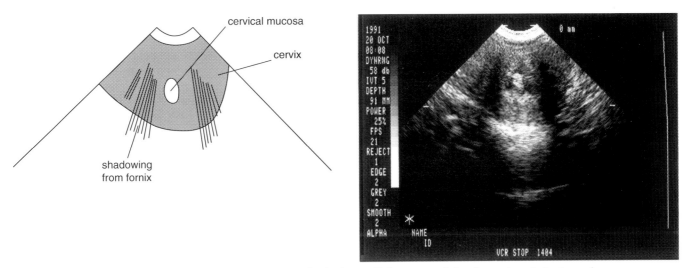

Figure 15–51. In the coronal transvaginal plane of the true pelvis, the anteverted uterus is sectioned transversely. Shadowing from the vaginal fornices is identified at the level of the cervix. Transvaginal sonography provides more detailed visualization of the cervical canal and mucosa.

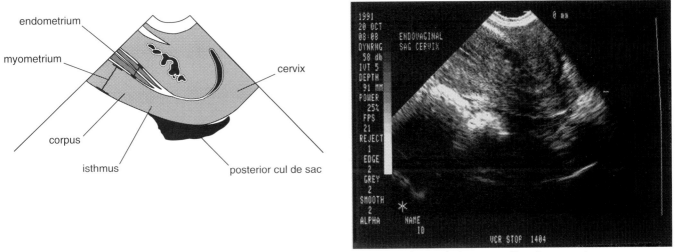

Figure 15–52. This sagittal transvaginal image demonstrates the cervix in an anteflexed uterus. A small quantity of anechoic fluid is seen in the posterior cul de sac. Note that the uterus bends forward at the level of the isthmus.

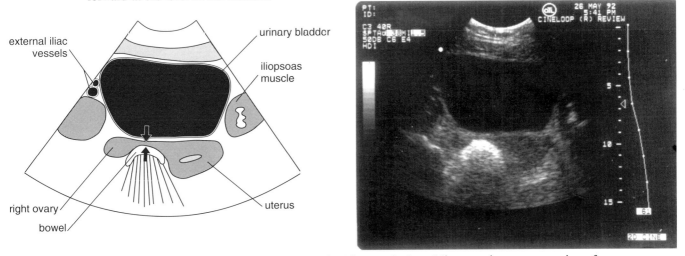

Figure 15–53. In the transverse transabdominal image, the broad ligament is seen as a region of low level echoes extending laterally from the uterine cornu toward the ovary (shown by arrows). The fallopian tube cannot be clearly distinguished.

Ovaries

The ovaries are located along the posterior aspect of the broad ligaments within the adnexal spaces of the true pelvis. These organs are most commonly identified lateral to the uterine fundus. The ovaries are slightly hypoechoic and more heterogeneous compared with the uterine myometrium. During reproductive years, small anechoic follicles are often visualized within the ovaries.

The ovaries are located along the lateral pelvic walls, medial to the iliopsoas muscles and external iliac vessels. The internal iliac vessels lie posterior to the ovaries. Sonographically, the vascular structures of the pelvis are anechoic and tubular. Sagittal views of the ovary with corresponding measurements are demonstrated in Figures 15–54 and 15–55. Transverse views of the ovary with a corresponding measurement are demonstrated in Figures 15–56 and 15–57.

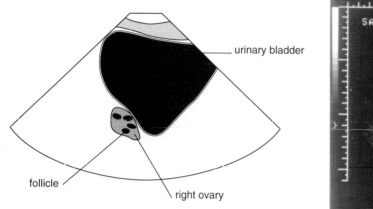
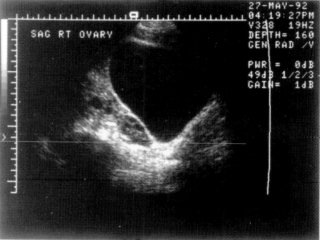

Figure 15–54. The almond shape of the ovary is apparent in this sagittal transabdominal image. The ovaries appear hypoechoic compared with the uterine myometrium, and several small anechoic follicles are seen within the ovary.

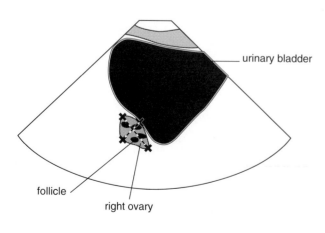
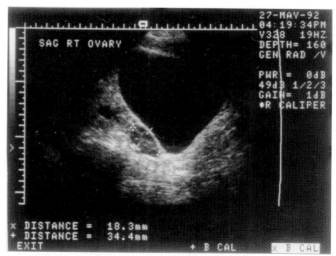

Figure 15–55. The length and thickness of the ovary are measured in the sagittal plane. The length is taken at the longest dimension of the ovary. The anteroposterior thickness is measured perpendicular to the length.

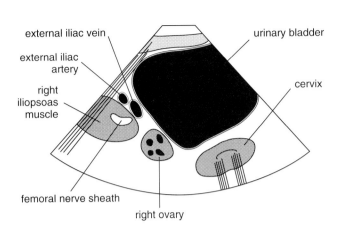

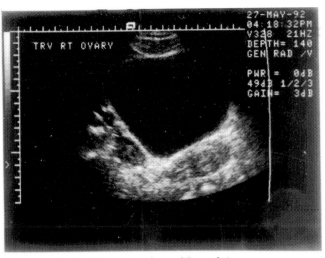

Figure 15–56. The transverse transabdominal image demonstrates the anatomic position of the ovary relative to its surrounding structures. The iliopsoas muscle and external iliac vessels are seen lateral to the right ovary. The uterus is seen medial to the right ovary. In this woman, the right ovary is located lateral to the cervix. More often, the ovary will be identified lateral to the uterine corpus or fundus.

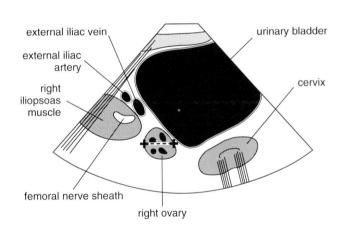

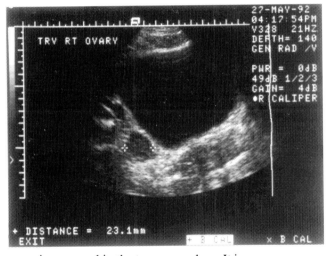

Figure 15–57. Transabdominally, the width of the ovary is measured in the transverse plane. It is also possible to measure the anteroposterior thickness of the ovary in this plane, perpendicular to the width.

Ovarian size and shape vary considerably throughout the ovulatory cycle. Follicles developing within the ovary are anechoic and vary in both size and number. The anechoic pattern of a follicle is due to visualization of the fluid-filled follicular antrum. (See Figures 15–58, 15–59, and 15–60.) The oocyte and cellular layers of the developing follicle cannot be identified. The cumulus oophorus of the secondary follicle can occasionally be seen as a thin echogenic crescent along the wall of the follicular antrum. (See Figure 15–61.) A mature graafian follicle is anechoic, with smooth walls, and measures approximately 18 to 22 mm in size. Acoustic enhancement is often seen posterior to the ovary due to the cystic nature of the follicles. The graafian follicle is commonly referred to as the **dominant follicle**. (See Figure 15–62.)

Following ovulation, the follicular fluid of the ruptured graafian follicle drains into the peritoneal cavity and can be seen in the pouch of Douglas. Fluid in the posterior cul de sac appears anechoic and molds to the shape of surrounding structures. Acoustic enhancement can usually be seen posterior to this fluid collection. (See Figures 15–30, 15–52, and 15–66.)

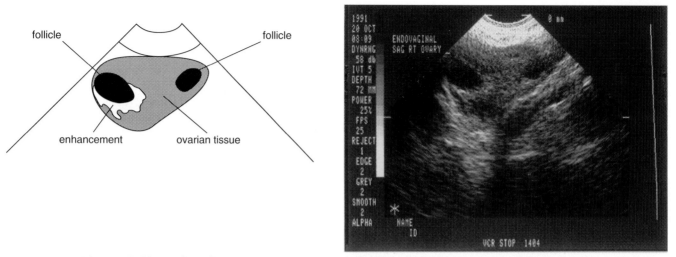

Figure 15–58. This sagittal transvaginal image of the right ovary demonstrates normal ovarian parenchyma and two developing follicles. Moderate acoustic enhancement is seen posterior to the larger follicle.

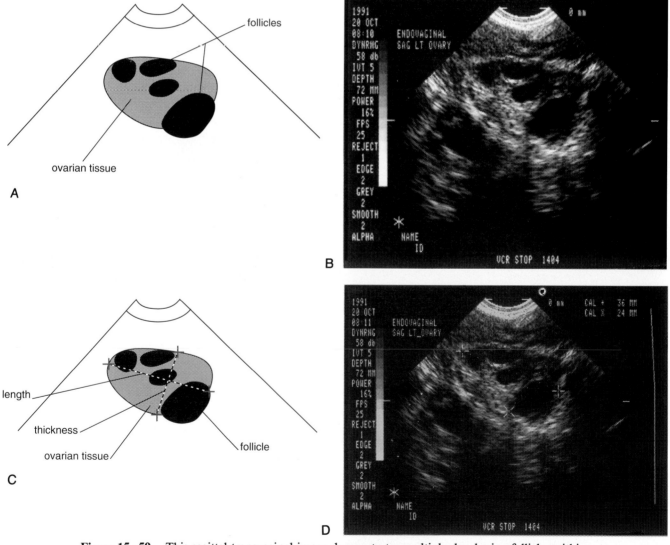

Figure 15–59. This sagittal transvaginal image demonstrates multiple developing follicles within the ovary. The length and anteroposterior thickness of the ovary are measured in *C* and *D*. Enhancement is seen posterior to the ovary due to the fluid-filled follicles.

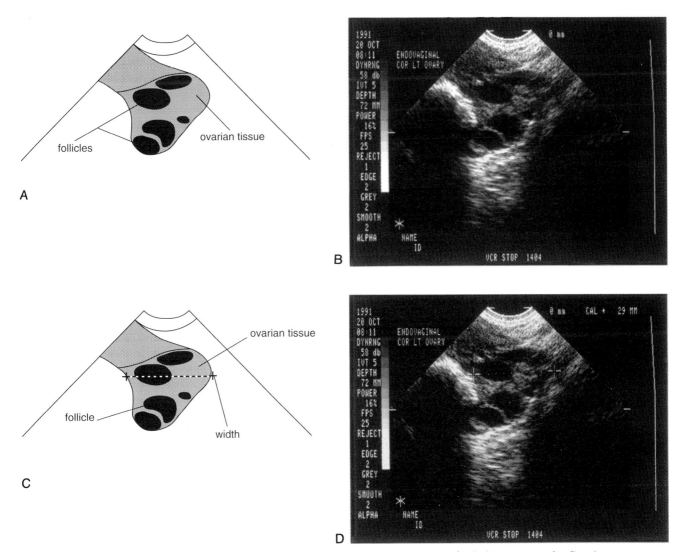

Figure 15–60. The ovarian width is measured in the coronal transvaginal plane, as seen in *C* and *D*. Individual follicles would be measured in the same three-dimensional manner as the ovary itself.

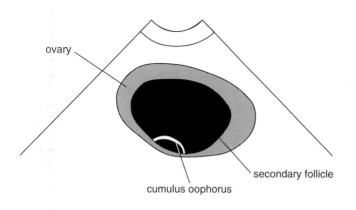

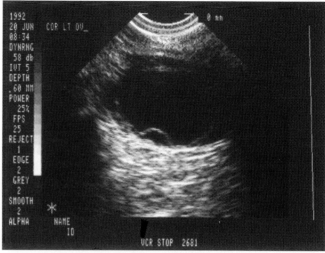

Figure 15–61. This coronal transvaginal image demonstrates the cumulus oophorus as a thin hyperechoic crescent along the wall of the mature follicle. The secondary oocyte is contained within the cumulus oophorus.

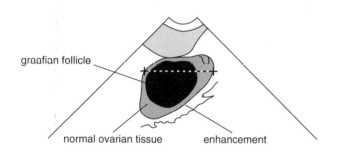

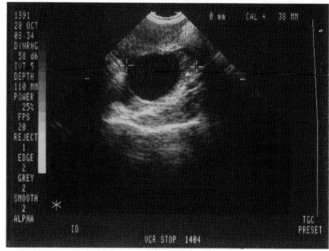

Figure 15–62. This coronal transvaginal image demonstrates a mature graafian follicle within the ovary. Sonographically, the graafian follicle is anechoic, smooth walled, and round or oval in shape. The mature follicle is usually 18 to 22 mm in size and exhibits posterior enhancement.

Immediately postovulation, the corpus luteum is irregular in shape and contains internal echoes due to hemorrhage. These internal echoes vary in appearance from multiple fine septations to diffuse, homogenous low level echoes. (See Figures 15–63 and 15–64.) This central blood clot may become completely anechoic over time, at which point the corpus luteum resembles the sonographic appearance of a mature follicle. Eventually, the corpus luteum regresses, leaving a small amount of scar tissue in the ovary, called the corpus albicans. (See Figure 15–65.) The corpus albicans is occasionally seen as an echogenic focus within the ovarian stroma. Transvaginal sonography provides excellent definition of the ovaries and the follicular structures.

The ovaries may be situated anywhere within the adnexal regions, including the posterior cul de sac. They may also be found superior to the uterine fundus. The ovaries are secured posterior to the broad ligaments and thus cannot be situated anterior to the uterus or between the uterus and the urinary bladder.

Pelvic Bowel

Loops of small bowel resting within the pelvic cavity appear heterogeneous and hyperechoic, and demonstrate peristaltic activity. The small intestine is displaced superiorly by the distended urinary bladder during transabdominal ultrasound examination. In transvaginal imaging, these loops of bowel can be seen in peristalsis around the uterus and ovaries. Gas in the small intestine can occasionally obscure visualization of the ovaries.

The sigmoid colon and rectum do not demonstrate peristalsis. The sonographic appearance of these structures is variable, depending largely on filling stages. The colon and rectum typically appear echogenic with posterior shadowing due to gas and fecal material. They can

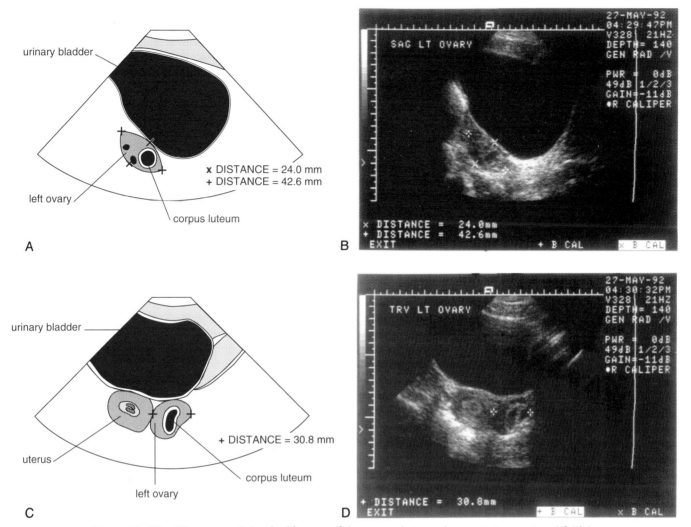

Figure 15–63. These transabdominal images of the corpus luteum demonstrate a ruptured follicle in both the sagittal (*A*, *B*) and transverse planes (*C*, *D*). Following ovulation, the walls of the follicle are irregular, and low level echoes are seen within this developing corpus luteum.

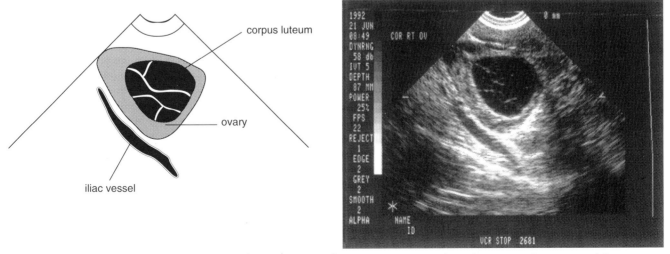

Figure 15–64. The sonographic appearance of the corpus luteum is variable. In this coronal transvaginal image, the corpus luteum contains multiple fine septations.

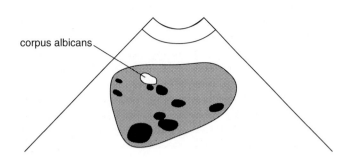

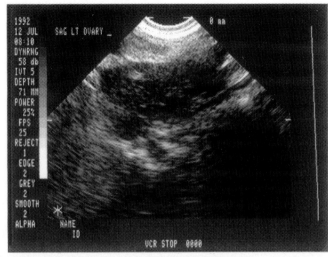

Figure 15-65. The corpus albicans is the remaining scar tissue in the ovary following regression of the corpus luteum. This sagittal transvaginal image demonstrates the corpus albicans, which appears as a highly echogenic foci within the ovary.

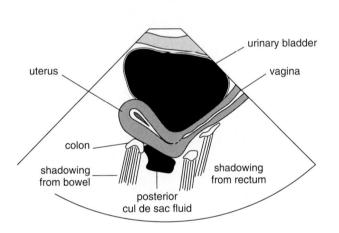

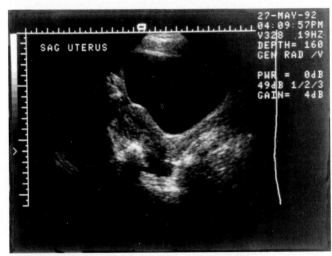

Figure 15-66. The rectum and sigmoid colon of the pelvic bowel are often seen in the sagitttal transabdominal image. The rectum appears hyperechoic, posterior to the vagina. The sigmoid colon has a similar appearance and lies posterior to the uterus. A small quantity of anechoic fluid is seen in the posterior cul de sac; this is a frequent finding following ovulation.

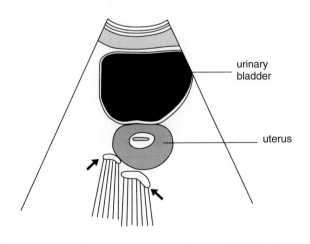

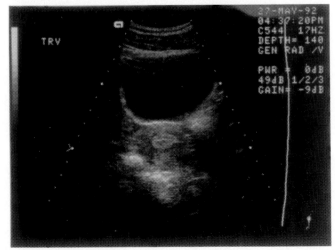

Figure 15-67. This transverse transabdominal image of the bowel also demonstrates the sigmoid colon (shown by arrows) posterior to the uterus.

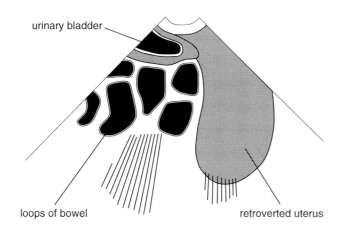

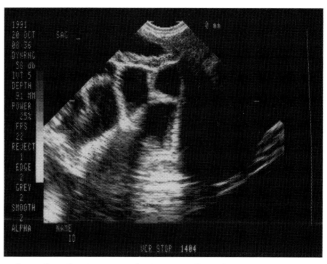

Figure 15–68. Peristaltic loops of small bowel are often visualized transvaginally. In this sagittal image, the uterus is moderately retroverted. Loops of bowel are resting in the anterior cul de sac.

be identified posterior to the uterus and vagina. (See Figures 15–66, 15–67, and 15–68.)

Pelvic Skeleton

Sonography is not a modality of choice for evaluating osseous structures. On the other hand, the distinctive sonographic appearance of the pelvic skeleton creates useful landmarks. The lumbar and sacral spine form the posterior boundary of the true pelvis. The vertebral bodies are highly echogenic with posterior acoustic shadowing. The iliac crests can be identified as highly echogenic linear structures with posterior shadowing. These crests are seen in the near field of a transabdominal image when scanning along the superolateral aspect of the pelvis. (See Figures 15–69 and 15–70.)

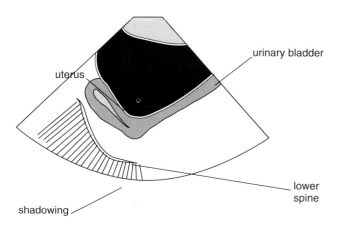

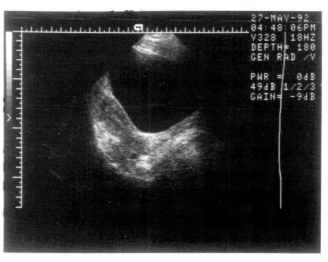

Figure 15–69. The lower vertebral spine is seen in the far field of a midsagittal plane of the true pelvis. The vertebral bodies appear hyperechoic with posterior shadowing.

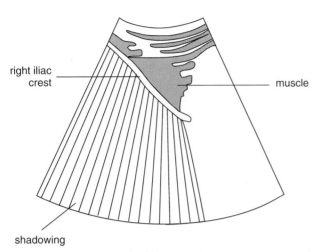

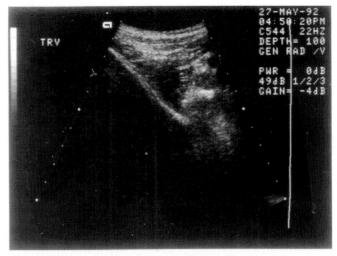

Figure 15–70. The iliac crest is easily identified as a hyperechoic structure in the near field of this transverse transabdominal image. As with the vertebral spine, this bone creates acoustic shadowing, so that structures posterior to the bone are not visualized.

SONOGRAPHIC APPLICATIONS

Pelvic sonography is often used in assessing the size and shape of the uterus and the ovaries. Ultrasound is used in diagnosing congenital uterine anomalies, uterine and ovarian masses, and pelvic inflammatory processes.

Ultrasound aids in evaluating ovarian masses in the pediatric through the geriatric populations. This diagnostic tool is helpful in differentiating physiologic changes in the ovary from ovarian neoplasms. It is possible to characterize the cystic or solid composition of pelvic masses through ultrasound. This modality is more limited, however, in providing definitive diagnoses of the benignity or malignancy of such masses.

Color flow and **spectral Doppler** are valuable tools in assessing blood flow to the ovaries and to ovarian masses. During the normal ovulatory cycle, the functional ovary receives greater vascular perfusion between days 9 and 28 of the menstrual cycle. This is reflected in a lower resistance Doppler waveform in the ovary producing the dominant follicle.[4] A low resistance waveform has a high amount of diastolic flow.

Doppler assessment of arteries supplying malignant pelvic tumors commonly exhibits low resistance waveforms. Benign neoplasms are generally supplied by higher resistance vessels. Clinical studies utilizing transvaginal color flow Doppler and spectral Doppler suggest great potential for differentiating benign from malignant tumors using these techniques. (See Figure 15–71.)

Ultrasound plays a significant role in diagnosing and

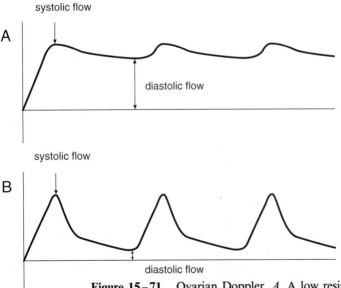

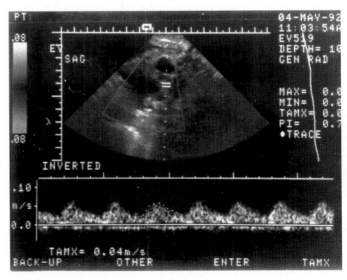

Figure 15–71. Ovarian Doppler. *A*, A low resistance waveform, obtained in the ovarian artery. Low resistance vessels exhibit a high amount of flow during diastole. *B*, An ovarian artery with higher resistance. *C*, Doppler signal obtained from a malignant ovarian tumor. The low resistance of this vessel is reflected in the low pulsatility index of 0.79.

managing infertility. Pelvic sonography is used in assessing contributing causes of infertility such as endometriosis, congenital anomalies, myomata, and pelvic inflammatory disease. Transvaginal sonography is routinely employed in monitoring follicular development, particularly in patients undergoing hormone therapy. Follicular size, endometrial thickness and echopattern, and visualization of the cumulus oophorus are important predictive factors of ovulation. Ultrasound guidance is also particularly important for ovum retrieval prior to **in vitro fertilization**.

An additional application of pelvic sonography is in detecting *intrauterine contraceptive devices (IUDs, IUCDs)*. While IUDs are seldom used in the United States, their use is widespread in many other parts of the world. Figure 15–72 demonstrates four common types of IUDs. These devices generally appear highly echo-

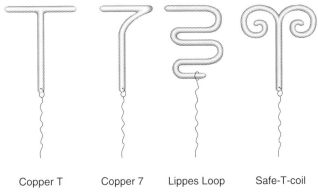

Copper T   Copper 7   Lippes Loop   Safe-T-coil

Figure 15–72. Intrauterine contraceptive devices.

genic with varying degrees of posterior acoustic shadowing. Figures 15–73, 15–74, and 15–75 demonstrate the typical sonographic patterns of IUDs.

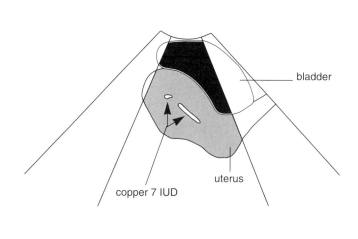

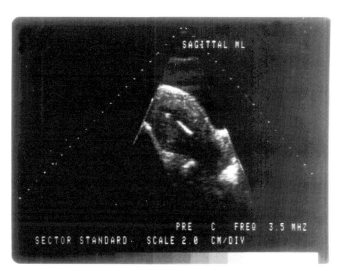

Figure 15–73. The Copper Seven IUD is easily visualized in a sagittal view of the uterus. This device is highly echogenic and rests within the endometrial cavity.

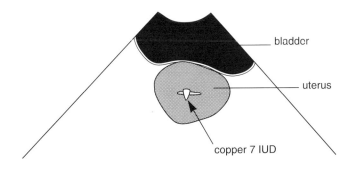

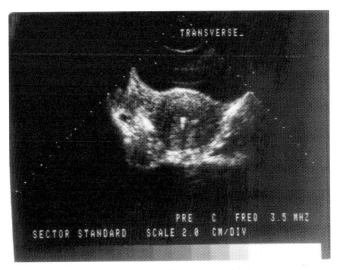

Figure 15–74. This image demonstrates the Copper Seven IUD in a transverse transabdominal scan.

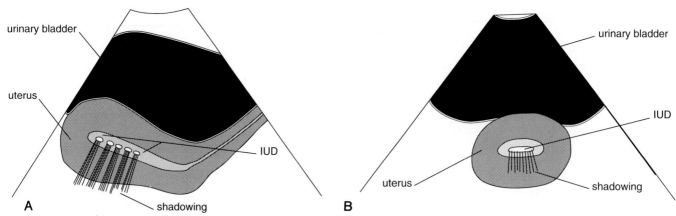

Figure 15–75. *A*, A sagittal plane through the Lippes Loop IUD has the distinct appearance of five echogenic foci spaced in a line within the endometrial canal. *B*, A transverse plane may depict a longer segment of the device. Posterior shadowing is frequently seen with IUDs.

NORMAL VARIANTS

Variations in uterine position are shown in Figure 15–1. Some were illustrated in transvaginal images earlier in this chapter. It is important to be able to recognize variations in uterine position both transvaginally and transabdominally. Figure 15–76 demonstrates a sagittal

transabdominal view of the retroverted uterus. Because of the posterior position of the retroverted uterine fundus, it is more difficult to evaluate the uterine echotexture. Figure 15–77 is a schematic drawing of the retroflexed uterus imaged in a sagittal transabdominal plane.

When the bladder is fully distended, both the ante-

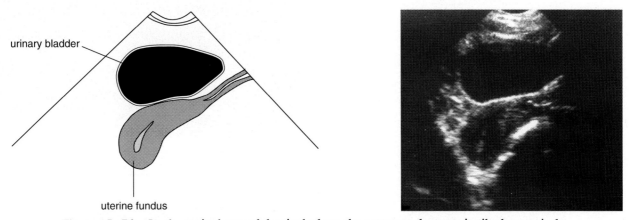

Figure 15–76. In the sagittal transabdominal plane the retroverted uterus is tilted posteriorly, toward the posterior cul de sac.

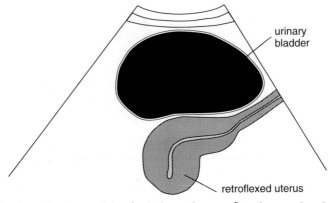

Figure 15–77. In the sagittal transabdominal plane, the retroflexed uterus bends more posteriorly, with flexion occurring at the isthmus.

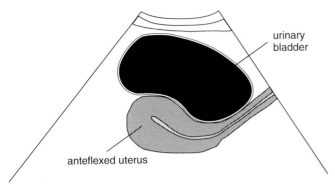

Figure 15–78. In the sagittal transabdominal plane, the anteflexed uterus slightly indents the urinary bladder.

The Bicornuate Uterus

Incomplete fusion of the Müllerian ducts can result in partial duplication of the uterus. The bicornuate uterus is recognized sonographically by the presence of two endometrial canals. The endometrial canals usually communicate at the level of the cervix. This congenital anomaly is best appreciated in the transverse plane. Figure 15–79 demonstrates a transverse transabdominal image of a bicornuate uterus. A gestational sac is seen in the right horn of the uterus. Myometrial tissue is seen separating the two endometrial canals of the uterus.

Post Hysterectomy

Pelvic sonography is useful in evaluating ovaries in women who have undergone hysterectomy. In the absence of the uterus, the ovaries typically rest within the posterior cul de sac. Figure 15–80 is a schematic drawing of the transabdominal midsagittal plane post hysterectomy.

verted and anteflexed uterus are pushed posteriorly. Consequently, it is difficult to differentiate these positions transabdominally. Figure 15–78 demonstrates the slight anterior flexion of the isthmus as seen transabdominally.

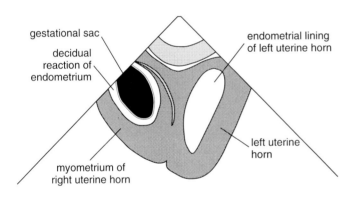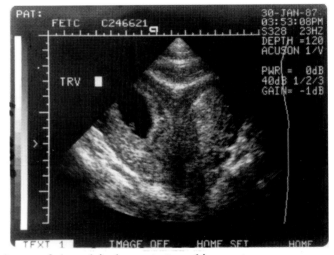

Figure 15–79. This transverse transabdominal image of the pelvis demonstrates a bicornuate uterus containing a gestational sac within the right endometrial cavity. The gestational sac is anechoic and is surrounded by the hyperechoic decidual reaction of the endometrial lining. Myometrial tissue separates the endometrial canals of the left and right uterine horns.

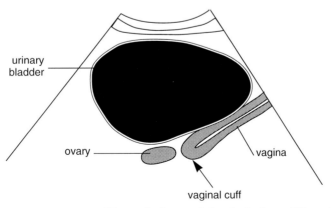

Figure 15–80. Post hysterectomy. The sagittal transabdominal plane of the pelvis posthysterectomy. The vaginal cuff is seen and the uterus is absent. The ovaries can often be identified in the posterior cul de sac.

REFERENCE CHARTS

Associated Physicians

Gynecologist: A physician specializing in female reproduction, including physiology, endocrinology, and diseases of the genital tract.

Endocrinologist: A physician specializing in the physiologic and pathologic association of hormonal secretions of the body.

Obstetrician: A physician specializing in the medical care of pregnant women.

Radiologist: A physician specializing in the administration and interpretation of diagnostic medical imaging.

Common Diagnostic Tests

Computed Tomography and Magnetic Resonance Imaging: CT and MRI are both extremely important diagnostic tools in evaluating the female pelvis. Improvements in contrast agents continue to enhance the superior tissue characterization of these modalities. These tests are performed by trained technologists and interpreted by radiologists.

Laparoscopy: An endoscopic procedure performed under local or general anesthesia in which a telescopic instrument is inserted into the abdominal cavity from the area of the navel. The laparoscope can be manipulated in order to visualize the abdominal or pelvic organs. This test is performed and interpreted by a gynecologist.

Hysteroscopy/salpingoscopy: An endoscopic procedure in which a telescopic instrument is inserted through the vagina and into the uterus. This test allows visualization of the interior uterine walls. This technique can also be used to visualize the fallopian tubes. These tests are performed and interpreted by a gynecologist or a similarly trained physician.

Hysterosalpingography: A radiologic examination of the uterus and fallopian tubes following dye (contrast agent) administration. Tubal blockage and structural abnormalities of the uterus can be diagnosed. This procedure is performed and interpreted by a radiologist.

Laboratory Values

Human Chorionic Gonadotropin (hCG): A highly accurate blood pregnancy test. This hormone is produced by the placental trophoblastic cells and plays an important role during the first trimester of pregnancy.

Leukocytosis: An abnormally high serum white blood cell count (exceeding 10,000 per mm³). This condition is indicative of an infectious process (such as pelvic inflammatory disease).

Estrogen/Progesterone: These hormones are produced by the ovary during the normal menstrual cycle. Serum concentrations of these hormones can be useful in evaluating ovulatory function.

Normal Measurements

	Length	×	Thickness	×	Width
Adult Uterus:	8 cm	×	3 cm	×	5.5 cm
Adult Ovary	2.5–5 cm	×	0.6–2.2 cm	×	1.5–3 cm
Postmenopausal Ovary	2 cm	×	1 cm	×	2 cm
Adult Ovarian Volume	approximately 6 to 13 cc				

Vasculature

Uterine Vasculature:

Aorta—common iliac artery—uterine—internal iliac artery—uterine artery—arcuate arteries—radial arteries—straight arteries—spiral arteries—spiral veins—straight veins—radial veins—arcuate veins—uterine vein—internal iliac vein—common iliac vein—inferior vena cava.

Ovarian Vasculature:

PATHWAY ONE. Aorta—common iliac artery—internal iliac artery—uterine artery—ovarian branch of uterine artery—ovarian branch of uterine vein—uterine vein—internal iliac vein—common iliac vein—inferior vena cava.

PATHWAY TWO. Aorta—right ovarian artery—right ovarian vein—inferior vena cava *or* aorta—left ovarian artery—left ovarian vein—left renal vein—inferior vena cava.

Affecting Chemicals

Birth Control Pills: Estrogen and progestin provide a highly effective form of birth control. These medications mimic the hormonal conditions of pregnancy, resulting in an anovulatory state.

Diethylstilbestrol (DES): A synthetic estrogen commonly administered to pregnant women from the late 1940s to the early 1970s. This medication was thought to reduce the risks of spontaneous abortion. DES was taken off the market after it was discovered to cause multiple problems involving the reproductive organs of offspring exposed to the drug in utero. A small, irregular, T-shaped uterus is a common malformation associated with DES exposure.

Menotropins (Pergonal), Urofollitropin (Metrodin), Clomiphene Citrate (Clomid): Medications commonly prescribed in infertility to stimulate follicular maturation and induce ovulation.

References

1. Gonen Y, Casper R: Prediction of implantation by the sonographic appearance of the endometrium during controlled ovarian stimulation for in vitro fertilization (IVF). In Vitro Fertilization Embryo Transfer 7(3):146–152, 1990.
2. Ueno, J, Oehninger S, Brzyski R, et al.: Ultrasonic appearance of the endometrium in natural and stimulated in-vitro fertilization cycles and its correlation with outcome. Hum Reprod 6:901–904, 1991.
3. Grunfeld L, Walker B, Bergh P, et al: High-resolution endovaginal ultrasonography of the endometrium: a noninvasive test for endometrial adequacy. Obstet Gynecol 78:200–204, 1991.
4. Taylor L, Burns P, Wells P, et al: Ultrasound Doppler flow studies of the ovarian and uterine arteries. Brit J Obstet Gynecol 92:240–246, 1985.
5. Bourne T, Campbell S, Steer C, et al: Transvaginal colour flow imaging: a possible new screening technique for ovarian cancer. Brit Med J 299:1367–1370, 1989.
6. Campbell S, Bhan V, Royston P, et al: Transabdominal ultrasound screening for early ovarian cancer. Brit Med J 299:1363–1366, 1989.

Bibliography

Corson S: Conquering Infertility, a Guide for Couples (rev. ed.). New York, Prentice Hall, 1983.

Ferner H, Staubesand J (eds.): Sobatta's Atlas of Human Anatomy, vol 2. Baltimore, Urban & Schwarzenberg, 1983.
Fleischer A, Rodgers W, Rao B, et al: Assessment of ovarian tumor vascularity with transvaginal color Doppler sonography. J Ultrasound Med 10:563–568, 1991.
Kurjack A, Zalud I, Alfirevic Z, Jurkovic D: The assessment of abnormal pelvic blood flow by transvaginal color and pulsed Doppler. Ultrasound Med Biol 16(5):437–442, 1990.
Kurjack A, Zalud I, Jurkovic D, et al: Transvaginal color Doppler for the assessment of pelvic circulation. Acta Obstet Gynecol Scand 68:131–135, 1989.
Lev-Toaff A, Toaff M, Friedman A: Endovaginal sonographic appearance of a DES uterus. Ultrasound Med 9(11):661–4, 1990.
Netter F: Atlas of Human Anatomy. Summitt, NJ, CIBA-GEIGY, 1989–1991.
Sanders R: With the Sonographers of the Johns Hopkins Hospital. Clinical Sonography, a Practical Guide, 2nd ed. Boston, Little, Brown, 1992.
Van Gils A, Tham R, Falke T, Peters A: Abnormalities of the uterus and cervix after diethylstilbestrol exposure: correlation of findings on MR and hysterosalpingography. Am J Roentgenol 153(6):1235–1238, 1989.
Vieiralves-Wiltgen C, Engle F: Identification and management of DES-exposed women. Nurse Practitioner 13(11):15–20, 1988.
Waldroup L, Liu J: Sonographic anatomy of the female pelvis. In Berman, M (ed.). Diagnostic Medical Sonography, a Guide to Clinical Practice (vol. 1), Obstetrics and Gynecology. Philadelphia, JB Lippincott, 1991.

SECTION V

OBSTETRICS

Chapter 16

FIRST TRIMESTER OBSTETRICS

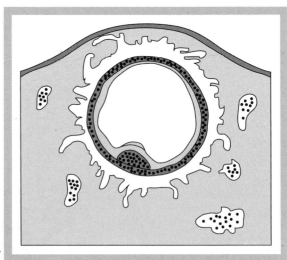

Implementation of the early human embryo. (From Guyton AC: Textbook of Medical Physiology, 8th ed. Philadelphia, WB Saunders, 1991, p 916.)

G. WILLIAM SHEPHERD

Objectives:

Describe the role of the female reproductive system in creating and supporting a developing embryo.

Describe the locations and functions of the early support tissues of the gestation.

Describe the early embryogenesis of the fetal organs and organ systems.

Describe the ultrasound appearance of the gestational sac and early embryo.

List the laboratory tests which may be performed during the first trimester and describe the information they supply.

Define the key words.

Key Words:

Alimentary canal
Amnion
Amniotic cavity
Amniotic fluid
Antiflexion

Antiversion
Biparietal diameter
Blastocyst
Chorion
Chorion frondosum
Chorion laeve
Chorionic villi
Corpus albicans
Corpus luteum
Crown-rump length (CRL)
Decidua
Decidua basalis
Decidua capsularis
Decidua vera
Decidual reaction
Double sac sign
Embryonic disk
Endometrium
Estrogen
Fetal pole
Follicle stimulating hormone (FSH)
Foregut
Gestational sac

Hindgut
Human chorionic gonadotropin (HCG)
Implantation
Inner cell mass
Lacunae
Luteinizing hormone (LH)
Mesencephalon
Midgut
Morula
Neurocrest
Neuroplate
Neurotube
Placenta
Primary yolk sac
Progesterone
Prosencephalon
Retroflexion
Retroversion
Rhombencephalon
Trophoblastic cells
Zygote

INTRODUCTION

Chapters 16, 17, and 18 describe the anatomy, physiology, embryology, and ultrasound appearance of the embryo (or fetus) and its support structures at various stages of pregnancy. The organs and organ systems are presented as individual units, while ultrasound images show the relationships among the organs. Chapter 18 describes some special situations and examinations which may arise during a pregnancy.

FEMALE REPRODUCTIVE SYSTEM

Preparation of the female reproductive organs for support of a pregnancy begins 14 days prior to conception. On the first day of the menstrual cycle, **follicle stimulating hormone (FSH)** is released by the anterior lobe of the pituitary gland. The presence of this hormone in the bloodstream initiates the process of follicle maturation. At this time the **ovary** makes moderate amounts of **estrogen**. On days 2 through 7 of the menstrual cycle, the follicle grows and produces increasing amounts of estrogen, which in turn stimulates the lining of the uterus (**endometrium**) and produces many new blood vessels. During days 7 through 12 the follicle nears maximum size (22 to 25 mm) and estrogen levels increase. During days 13 and 14 the high estrogen level in the bloodstream causes the release of **luteinizing hormone (LH)** from the anterior lobe of the pituitary gland. Luteinizing hormone causes the follicle to rupture, releasing the ovum. On days 14 and 15 the follicle is transformed into the **corpus luteum**, and produces **progesterone**. This hormone prepares the uterus for **implantation**. If fertilization does not occur by the twenty-first day of the menstrual cycle, the estrogen and progesterone levels will fall. The endometrium then outgrows its blood supply and sloughs off. On day 28, the last day of the period, the corpus luteum is much decreased in size and is now called the corpus albicans. The menstrual cycle then begins anew. The cyclic alteration of hormonal levels, the changes in the uterus, and the changes in the follicle will continue until

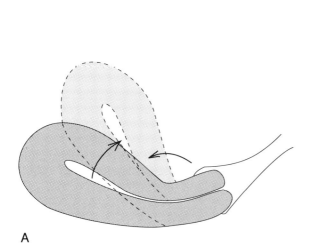

A

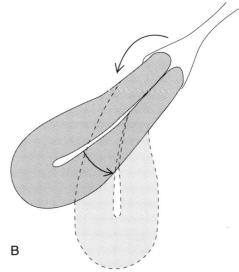

B

Figure 16–1. *A,* An antiverted uterus. The dotted line indicates the position of an antiverted antiflexed uterus. The arrows indicate the angles of antiversion and antiflexion. *B,* A retroverted uterus. The dotted line indicates the position of a retroverted retroflexed uterus. The arrows indicate the angles of retroversion and retroflexion.

the fertilized ovum, or **zygote**, is carried to the uterus or until cessation of menstruation (menopause).

It is important to recall, from Chapter 15, that the position of the uterus will affect the appearance of the early gestation during an ultrasound examination. The uterus may be tilted forward at the junction of the uterus and cervix, a position known as **antiversion**. Or it may be tilted in a posterior direction, or **retroversion**. The uterus may be tilted forward at the isthmus (or waist of the uterus), known as **antiflexion**. The uterus may be tilted away from the anterior wall of the abdomen at the isthmus, called **retroflexion**. The uterus may in fact be antiverted and retroflexed, antiverted and antiflexed, retroverted and antiflexed, or retroverted and retroflexed. These variations in uterine position are shown in Figure 16–1.

The ovaries and the fallopian tubes complete the female reproductive tract. The ovaries produce hormones and ova, and the fallopian tubes serve as the conduits by which fertilized ova or zygotes reach the endometrial lining of the uterus.

FERTILIZATION AND EARLY DEVELOPMENT

Fertilization usually takes place in the distal third of the fallopian tube on about day 15. The ovum, now referred to as a **zygote**, will divide and eventually form a cluster of 16 to 32 cells, the **morula**. The morula continues to grow and forms a **blastocyst** by day 20. The blastocyst is a fluid-filled cyst lined with **trophoblastic cells**. There is a clump of cells at one end, the **inner cell mass**. Implantation into the uterine lining usually occurs between days 20 and 23. Maternal endometrial cells adjacent to the blastocyst become modified to supply nourishment to the developing embryo. This change in the endometrium is the **decidual reaction**. There is a rapid proliferation of the **syncytiotrophoblastic** tissues (trophoblastic cells which contact the endometrium) during the fourth week. A primitive uteroplacental circulation is established early in implantation. Primary **chorionic villi** are formed, surrounded by pools of maternal blood called **lacunae**. Chorionic villi are finger-like projections of the outermost layer of embryonic tissue extending into the deciduate uterine tissues. These events are depicted in Figure 16–2.

During week 4, the inner cell mass changes dramatically. It forms an **embryonic disk**, an embryonic cavity, and a **primary yolk sac**. The primary yolk sac regresses by the end of week 4 and a secondary yolk sac forms between the **amnion** (the innermost membrane of the embryo) and the **chorion** (the outermost tissues of the embryo). Figure 16–3 demonstrates the relationships of the embryo, yolk sac, amnion, and chorion to one another.

At this point, week 5, a very small gestational sac exists in the uterus. The tissues that make up this sac are as follows: The **decidua** is the changed lining of the uterus during pregnancy. It is composed of several tissues, as follows. The **decidua basalis** is the thick decidua existing at the implantation site. The **decidua vera** is the decidua along the remainder of the uterine cavity, beside the implantation site. It is also called the **decidua parietalis**. The **decidua capsularis** is the thin decidua overlying the portion of the gestational sac facing the endometrial cavity. The **chorion** is the embryonic tissue lining the exterior of the gestational sac. The purpose of the chorion is to invade the decidua and establish nutrition for the embryo. The **chorion frondosum** is the portion of the chorion located at the implantation site. It consists of projecting fingers of tissue, the chorionic villi, which are actively invading the decidua of the uterus. The **chorion laeve** is the thin chorionic covering of the gestational sac facing the endometrial cavity. Figure 16–4 demonstrates the relationships of these early gestational tissues.

Two fetal membranes surround the embryo. The amnion is inside the sac and makes contact with the fluid surrounding the embryo and often with the fetus. The amnion consists of four connective layers and one epithelial layer. It is derived from primary embryonic ectoderm and is not a vascular membrane. The amnion will become the covering of the umbilical cord. The fluid and the embryo are enclosed by the amniotic membrane. The yolk sac lies outside this membrane, but inside the next membrane of the embryo called the chorion. The chorion is derived from trophoblastic ectoderm, the original layer of cells in the blastocyst. This membrane is vascular; it surrounds the amnion and the yolk sac. The chorion is juxtaposed to the endometrial cavity. The amnion and the chorion eventually fuse (usually after 16 weeks) and become closely associated.

The **amniotic fluid** is the liquid enclosed by the amnion which surrounds and bathes the embryo. This fluid has five important functions: (1) permits symmetrical growth of the embryo and fetus; (2) prevents adhesions from forming in the fetal membranes; (3) cushions the embryo and acts as a "shock absorber"; (4) helps to maintain proper temperature of the embryo; and (5) allows movement and thus development of muscle tone. The amniotic fluid may also have a function in fetal lung development.

Implantation of the embryo in the uterus initiates the early development of the **placenta**. The early invading chorionic tissues produce a hormone **human chorionic gonadotropin (HCG)**. This hormone stimulates the corpus luteum to grow and continues to produce progesterone. The corpus luteum will eventually reach approximately 4 cm in diameter in 8 to 9 weeks. It will then regress, disappearing at about 12 weeks. Figure 16–5 is an ultrasound image of a corpus luteum.

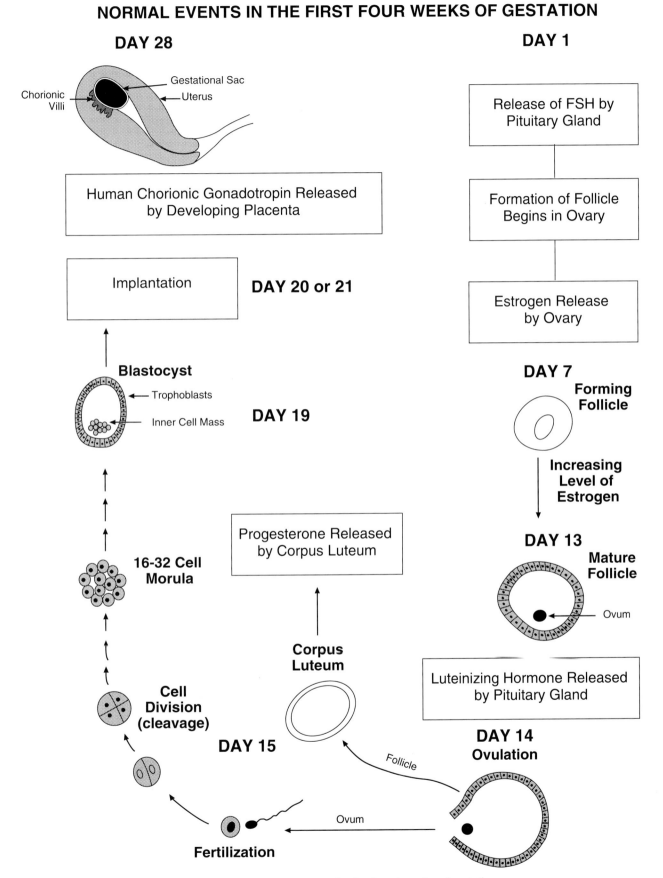

Figure 16–2. Normal events in the first 4 weeks of gestation.

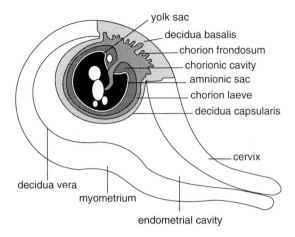

Figure 16-3. An 8- to 10-week gestational sac.

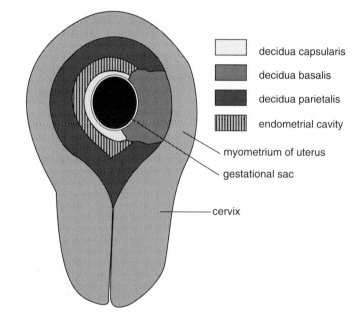

Figure 16-4. Decidual reaction associated with a 4- to 5-week gestational sac. The elements which produce the double sac sign are indicated.

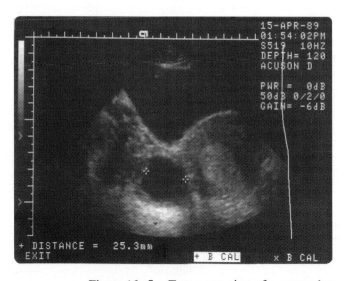

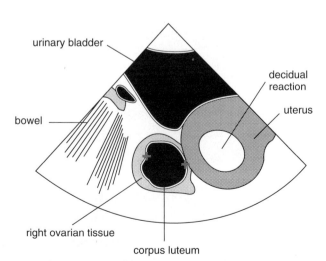

Figure 16-5. Transverse view of a corpus luteum cyst adjacent to a uterus with an early decidual reaction.

SONOGRAPHIC APPEARANCE OF THE EARLY GESTATION

The gestational sac has a distinct appearance in ultrasound at this time. It is known as the **double sac sign**. At a menstrual age of 5 weeks, a gestational sac may be seen before a yolk sac or embryo is visible. A normal sac should have a double sac sign. This sign distinguishes a pseudosac from the actual one. Two echogenic concentric rings are seen separated by a hyperechoic zone. The inner ring is the decidua capsularis plus the chorion laeve. The outer ring is the decidua vera. The darker zone separating these rings is probably due to a small amount of fluid in the endometrial cavity dividing these tissues. The bright rim is thicker at the implantation sight; it represents the decidua basalis and the chorion frondosum. Figures 16-6 and 16-7 show the double sac sign.

The secondary yolk sac will become visible at 5 to 6 weeks. (See Figure 16-8.) It may be possible to see the secondary yolk sac even though the **fetal pole** (embryo) is still not discernible. The yolk sac can serve as an aid in determining the viability of the pregnancy since a faint flickering motion may be visible adjacent to the yolk sac. This flicker probably represents neurologically active heart tissue. It is often seen before the embryo can be distinguished and will confirm viability despite the lack of visualization of the embryo per se. The yolk sac is about 5 to 6 mm at this stage.

The embryo should be visible by 6 weeks, earlier if endoscanning or transvaginal transducers are employed. The head and rump of the embryo will become discernible at 7 to 9 weeks depending on the type of equipment used, the body habitus (size of the woman), and, of course, the skill of the sonographer.

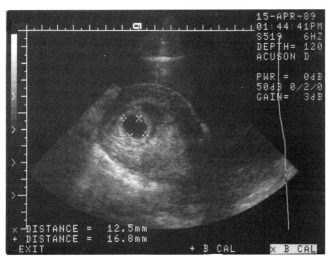
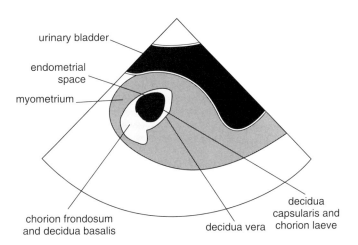

Figure 16-6. Longitudinal view of a 5-week gestational sac.

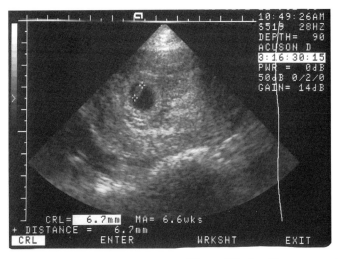
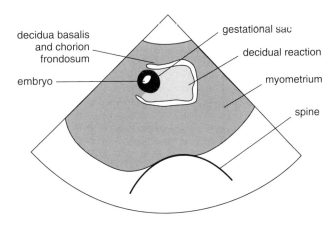

Figure 16-7. Transverse view of a 5-week gestational sac.

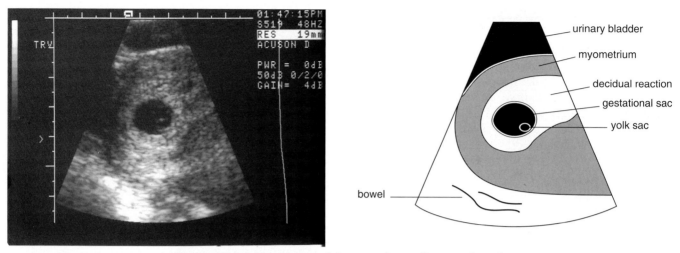

Figure 16–8. Appearance of the secondary yolk sac at 6 weeks.

SONOGRAPHIC MEASUREMENTS OF THE EARLY GESTATION

At this point in the pregnancy two important measurements are determined by ultrasound. The distance from the top of the head to the bottom of the rump is called the **crown-rump length**. Figure 16–9 demonstrates this measurement. This length can be used to accurately determine the age of the gestation. It is accurate to within 4 days of the actual age if done correctly. Thus, measurements made during the late first trimester are more dependable than later measurements in dating a pregnancy. Every gestation begins as a single cell but eventually individual differences in growth rate give rise to a range of sizes, all of which are normal for a given gestational age. Early in the pregnancy these individual differences are much less pronounced than they are later and therefore more reliable.

Another measurement that can be used to date the pregnancy, particularly before the embryo can be visualized, is the average sac diameter. This is the measurement from the inside borders of the gestational sac; the average length, width, and height are measured and divided by 3. Figure 16–10 demonstrate these measurements. The average sac diameter can be used to date the gestation in early embryos and to determine whether adequate fluid is present later on when the crown-rump measurement may be obtained. There should be a good correlation between the age determined by sac size and the gestational age determined by the crown rump. Viability of the pregnancy is evident by the observation of embryonic heart activity, which often may be seen as early as 5.2 weeks with transvaginal scanning. Heart motion should certainly be seen by 7 weeks with transabdominal scanning, except in instances in which a woman's size may inhibit clear visualization of the embryo.

As the primitive placenta is forming in the uterus and

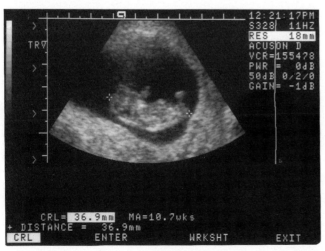

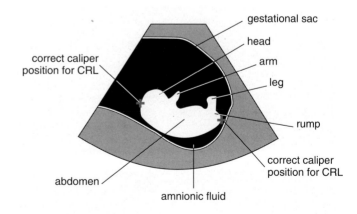

Figure 16–9. The crown rump measurement in a 10.5-week embryo.

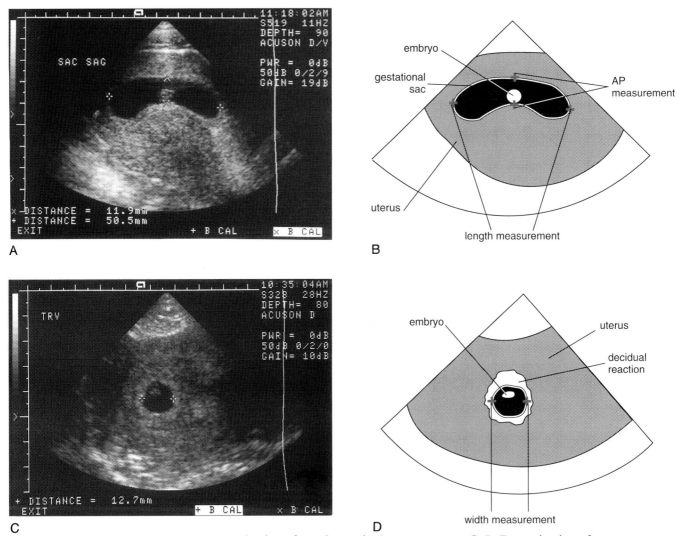

Figure 16-10. *A, B,* Determination of sac size: sagittal measurements. *C, D,* Determination of sac size: transverse measurement.

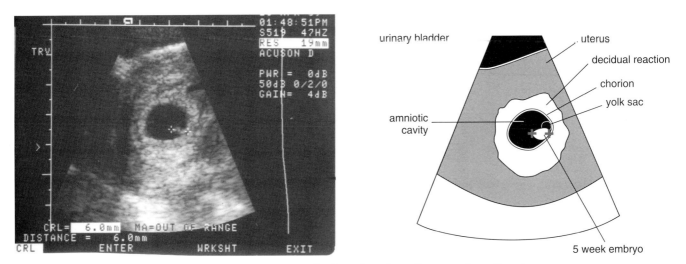

Figure 16-11. Appearance of a 5-week embryo (between the calipers).

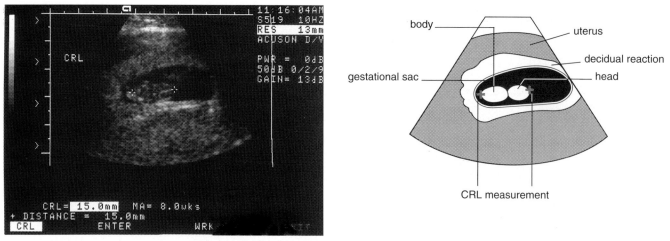

Figure 16–12. Appearance of a 7- to 8-week embryo.

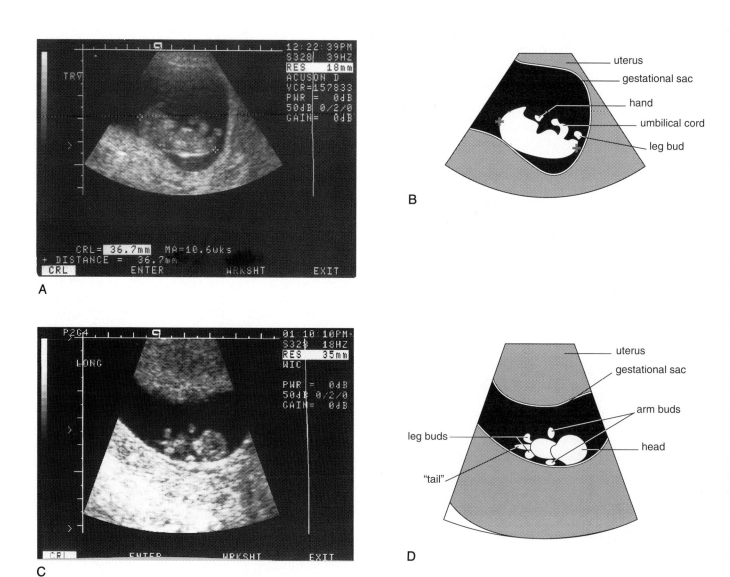

Figure 16–13. *A, B,* Appearance of a 10- to 11-week embryo. *C, D,* A 9.5 week embryo. All four developing limbs can be seen. Note that the caudate pole (tail) of the embryo protrudes beyond the limbs. This is normal for this age.

the corpus luteum is decreasing in size, the embryo itself is undergoing some marked changes and is increasing dramatically in size. At 5 to 6 weeks the fetal pole (or embryo) is barely evident with transabdominal scanning. At this point, it is about 5 mm in length, ovoid or shapeless, and hugs the wall of the gestational sac. (See Figure 16–11.) By the seventh week, the embryo is close to 1 cm in length and is beginning to assume a shape which reveals the end containing the head at one end and the rump at the other. (See Figure 16–12.) Cardiac activity can clearly be seen in the area of the future fetal thorax. It is also possible, as early as 7 weeks, to discern some slight gross motion of the fetus. Fetal limb buds should be seen by 8.5 to 9.5 weeks of gestation, and more pronounced development of the limbs is clear by the end of the first trimester. (See Figure 16–13.)

EMBRYOLOGY OF INDIVIDUAL ORGAN SYSTEMS

Most of the organs and systems of the adult have been developed and correctly positioned as early as 10 menstrual weeks of age.[2] At this point in time the embryo has progressed to the fetal stage. Thus, in the 8 weeks since conception, or 10 weeks by menstrual dates, the embryo has been transformed from a single cell to an organism which now has a **neurocranial axis**, a **cardiovascular system**, a **gastrointestinal system**, a **urogenital system**, and a **primitive skeleton** and **muscles**. Although all of these tissues and organs are present, it is impossible to visualize them with the available ultrasound technology. Transvaginal ultrasound may make it possible to visualize some organs and organ systems prior to 10 weeks of development, and it is probable that improvements in ultrasound technology may render many organ systems visible to ultrasound as early as 9 to 12 weeks of menstrual age. It is important therefore to have a basic understanding of the embryological development of these systems.

Early Embryology of the Central Nervous System

The **neuroplate**, the most primitive component of the neurological axis, develops in 2.5 to 3 weeks after conception or at 4 to 5 menstrual weeks. This plate will form the **neurocrest** and **neurotube**. The neurotube will eventually form the brain and spinal cord. By the sixth menstrual week, the primitive embryonic brain consists of three segments: the forebrain (the **prosencephalon**), the midbrain (the **mesencephalon**), and the hindbrain (the **rhombencephalon**). The forebrain will eventually become the cerebrum and lateral ventricle. The thalamus will also develop from the forebrain. The midbrain will become the midbrain in the adult and it will also form

the aqueduct of Sylvius. The hindbrain will develop into the pons, medulla, and the cerebellum of the adult. It will also form the fourth ventricle.

The posterior portion of the neurotube will develop in the fetal spine and spinal cord. This tube is closed from anterior-posterior ends by the sixth week of development. Mineralization of the fetal spine does not begin until 8 weeks of development.[3]

Sonographic Appearance of the Early Central Nervous System

At 10 weeks' gestation, the brain appears as an anechoic, fluid-filled mass. By 12 weeks, however, two hyperechoic structures can be seen within the fetal skull. These structures represent the choroid plexus—structures which produce the cerebrospinal fluid in the embryo. The developing cerebral cortex is present at this time as a ring of hypoechoic tissue surrounding the choroid plexus; however, it is normally not visible during ultrasound examination prior to 12 weeks' menstrual age.[4]

Visualization of the spine by ultrasound is not possible before the second and third trimester. While both the fetal brain and fetal spine are difficult (if not impossible) to visualize during the first trimester, the fetal skull can be detected during ultrasound examination as early as 11 or 12 weeks. The presence of a visible fetal skull at 12 weeks allows the sonographer to obtain two other important measurements: the **biparietal diameter (BPD)** and the fetal head circumference (HC). Both are discussed in Chapter 17.

Early Embryology of the Embryonic Heart

The embryonic heart begins as two tubes which eventually fuse along their midlines to form a very primitive tubular heart. Initially this heart is required only to move blood across the circulatory system of the yolk sac. Later in the first trimester, the four-chambered heart is formed from the simple tubular heart by a series of folds and fusions of tissues in the tubular pump. This minute four-chambered heart now pumps fetal blood throughout the growing embryo and its attendant placenta. A detailed description of the embryologic heart is found in Chapter 22.

Sonographic Appearance of the Heart

Pulsations in the tubular heart may be seen as early as 5.2 weeks' menstrual age if transvaginal ultrasound technology is employed.

Embryonic heart activity is often noted as early as 6.5 weeks when a transabdominal ultrasound examination is performed.[5] Cardiac activity should be noted by 7 weeks in most pregnancies if the embryo is viable. The structural components of the fetal heart cannot be visualized with ultrasound until the second trimester. Normal anatomy of the fetal heart is discussed in Chapter 17.

Early Embryology of the Lungs

As the primary yolk sac regresses and the embryo elongates, a long hollow tube is formed on the anterior surface of the embryo. This tube will become the **alimentary canal**. The canal is the rudimentary gastrointestinal system and forms other organs. The fetal lungs begin development as small paired buds arising from the anterior surface of the most superior portion of this tube. The fetal lung buds are present at about 5 weeks of gestational age and form numerous branching buds which grow and increase in number until 17 weeks of gestation.

Sonographic Appearance of the Lungs

It is not until midway in the second trimester that the fetal lungs are visible with ultrasound.

Early Embryology of the Abdominal Organs

The fetal gastrointestinal system arises from the alimentary canal when the primary yolk sac regresses and the embryo elongates, forming a small hollow tube running the length of the embryo in an anterior position. This canal divides into the **foregut** (the most superior end), the **midgut**, and the **hindgut** (the most inferior end). The foregut will eventually give rise to the pharynx, the esophagus, the stomach, and the proximal duodenum. It will also give rise through outpouching to the liver and pancreas. The midgut will give rise to the small intestine and a portion of the colon. The hindgut will eventually develop into the distal colon, rectum, and portions of the bladder. During the eighth to eleventh weeks of preg-

nancy (menstrual dates), the small bowel usually herniates out of the embryo at the base of the umbilical cord. This is a normal event, but the bowel should retract into the embryo by 12 weeks of development.

Sonographic Appearance of the Abdominal Organs

Figure 16–14 is an ultrasound image of a 10.5 week embryo in which a small bulge in the proximal umbilical cord can be seen. This bulge represents a small amount of fetal bowel which has herniated into the cord. Fetal intestinal activity does not begin until the eleventh week of development and fetal swallowing usually does not begin until the twelfth week of development.[6] Therefore, the fetal stomach cannot be visualized with ultrasound until the early second trimester.

Early Embryology of the Fetal Genitourinary System

Functional fetal kidney tissue does not appear until approximately 10 menstrual weeks. The production of fetal urine does not occur until early in the second trimester.[7] The kidneys and bladder are discussed in Chapter 17.

Sonographic Appearance of the Genitourinary System

The fetal kidneys and fetal bladder are not imaged adequately by ultrasound during the first trimester. Fetal sex organs are not visible until at least 15 weeks of development and consequently are discussed in Chapter 17.

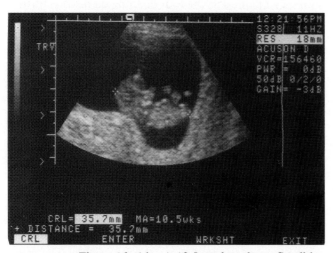
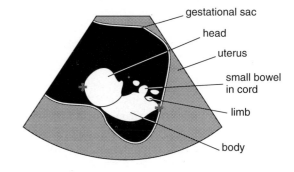

Figure 16–14. A 10.5-week embryo. Small bowel has herniated into the base of the umbilical cord. The small bowel will migrate back into the embryonic abdomen in a few days.

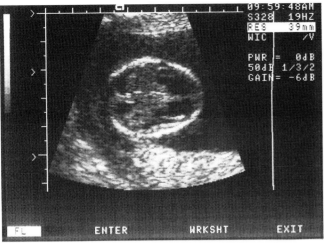
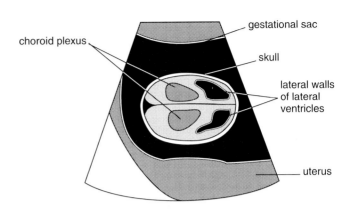

Figure 16–15. Appearance of a 12-week fetal skull. The choroid plexus is present.

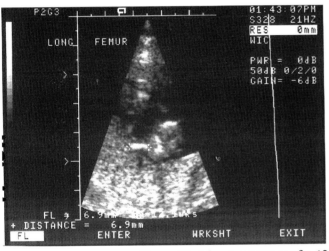
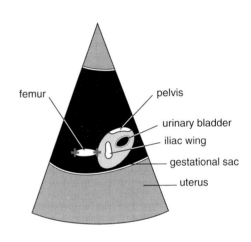

Figure 16–16. Appearance of a 12-week fetal femur (between the calipers).

Embryology of the Fetal Skeleton

As mentioned earlier, mineralization of the fetal spine does not begin until 8 weeks, as is also the case with other elements of the fetal skeleton. The fetal skull and femur are adequately mineralized by 11.5 to 12 weeks.

Sonographic Appearance of the Early Skeleton and Limbs

Mineralization of fetal bones allows their visualization by ultrasound. The fetal skull and femur can be visualized by the eleventh to twelfth week of gestation. Figures 16–15 and 16–16 represent ultrasound images of a 12-week fetal skull and femur, respectively. Fetal limbs can be imaged as buds as early as 8 to 9 weeks of gestational age, and fetal limb movement can be seen as early as 10 to 12 weeks of gestation. In fact, slight twitching or somatic movement can be seen in embryos as small as 7 mm in length or about 7 weeks of gestational age.

CONCLUSIONS ABOUT EARLY DEVELOPMENT

The first 10 weeks of gestation represent the embryonic period of development. This is the time in which tremendous changes in cellular architecture and embryonic architecture occur. A single fertilized ovum develops into essentially all of the future tissues of the fetus. Unfortunately, the small size of the embryo and ultrasonic characteristics of these organs and organ systems render them undetectable to ultrasound at this early developmental stage. It is possible that developments in ultrasound technology (primarily higher frequency transducers) may allow visualization of some of these organ systems prior to 12 weeks of gestation.

SONOGRAPHIC APPLICATIONS

Indications for Ultrasonography during the First Trimester

Ultrasonic examinations of the uterus are becoming more and more commonplace. There are many possible medical indications for a woman to receive a sonogram during the first trimester. Ten of the most common indications are as follows: (1) vaginal bleeding — to determine the viability of the gestation or to rule out an ectopic pregnancy; (2) pain — to rule out a mass, an abruption, or an ectopic pregnancy; (3) large for dates — to rule out a mass, multiple gestation, fetal anomaly, or incorrect menstrual history; (4) small for dates — to rule out fetal death, a fetal anomaly, incorrect menstrual history, or an ectopic pregnancy; (5) unknown date — to determine the correct gestational age especially in a woman who may receive a repeat cesarean section; (6) substance abuse — to rule out fetal anomalies and determine the growth rate of the fetus (also indicated relative to certain prescription drugs during early pregnancy); (7) intrauterine contraceptive device — the presence of an IUD can complicate a pregnancy; (8) trauma — to determine fetal well-being; (9) history of miscarriage — to determine the viability of the gestation; (10) history of multiple gestations, or for a woman attending a fertility clinic — to rule out multiple gestations.

SAFETY CONSIDERATIONS

In 1984 a fact-finding panel of the National Institutes of Health issued guidelines for ultrasound examinations during pregnancy. It includes 29 indications for obstetric ultrasound. However, the panel did not endorse routine ultrasound screening in pregnant women, based on the fact that there is not enough evidence to demonstrate that the clinical benefits of such screening would outweigh the economic, legal, and psychological costs involved. The panel stated that there is no evidence to indicate that either the woman or the fetus is harmed during these studies.[8]

CONCLUSION

The first trimester ultrasound examination generates information which is useful in managing the pregnancy. Menstrual age of the gestation can be determined easily within 4 to 5 days during the first trimester by ultrasonic measurements. The number, position, and viability of

the embryo are also quickly accessed. Adnexal masses and the presence or absence of hemorrhage in the area of the gestational sac are quickly determined. Thus, while ultrasound does not clearly visualize the internal architecture of the first trimester embryo it does indicate the state of health of the embryo and the gestational sac. Moreover, the pregnancy can be accurately dated when ultrasound examination is performed during the first 12 weeks.

REFERENCE CHARTS

Associated Physicians

Obstetrician and/or Gynecologist: Manages the preterm care of both women and fetus, and delivers the fetus. The physician is responsible for care of the infant in the first few minutes of life.

Radiologist/Sonologist: Interprets the ultrasound image of the fetus, uterus, and adnexa.

Fertility Specialist: Specializes in treating disorders of the female reproductive system.

High-risk Obstetrician: Specializes in the preterm management of women whose pregnancies are at high risk due to various medical problems or in whom an identified risk might endanger her or her fetus.

Common First Trimester Tests

Pregnancy Test (Urine): This rapid test of a woman's urine determines the existence of pregnancy. It is usually performed by a laboratory technician and interpreted by a pathologist or an obstetrician.

Beta HCG: This blood test quantitates the serum level of human chorionic gonadotropin. The blood level of this hormone is used to estimate the age of the gestation. This test is usually performed by a laboratory technician and interpreted by a pathologist or an obstetrician.

Maternal/Paternal Blood Typing: This test determines whether the parents are Rh positive or negative. It is more important for subsequent pregnancies than for the first pregnancy. This test is usually performed by a laboratory technician and interpreted by a pathologist or an obstetrician.

Measurements Assessed during the First Trimester

Average Sac Size: Length + Height + Width/3

Crown-Rump Length (CRL): Maximal length of the embryo from head to rump.

Laboratory Values

Values change from week to week and are different for each test.

Vasculature

Nonapplicable.

Affecting Chemicals

Nonapplicable.

References

1. Robinson HP, Fleming JEE: A critical evaluation of sonar crown-rump length measurements. Brit J Obstet Gynecol 82:703–708, 1975.
2. Lyons EA, Levi CS: Ultrasound in the first trimester of pregnancy. In Callen PW (ed.): Ultrasonography in Obstetrics and Gynecology. Philadelphia, WB Saunders, 1982.
3. Cochlin DL: Ultrasound of the fetal spine. Clin Radiol 33:641–650, 1982.
4. Cyr DR, Mack LA, Nyberg DA: Fetal rhombencephalon: normal ultrasound findings. Radiology 166:691–692, 1988.
5. Rempen A: Diagnosis of viability in early pregnancy with vaginal sonography. J Ultrasound Med 9:711–716, 1990.
6. Pritchard JA: Fetal swallowing and amniotic fluid volume. Obstet Gynecol 18:606–610, 1966.
7. Grannum PA: The genitourinary tract. In Nyberg, DA, Mahoney BS, Pretorius DH (eds.): Diagnostic Ultrasound of Fetal Anomalies, St. Louis, Mosby-Year Book, 1990.
8. National Institutes of Health Consensus Development Conference. U.S. Government Printing Office, Washington, D.C., 1984.

Chapter 17

SECOND AND THIRD TRIMESTER OBSTETRICS

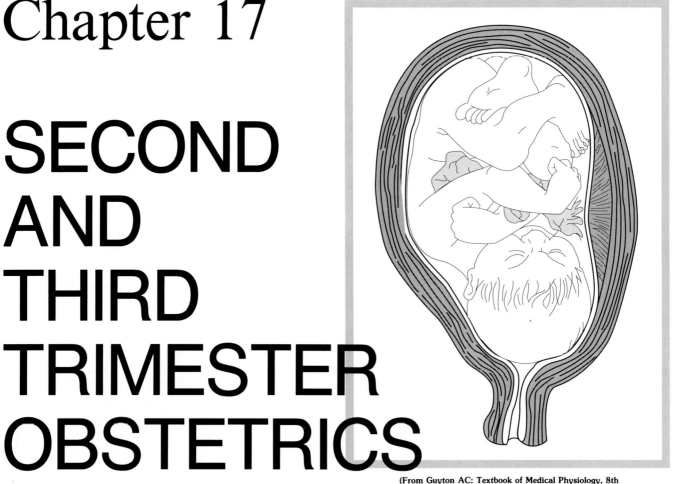

(From Guyton AC: Textbook of Medical Physiology, 8th ed. Philadelphia, WB Saunders, 1991, p 924.)

G. WILLIAM SHEPHERD

Objectives:

Describe the role of the placenta in supporting the gestation.

Describe the organs that become visible during the second trimester and describe their sonographic appearance.

Describe the sonographic measurements of the fetus performed during the second and third trimesters.

Define the key words.

Key Words:

Aqueduct of Sylvius
Arachnoid layer

Basal layer
Biparietal diameter
Brachiocephalic
Cavum septum pellucidum
Cephalic index
Cerebral peduncles
Cerebrospinal
Chorionic plate
Cisterna magna
Cisterns
Cotyledons
Dolichocephalic
Ductus arteriosus
Ductus venosus
Dura mater

INTRODUCTION

The second and third trimesters of the pregnancy are a period of growth and maturation of the organs and organ systems which formed during the first trimester. By the twelfth week most of these organs which formed during the first trimester are located in their final anatomical positions. Thus, the first trimester can be termed "a trimester of differentiation and development" and the second and third trimesters may be referred to collectively as "trimesters of growth and maturation."

EMBRYOLOGY OF THE PLACENTA

The tremendous amount of growth which occurs during the second and third trimesters is highly dependent on the ability of the fetus to acquire nutrients and oxygen. It is also highly dependent on fetal ability to remove the waste products of metabolism. The organ which accomplishes these tasks is the placenta.

The early placenta is composed of the decidua basalis and the chorion frondosum. The chorion frondosum forms chorionic villi, which are small finger-like projections of embryonic tissue. Surrounding these embryonic projections is maternal tissue called the lacunar network. The **lacunar network** is a tissue extremely rich in small blood vessels and which, after contact with the trophoblastic cells of the villi, breaks down and forms small pools of maternal blood, or **lacunae**. It is the contact of the embryonic circulatory system with the maternal lacunae that facilitates the transfer of oxygen and metabolites to the developing fetus, and the transfer of carbon dioxide and waste products from the developing fetus.

Each chorionic villus branches to form groups of villi. Large groups of villi are known as **cotyledons**, and groups of cotyledons form between one and five lobules. As the fetus increases in size so do its requirements for nutrition and waste product removal. The placenta also increases in size to keep up with this increasing demand. At 12 weeks, the placenta is between 1 and 2 cm in thickness. By 40 weeks of gestation, the placenta may be between 2.5 and 4 cm in thickness.[1] The diameter of a term placenta can be as much as 20 cm.[2] Figure 17–1 represents an ultrasound image of a placenta at 18 weeks' gestational age.

The placenta may be divided into three basic areas: (1) The **chorionic plate** is the portion toward the inside of the sac (touching the amniotic membrane); (2) the **basal**

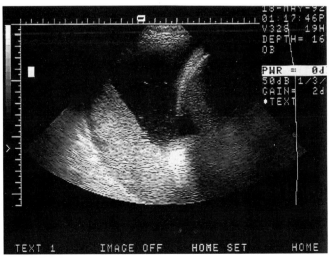
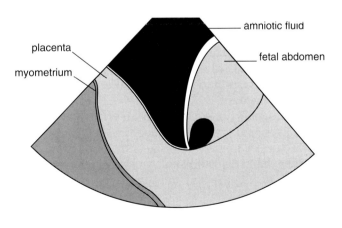

Figure 17–1. The placenta in an 18-week gestation.

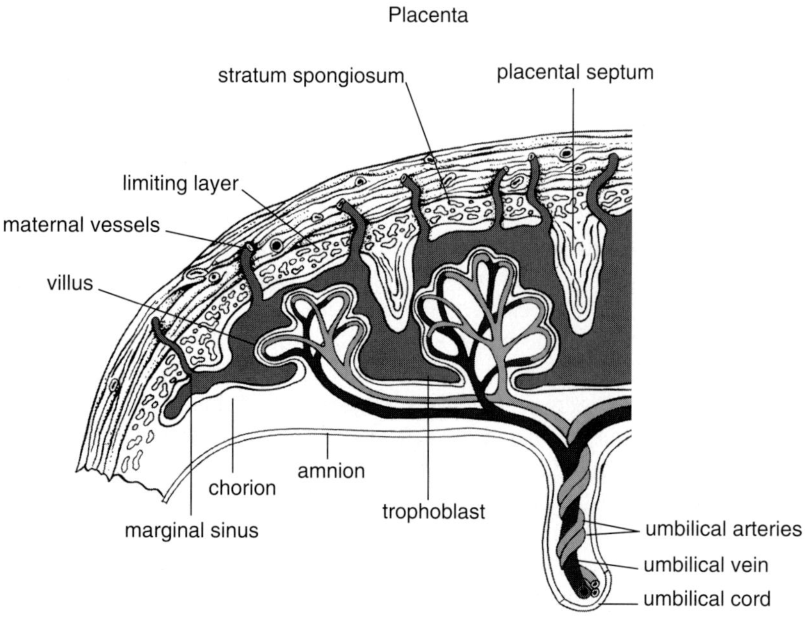

Figure 17-2. Maternal-fetal circulatory pattern in the placenta.

layer (base plate) is that portion on the outside (touching the uterus); and (3) the **placental substance** is the placental material between the basal layer and the chorionic plate. The placenta is composed of cotyledons and lobules; although it may appear to be homogeneous, on ultrasound examination it is seen to be separated by functional circulatory groups. Small venules course through the substance of the placenta, becoming progressively larger as they converge, eventually forming a single umbilical vein. Conversely, two umbilical arteries enter the substance of the placenta and progressively divide with the villi to form even smaller vessels. The umbilical cord, which connects the fetus to the placenta, is formed by the two umbilical arteries and a single umbilical vein. The covering of the cord is formed by the amniotic membrane. At term, the cord is approximately 50 to 60 cm in length.

The enormous circulatory surface provided by the many fetal and maternal blood vessels allows nutrients and metabolic waste products to be exchanged in the placenta. Carbon dioxide is at a much higher concentration in the fetal blood and thus tends to move into the maternal blood. Oxygen is at a much higher level in the maternal bloodstream and thus moves into the fetal blood. The placenta thus functions as an organ of respiration for the fetus.

The placenta also functions as an endocrine gland. It produces human chorionic gonadotropin (HCG), which communicates to the rest of the body that a gestation is present within the uterus. The maternal blood, which supplies the oxygen and nutrients and removes waste products and carbon dioxide, arrives at the placenta via the **spiral arterioles**. These blood vessels coil their way up to the base of the placenta from the endometrial layer of the uterus. Figure 17-2 depicts the maternal placental circulation and the parts of the placenta.

SONOGRAPHIC APPEARANCE OF THE PLACENTA

Early in the pregnancy, the placenta is seen as a thickening inside the gestational sac, and is fairly uniform in echogenicity. However, an area of sonolucency may be seen on its fetal surface. This represents the cord insertion site. Figure 17-3 depicts an ultrasound image of the cord insertion site. Anechoic tubular structures may also be seen on the uterine surface of the placenta. These structures represent the marginal veins. An image of these veins is shown in Figure 17-4. Small anechoic areas within the substance of the placenta represent maternal venous lakes or lacunae. It is often possible to see a swirl-like motion within these lakes. This presumably represents very slow circulation of maternal blood. A prominent venous lake is shown in Figure 17-5.

The sonographic appearance of the placenta may change during the last few weeks of the pregnancy. This change in ultrasound appearance is normal, but may occur too early. A system of grading a placenta's ultrasound appearance, developed by Grannum et al in 1979, is in wide use.

There are four categories of placental classification: (1) Grade 0: This configuration represents all normal first and second trimester placentas. A Grade 0 placenta has a smooth chorionic plate, a substance which is devoid of focal hyperechoic areas, and a basal layer which is free of hyperechoic densities as well. This placenta may be found at any time during the pregnancy, even up to 40 weeks, and is considered normal. (2) Grade I: The chorionic plate shows some subtle indentation. The substance of the placenta has a few scattered, bright echoes. No echoes can be seen in the basal layer of a Grade I placenta. These placental findings may appear as normal changes at any time after 34 weeks of development. (3)

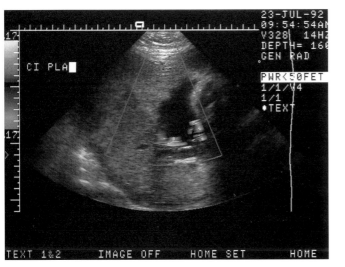
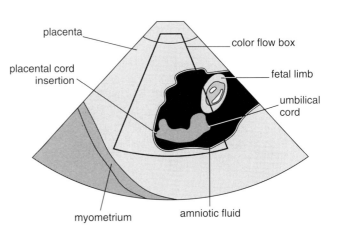

Figure 17–3. Color flow demonstration of the placental cord insertion site. (See Color Plate 7 at the back of this book.)

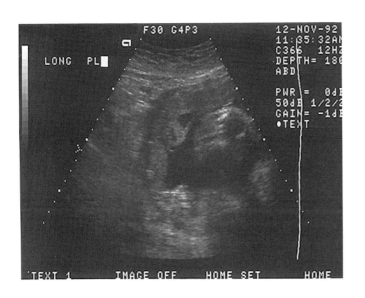
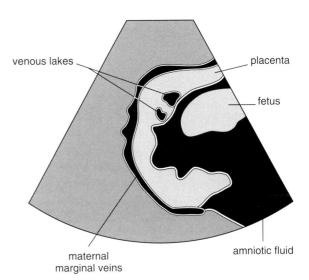

Figure 17–4. Maternal marginal veins below the placenta in a 25-week gestation.

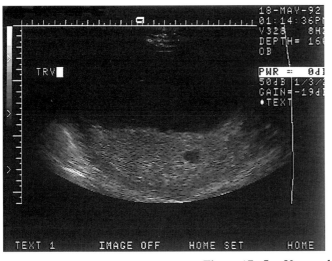
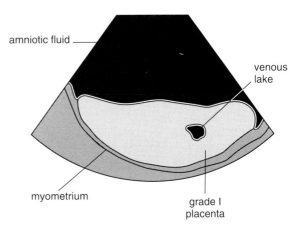

Figure 17–5. Venous lake in a 32-week gestation.

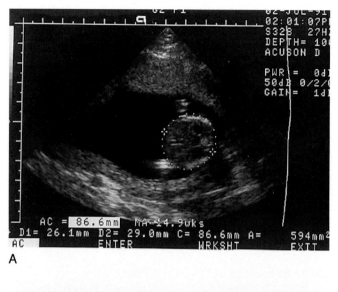

A

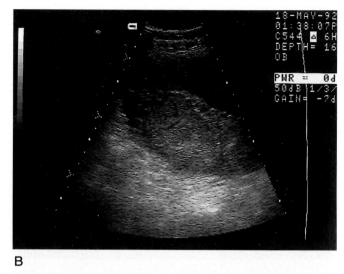

B

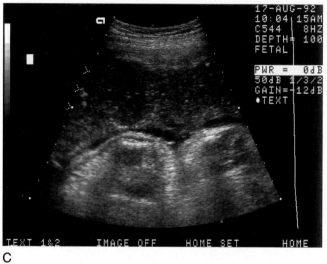

C

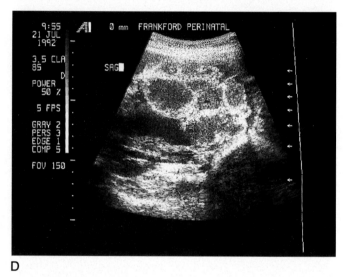

D

PLACENTAL GRADING

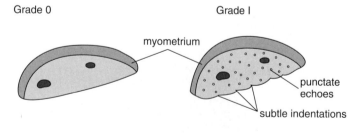

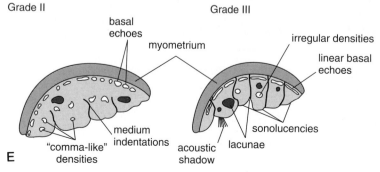

E

Figure 17–6. *A,* Image of a Grade 0 placenta; *B,* Image of a Grade I placenta; *C,* Image of a Grade II placenta; *D,* Image of a Grade III placenta; *E,* Placental grading.

Grade II: This category of placentas has comma-like indentations in the chorionic plate. The substance of the placenta contains scattered, bright echoes. The basal plate in a Grade II placenta contains a few linear hyperechoic densities. A Grade II placenta may be normal and may be seen at any time after 36 weeks of development. (4) Grade III: A Grade III placenta has indentations in the chorionic plate, which now extends as far as the basal layer, dividing the placenta into segments. The substance of the placenta may contain both bright echoes and sonolucent areas. The bright echoes will be much larger than the small, scattered densities seen in the Grade I placenta, and may have acoustic shadows behind them. The basal layer of a Grade III placenta has very long hyperechoic linear echoes and may, in very advanced stages, become an unbroken line. Representative ultrasound images and drawings of each of the four placental grades are shown in Figure 17–6.

Initially it was believed that the placental grading system, which essentially measures amounts of calcification within the aging placenta, could be used as a means to date a gestation.[3] It is now known that dating the gestation by placental grading techniques is highly inaccurate.[4] However, there is a distinct relationship between the age of the gestation and the grade of the placenta. The appearance of a Grade I placenta (if it occurs at all) should occur after 34 weeks. A Grade II should appear after 36 weeks and a Grade III placenta should appear after 38 weeks. Appearance of these grades before the stated times may indicate a problem.

The position of the placenta relative to the internal cervical os is extremely important and should always be documented during an ultrasound examination during the second and third trimesters. **Placenta previa** occurs when any portion of the internal cervical os is obstructed by part of the placenta. There are three types of placenta previa: Total (or complete) placenta previa occurs when the entire cervical os is obstructed by an overlying placenta. It may be associated with vaginal bleeding, and usually requires cesarean section, since vaginal delivery would be extremely dangerous to the fetus and possibly to the mother as well. A partial (or incomplete) previa occurs when a portion of the cervical os is blocked by the overlying placenta. This condition is also associated with vaginal bleeding and also necessitates cesarean section. Marginal previa exists when the placenta extends up to but not above the internal cervical os. These patients usually are followed by examinations during the final weeks of the pregnancy. Placenta previa is the most common cause of vaginal bleeding during the second and third trimesters. Occasionally, the term low-lying placenta (or potential placenta) may be used by a radiologist. The term describes a placenta that ends within a few millimeters of the internal cervical os. A follow-up ultrasound examination is usually performed for these patients and quite often the placenta will appear to have moved upward in the uterus. Of course, the placenta itself cannot move from one position to another, but the lower uterine segment can stretch as the uterus is pushed upward by the growing fetus.

There are three causes of placenta previa: (1) a low-lying placenta in a normal uterus; (2) a low-lying placenta due to the presence of a fibroid tumor superior to the implantation site; and (3) a vascular malformation which allows placental formation in only the lower portion of the uterus.

EMBRYOLOGY OF FETAL MEMBRANES

The fetus and the placenta are surrounded by fetal membranes. The chorion surrounds both the fetus and the outside of the placenta. The amnion surrounds the fetus and is in contact with the fetal side of the placenta. The amnion also covers the umbilical cord. A normal variation of fetal membranes, **chorioamniotic separation**, may occur during the pregnancy. It is of no clinical consequence and is considered a normal finding.

SONOGRAPHIC APPEARANCE OF FETAL MEMBRANES

Early in the gestation, the chorion and amnion appear as separate membranes, as shown in Figure 17–7. Sepa-

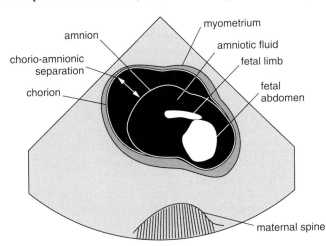

Figure 17–7. Chorioamnionic separation in a 14-week gestation.

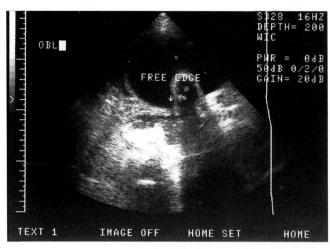

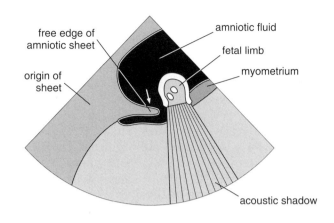

Figure 17–8. Free edge of an amniotic sheet (*arrow*) in a 30-week gestation.

ration of these membranes persists until about 16 menstrual weeks, when the amnion normally fuses with the chorion. Ultrasound examination of fetal membranes is especially important in the case of twin pregnancies (discussed in Chapter 18).

Intrauterine synechiae (or **amniotic sheets**) are sometimes observed during the course of a normal ultrasound examination. These structures represent four layers of membrane which have protruded into the amniotic fluid.[5] The two outside layers of the amniotic sheet consist of amnion; the two inside layers, of chorion. (See Figure 17–8.)

EMBRYOLOGY OF AMNIOTIC FLUID

Amniotic fluid is the liquid enclosed by the amnion which surrounds and bathes the fetus. This fluid has five functions: (1) it permits symmetrical growth; (2) it prevents adhesions; (3) it cushions the embryo and protects it from shock; (4) it moderates temperature; and (5) it allows movement and the development of muscle tone. Amniotic fluid also has a role in lung maturation. The quantity of amniotic fluid in the uterus during pregnancy increases in almost a linear manner until about 34 weeks of gestation. At that point in time, the volume of fluid begins to decrease considerably until delivery.[6] The chemical composition of amniotic fluid is influenced by materials diffusing across the fetal skin and placenta, and by the fetal digestive tract and urinary system.[7] Amniotic fluid is swallowed by the fetus as it passes through the fetal gastrointestinal system. Much of this fluid is absorbed by the gastrointestinal tract, then recirculates through the fetal kidneys and bladder. The volume of amniotic fluid depends on the balance between its absorption and its production.

The fetal effect on amniotic fluid volume increases with the pregnancy. During the third trimester, fetal kidneys may produce between 600 and 800 ml of fluid per day; near term, the fetus may swallow up to 450 ml of

fluid per day.[7] Thus, the volume of amniotic fluid reflects the state of fetal well-being. In fact, many fetal abnormalities are associated with marked increases or decreases in the volume of amniotic fluid. **Polyhydramnios** is the presence of excessive amniotic fluid within the uterus.

EMBRYOLOGY OF THE CARDIOVASCULAR SYSTEM

The circulatory system of the fetus differs from that of the neonate. The umbilical vein enters from the umbilical cord and courses from the midline abdominal wall posteriorly and slightly cephalad into the liver, where it becomes the **portal sinus** and the portal vein. The portal vein then bifurcates at the **ductus venosus** (which flows directly into the vena cava) and the right portal vein. These three vessels carry oxygenated blood from the placenta to the fetus. The ductus venosus allows some of the blood to move directly to the fetal heart. The ductus venosus is temporary and closes off shortly before birth, but remains as a ligament. The portal sinus remains patent (open) and becomes the proximal portion of the left portal vein. The fetal heart allows blood to move from right to left in the atrial chambers via the foramen ovale. This valve may remain patent after birth, but is held closed by the normal pressure gradient between left and right atria. The pulmonary artery and the aorta are connected by the **ductus arteriosus**. This vessel allows blood to move from the pulmonary artery to the aorta. The fetal lungs do not have a respiratory function and therefore do not require large quantities of blood. The ductus arteriosus will close at (or shortly after) birth.

Most of the fetal blood will return to the placenta via two umbilical arteries, which arise from the iliac arteries. However, some of the blood does bypass the umbilical arteries to oxygenate and nourish the lower extremities of the fetus.

SONOGRAPHIC APPEARANCE OF THE CARDIOVASCULAR SYSTEM

The fetal heart can be visualized as a four-chambered structure as early as 15 weeks and certainly by 20 weeks.

A four-chamber view can be obtained by tilting the transducer cephalad (with respect to the fetus) from the abdominal measurement plane. (See Figure 17–9.) The chambers should appear relatively symmetric, and a division between the chambers (the atrial and ventricular

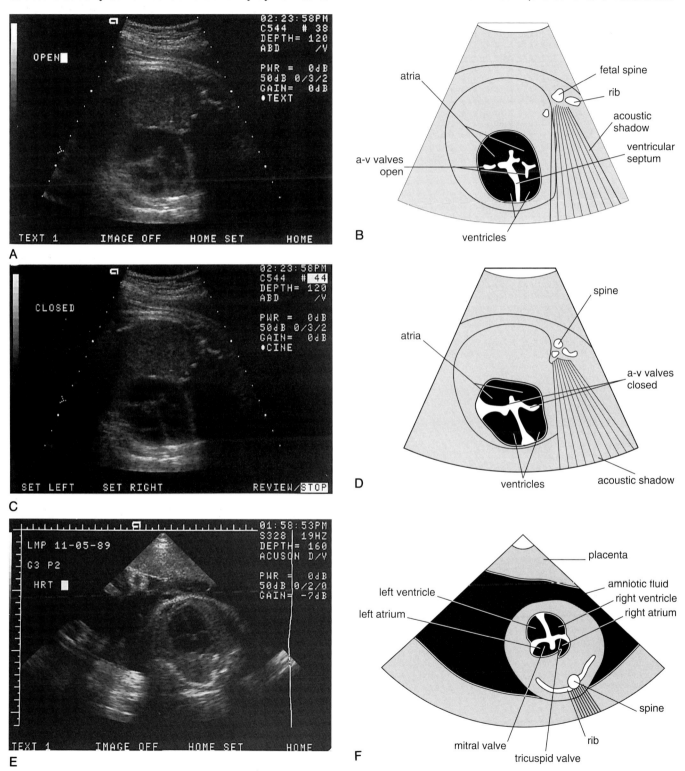

Figure 17–9. *A, B,* A 33-week fetal heart with the atrioventricular (a-v) valves open; *C, D,* A 33-week fetal heart with the atrioventricular valves closed; *E, F,* Classic four-chamber heart view in a 34-week gestation.

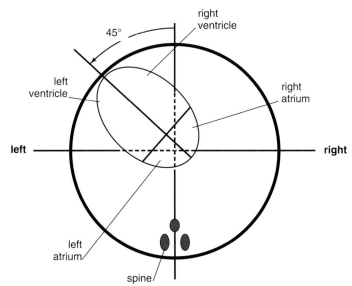

Figure 17–10. Position of the fetal heart.

septa) should be broken only at the **foramen ovale**. The heart should be seen on the left side, and no fluid collections in the chest should be seen. The axis of the heart should be tilted approximately 45 degrees to the anteroposterior axis of the fetal thorax and pointed to the left. (See Figure 17–10.) Sometimes it is necessary to image the ventricles and atria separately because of fetal position. Figure 17–11 shows the ultrasound appearance of the ventricles and atria when imaged in this manner.

A normal three-vessel cord presents on ultrasound examination as a large circular vein and two smaller circular umbilical arteries when viewed in cross-section. This view is sometimes referred to as the Mickey Mouse view; the umbilical vein looks like Mickey's head and the umbilical arteries look like his ears. (See Figure 17–12.)

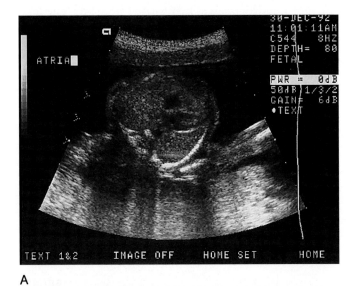

A

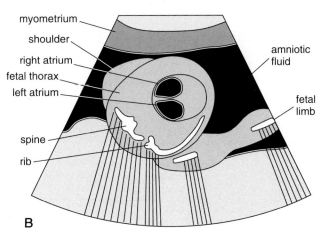

B

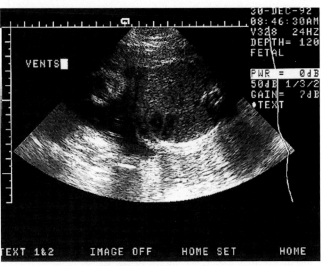

C

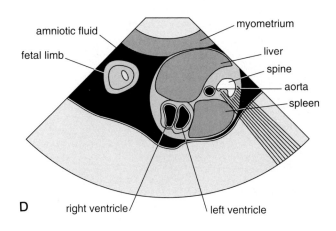

D

Figure 17–11. *A, B,* Atria of a 27-week fetal heart; *C, D,* Ventricles of a 27-week fetal heart.

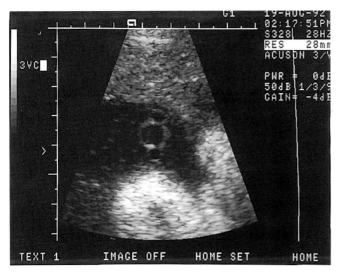

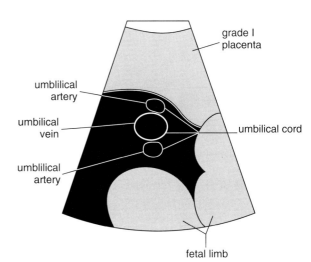

Figure 17-12. Appearance of the three-vessel cord.

EMBRYOLOGY OF THE FETAL LUNGS

The lungs begin development as small paired buds branching off the primitive alimentary canal. These buds increase in size, and multiple diverticula (outpouchings) form until about 17 weeks of gestation. The primitive lungs mature and become capable of functioning sometime after 25 weeks' gestation. The ability of the lungs to function can be measured by monitoring the LS ratio, to be described in Chapter 18. The lungs grow until they nearly fill the thoracic cavity.

The fetal lungs cannot be visualized by ultrasound until the middle of the second trimester. They will appear as medium gray, homogeneous structures within the fetal thorax. The position, shape, and axis of the fetal heart give information about the presence or absence of fetal lung masses. In a vertex lie, if one imagines a clock superimposed upon the four-chamber heart view, with the fetal spine at 6 o'clock, the right side of the fetal thorax at 3 o'clock, and the left side of the thorax at 9 o'clock, the sternum will be seen at 12 o'clock. The fetal heart normally points to approximately 10:30 in this representation.

The fetal diaphragm can be seen during a routine second or third trimester ultrasound examination. A longitudinal view of the fetal thorax should show the slightly hyperechoic line separating the liver or spleen from the thorax, as shown in Figure 17-13. This line should be slightly concave, with the cup-like portion opening toward the abdomen and the arched position pointing toward the thorax. It is not unusual to see this hyperechoic line move with fetal respiration, especially during the latter half of the third trimester.

EMBRYOLOGY OF THE NEUROCRANIAL AXIS

The central nervous system consists of the brain and the spinal cord. It arises from the posterior surface of the embryo (ectoderm). A linear depression is formed along

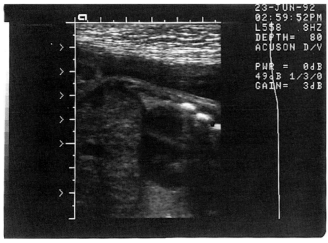

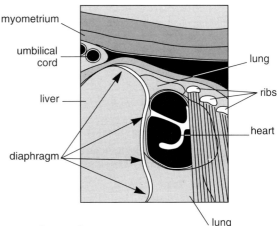

Figure 17-13. Diaphragm in a 27-week gestation.

the midline of the early embryo. The borders of the depression fold over to form the **neurotube** (described earlier, in Chapter 16). The neurotube gives rise to the spinal cord and the brain. Closure of this tube begins in midembryo and continues in both cephalad and caudad directions, completing the cephalad first. The brain is composed of three elements: the brain stem, the cerebellum, and the cerebrum. These elements are surrounded by membranes known as the **meninges**, which also surround the spinal cord. The brain and spinal cord also have an elaborate system of circulation composed of **ventricles**, **cisterns**, and **sinuses**. The brain stem is composed of the medulla, pons, midbrain, thalamus, and hypothalamus. It is a continuation of the spinal cord and is the base of the brain. The medulla oblongata is closest to the spinal cord and is responsible for control of respiration, heart rate, blood pressure, and certain involuntary reflexes (sneezing, coughing, and so on). The pons is located between the medulla and the cerebellum and helps to control respiration. The pons also transmits signals from the spinal cord to the cerebellum and cerebrum. The pons is anterior to the cerebellum, inferior to the cerebrum, and superior to the medulla. The midbrain sits between the pons and the thalamus. It relays signals from one part of the brain to another and controls head and eye movements. The thalamus and hypothalamus are superior to the midbrain and lie within the cerebrum. The thalamus is a relay system for cerebral impulses. The hypothalamus is the communication relay between the nervous system and the endocrine system.

The cerebellum is posterior and superior to most of the brain stem and is composed of two lateral halves. The cerebellum helps to coordinate movements, balance, and posture. A small central lobe, the vermis, relays information between the two hemispheres of the cerebellum.

The cerebellum is the largest component of the brain and is composed of five lobes: parietal, temporal, occipital, frontal, and insula (or isle of Reil), the only lobe not named for an overlying bone. The cerebrum is divided into two lateral hemispheres by the cerebral (or callosal) fissure. These hemispheres are connected by the corpus callosum. The parietal and temporal lobes are separated by the sylvian fissure. The insula lies in a central location deep in the cerebrum between the sylvian fissures.

The meninges are membranes which cover the brain and spinal cord. They are composed of three layers. The **dura mater** is the outermost layer and functions as a tough protective cover. The **arachnoid layer** is a fibrous cobweb-like structure and is the thin middle layer. The **pia mater** is a delicate and highly vascularized inner layer which closely follows the contours of the brain and spinal cord. The meninges not only provide protection for the central nervous system, but also facilitate cerebrospinal fluid movement from the subarachnoid space to the dural sinuses. The dura mater is actually two layers. The thicker outer layer is firmly adherent to the bones of

the skull. The thin inner layer follows the basic curvature of the brain, and reflections of this layer together with the arachnoid and pia mater layers serve to separate the structures of the brain. The **falx cerebri** is one example of these reflections. At the area where the reflection begins (where the outer and inner layers first separate), there is a small space. Collectively these spaces are known as the dural sinuses.

Cerebrospinal fluid (CSF) is similar to plasma in chemical composition except for the concentration of sodium ions, which is much higher in CSF. CSF fills the central canal of the spinal cord, the ventricles of the brain, and the subarachnoid space. It also is present within the cisterns of the brain. CSF acts as a protective cushion encasing the brain and spinal cord, and regulates the pressure within the spaces that it fills. CSF may also have a metabolic role; however, this role is not clearly defined.

Ventricles of the brain are part of a system which helps manufacture and distribute CSF. Four ventricles constitute this system. There are two **lateral ventricles**, one in each cerebral hemisphere. The lateral ventricles are the first and second ventricles. The **third ventricle** is found in the midline of the head and is located centrally in the thalamus. The **fourth ventricle** is also found in the midline of the brain, in a more posterior location. The lateral ventricles contain five regions; the frontal horns (most anterior), the lateral bodies (most superior), the occipital horns (most posterior), the temporal (most lateral), and the atria (the juncture of the temporal and occipital horns with the body of the lateral ventricle). The lateral ventricles are connected to the third ventricle by a tubular structure known as the **foramen of Monro**, which runs from the juncture of the frontal horn and body of the lateral ventricle to the roof of the third ventricle. The third ventricle is connected to the fourth ventricle by a long tubular structure known as the **aqueduct of Sylvius**. The fourth ventricle is connected to the central canal of the spinal cord laterally by two ducts, the **foramina of Luschka**, and medially by a single **foramen of Magendie**. All the ventricles are connected with one another, the central spinal canal, and the subarachnoid space.

Two large areas of choroid plexus are found on the floor of the lateral ventricles. Choroid plexus is also found in the third and fourth ventricles. Choroid plexus is a highly vascularized tissue which is related to the pia mater that secretes CSF, which appears anechoic. CSF flows from the lateral ventricle to the third and fourth ventricles, to the subarachnoid space, to the dural sinuses, where it is absorbed in the venous bloodstream. The subarachnoid space (the space between the pia mater and the arachnoid layer) is very small in most areas, but in certain areas it is enlarged, and CSF will pool. These areas are called cisterns. The lumbar cistern is the largest of these spaces and is found in the distal end of the spine. Other such cisterns are found in various locations within the brain. The largest of these cisterns is the **cisterna magna**, which is located at the base of the cerebellum in a posterior location within the skull.

The circulatory system of the brain is supplied by two internal carotid arteries and two vertebral arteries. The vertebral arteries join in the inferior and posterior portion of the brain to form basilar arteries, which enter the circle of Willis. The internal carotid arteries enter the circle laterally and inferiorly. The middle cerebral arteries arise laterally from the circle of Willis and course medially to the sylvian fissures. Paired anterior and posterior cerebral arteries also arise from this circle. The veins draining the brain are all tributaries of the dural sinuses and drain into the internal jugular veins.

The spine is a continuation of the brain stem. It contains a nerve bundle floating in CSF and covered by meninges. The CSF in the spinal column freely communicates with the CSF in the cranium.

SONOGRAPHIC APPEARANCE OF THE NEUROCRANIAL AXIS

Most of the components of the central nervous system described can be visualized during an ultrasound examination performed on a fetus of 15 weeks' gestation or greater. The lateral ventricles, choroid plexus, thalamus, falx cerebri, cerebellum, and cerebrum should all be visualized at this time. Another structure, the **cavum septum pellucidum**, can also be visualized. This is a small fluid-filled midline space, which arches directly atop the thalamus. The falx cerebri is a reflection of the membrane which covers the brain. This membrane is seen at right angles to the sound beam in the axial plane, as a bright echoic line which divides the cerebrum into right and left halves. The falx should be seen to divide the cerebrum into equal halves. The thalamus is a diamond-shaped area seen in the center of an axial section taken through the temporal lobe of the brain. The thalamus

appears as a structure with medium to low level echoes. The thalamus is divided into two equal sections by a hyperechoic line, the third ventricle, which extends upward into the space between the two halves. At times a very small quantity of fluid, which appears anechoic, can be seen giving this structure a slit-like appearance. The cavum septum pellucidi is another anechoic, fluid-containing structure seen in the midline of the brain at a temporal level in the axial scanning plane. This structure contains more fluid than the third ventricles. It is located forward of the thalamus and appears as two small bright lines parallel to the falx.

An axial scanning plane just above the level of the thalamus should show three hyperechoic lines parallel with the long axis of the head. The middle of these three lines is the falx cerebri. It should be seen to bisect the head left to right. Lateral to the falx are two bright lines. These represent the lateral borders of the lateral ventricles (LV). The distance from the falx to either of the lines should be approximately one third the distance from the falx to one side of the calvarium (skull) or less.[8] Figure 17–14 is an ultrasound image of normal lateral ventricles. Prior to 18 weeks of gestation, the ventricles fill most of the skull, and this rule does not apply, but should hold beyond 18 weeks of gestation.

The posterior portion of the brain can be visualized in an axial scanning plane inferior to the thalamus. The cerebellum should appear symmetric and of medium to low echogenicity. The cisterna magna may be seen in a posterior position with respect to the cerebellum. It has an anechoic appearance because it is filled with CSF. The cerebellum in a 19-week fetus is shown in Figure 17–15.

In the third trimester, it is possible to visualize symmetric vascular pulsations within the cerebrum. The choroid plexus appears as a hyperechoic collection of minute tubules lying just below the level at which the

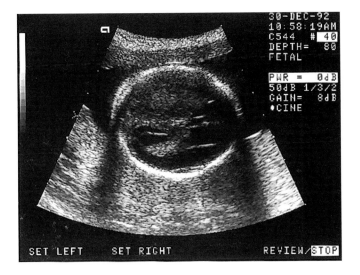

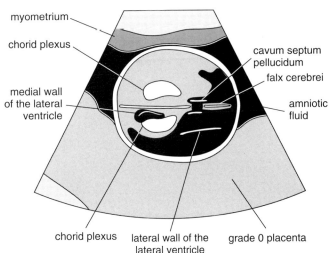

Figure 17–14. Lateral ventricles in an 18-week gestation.

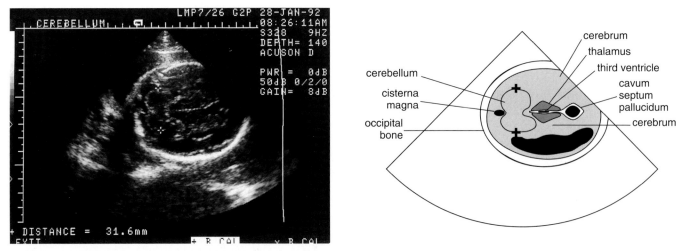

Figure 17–15. Cerebellum in a 19-week gestation.

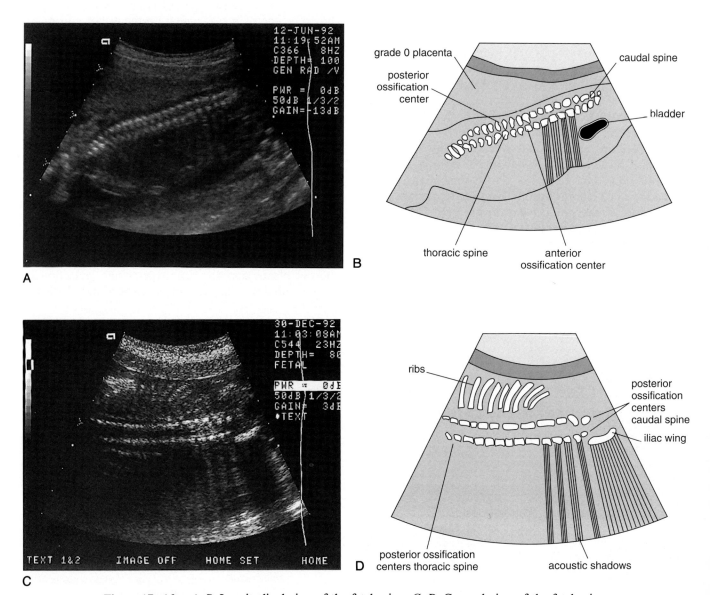

Figure 17–16. *A, B,* Longitudinal view of the fetal spine; *C, D,* Coronal view of the fetal spine.

lateral ventricles are measured. These structures are bright, drumstick-shaped areas on either side of the falx cerebri in the posterior portion of the head just below the level of the lateral ventricle body.

The fetal spine is clearly visible by 15 or 16 weeks of development, or even earlier depending on the mother's habitus, the quality of the ultrasound unit, and the position of the fetus. The normal posterior ossification centers of each vertebra are seen as two closely spaced hyperechoic foci, which may or may not give acoustic shadows. (See Figure 17–16.) Several vertebrae imaged at once appear as two rows of closely spaced reflectors when imaged in a longitudinal plane. These two rows are roughly parallel, but they are wider in the cervical and lumbar regions and narrower in the sacral region. The anterior ossification center of the vertebrae is equidistant from the two posterior ossification centers. In a transverse plane, these echoes are parallel or actually converge

toward each other. The skin covering the vertebrae is best seen in the transverse plane, while the spinal cord itself can best be seen between the vertebrae in a longitudinal plane. It is important to image the spine in both scanning planes. Coronal images (see Figure 17–16 C and D) show the parallel rows of the posterior ossification centers, while near-sagittal planes show one row of posterior ossification centers and one row of anterior ossification centers. The normal tapering of the spine in the sacral area is best seen in sagittal planes as shown in Figure 17–17 A and B.

It is also important to include a transverse image at the level of the iliac wing (see Figure 17–17 C and D), since this is a common site of spinal defects.[9] The spine should be imaged in its entirety in longitudinal planes; transverse images of the spine should be included in ultrasound examinations during the second and third trimesters.

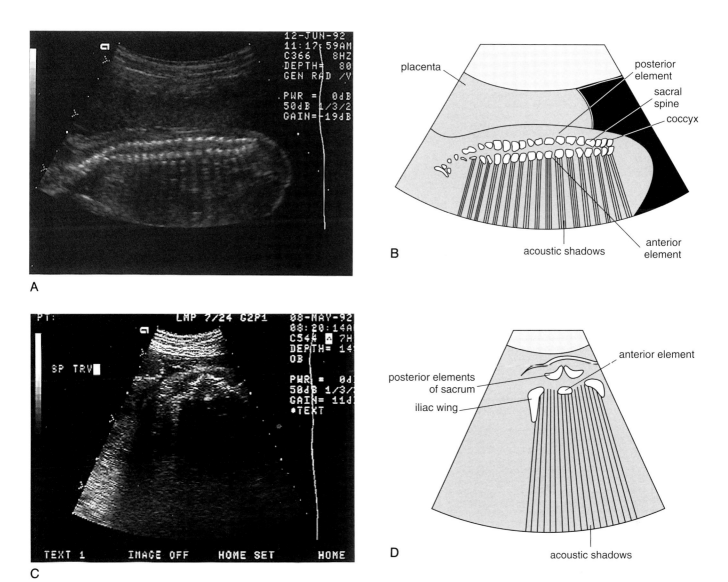

Figure 17–17. A, B, Longitudinal view of the sacral spine; C, D, Transverse view of the sacral spine.

EMBRYOLOGY OF THE ABDOMINAL ORGANS

Fetal intestinal peristalsis begins by 11 menstrual weeks of development and fetal swallowing commences within a few days of the start of peristalsis.[10] The fetus swallows small amounts of amniotic fluid early in the second trimester and thus it is possible to visualize the fluid-filled fetal stomach as early as 12 weeks into the pregnancy. Figure 17–18 shows the ultrasound appearance of a fluid-filled fetal stomach early in the second trimester.

During the mid- to late second trimester, fetal **meconium** will accumulate in the bowel, which serves as an accumulation point for this fetal waste material. The liver, pancreas, and spleen form as diverticula off the primitive alimentary tube. The fetal liver is the site of production of red blood cells and is proportionately much greater in size in the fetus than in the adult. The left lobe of the fetal liver is the first site to receive oxygenated blood from the placenta and is larger propor-

tionately in the fetus than it will be in the adult. It is the large size of the fetal liver that forces the diaphragm upward into the thorax and causes the fetal heart to be in a nearly horizontal plane.

SONOGRAPHIC APPEARANCE OF THE ABDOMINAL ORGANS

The fetal small and large intestines may appear as either hyper- or hypoechoic structures depending on their contents when imaged. Figure 17–19 shows one type of ultrasound appearance of fetal large and small bowel. Gas is not seen; however, cells and debris from the amniotic fluid may appear as hyperechoic contents, and conversely, amniotic fluid accumulating in the bowel appears hypoechoic.[11] The varied appearance of fetal bowel during pregnancy makes evaluation by ultrasound still images difficult and not very useful clinically. Real-time observations are helpful.

A transverse section through the fetal mid-abdomen

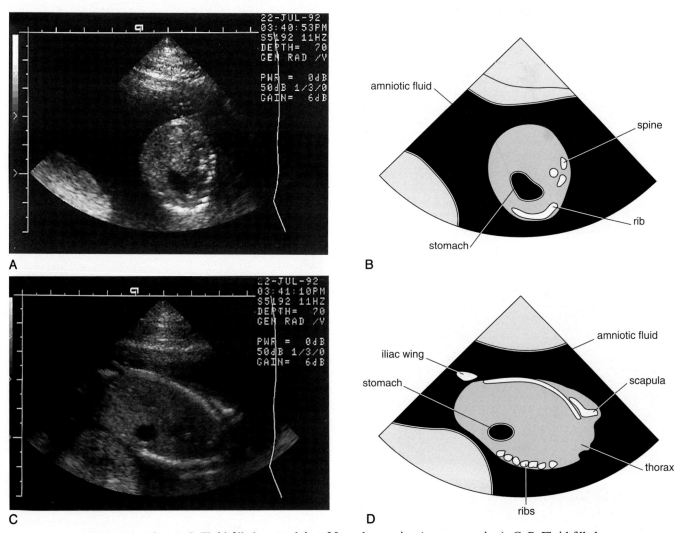

Figure 17–18. *A, B,* Fluid-filled stomach in a 35-week gestation (transverse view); *C, D,* Fluid-filled stomach in a 35-week gestation (longitudinal view).

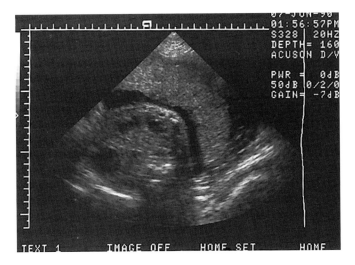
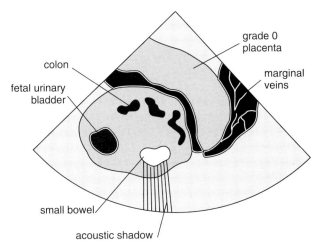

Figure 17–19. Fetal bowel in a 30-week gestation.

will demonstrate an anechoic structure on the left, representing the fluid-filled fetal stomach, and a medium reflective structure occupying most of the fetal abdomen representing the fetal liver as shown in Figure 17–20. The fetal spleen may also be seen in a location posterior and lateral to the fetal stomach (see Figure 17–20). It is possible during ultrasound examination in the second half of the second trimester (and throughout the third trimester) to see a small drumstick-shaped organ on the right side of the fetus. The is the fetal gallbladder, which is shown in Figure 17–21. It is also possible to see the umbilical vein coursing through the fetal liver. The vein's course is nearly perpendicular to the axis of the fetus as it nears its bifurcation point within the liver. Because of this, it is possible to see a fairly lengthy segment of the vein in a pure transverse plane taken at a level of the fetal stomach. The bifurcation of the fetal umbilical vein is shown in Figure 17–22. The cord insertion into the abdomen is shown in Figure 17–23.

The umbilical vein, fetal stomach, transverse spine, and fetal liver are important landmarks for measurement of the fetal abdominal diameter or abdominal circumference (described later in this chapter). The fetal spleen is similar in echogenicity to the fetal liver throughout the second and third trimesters. The fetal large bowel will enlarge as the pregnancy progresses and it fills with meconium.

Occasionally, fetal colon which has grown due to the presence of meconium has been mistaken by sonographers for fluid-filled abnormalities such as ovarian cysts, renal cysts, atresic fluid-filled small bowel, or abdominal masses.[11] The fetal colon is in the same anatomical position as in the adult and careful examination of suspected abnormalities in both longitudinal and transverse planes should eliminate this confusion. The transverse portion of the fetal colon is shown in Figure 17–24.

Assessment of the fetal abdomen is relatively easy

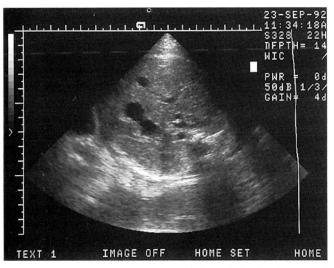
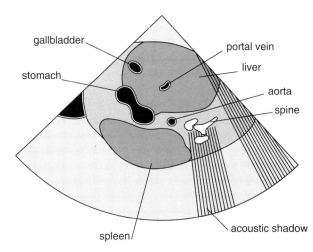

Figure 17–20. Liver and spleen in a 27-week gestation.

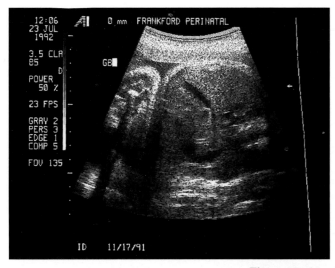

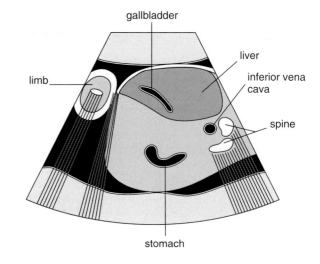

Figure 17–21. Fetal gallbladder.

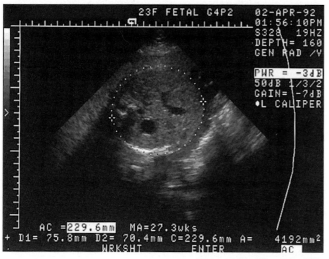

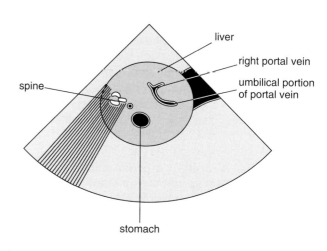

Figure 17–22. Umbilical portion of the portal vein.

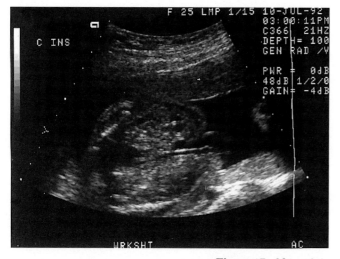

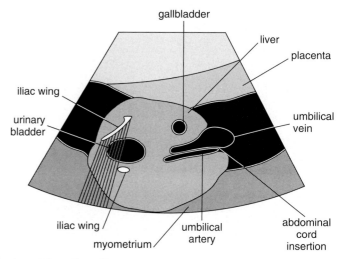

Figure 17–23. Abdominal cord insertion site.

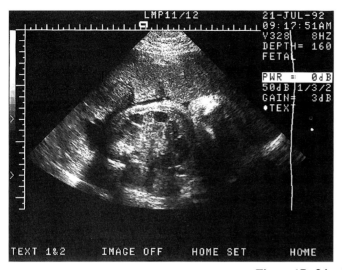

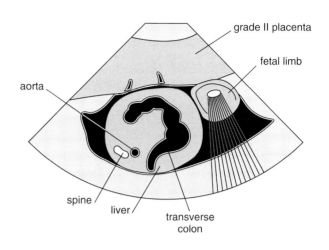

Figure 17–24. Transverse colon.

when compared with assessment of the adult abdomen. The fetus has no overlying bowel gas or large body wall to prevent visualization of its contents. As ultrasound imaging technology improves, it is probable that additional abdominal structures will be detectable during ultrasound examinations.

EMBRYOLOGY OF GENITOURINARY ORGANS

The fetal genitourinary system consists of the urinary bladder, ureters, urethra, and genitalia. The bladder and ureters are formed at approximately 6 menstrual weeks of development. The kidneys, which form in association with urethral buds, develop between 7 and 9 weeks of gestation and become functional at approximately 10 weeks of menstrual age.[12]

SONOGRAPHIC APPEARANCE OF THE GENITOURINARY SYSTEM

It is sometimes possible to visualize the fetal bladder as early as 13 weeks, but evaluation at this early age is unreliable. By 15 weeks' menstrual age, over 90 percent of all fetal bladders can be visualized.[13] In general, if the fetal bladder is not visualized by 15 or 16 weeks, a follow-up ultrasound examination will be ordered later in the pregnancy to document the presence of a fetal bladder and thus confirm fetal kidney function. Figure 17–25 demonstrates the ultrasound appearance of a fluid-filled fetal urinary bladder.

The fetal kidneys can be visualized as early as 15 weeks. Fetal kidneys cannot be reliably detected, however, until 20 weeks of gestational age.[13] The age at which the fetal kidney can be detected depends on the quality of the ultrasound unit, the ability of the sonog-

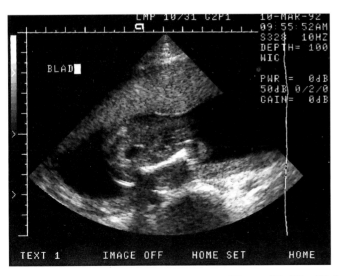

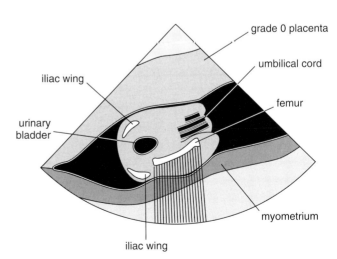

Figure 17–25. Fluid-filled urinary bladder.

rapher, the size of the woman, and the position of the fetus. By approximately 20 menstrual weeks, the internal anatomy of the fetal kidneys can be appreciated.

The renal capsule, renal pyramids, slit-like renal sinus, and, occasionally, a hyperechoic dilated renal collecting system can all be visualized with careful scanning tech-niques (Figure 17–26). The fetal kidneys grow at a rate that keeps them proportionately equal to the other devel-oping fetal structures. In general, the length of the fetal kidneys may be represented by the length of four to five vertebrae of the fetus.[14] The ratio of kidney diameter to the diameter of the fetal abdomen should remain be-

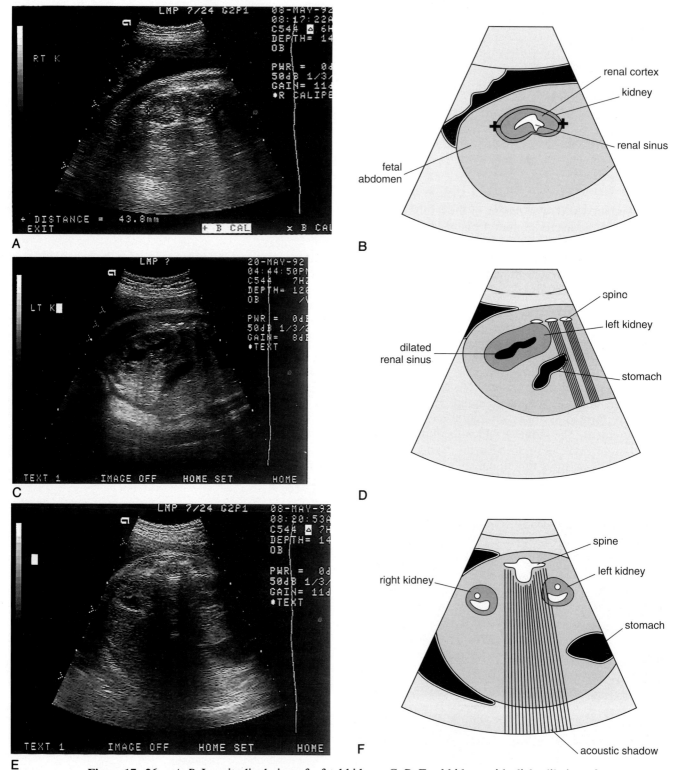

Figure 17–26. *A, B,* Longitudinal view of a fetal kidney; *C, D,* Fetal kidney with slight dilation of the collecting system; *E, F,* Transverse view of fetal kidneys.

tween 0.27 and 0.23 during the gestation.[15] The fetal bladder also grows in proportion to the rest of the fetus during the remainder of pregnancy and its size depends on the degree of filling. A normal fetal bladder should empty and fill once during a 30-minute sonographic examination.[13]

The fetal adrenal glands may be visualized as early as 10 menstrual weeks. These structures appear as medium echoic structures superior to the fetal kidneys. Careful high-resolution scanning of the fetal adrenal glands may reveal a central hyperechoic line and a hyperechoic capsule. Figure 17–27 demonstrates the relationship of the adrenal glands to the fetal kidney. The fetal adrenal glands are sometimes confused with the fetal kidneys early in the pregnancy; however, they are located more superiorly and their internal architecture is not similar to that found in the fetal kidney.

The fetal vagina or penis and scrotum may be visualized after 20 weeks of development and certainly should be distinguishable by 26 weeks. The testicles normally descend to the scrotum by 28 to 34 weeks.[16] The fetal labia may be detectable as early as 17 or 18 menstrual weeks. Figure 17–28 displays the ultrasound appearance of both female (A, B) and male (C, D) external genitalia in utero. The fetal ovaries are usually not visualized unless ovarian cysts are present. The fetal uterus or prostate is not generally evaluated during an ultrasound examination.

Ultrasound examination of the perineum of a female fetus should demonstrate the labia of the external genitalia. These structures appear as two small buds protruding from the perineum separated by a hyperechoic line. The female labia may be visualized as early as 17 or 18 menstrual weeks and generally can be consistently demonstrated only at 24 weeks or more. The male scrotum may appear empty prior to 20 weeks of menstrual age since the testicles may not descend before this time. If the scrotum is visualized after the testicles have descended, it is not unusual for small hydroceles (fluid collections) to be seen bilaterally.[16] The fetal penis may

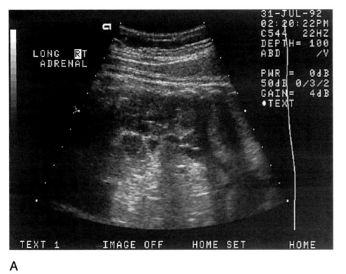

A

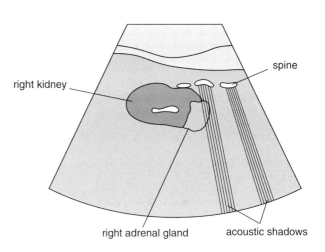

B

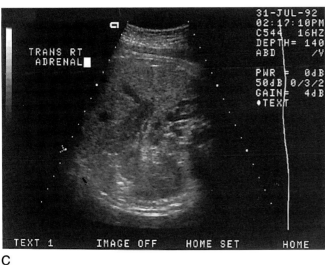

C

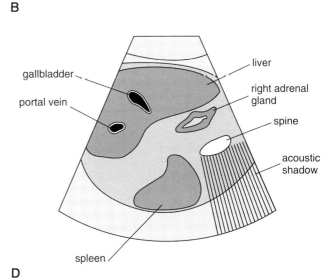

D

Figure 17–27. *A, B,* Longitudinal section of a fetal adrenal gland; *C, D,* Transverse section of a fetal adrenal gland.

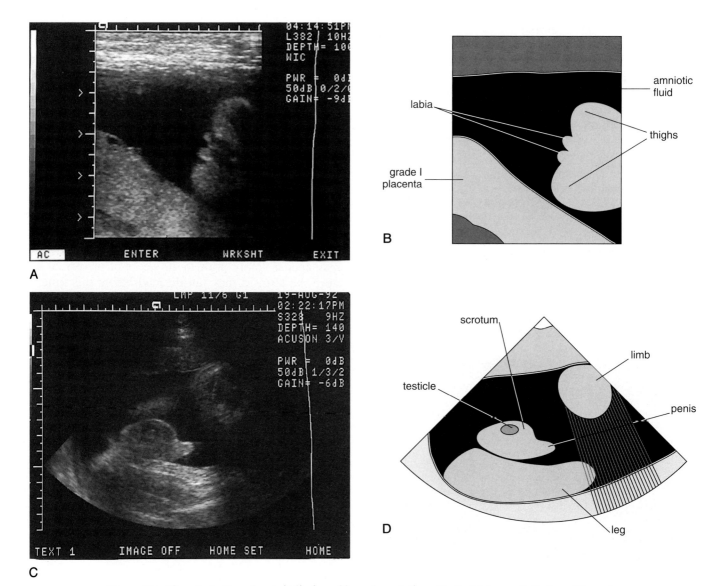

Figure 17-28. *A, B,* Female genitalia in a 32-week gestation; *C, D,* Male genitalia in a 30-week gestation.

be visualized as a medium echogenic structure extending from the perineum. Determination of sex depends on the visualization of either the female labia or the male scrotum. Assignment of sex should not be made on the basis of the presence or absence of a fetal penis. The penis may be quite small and not visualized, suggesting the presence of a female fetus, or a female clitoris may suggest the presence of a small penis. Thus, if the gender of the fetus is to be determined, the sonographer must be able to distinguish between the labia and scrotum.[17]

EMBRYOLOGY OF THE FETAL SKELETON

The fetal skeleton is completely formed and positioned by about 10 weeks' gestational age. The bones continue to grow and accumulate minerals (ossify) throughout the second and third trimesters. The fetal skull and femur are the first components to ossify followed by portions of the spine, rib cage, and the short bones of the extremities and the pelvic bones. The bones of the hands and feet (metacarpal and metatarsal) ossify during the early second trimester. The smallest bones of the hand and feet (carpals and tarsals) may continue to ossify up to birth.[18]

SONOGRAPHIC APPEARANCE OF THE FETAL SKELETON

The fetal skeleton, fetal limbs, and fetal digits can be seen during the second and third trimesters with ultrasound examination. (See Figure 17-29.) The echogenicity of the fetal skeleton is an indication of the degree of mineralization that has taken place within the developing bones. Acoustic shadowing of the larger fetal bones

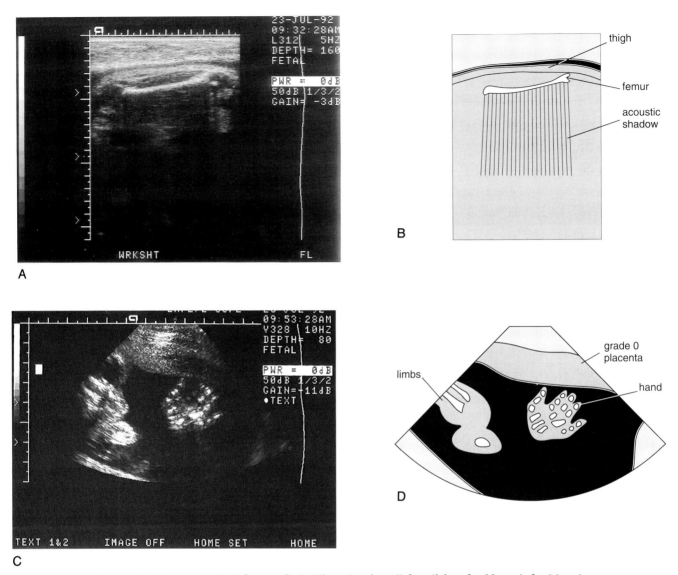

Figure 17–29. *A, B,* Fetal femur; *C, D,* View showing all five digits of a 33-week fetal hand.

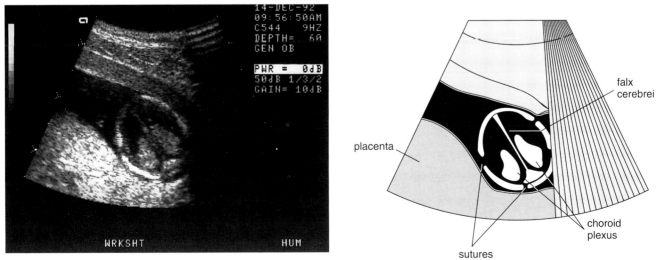

Figure 17–30. Sutures of the skull.

should be evident during the second and third trimester ultrasound examinations. A complete fetal cranium is seen at 12 weeks' gestation, as are the cranial sutures. (See Figure 17-30.) A complete fetal cranium should be evident at 12 weeks of development.

SONOGRAPHIC MEASUREMENTS OF THE FETUS

High-resolution ultrasonography allows visualization of the fetus with great detail and clarity. It is now possible to measure internal organs, fetal bones, portions of the fetal organs, and fetal body parts. However, in a routine ultrasound examination there are several measurements which should always be performed and which offer the clinician significant information about the growth rate of the fetus, and thus its fitness.

Certain measurements of the fetal head should be made. After about 12 weeks of development it is possible to accurately measure the diameter of the fetal skull. This measurement is known as the **biparietal diameter (BPD)**. (See Figure 17-31.) This is a measurement from the leading edge of the near-field parietal bone (the outside surface) to the leading edge of the far-field parietal bone (the inside surface). It is performed at a scanning plane which contains several specific intracranial markers. Four brain structures should be visualized at this level: (1) the falx cerebri, (2) the thalamus, (3) the cavum septum pellucidum, and (4) the third ventricle. The falx cerebri is the reflection of the meninges dividing the cerebrum into two equal halves. This membrane should be at right angles to the sound beam and thus produce a bright echogenic line which is located in a central position within the skull. At the level for the BPD measurement, the falx cerebri should not extend completely from front to back. The thalamus is a medium to low level echoic diamond-shaped structure in the center of the section. The thalamus is divided equally into right and left halves by a hyperechoic line, or slit. This slit represents the third ventricle. The cavum septum pellucidum is an anechoic fluid-containing structure located in the midline of the section in the frontal region. This structure contains more fluid than the third ventricle and is anterior to the thalamus. It appears as an anechoic, fluid-containing zone, bordered by two small hyperechoic lines. Visualization of these four structures assures not only that the correct level is being used for the BPD measurement, but also that the correct tilt has been selected. Figure 17-31 shows the correct plane for a BPD measurement.

Once the correct plane for the BPD has been imaged, the same image can be used for other measurements of the fetal head. The caliper at the leading edge of the far parietal bone is moved to the outside edge. This measurement becomes the outer to outer measurement of the fetal head. It is used with the **occipital-frontal diameter (OFD)** to calculate the **cephalic index (CI)**. The OFD is the outer to outer back to front diameter of the fetal head. (See Figure 17-32 B and C for the position of the OFD.) The CI equals the BPD (outer to outer) divided by the OFD. The CI should be between 0.72 and 0.86.[19] Another measurement at this level is the head circumference, which is a tracing of the outer edge of the fetal skull at the level of the BPD. This measurement is shown in Figure 17-32 D and E. If the cephalic index is above 0.86, the head is wider than average, or **brachiocephalic**. If the cephalic index is under 0.72, the head is narrower than average, or **dolichocephalic**. The head circumference is usually used for dating the pregnancy when the cephalic index is abnormal. Charts are available which correlate the values for BPDs or HCs with estimated gestational age. Occasionally, it is not possible to obtain an image at the appropriate level, and a measurement at a slightly lower level of the fetal head must be used. In this image the **cerebral peduncles** can be visualized. These structures lie directly below the fetal thalamus. The cerebral peduncles are smaller than the thalamus and are slightly more echoic and rounder than the thalamus. Charts are available which correlate HC and BPD measurements with gestational age.[19,20]

There are two ways to measure the fetal abdomen: (1) Two perpendicular diameters of the fetal abdomen are measured, and the average diameter is calculated by dividing the sum of these diameters by two; (2) the abdominal circumference is measured directly. This circumference can also be calculated from the average diameter by multiplying this number by pi, or 3.14. Measurement of the circumference of the fetal abdomen is the more accurate method, but not all ultrasound instruments have the ability to trace or draw ellipses. Three landmarks are used to select the correct scanning plane for the abdominal measurements. (See Figure 17-33.) First, the fetal spine should appear as three bright

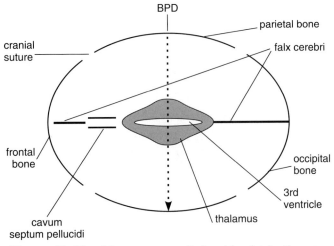

Figure 17-31. Measurement of the biparietal diameter (BPD).

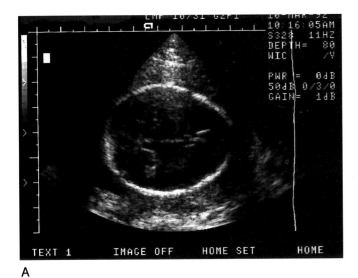

A

echogenic reflectors. These are the ossification centers of the vertebrae. There may be acoustic shadowing from these elements, but this is not always the case. Second, the anechoic fluid containing the fetal stomach should be seen on the fetal left in the correct plane for measuring the fetal abdomen. The size of the fetal stomach will vary, but it should appear anechoic. The fetal abdomen should appear round or nearly round in a correct measurement. The umbilical vein, the third marker for an abdominal measurement, should be seen coursing within the fetal liver. The walls of the umbilical vein appear as short, bright echogenic linear structures about one third to one half the distance to the center of the fetal abdomen. Ideally, the division of the umbilical vein into the left and right portal veins should be seen. The umbilical vein and portal veins are both anechoic. Figure 17–34 illustrates the correct images for measuring the abdominal circumference and abdominal diameter, respectively.

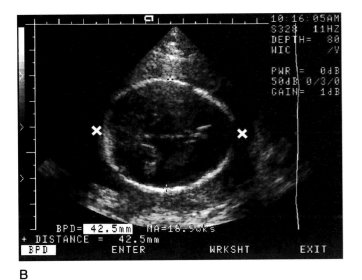

B

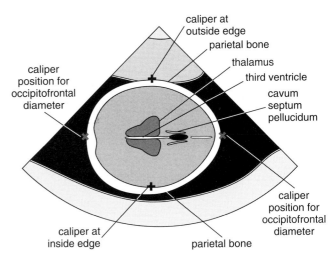

C

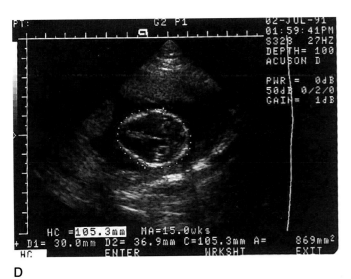

D

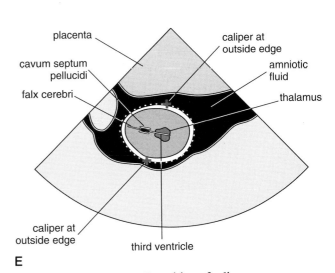

E

Figure 17–32. *A*, Image for a BPD; *B*, *C*, position of calipers for OFD and *D*, *E*, position of calipers for BPD (outer to outer).

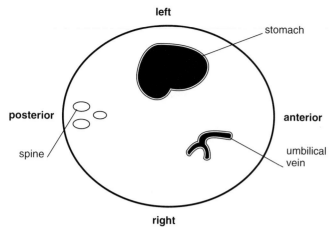

Figure 17–33. Level for abdominal measurement.

Several potential problems may occur when measuring the fetal abdomen. The fetal gallbladder may resemble the umbilical vein; however, this structure cannot be traced through the abdominal wall and is usually to the right side of the abdomen. The umbilical vein is almost always in a midline position. At times the fetal stomach cannot be visualized and it is necessary for the sonographer to wait for the fetus to swallow additional amniotic fluid or to measure the abdomen using only two of the previously described landmarks. The correct identification of the umbilical vein is now critical to achieve correct measurement. If the average diameter measurement method is used to assess the fetal abdomen, two perpendicular outside diameters should be selected; the average diameter should be calculated from these. Charts are available which report estimated gestational age with respect to either abdominal diameter or abdominal circumference.[21]

The fetal femur can be measured as early as 12 weeks of development.[22] This bone is measured end to end across any curve in the bone. The femur is located first by imaging the iliac wings and bladder, then moving the transducer to a position which images the entire length of the femur. Ideally, the femur should be perpendicular or nearly perpendicular to the sound beam. Care should be taken to avoid including the patella in the measurement. Figure 17–35 demonstrates the measurement of a fetal femur. Both femurs should be measured and if the femur lengths do not agree with head or abdominal measurements, humeri and possibly the short bones should also be measured. Charts are available which correlate estimated gestational age with femur length, humerus length, and even tibial and fibular lengths.[22,23]

Charts are available (in some cases built directly into the ultrasound unit's software) which correlate estimated gestational age with the measurements discussed earlier. Another chart is available which estimates fetal weight

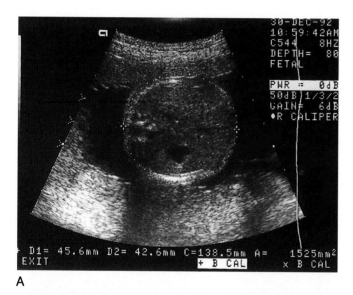

A

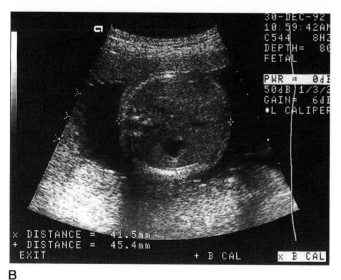

B

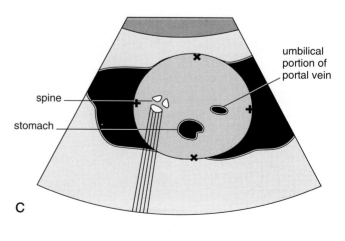

C

Figure 17–34. *A,* Ultrasound of an abdomen for a circumference measurement (22-week gestation); *B, C,* position of calipers for average abdominal diameter measurements.

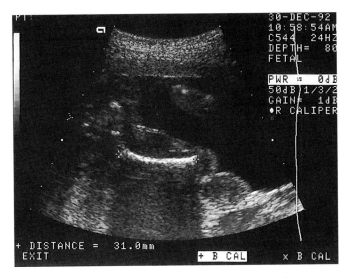

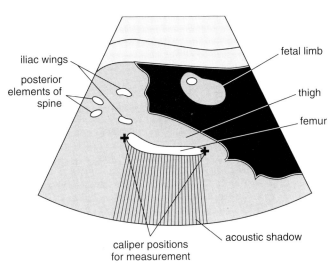

Figure 17–35. Measurement of a femur.

based on abdominal diameter and femur length[24] or abdominal circumference and head circumference.[25] At times, it is necessary to measure the fetal cerebellum, heart, cisterna magna, or even the circumference of the fetal thorax. These special measurements will be discussed in Chapter 18. The American Institute for Ultrasound in Medicine has published guidelines giving the views which should be obtained during second and third trimester ultrasound examinations.[26]

References

1. Hoddick WK, Mahoney BS, Callen PW et al: Placental thickness. J Ultrasound Med 4:479–482, 1985.
2. Blecker OP, Kloosterman GJ, Breur W et al: The volumetric growth of the human placenta. A longitudinal ultrasonic study. Am J Obstet Gynecol 149:512–517, 1977.
3. Petrucha RA, Platt LD: Relationship of placental grade to gestational age. Am J Obstet Gynecol 144:733, 1982.
4. Hopper KD, Komppa GH, Williams BP, et al: A reevaluation of placental grading and its clinical significance. J Ultrasound Med 3:161–266, 1984.
5. Mahoney BS, Filly RA, Callen PW: The amniotic band syndrome and potential pitfalls. Am J Obstet Gynecol 152:63–68, 1985.
6. Queenan JT, Gadow EC: Polyhydramnios: Chronic versus acute. Am J Obstet Gynecol 108:349–355, 1970.
7. Abramovich DR, Garden A, Jandial L, et al: Fetal swallowing and voiding in relation to hydramnios. Obstet Gynecol 54:15–20, 1979.
8. Robinson HP, Hood VD, Adam AH, et al: Diagnostic ultrasound: early detection of fetal neural tube defects. Obstet Gynecol 56:705–710, 1980.
9. Lindfors, KK, McGahan JJP, Tennant FP, et al: Mid-trimester screening for neural tube defects: correlation of sonography with amniocentesis results. Am J Radiol 149:141–145, 1987.
10. Nyberg DA, Mack LA, Patten RM et al: Fetal bowel: normal sonographic findings. J Ultrasound Med 6:3–8, 1987.
11. Suhas G, Paruleskar G: Sonography of normal fetal bowel. J Ultrasound Med 10:211–220, 1991.
12. Moore KL: The urogenital system in the developing human: clinically oriented embryology, 4th ed. Philadelphia, WB Saunders, 1988, 246–285.
13. Clautice-Engle T, Pretorius DH, Budorick NE: Significance of nonvisualization of the fetal urinary bladder. J Ultrasound Med 10:615–618, 1991.
14. Mahoney B: The genitourinary system. In Callen PW (ed.): Ultrasonography in Obstetrics and Gynecology, 2nd ed. Philadelphia, WB Saunders, 1988, 256.
15. Grannum PT, Bracke M, Silverman R, et al: Assessment of fetal kidney size in normal gestation by comparison of ratio of kidney circumference to abdominal circumference. Am J Obstet Gynecol 136:249–254, 1980.
16. Zafaranloo S, Gerard PS, Wise G: Sonographic assessment of fetal male genitalia. J Diagn Med Sonog 7:205–207, 1991.
17. Cooper C, Mahoney BS, Bowie JD, et al: Prenatal ultrasound diagnosis of ambiguous genitalia. J Ultrasound Med 4:4433–4436, 1989.
18. Mahoney BS: The extremities. In Nyberg DA, Mahoney BS, Pretorius DH (eds.) Diagnostic Ultrasound of Fetal Anomalies: Text and Atlas. St. Louis, CV Mosby, 1990, 492–562.
19. Hadlock FP, Deter RL, Harrist RB, et al: Fetal head circumference: relation to menstrual age. Am J Roentgenol 138:649–653, 1982.
20. Chervenak FA, Jeanty P, Cantraine F, et al: The diagnosis of fetal microcephaly. Am J Obstet Gynecol 149:512–517, 1984.
21. Deter RL, Harrist RN, Hadlock FP, et al: Fetal head and abdominal circumference II: Critical reevaluation of the relation to menstrual age. J Clin Ultrasound 10:365–372, 1982.
22. Warda AH, Deter RL, Rossavik IK, et al: Fetal femur length: a critical re-evaluation of the relationship to menstrual age. Obstet Gynecol 66:69, 1985.
23. Merz E, Mi-Sook KK, Pehl S: Ultrasonic mensuration of fetal limb bones in the second and third trimesters. J Clin Ultrasound 15:175–183, 1987.
24. Hadlock FP, Harrist RB, Carpenter RJ, et al: Sonographic estimation of fetal weight. Radiology 150:535–540, 1984.
25. Warsof ST, Gohari P, Berkowitz RL, et al: The estimation of fetal weight by computer assisted analysis. Am J Obstet Gynecol 128:881, 1977.
26. Leopold GR: Antepartum obstetrical ultrasound examination guidelines. J Ultrasound Med 5:241–242, 1986.

Chapter 18

OBSTETRIC SONOGRAPHY/ SPECIAL SITUATIONS

G. WILLIAM SHEPHERD

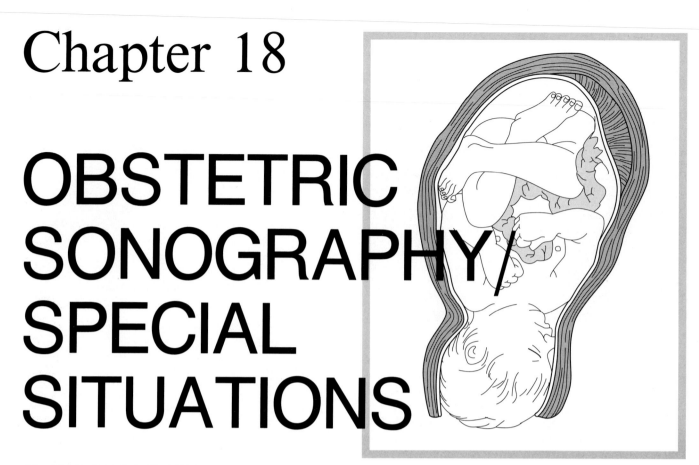

(From Guyton AC: Textbook of Medical Physiology, 8th ed. Philadelphia, WB Saunders, 1991, p 924.)

Objectives:

Define amniocentesis and its purpose.

Describe chorionic villus sampling (CVS) and its purpose.

Describe how biophysical profiles are scored.

Describe the indications for a biophysical profile.

Describe the three types of identical twins that occur in certain pregnancies.

Define the key words.

Key Words:

Alpha-fetoprotein (AFP)
Amniocentesis
Biophysical profile
Chorionic villus sampling (CVS)
Diamniotic-monochorionic twins

Dichorionic-Diamniotic twins
Dizygotic twins
Fraternal twins
L-S ratio
Monochorionic-monoamniotic twins
Monozygotic twins
Nonstress test
Umbilical cord doppler

INTRODUCTION

The two preceding chapters gave an overview of the anatomy, physiology, and sonographic appearance of the developing fetus and its support structures. The measurements described are sufficient for most pregnancies. Sometimes an extraordinary situation presents itself and requires additional ultrasound procedures or ultrasound-guided procedures. This chapter addresses those higher-risk pregnancies.

ASSESSING FETAL WELL-BEING

The Biophysical Profile

There are times when it is necessary for a clinician to determine whether or not a fetus is in distress. In order to assess the well-being of the fetus, a **biophysical profile** is usually ordered. It is a test which measures fetal well-being.[1] This test is extremely sonographer dependent, since movement is not captured on still images. Several parameters are followed during this examination, which is timed and cannot exceed 30 minutes in length. The first parameter is gross fetal movement, which consists of the extension or flexion of an arm or leg, arching of the back or neck, or twisting of the trunk. If two such movements are observed during a 30-minute period, two points are allotted. A second parameter is fetal tone or fine motion. Fetal tone consists of finger or toe movement, and at least two such movements should be visualized during a 30-minute examination. Two points are assigned if the movements occur. Next, fetal respiration is measured; at least 60 seconds of respiration should be seen during the examination. Fetal respiration is visualized by seeing the fetal diaphragm move upward and downward or by observing the kidneys moving past vertebrae as they are pushed upward by the spleen or liver, and ultimately the diaphragm. If at least 60 seconds of respiration are observed, another two points are assigned. The final category is the quantity of amniotic fluid. At least one pocket having an average diameter of 1 cm should be visualized within the uterus.

In some hospitals, other methods of assessing amniotic fluid are used, for example, the four-quadrant analysis: In this method, the anteroposterior diameter of the largest pocket in each of the four quadrants is measured and they are then totalled. The sum should equal at least 8 cm for the full two points to be assigned. This criterion is based on the amniotic fluid index (AFI) method developed by Phelan et al.[2] The maximum score for the ultrasound portion of the biophysical profile is eight points. Two additional points may be added if a **nonstress test** is successfully completed. The test measures spontaneous heart rate accelerations by means of a continuous wave Doppler heart monitor and strip chart.

The biophysical profile is summarized in Table 18–1. A total of eight or 10 points means unqualified passing. A score of six usually will be followed by a second biophysical profile within 24 hours. In most cases a score of four or less will be followed by induction of labor or a cesarean section, if possible. The indications for performing a biophysical profile include intrauterine retardation of growth, maternal diabetes, preterm labor, a failed nonstress test, an irregular heart rate, oligohy-

TABLE 18–1   Biophysical Profile Scoring

	CRITERION	SCORE (pts)
Part I Nonstress test	2 accelerations of 15 beats per minute in 30-min test	2
Part II Ultrasound Examination Gross movement	3 separate flexions and extensions in 30-min examination	2
Tone	1 episode of fetal opening and closing of hand or clenching of foot in 30-min examination	2
Respiration	At least 60 seconds of fetal breathing in 30-min examination	2
Fluid	At least 1 pocket of amniotic fluid of at least 1 cm in 2 dimensions	2
	Unqualified pass	8 or more
	Maximum total	10

Data from Manning EA, Platt LD, Sipos L: Antenatal fetal evaluation: development of a fetal biophysical profile. Am J Obstet Gynecol 136:787–795, 1980.

dramnios, a prematurely aged placenta, a postdates pregnancy, no sensation of fetal movement, or any other condition which places the fetus at high risk.

Doppler Examination

Umbilical cord Doppler is a relatively recent examination technique which measures the resistance to blood flow within the placenta. The Doppler signal from the umbilical artery is obtained with continuous wave, or in some cases, pulse wave, Doppler. The spectrum of the signal is analyzed to determine the diastolic flow. The extent of diastolic flow is directly related to the flow resistance of the placenta. There is good correlation between the absence of effective diastolic flow and a poor outcome.[3] In some institutions a poor high resistance flow pattern will increase the likelihood of an induced delivery. The thought is that the damage to the fetus may be minimized by its removal from an inadequate environment.

The use of umbilical cord Doppler measurements is increasing. A graph has been developed which presents the uppermost normal systolic to diastolic flow rate ratio at various stages of development.[4] Doppler measurements may also be used to assess maternal circulation to the uterus. During pregnancy the uterine arteries have very low pulsatility and may appear almost as venous signals when the Doppler wave form is examined. However, a modest cardiac pattern should be obtained. Examples of umbilical artery and maternal uterine artery Doppler wave forms are presented in Figures 18–1, and 18–2. It is possible that in the near future ultrasound Doppler techniques will be used to assess not only umbilical arteries and uterine arteries but arteries within the fetus as well.[5,6]

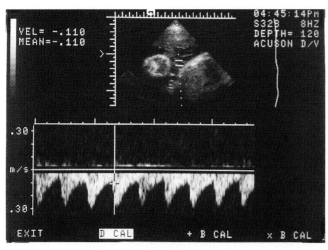

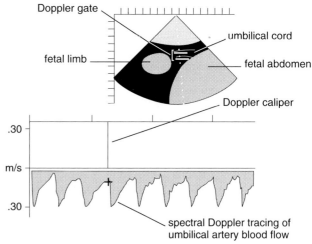

Figure 18-1. Ultrasound pulsed Doppler interrogation of the umbilical artery. This is a normal low resistance wave form.

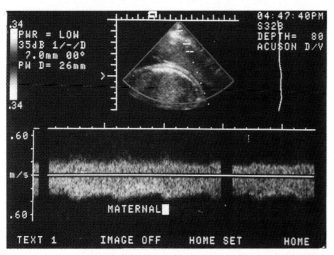

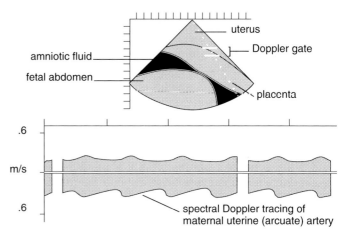

Figure 18-2. Ultrasound pulsed Doppler interrogation of uterine circulation during the third trimester. The wave form on top of the line is a venous signal. The wave form under the line is that of a uterine artery. Note their similarity. The artery has a very low pulsatility.

Assessing Lung Maturity

Occasionally it is necessary to perform **amniocentesis** late in the pregnancy. Amniocentesis is the removal of a small quantity of amniotic fluid from the sac surrounding the fetus. Quite often amniocentesis is done with ultrasound guidance, particularly late in the pregnancy when smaller, more localized fluid pockets are generally present. The amniotic fluid can be tested to detect two chemicals: lecithin and sphingomyelin. The ratio of lecithin to sphingomyelin, the **L-S ratio**, measures the degree of fetal lung development.[7] It does not make sense to remove the fetus from an environment, even though the fetus is under some stress, to an environment in which it cannot survive. Evaluation of the L-S ratio allows the clinician to decide whether or not an emergency delivery can be performed.

ASSESSING GENETIC AND DEVELOPMENTAL WELL-BEING

Genetic Amniocentesis

Certain invasive obstetric procedures require ultrasound guidance, or are safer and quicker with it. One of these—amniocentesis to determine the L-S ratio—has already been described. Amniocentesis may also be performed at an earlier time in the gestation in order to collect amniotic fluid for genetic assessment. Genetic amniocentesis is usually performed between 15 and 17 weeks of gestational age. In some hospitals, this procedure is done as early as 13 weeks. Although it is considered experimental, in this method the amniotic fluid is analyzed to determine its biochemical components. One component, **alpha-fetoprotein (AFP)** is a protein whose concentration increases beyond normal limits when certain defects are present. A portion of the amniotic fluid is cultured for a period of 2 to 4 weeks, and a chromosomal analysis of the amniotic cells is done. Of particular interest is the karyotype (a chromosomal map) to detect Down's syndrome. Many other genetic abnormalities can be detected by this procedure, and the list is growing as research continues. Also, through research in molecular biology, molecular probes have been devised which can detect a great number of genetic disorders, and which will give test results in a shorter period of time than other conventional cell culture and chromosomal banding techniques. Some of the major indications for amniocentesis include: (1) maternal age of 35 or older (these women are at higher risk for giving birth to infants with Down's syndrome; (2) history of a genetic disorder in the family; (3) elevated maternal serum AFP; (4) decreased maternal serum AFP (risk of delivering a Down's syndrome infant); (5) suspicious findings on an ultrasound examination.

Ultrasonography plays several roles during the amniocentesis procedure. The gestational age is determined, as are the viability of the fetus and its position. The size of the pocket of amniotic fluid is also noted by ultrasound, as is the position of the placenta and any changes in the position of the fetus. After these ultrasound determinations have been made, the doctor or nurse will prepare the maternal abdomen with sterile washes. In some institutions a sterile needle will be affixed to the ultrasound transducer. In others, the sonographer or sonologist will place a sterile cover over the transducer and visualize the amniocentesis needle as it is inserted "freehand" (i.e., needle not attached to transducer) within the amniotic sac. During the procedure, the sonographer observes the area in which the fluid is being collected. Following the procedure, the sonographer makes sure the fetus is viable and that any visible hemorrhage that may have been caused by the procedure has ceased. The sonographer should be alert for the occurrence of abrupt maternal or fetal movement, and should follow standard sterile techniques.

Certain risks are associated with amniocentesis and they must be weighed against the advantages. Slow leakage of amniotic fluid has occurred in a very limited number of cases following amniocentesis.[8] The insertion of the needle can induce premature labor.[8] Inadequate sterile technique may lead to amnionitis, an infection of the gestational sac, which can be life-threatening to the fetus as well as to the mother.[9] Hemorrhage from the placenta may occur if a transplacental approach is required to collect amniotic fluid. The fetus may be injured by the needle if the fetus suddenly moves into the pocket where the fluid is being collected. In general, injury due to fetal movement is very slight; however, care must be taken to avoid collecting in a pocket which contains considerable umbilical cord or the fetal head or thorax.[9]

Chorionic Villus Sampling (CVS)

Ultrasonography also plays a role in **chorionic villus sampling (CVS)**. CVS is another means of collecting tissue for genetic analysis, using early placental tissue buds or chorionic villi. The cells in the villi are growing rapidly, thus there are many more mitotic figures (visible chromosomes) as compared with the cells obtained with genetic amniocentesis. Thus, culturing of the tissue is not required, so the analysis can be done immediately after the procedure. The results are available to the mother usually within a week. The procedure is done at menstrual age of about 10 weeks. It is performed by a physician under transabdominal ultrasound guidance. The entire procedure usually requires about 15 minutes. As in genetic amniocentesis, ultrasound is used prior to the procedure to determine fetal viability, to obtain an occurate gestational age, and to rule out abnormalities.

There are several advantages for using CVS as opposed to amniocentesis. Results are available much earlier than in amniocentesis, and this confers the psychological advantage of a less stressful waiting period. If the woman desires an abortion, it can be done by 12 weeks' gestation. There is less risk to her if the abortion is done at this point rather than at 18 or 19 weeks, the usual age following genetic amniocentesis. This test can be done earlier in the pregnancy and thus offers a greater advantage to a woman who is at high risk for giving birth to an abnormal infant.

CVS does carry certain risks. Following the procedure, spontaneous bleeding or even spontaneous abortion can occur. Spontaneous abortion has been estimated to occur in approximately 1 percent of CVS procedures.[10] Theoretically, the procedure could cause an abruption; however, this has never been reported to my knowledge. Chorioamnionitis could occur if a pathogen is introduced through the vagina.

In general, the loss rate due to CVS is extremely low. CVS does not detect nongenetic defects such as spina bifida or abdominal wall defects, and a follow-up ultrasound examination is usually recommended later in the pregnancy when such defects may be detectable. The viability of the fetus is always confirmed following CVS.

CVS requires ultrasonic guidance. Generally the physician will try to collect the chorionic villi through a small catheter inserted through the vagina. However, a fundal placenta or fibroids in the lower uterine segment may necessitate a transabdominal needle approach. In both cases, ultrasound guidance informs the clinician when the top of the collecting device is in place and an area rich in chorionic villi has been reached.

Other Ultrasound-Guided Procedures

Ultrasound guidance is also used to help the physician when collecting umbilical cord blood from the fetus or when transfusing the fetus.[11,12] (These procedures are performed in the course of certain abnormal pregnancies and are beyond the scope of this chapter.) The ultrasonographer plays an ever-increasing role in invasive procedures.

EMBRYOLOGY OF MULTIPLE PREGNANCIES

Multiple pregnancies involve special ultrasound techniques as well as special risk factors. The usual indication of a multiple pregnancy is "large for dates" or a family history of twins. The family history may indicate a tendency for release of multiple ova (fraternal twins) or a tendency for the early embryo to divide (identical twins). The use of fertility drugs also increases the possibility of a multiple pregnancy.

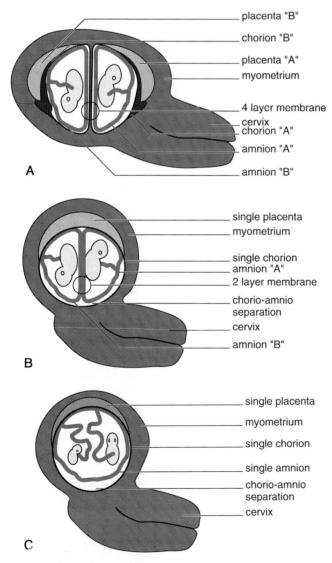

A

placenta "B"
chorion "B"
placenta "A"
myometrium
4 layer membrane
cervix
chorion "A"
amnion "A"
amnion "B"

B

single placenta
myometrium
single chorion
amnion "A"
2 layer membrane
chorio-amnio separation
cervix
amnion "B"

C

single placenta
myometrium
single chorion
single amnion
chorio-amnio separation
cervix

(note: dischordant growth)

Figure 18–3. *A*, Depiction of diamnionic-dichorionic twins. *B*, Diamnionic-monochorionic twins. *C*, Monoamnionic-monochorionic twins.

Identical twins are referred to as **monozygotic twins**, which develop from a single fertilized egg, or zygote.

There are three types of monozygotic twins. They are classified according to the time at which the embryo divides. **Dichorionic-diamniotic twins** are produced by the division of an embryo before both the chorion and amnion have been determined embryologically. This is before the embryo is 4 days old in relation to conception or before approximately 18 days based on the last menstrual period. The embryo is at the morula stage at this time, and consists of 32 to 64 cells. Each embryo will have an individual placenta and amniotic sac.

Diamniotic-monochorionic twins develop when the embryo divides sometime after 4 days postconception, but before 7 days postconception, between menstrual age of 18 and 21 days. The embryo is a blastocyst at this point of development. Each embryo will have an individual sac, but the two embryos will share a common placenta. The amniotic cavity has not formed at the time of division, while the chorion has already developed.

Monochorionic-monoamniotic twins occur when the division takes place between 3 and 4 menstrual weeks of age. The embryos will reside within a single amniotic sac and will share a common placenta. The division of the embryo occurs just prior to the formation of the embryonic disk. The three types of monozygotic twins are depicted in Figure 18–3. If the embryo divides after the menstrual age of 4 weeks, conjoined (or "Siamese") twins can result. This is very rare. The later the division of the embryo, the greater the number of shared organs.

Fraternal twins (or **dizygotic twins**) result when ovulation produces two eggs, and each is fertilized and implanted. There are then totally separate embryo sacs and placentas. Dizygotic twins are similar to diamniotic-dichorionic monozygotic twins.

SONOGRAPHIC APPLICATIONS IN MULTIPLE PREGNANCIES

There are special considerations in ultrasound examination of a twin pregnancy. The sonographer must determine, if possible, whether the developing embryos, or fetuses, reside in a single sac or are separated by a membrane. The appearance of a dichorionic-diamniotic monozygotic pregnancy will be identical to that of a dizygotic pregnancy. Both will involve two complete embryos, two complete sacs, and two separate placentas. Quite often, later in the pregnancy, the borders of the placentas will move close to each other and may finally fuse, making the determination of monochorionic or dichorionic pregnancy difficult if not impossible. If the fetuses are of opposite sexes, then a diagnosis of fraternal (or dizygotic) twins can be made. If, however, the twin fetuses are of the same sex, they could be either identical or fraternal, and only genetic analysis can determine the type prior to delivery. In a diamniotic pregnancy, whether placentas are or are not shared, a membrane should be seen separating the fetuses. The thickness of this membrane can indicate whether the pregnancy is mono- or dichorionic. The membrane separating diamniotic-monochorionic fetuses is two layers thick, consisting of two amnions only, one from each fetus. The membrane separating diamniotic-dichorionic fetuses is four layers thick, that is, two amnions plus two chorions.

THE EXPANDING ROLE OF SONOGRAPHY

This chapter presented an overview of several high risk conditions associated with pregnancy. All of them require extensive use of ultrasound examination or ultrasound guidance during invasive procedures. The role of the sonographer in the high risk obstetric laboratory is one of high responsibility, and a high degree of professionalism is required. The high risk obstetric laboratory is an exciting environment, but requires a thorough knowledge of normal and abnormal fetal anatomy. As new clinical management procedures evolve for handling high risk pregnancies, the role of ultrasound is sure to grow. Recently, fetal surgical procedures have been carried out with a high degree of success. These procedures require the use of ultrasound for, first, detecting the anomaly, and second, for locating an incision point within the uterus for extracting the fetus for surgery. The postsurgical period also requires ultrasound examination of the surgical site. The use of ultrasound in managing high risk pregnancies and in providing guidance during fetal surgery is sure to increase the demand for highly qualified sonographers.

REFERENCE CHART

Ultrasound-Guided Invasive Procedures

Amniocentesis to determine lung maturity
Genetic amniocentesis
Chorionic villus sampling
Umbilical blood collection and transfusion
Fetal surgery

References

1. Manning EA, Platt LD, Sipos, L: Antenatal fetal evaluation: development of a fetal biophysical profile. Am J Obstet Gynecol 136:787–795, 1980.
2. Phelan JP, Smith CV, Broussard P: Amniotic fluid volume assessment with the four-quadrant technique at 36–42 weeks gestation. J Reproduct Med 32:540–542, 1987.
3. Rochelson B, Schulman H, Farmakides G, et al: The significance of absent end-diastolic velocity in umbilical artery velocity waveforms. Am J Obstet Gynecol 156:1213–1218, 1987.
4. Meizner I, Katz M, Lunenfeld E, et al: Umbilical and uterine flow velocity waveforms in pregnancies complicated by major fetal anomalies. Prenatal Diag 7:491–496, 1987.
5. Huhta JC, Strasburger JF, Carpenter RJ, et al: Pulsed Doppler fetal echocardiography. J Clin Ultrasound 13:247–254, 1985.
6. Reed KI, Meijboom EJ, Sahn DJ, et al: Cardiac Doppler flow velocities in human fetuses. Circulation 73:41–46, 1986.
7. Gluck L, Kulovich MV: Lecithin sphingomeyelin ratios in amniotic fluid in normal and abnormal pregnancy. Am J Obstet Gynecol 115:539, 1973.
8. Tabor A, Phillip J, Madsen M, et al: Randomized controlled trial of genetic amniocentesis in 4,606 low-risk women. Lancet 1:1287–1292, 1986.
9. Creasman WT, Lawrence RA, Thiede HA: Fetal complications of amniocentesis. JAMA 204:91, 1968.
10. Crane JP, Beaver HA, Cheung SW: First trimester chorionic villus sampling versus mid-trimester genetic amniocentesis: preliminary results of a controlled prospective trial. Prenatal Diag 8:355–356, 1988.
11. Cooperberg PL, Carpenter CW: Ultrasound as an aid to intrauterine transfusion. Am J Obstet Gynecol 128:239–241, 1977.
12. Grannum PT, Copel JA, Plaxe SC, et al: In utero exchange transfusion by direct intravascular injection in severe erythroblastosis fetalis. N Engl J Med 314:1431–1434, 1986.

SECTION VI

SMALL PARTS SONOGRAPHY

Chapter 19

THYROID AND PARATHYROID GLANDS

WAYNE C. LEONHARDT

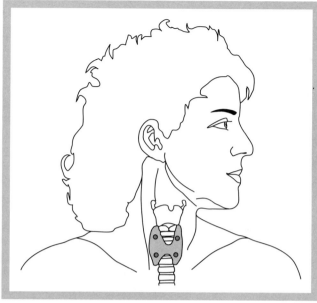

Thyroid and parathyroid glands. (From Guyton AC: Textbook of Medical Physiology, 8th ed. Philadelphia, 1991, p 810.)

Objectives:

Label thyroid, parathyroid gland anatomy, and relevant adjacent anatomic structures in schematic drawings.

Describe normal embryologic development of the thyroid and parathyroid glands.

Describe the sonographic appearance of the normal thyroid, parathyroid glands, and relevant adjacent anatomic structures in the neck on sectional sonograms.

Describe pertinent sonographic terminology of the thyroid, parathyroid glands, and relevant adjacent anatomic structures in the neck.

Describe the physiology of the thyroid and parathyroid glands.

Describe various shapes of normal parathyroid glands.

Describe ectopic locations of parathyroid glands.

Describe clinical laboratory tests, related diagnostic tests, normal laboratory values, and associated physicians in the work-up of thyroid and parathyroid glands.

Describe the sonographic indications with reference to the thyroid and parathyroid glands.

Describe key words associated with thyroid function and anatomy, parathyroid gland function and anatomy, and relevant adjacent anatomic structures in the neck.

Define the key words.

Key Words:

Aberrant parathyroid glands
Acoustic walls
Adrenal gland
Alkaline phosphatase
Anechoic
Attenuation
Basal metabolic rate (BMR)
Calcitonin
Carotid bulb
Carotid sheath
Chloride
"Cold nodule"
Colloid
Colloid follicle
Computed tomography (CT)
Cricoid cartilage
Echogenic
Ectopic parathyroid glands
Endocrine gland
Endocrinologist
Entodermal diverticulum
Foramen cecum
"Hot nodule"
Hypercalcemia
Hyperechoic
Hyperfunctioning nodule
Hyperparathyroidism
Hyperplasia
Hyperthyroidism
Hypocalcemia
Hypoechoic
Hypothalamus
Hypothyroidism
Inferior thyroid artery
Inferior thyroid vein
Infrahyoid muscle
Inhomogeneity
Internal jugular vein
Interventional radiologist
Isthmus
Longus colli muscle
Magnetic resonance imaging (MRI)
Major neurovascular bundle
Minor neurovascular bundle

Nuclear medicine technologist
Omohyoid muscle
Ovaries
Parathormone
Parathyroid adenoma
Parathyroid gland
Parathyroid hormone
Pathologist
Pharyngeal pouches
Phosphate excretion
Phosphorus
Pituitary gland
Primary hyperparathyroidism
Primordia
Protein
Pyramidal lobe
Radioactive iodine uptake (RAI)
Radioimmunoassay
Radiologic technologist
Radiologist
Recurrent laryngeal nerve
Scintigraphy
Serum calcium
Serum protein
Sonographer
Sonologist
Spatial resolution
Sternocleidomastoid muscle
Sternohyoid muscle
Sternothyroid muscle
Strap muscles
Superior thyroid artery
Superior thyroid vein
Surgeon
Sympathetic ganglia vasomotor
Technetium-99 pertechnetate
Technetium-99 sestamibi
Testes
Thallium-201
Thallous chloride
Thymus
Thyroglobulin
Thyroglossal cyst
Thyroglossal duct
Thyrohyoid
Thyroid gland
Thyroid plexus
Thyroid stimulating hormone (TSH)
Thyrotropin
Thyrotropin releasing factor
Thyroxine (T4)
Triiodothyronine
T3 resin uptake
Uric acid
Vasomotor

THYROID GLAND

INTRODUCTION

The thyroid gland is an endocrine gland (one of the ductless glands, which release their secretion into the blood) consisting of two lateral lobes and a connecting portion called the **isthmus.** (See Figure 19–1.) It secretes three significant hormones: thyroxine (T4), triiodothyronine (T3), and calcitonin, which affect body metabolism, growth, and development.

PRENATAL DEVELOPMENT

The thyroid gland arises from a median, sac-like **entodermal diverticulum** (the thyroid sac) which begins to thicken during the third week of embryologic development. It arises at the level of the first and second **pharyngeal pouches** (epithelial entodermal-lined cavities that give rise to a number of vital organs within the embryo) of the ventral wall of the pharynx.[1,2] The stalk between the thyroid and the tongue is called the **thyroglossal duct.** It opens in the embryo at the **foramen cecum,** located at the base of the tongue.[3] The thyroglossal duct atrophies by the sixth week of embryonic development, and by the eighth week thyroid follicles begin to form. They acquire **colloid** by the third month of development. The thyroglossal duct normally closes after birth. If it persists, cysts, fistulas, or an accessory pyramidal lobe may develop.[1,3]

Aberrant thyroid tissue may be found anywhere along the path of the thyroid gland. The descent begins at the level of the foramen cecum to the first tracheal ring. (See Figure 19–2.) The lingual type accounts for 90 percent of ectopic thyroids.

LOCATION

The **thyroid** is composed of right and left lobes connected by an isthmus. It is a superficial structure which lies below the larynx and anterior to the trachea. The isthmus unites the lower third of the lobes at the level of the second, third, and fourth tracheal rings. (See Figure 19–1.) The general shape of the thyroid gland is that of a U or a low-slung H. (See Figure 19–3.) In the latter, the cross bar represents the isthmus, and the vertical bars represent two conical lateral (right and left) lobes, blunted below and tapered above. In the traverse plane the thyroid gland has a horseshoe appearance. (See Figure 19–1.)

In cross-section, the thyroid is outlined laterally by the **common carotid artery (CCA)** and the **internal jugular vein (IJV)**; medially by the **trachea (T),** anterolaterally by the infrahyoid or strap muscles and sternocleidomastoid muscles.[4] Infrahyoid muscles are double-layered muscle planes located anterior to the neck, superficial to the larynx, trachea, and thyroid gland. They include the **sternohyoid (SH), sternothyroid (ST), omohyoid (OH),** and **thyrohyoid (TH).** The **longus colli muscle (LCM), esophagus (E),** and **minor neurovascular bundle (MNB),** consisting of the inferior thyroid artery and recurrent laryngeal nerve, mark the posterior border of the thyroid.[4,6] (See Figure 19–1.) The **major neurovascular bundle (MNB)** consists of the common carotid artery, internal jugular vein, and the vagus nerve. It is encased by the **carotid sheath,** which consists of areolar tissue.[5,6]

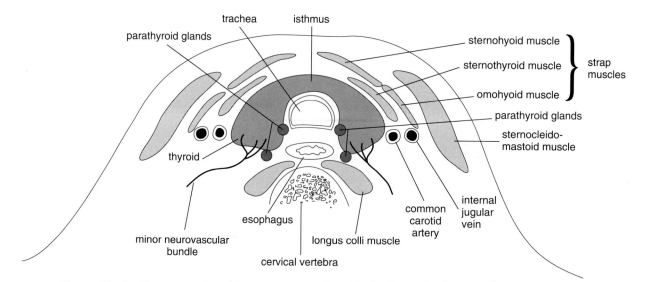

Figure 19–1. Transverse thyroid anatomy, parathyroid glands, and relevant adjacent structures. Shaded circles represent normal location of parathyroid glands.

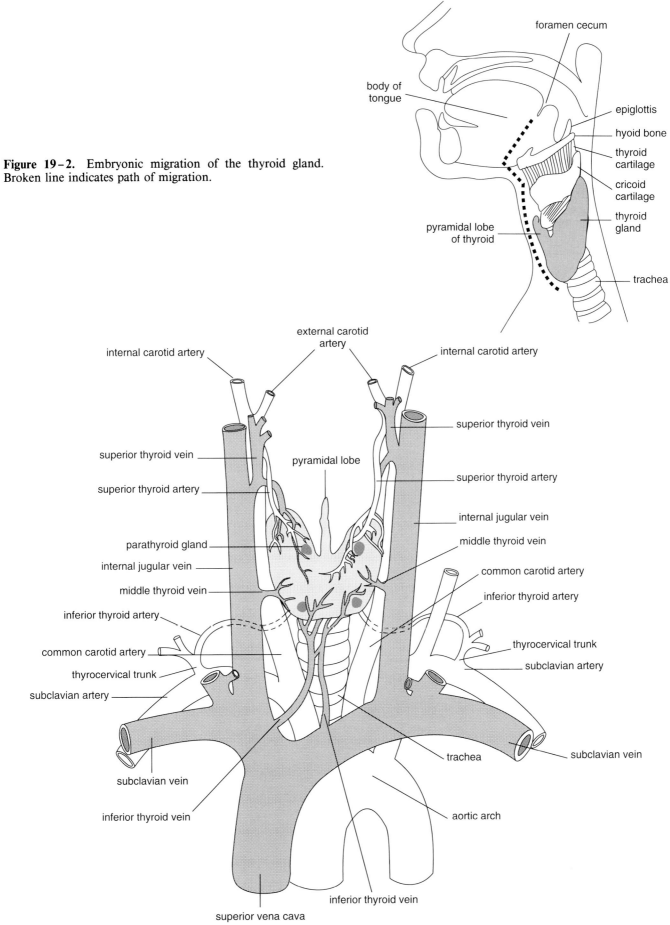

foramen cecum

body of tongue

epiglottis

hyoid bone

thyroid cartilage

cricoid cartilage

thyroid gland

pyramidal lobe of thyroid

trachea

Figure 19-2. Embryonic migration of the thyroid gland. Broken line indicates path of migration.

external carotid artery

internal carotid artery

internal carotid artery

superior thyroid vein

superior thyroid vein

pyramidal lobe

superior thyroid artery

superior thyroid artery

internal jugular vein

parathyroid gland

middle thyroid vein

internal jugular vein

common carotid artery

middle thyroid vein

inferior thyroid artery

inferior thyroid artery

thyrocervical trunk

common carotid artery

subclavian artery

thyrocervical trunk

subclavian artery

subclavian vein

subclavian vein

trachea

inferior thyroid vein

aortic arch

superior vena cava

inferior thyroid vein

Figure 19-3. Frontal view of the thyroid and parathyroid regions. Dark circles, normal parathyroid locations.

SIZE

The size and weight of the thyroid gland vary with sex and age. In general, the thyroid is larger in women than in men and increases in size with increasing age. The average weight of the thyroid is approximately 25 to 35 grams. The adult thyroid gland measures approximately 4 to 6 cm in length, 2.0 to 3.0 cm in anteroposterior diameter, and 1.5 to 2 cm in width. (See Figures 19-4 and 19-5.) The isthmus measures approximately 2 to 6 mm in anteroposterior diameter.[7] (See Figure 19-6.) In infants and children, the gland measures approximately 2 to 3 cm in length, 0.2 cm to 1.2 cm in anteroposterior diameter, and 2 to 3 cm in width.[8] (See Figures 19-4, 19-5, and 19-6.)

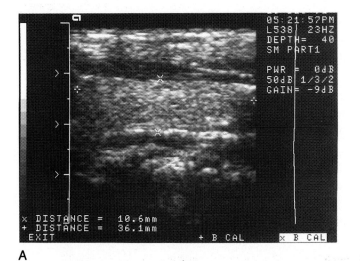

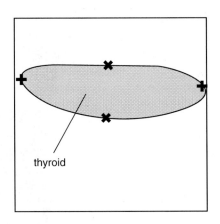

Figure 19-4. *A*, Longitudinal section of thyroid gland. *B*, Caliper placement measuring the length and AP (anterior/posterior) diameter. Note position of calipers (x, +).

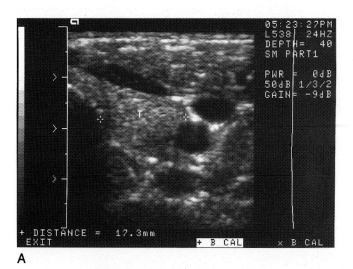

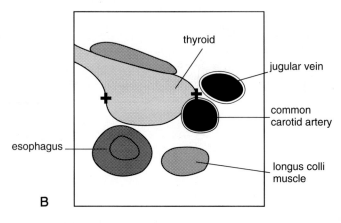

Figure 19-5. *A*, Transverse section. *B*, Measurement of left lobe of thyroid gland. Note placement of calipers.

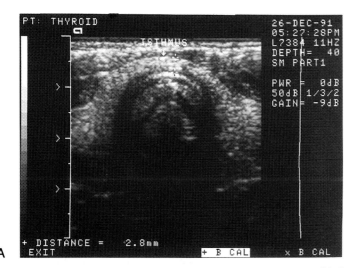

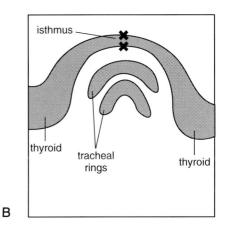

Figure 19-6. *A*, AP measurement of isthmus. *B*, Transverse section.

GROSS ANATOMY

The thyroid gland is composed of right and left lobes connected by an isthmus. It is covered by two thin layers of connective tissue. The first layer is the pretracheal fascia, or false thyroid capsule, which surrounds the gland. The second layer is the true thyroid capsule, adherent to the gland surface. Thyroid parenchyma is composed of follicles (glandular epithelium and colloid), connective tissue, stroma, blood vessels, nerves, and lymphatics.[13,14]

PHYSIOLOGY

The thyroid plays a major role in growth and development, and regulates basal metabolism by the synthesis, storage, and secretion of thyroid hormones.[9] As mentioned, it produces and secretes three hormones: **triiodothyronine (T3)**, **thyroxine (T4)**, and **calcitonin**. The secretion of these hormones is regulated by the **hypothalamus** and the **pituitary gland**. Thyroid secretion is primarily controlled by **thyroid stimulating hormone (TSH)** secreted by the anterior pituitary gland.[9-11] Thyroxine is the primary hormone (90 percent) secreted by the thyroid. Triiodothyronine represents a small portion (approximately 10 percent).[12]

Calcitonin is secreted by the **parafollicular cells (C cells)** of the normal thyroid. Its primary function is to decrease blood calcium levels, preventing hypercalcemia. This hormone works the opposite of parathormone, discussed later in this chapter. Plasma calcitonin concentration level is elevated in a number of conditions; more importantly, it is elevated in the majority of patients with medullary thyroid carcinoma.[11] The thyroid is composed of follicles filled with **colloid**, which is secreted by cuboidal epithelioid cells lining the periphery of the follicle. Colloid consists mainly of a glycoprotein, thyroglobulin, which contains thyroid hormones within its molecule. When thyroid hormone is needed, thyroid stimulating hormone (TSH), or **thyrotropin**, secreted by the anterior pituitary gland, triggers the release of hormones into the bloodstream.[12] The secretion of TSH is regulated by the thyrotropin-releasing factor, produced by the hypothalamus. The level of thyrotropin-releasing factor is controlled by the **basal metabolic rate (BMR)**. A decrease in BMR results from a low concentration of thyroid hormones, causing an increase in **thyrotropin-releasing factor**. This causes an increase in TSH secretion and an increase in the release of these hormones. Once the blood level of hormones is returned to normal, the BMR stabilizes and TSH secretion ceases.[9,11]

BLOOD SUPPLY

The thyroid is a highly vascular gland. Its blood supply consists of paired superior and inferior thyroid arteries and veins, and often middle thyroid veins. The **superior thyroid artery** is the first branch of the external carotid artery. It runs downward and forward to the apex of the lateral lobe. The **inferior thyroid artery** is the largest branch of the thyrocervical trunk of the subclavian artery. It ascends to the inferior pole of the gland. Superior thyroid veins accompany the superior thyroid arteries. **Superior thyroid veins** arise above the anterolateral surface of the gland, cross the common carotid artery, and empty into the internal jugular veins above the thyroid cartilage. Inferior thyroid veins arise in the venous plexus of the thyroid gland, communicate with the superior and middle thyroid veins, and empty into the left and right innominate veins. The **middle thyroid veins** arise from the venous plexus on the lateral surface of the gland, and empty into the lower end of the jugular vein.[5] (See Figure 19-3.)

SONOGRAPHIC APPEARANCE

The normal thyroid gland is uniformly echogenic, with medium level echoes similar to those of the liver and testes.[15,16] (See Figure 19–4.) Branches of the inferior and superior thyroid arteries and veins appear as 1- to 2-mm **anechoic** tubular structures. (See Figure 19–7.) Color Doppler sonography is helpful in identifying intra- and extrathyroidal arteries and veins. On transverse images, the common carotid artery and internal jugular vein are seen as circular anechoic areas adjacent to the lateral border of the thyroid gland. The neck muscles (infrahyoid, sternocleidomastoid, and longus colli) are **hypoechoic** relative to the thyroid gland. (See Figure 19–8.) In transverse section the longus colli muscle is triangular. The esophagus in transverse section is visualized slightly to the left of midline, adjacent to the trachea, and appears hypoechoic with an echogenic center representing mucosa. (See Figure 19–9.) Within the sagittal plane of imaging the infrahyoid and sternocleidomastoid muscles are anterior to the thyroid and the longus colli muscle is posterior.[4,9] (See Figure 19–10.)

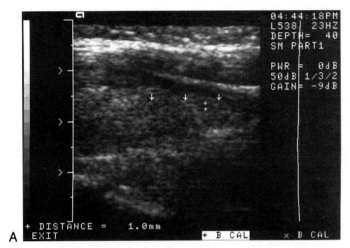

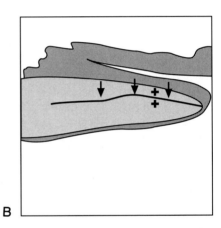

Figure 19–7. *A*, Longitudinal section of thyroid gland; 1- to 2-mm tubular structure (*arrows*) represents intrathyroidal artery or vein. *B*, Calipers measuring linear tubular structure.

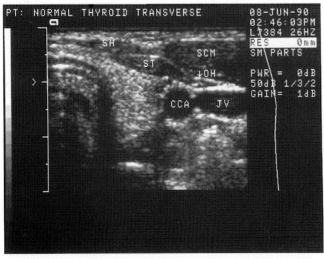

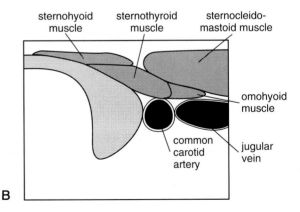

Figure 19–8. *A* and *B*, Transverse section of thyroid gland and relevant adjacent anatomic structures.

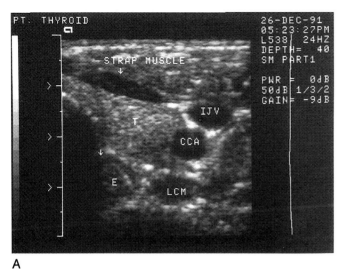
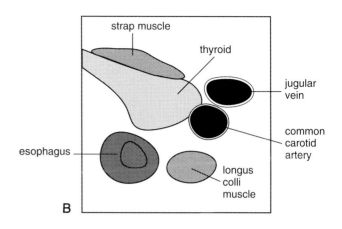

Figure 19-9. *A*, Transverse section of left lobe of thyroid gland. *B*, Note anatomic relationship and shape of esophagus; longus colli muscle.

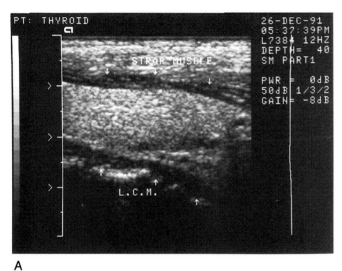
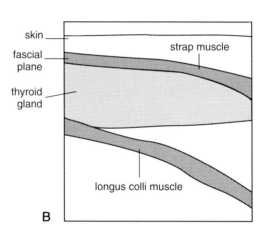

Figure 19-10. *A*, Longitudinal section of strap muscle and longus colli muscle. *B*, Note relationship to thyroid gland.

SONOGRAPHIC APPLICATIONS

"Cold nodule" nonfunctioning nodule on scintigraphy
Ultrasound guidance (fine needle aspiration)
Determining the nature of a neck mass (size, shape, location, and echogenicity)
Detecting an occult carcinoma
Detecting recurrent carcinoma after thyroidectomy
Screening patients with histories of head and neck irradiation
Monitoring the size of nodules under treatment (thyroid suppression therapy)
Determining the size of a nodule
Delineating a thyroid nodule during pregnancy

NORMAL VARIANTS

An accessory lobe called the **pyramidal lobe** is present in approximately 15 to 30 percent of the population. It extends cephalad from the isthmus and ascends as far as the hyoid bone. A pyramidal lobe may extend from the right or left side of the isthmus; however, it arises more frequently on the left.[9] (See Figure 19-3.) Other variations include absence of the isthmus, asymmetry (right lobe may be twice the size of the left lobe), or absence of lateral lobes. Complete absence of the gland or failure of the gland to function is seldom noticed until a few weeks after birth, because the fetus is supplied, through the placenta, with sufficient maternal thyroid hormone to permit normal development.[1]

REFERENCE CHARTS

Associated Physicians

Surgeon: Specializes in surgery, a branch of medicine which treats diseases, deformities, and injuries by operative methods.

Endocrinologist: Specializes in medical diseases of the endocrine system. Principal endocrine glands include the thyroid, parathyroid, adrenal, pituitary, testes, and ovaries.

Radiologist: Specializes in the diagnostic interpretation of imaging modalities that assess thyroid and parathyroid abnormalities.

Interventional Radiologist: Specializes in invasive radiographic procedures for diagnosis and treatment.

Pathologist: Specializes in the interpretation of tissue biopsies and blood tests.

Common Diagnostic Tests

Evaluation of the thyroid gland requires both physiologic and morphologic information in the treatment of thyroid disease. Various diagnostic tests available to achieve diagnostic efficacy include scintigraphy (radionuclide scanning), high resolution sonography, computed tomography (CT), magnetic resonance imaging (MRI), and aspiration biopsy.

Scintigraphy: Scintigraphy is the most common screening technique used in conjunction with ultrasound for the evaluation of thyroid function and morphology.[17] A radioactive tracer (iodine or technetium 99) is administered that targets the thyroid gland. It is monitored and photographed to assess thyroid function and differentiate between normal and abnormal thyroid tissue. This test is performed by a **nuclear medicine technologist**. Interpretation of the test is by the **radiologist**. The **spatial resolution** of this technique makes it difficult to delineate and characterize small nodules.[4] Multiple nodules may be present within the gland when scintigraphy indicates only a solitary nodule.[17] Nonfunctioning nodules are designated "**cold**," and may represent a number of benign conditions.[16] The probability of a cold nodule being malignant in a multinodular gland is approximately 1 to 6 percent.[15] **Hyperfunctioning nodules** are designated "**hot.**"[16]

Ultrasound: Ultrasound uses high frequency sound waves to image and characterize thyroid parenchyma and adjacent anatomic structures. Cross-sectional and sagittal images are obtained of the thyroid gland and relevant anatomy to differentiate normal from abnormal echo patterns. Ultrasound is the most definitive imaging technique for determining whether a lesion is cystic or solid and whether it is intrathyroid or extrathyroidal. It is excellent for localizing nodules for aspiration biopsy. In selected cases ultrasound biopsy can eliminate the need for surgery.[18] Penetration is limited when evaluating the retrotrachea and substernal regions because **acoustic wall**s or air-containing structures such as the trachea and the lung preclude through sound transmission. This test is performed by a **sonographer** and **sonologist**. Interpretation of the test is by the sonologist.

Computed Axial Tomography (CT Scan): CT images the thyroid gland and adjacent anatomy in cross-section. A contrast material is usually administered to differentiate between pathology and normal anatomy. CT is less specific than sonography for establishing the cystic nature of nodules. However, it overcomes sound penetration limitations and provides anatomic definition in the substernal and retrotracheal regions. CT, like magnetic resonance imaging (MRI), is useful in assessing the overall extent of a mass. Less desirable features of CT imaging include streak artifacts from the shoulder girdle, use of intravenous iodinated contrast material, and exposure to ionizing radiation. This test is performed by a radiologic technologist. Interpretation of the test is by the radiologist.

Magnetic Resonance Imaging (MRI): MRI involves magnetism and radio waves. It provides multiplane imaging and may provide a contrast scale between normal and pathologic thyroid anatomy and adjacent anatomic structures. This technique permits excellent delineation of anatomic structures in the neck and thorax. For example, blood vessels are easily identified from adjacent lymph nodes. MRI is an excellent imaging modality for monitoring disease processes pre- and post-therapy.[18] This test is performed by a radiologic technologist. Interpretation of the test is by the radiologist. CT and MRI are particularly useful when thyroid tissue extends into the mediastinum and cervical region.[17]

Fine Needle Aspiration: Fine needle aspiration may provide the definitive diagnosis of thyroid nodules. With sonographic guidance, lesions a few millimeters in size can be biopsied. Such biopsies are easy to perform and well tolerated by the patient. With an experienced pathologist, a diagnostic sensitivity of 96 percent can be achieved.[18] Complications are unusual, a small hematoma being the most common. This procedure is performed by a radiologist, an endocrinologist, or a surgeon. Interpretation of the test is done by a pathologist.

Laboratory Tests

Thyroid hormone production is modulated by a feedback control mechanism effected through the hypothalamus and the pituitary gland. Thyrotropin (TSH), secreted by the anterior pituitary, controls thyroid hormone production.[11] Several laboratory tests are done to evaluate thyroid function. No one clinical test can be used alone to diagnose hypo- or hyperthyroidism. Common tests include T4, T3, TSH (thyroid stimulating hormone), T3 resin uptake, and RAI (radioactive iodine uptake).[19] The following laboratory tests are performed by a licensed laboratory technologist. Interpretation of the tests is done by the pathologist.

Thyroxine: Thyroxine (T4), with four iodine atoms, is the most abundant thyroid hormone produced. T4 is commonly used for screening and follow-up of patients whose diagnosis is either hypo- or hyperthyroidism. The test measures both free thyroxine and the portion carried by the thyroid binding plasma protein. T3 (triiodothyronine) contains three iodine atoms and represents a small portion of thyroid hormone, but it is more potent than T4. Both T3 and T4 can also be measured indirectly by **radioimmunoassay**. This is a very sensitive method of determining the concentration of hormones in blood plasma. A venous blood sample is drawn and "tagged" with specific radioactive substances that specifically bind with either T3 or T4.[19,20] The amount of radioactivity measured indirectly indicates the concentration of thyroid hormone indirectly. Increased levels of T3 and T4 are associated with hyperthyroidism, while decreased levels indicate **hypothyroidism**.[19,20]

T3 Resin Uptake: The T3 resin uptake test measures the amount of T4 indirectly by measuring the amount of T3 that can be attached to the proteins that bind the thyroid hormones. The resin uptake test measures the amount of T3 remaining and free to bind to the resin added to the blood sample. A measured amount of radioactive tagged T3 and resin is added to a sample of the patient's blood. The resin is placed in a test tube to absorb any of the radioactive-tagged T3 that cannot be taken up by the thyroid binding globulin in the blood sample. Increased T3 into the resin indicates hyperthyroidism; decreased T3 into the resin indicates hypothyroidism.

Thyroid Stimulating Hormone: TSH (thyroid stimulating hormone) or thyrotropin, produced by the pituitary gland, controls the serum levels of the thyroid hormones.[19] Measurement of TSH is useful in determining whether hypothyroidism is due to primary hypofunction of the thyroid gland (intrinsic thyroid disease) or to secondary hypofunction of the anterior pituitary gland, caused by insufficient stimulation by the pituitary.[19,20]

TSH also measures a patient's response to thyroid medication, particularly one with primary hypothyroidism, and pituitary hypothyroidism.[16]

Radioactive Iodine Test: The radioactive iodine (RAI) uptake test evaluates thyroid function by measuring the amount of orally ingested 123I or 131I that accumulates in the thyroid gland after 6 and 24 hours. The largest portion of iodine is transported via the circulatory system to the thyroid gland. An external counting probe (gamma detector) measures the radioactivity in the thyroid as a percentage of the original dose, indicating the ability of the gland to trap and retain iodine. The normal range is about 10 to 15 percent at 6 hours and 15 to 30 percent at 24 hours[19,20] This test is performed by a nuclear medicine technologist. Interpretation of the test is done by the radiologist.

Laboratory Values

Resin T3 Uptake (RT$_3$ U) (Specimen S): 25–35 percent.
Thyroid–Stimulating Hormone (Specimen S): 5–10 u U/ml.
Thyroxine (T4) (Specimen S): 4.5–13$_{ug}$/dl.
Triiodothyronine: 75–195 ug/dl (pregnancy and oral contraceptives tend to increase values).

Normal Measurements

Adult Thyroid Gland: 4–6 cm in length, 2–3 cm in anteroposterior diameter, 1–2 cm in width.
Isthmus: 0.2–0.6 cm in anteroposterior diameter.
Infants and Young Children: 2–3 cm in length, 0.2–1.2 cm in anteroposterior diameter, 1–1.5 cm in width.

Vasculature

Superior Supply: External carotid artery—superior thyroid artery—superior thyroid veins—internal jugular veins.
Inferior Supply: Thyrocervical artery—inferior thyroid artery—inferior thyroid veins—middle thyroid veins—right and left innominate veins.

Affecting Chemicals

Thyroid Stimulating Hormone (TSH): Stimulates the thyroid to make and release thyroid hormones.

PARATHYROID GLANDS

INTRODUCTION

Parathyroid glands are small encapsulated oval bodies attached to the posterior surfaces of the lateral lobes of the thyroid gland. Most people have four symmetric parathyroid glands. (See Figures 19–1 and 19–3.) Parathyroid glands secrete parathyroid hormone. Their primary function is to maintain homeostasis of blood calcium levels by promoting calcium absorption, thereby preventing hypocalcemia.

PRENATAL DEVELOPMENT

The parathyroid glands develop from the third and fourth pharyngeal pouches, epithelial entodermal-lined cavities that give rise to a number of vital organs. Parathyroid-3 tissue descends and rests on the dorsal surface of the thyroid gland and forms the inferior parathyroid gland. It originates from the third pouch in conjunction with the thymic **primordium** in the fifth embryonic week. These **primordia** lose their connection with the pharyngeal wall and migrate together caudally to lie in a lower position in the neck. Parathyroid-4 loses its contact with the wall of the pharynx and attaches to the caudally migrating thyroid. It eventually rests on the dorsal surface of the upper thyroid gland and forms the superior parathyroid gland.[3] (See Figure 19–11.)

The **thymus** descends to the thorax and lies behind the sternum and anterior to the pericardium and great vessels.

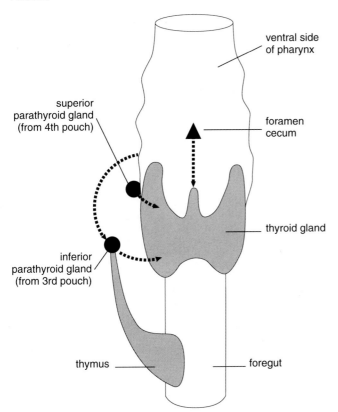

Figure 19–11. Migration of the thymus and parathyroid glands.

LOCATION

The **parathyroid glands** are typically located posterior to the thyroid gland. Superior parathyroid glands are situated more posteriorly and medially than inferior parathyroid glands. They normally lie at the level of the lower border of the **cricoid cartilage**.[18,21] Inferior parathyroid glands are situated more anteriorly than superior parathyroid glands. They are found on the posterior lateral surface of the thyroid gland, anterior and medial to the **recurrent laryngeal nerve** and **inferior thyroid artery**. Inferior parathyroid glands may also be imbedded within the thyroid tissue.[18] Earlier, this chapter outlined the normal anatomic relationship among the thyroid, common carotid artery, internal jugular vein, longus colli muscle, esophagus, and strap muscles. (See Figure 19–1.) In the transverse plane, key anatomic structures used to localize parathyroid adenomas are the longus colli muscle, thyroid lobe, common carotid artery, and the internal jugular vein. The area between this anatomic triangle should be free of any masses. The minor neurovascular bundle is the only anatomic structure which lies in this region and measures 5 mm in diameter. When a mass measures greater than 5 mm in diameter it is suspected to be a parathyroid adenoma.[6,21]

SIZE

Normal parathyroid glands measure approximately 5 to 7 mm in length, 3 to 4 mm in width, and 1 to 2 mm in thickness ($5 \times 3 \times 1$ mm). They weigh less than 65 mg excluding surrounding fat.[5,18]

GROSS ANATOMY

Parathyroid glands are composed of masses of chief cells, with some wasserhelle (water-clear) and oxyphil cells arranged in a columnar fashion.[21] The color of parathyroid glands varies from light yellow in older patients to a reddish or light brown in young patients.[18]

The shape of parathyroid glands varies, they are generally oval, bean shaped, or spherical (83 percent), or sometimes elongated (11 percent), bilobated (5 percent), or multilobated (1 percent). (See Figure 19–12.) Abnor-

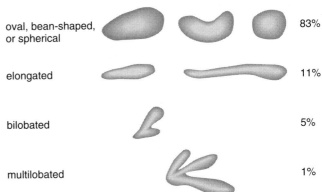

Figure 19–12. Parathyroid gland variations.

mal parathyroid glands range in size from 5 mm (small) to 45 × 32 × 18 mm (giant).[18,23]

PHYSIOLOGY

Parathyroid glands secrete **parathyroid hormone**, also called **PTH** or **parathormone**. Their primary function is to help maintain homeostasis of blood calcium concentration by promoting calcium absorption into the blood, preventing **hypocalcemia**. When serum calcium levels are low, the parathyroid hormone raises serum calcium by releasing calcium from the bone, increasing calcium absorption in the gut, and decreasing renal calcium by decreasing renal **phosphate excretion**.[18,21,22]

BLOOD SUPPLY

The superior and inferior parathyroid glands are supplied by separate small branches of the superior and inferior thyroid arteries and by branches from the longitudinal anastomoses between these vessels. (See Figure 19–3.) Venous drainage is into the **thyroid plexus** of the veins. The lymphatic channels drain with those of the thyroid gland. The nerve supply is abundant; it arises from the thyroid branches of the cervical **sympathetic ganglia** and is **vasomotor** in function.[5]

SONOGRAPHIC APPEARANCE

Normal parathyroid glands are usually not seen by ultrasound, but occasionally a single gland may be identified as a flat hypoechoic structure posterior to the thyroid gland and anterior to the longus colli muscle.[24] The typical sonographic appearance of a parathyroid adenoma is an oval or bean-shaped hypoechoic to anechoic structure without through transmission. It is virtually never more echogenic than the thyroid gland. With enlargement, changes may include lobulation, acoustic inhomogeneity, cystic degeneration, and occasional calcification.[23] Recent studies using color Doppler have relied on vascularity to differentiate thyroid lesions from parathyroid adenomas. Thyroid lesions tend to have some vacularity when only 5 mm in size. Parathyroid adenomas are avascular until they reach a size of 1 cm.[25] Earlier in this chapter the normal sonographic appearance of the thyroid and relevant adjacent anatomic structures was discussed.

It is of paramount importance to have a thorough understanding of the normal sonographic appearance of relevant anatomic structures in the neck, to avoid pitfalls in imaging. Longitudinally, the longus colli muscle runs the length of the thyroid gland and is relatively hypoechoic compared to the thyroid. (See Figure 19–10.) In the transverse plane the longus colli muscle appears to be triangular. (See Figure 19–9.) Parathyroid adenomas commonly lie along the longus colli muscle posterior to the thyroid gland and sometimes are mistaken for the longus colli muscle, particularly when the glands are elongated. In the transverse plane, the internal jugular vein appears sonographically as a circular anechoic structure lateral to the common carotid artery. An anechoic parathyroid adenoma located medial to a collapsed jugular vein may be mistaken for a normal internal jugular vein. Transversely and slightly to the left of midline, the sonographic appearance of the esophagus is a circular hypoechoic structure with an echogenic center. It is located between the inferior lobe of the thyroid and the longus colli muscle and may be mistaken for a large parathyroid adenoma. (See Figure 19–9.)

SONOGRAPHIC APPLICATIONS

Patients newly diagnosed with hyperparathyroidism
Patients with hypercalcemia
Ultrasound guidance (fine needle aspiration)
Patients undergoing repeat neck exploration

NORMAL VARIANTS

Most people (about 80 to 85 percent) have four parathyroid glands located in a symmetric position.[18,21] Thirteen to 15 percent have more than five parathyroid glands, and 5 percent have only three glands. Eight to 85 percent of parathyroid glands are contiguous with the thyroid gland.[18] (See Figures 19–2 and 19–3.)

Ectopic Glands

Ectopic parathyroids account for approximately 15 to 20 percent of the total. About 10 to 15 percent are found within the thymus or perithymic tissues. Other aberrant locations include the carotid bulb and sheath (1 percent), the retroesophageal space (1 to 3 percent), and intrathyroidal (1 percent).[18] (See Figure 19–13.)

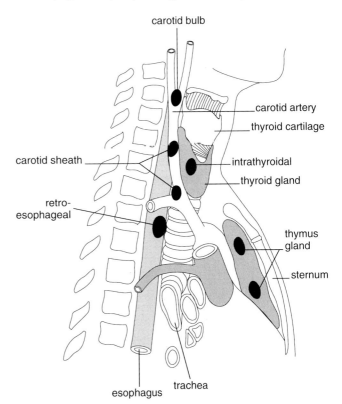

Figure 19–13. Lateral section of mediastinum and neck illustrating aberrant locations of parathyroid glands. Dark circles indicate aberrant locations: thymus gland, carotid bulb, retroesophageal, intrathyroidal, carotid sheath.

Associated Physicians

Surgeon: Specializes in surgery, a branch of medicine which treats diseases, deformities, and injuries by operative methods.

Endocrinologist: Specializes in medical diseases of the endocrine system. Principal endocrine glands include the thyroid, parathyroid, adrenal, pituitary, testes, and ovaries.

Radiologist: Specializes in the diagnostic interpretation of imaging modalities that assess thyroid and parathyroid abnormalities.

Interventional Radiologist: Specializes in invasive radiographic procedures for diagnosis and treatment.

Pathologist: Specializes in the interpretation of tissue biopsies and blood tests.

Common Diagnostic Tests

Several diagnostic tests are used to localize and evaluate parathyroid glands. These include high-resolution sonography (7.5 to 10.0 MHz), radionuclide imaging (scintigraphy using **thallium-201**, **thallous chloride**, and more recently, technetium 99-sestamibi), computerized tomography (CT), magnetic resonance imaging (MRI), and selective venous sampling.

Each of these techniques alone has a sensitivity of between 60 and 80 percent, and a specificity of between 90 and 95 percent in revealing abnormal parathyroid glands.[26] The combined use of ultrasound with either computed tomography, magnetic resonance, or radionuclide scanning raises the sensitivity to approximately 88 percent.[17]

Ultrasound: Ultrasound is the imaging modality recommended for the initial evaluation of patients with primary hyperparathyroidism who have not had surgery, and after elevated calcium levels and parathormone levels have been identified. High-resolution sonography (7.5 to 10.0 MHz) is performed in both longitudinal and transverse planes beginning at the sternal notch and progressing to the angle of the mandible in a search for abnormalities. Ultrasound is not a screening modality for parathyroid glands; there must be a clear indication for doing the examination, as **hypercalcemia**. This test is performed by a sonographer and sonologist. Interpretation of the test is done by the sonologist. Should ultrasound fail to identify abnormal parathyroid glands preoperatively or postoperatively, the combined use of either radionuclide scanning, computed tomography, or magnetic resonance is recommended to identify those glands in ectopic locations. The sensitivity of the other imaging techniques is superior to that of sonography in locating ectopic glands in the retroesophageal and substernal regions.[17] Ultrasound is a sensitive technique in verifying whether or not tissue consistent with a parathyroid gland exists in a particular aberrant location such as the carotid bulb or sheath.[26] Parathyroid aspiration biopsy under ultrasound guidance is often helpful in postoperative localization of parathyroid adenomas with a reported sensitivity of 91 percent.[18,27]

Scintigraphy: With scintigraphy, 20 mCi of Tc-99m MIBI (**Technetium sestamibi**) is administered intravenously and taken up by the patient's thyroid and parathyroid glands. Early (10-minute) and delayed (2-hour) images are compared. Technetium sestamibi "washes out" of the thyroid gland quickly, and focal uptake persists in abnormal parathyroid glands. The sensitivity of this technique ranges from 88 to 100 percent.[28] This test is performed by a nuclear medicine technologist. Interpretation of the test is by the radiologist.

Computed Axial Tomography (CT Scan): CT imaging of parathyroid glands occurs in the following sequence: contrast material is injected that helps distinguish the vasculature from other structures such as lymph nodes. Axial scans are performed from the base of the skull to the sternal notch at 5-mm increments. Abnormal parathyroid glands will be enlarged. This test is performed by a radiologic technologist. Interpretation of the test is by the radiologist.

Magnetic Resonance Imaging (MRI): MRI uses an anterior surface coil with increased detail to image parathyroid glands. Axial and sagittal views are taken from the base of the skull to the sternal notch at slice thicknesses of 4 to 5 mm. Abnormal parathyroid glands tend to have a high intensity signal in contrast to surrounding tissue. This test is performed by a radiologic technologist. Interpretation of the test is done by the radiologist. If the patient has had previous parathyroid surgeries which have failed to identify abnormal glands, or has had recurrent hyperparathyroidism with negative noninvasive test results, digital angiography followed by selective venous sampling is helpful. Selective venous sampling tends to lateralize the site of abnormal parathyroid glands by providing access to the venous system (primarily the superior, inferior, and middle thyroid veins) so that parathyroid hormone assays can be obtained to determine abnormal calcium levels. Because parathyroid adenomas may arise anywhere in the cervical and mediastinal regions, sampling may be necessary from the internal jugular veins inferiorly to the level of the renal veins. This test is performed by an interventional radiologist. Interpretation of the test is by the radiologist and a pathologist.

Serum Calcium: An elevated serum calcium level, or hypercalcemia, is usually a clue to hyperparathyroidism. Hypercalcemia can be life-threatening when serum calcium levels reach 14.5 mg/dl or higher. Most cases of primary hyperparathyroidism are diagnosed by documenting a simultaneous increase in blood levels of both bone calcium and parathyroid hormone (PTH). Other general laboratory tests used in the differential diagnosis of the hypercalcemic patient include phosphorus, alkaline phosphatase, uric acid, chloride, serum protein, urinalysis, and 24-hour calcium.[18] General laboratory tests are performed by a licensed laboratory technologist. Interpretation of the test is by a pathologist.

Urinary Calcium: Approximately 75 percent of patients with primary hyperparathyroidism have elevated urinary calcium levels. A low serum phosphorous level is seen in about 50 percent of patients. An increased serum phosphorous level in the absence of renal failure or excessive intake of phosphorus suggests a nonparathyroid cause of hypercalcemia. Alka-line phosphatase levels are elevated in about 10 percent of patients with primary hyperparathyroidism. Serum chloride levels are increased in about 40 percent of patients. Serum protein and serum uric acid levels are also increased in many patients.[18]

Laboratory Values

Alkaline Phosphorus (Specimen S): 1.5–4.5 Bodansky units/dl; 0.8–2.9 BLB units.

Calcium (Specimen S): Adult 8.4–10.2 mg/dl; child 8.8–10.7 mg/dl.

Chloride (CL): 98–106 mmol/L (specimen S); 110–250 mmol/L (CSF).

Phosphorus (Specimen S): 2.7–4.5 mg/dl.

Protein (Total): 6.5–8.3 g/dl (Specimen S); 0.5 percent of plasma (CSF).

Uric Acid (Specimen S): Male 3.5–7.2 mg/dl; female 2.6–6.0 mg/dl.

Normal Measurements

Adult Parathyroid Gland: 5–7 mm in length, 3–4 mm in width, 1–2 mm in thickness.

Vasculature

Superior Supply: External carotid artery—superior thyroid artery—superior thyroid veins—internal jugular veins.

Inferior Supply: Thyrocervical artery—inferior thyroid artery—inferior thyroid veins—middle thyroid veins—right innominate veins.

Affecting Chemicals

Parathormone (PTH): A hormone that affects parathyroid function and homeostasis.

References

1. Netter FH: The Thyroid and Parathyroid Glands. In Ciba Collection of Medical Illustrations. Endocrine system and selected metabolic diseases. vol. 4. Edison, NJ, Ciba Pharmaceutical, 1965, pp 41–73.
2. Willinsky RA, Kassel PW, Cooper HB, et al: Computed tomography of lingual thyroid. J Comput Assist Tomogr 11(1): 182–183, 1987.
3. Langman J: Special embryology, head and neck. In Medical Embryology, 4th ed. Baltimore, Williams & Wilkins, 1981, pp 268–297.
4. Butch J, Simeone JF, Mueller PR: Thyroid and parathyroid ultrasonography. Radiol Clin North Am 23: 57–71, 1985.
5. Woodburne RT: The head and neck. In Essentials of Human Anatomy, 3rd ed. New York, Oxford University Press, 1965, pp 77–89.
6. Cole-Beuglet C: Ultrasonography of thyroid, parathyroid, and neck masses. In Sarti DA, ed., Diagnostic Ultrasound, 2nd ed. Chicago, Yearbook, 1987, pp 608–655.
7. Odwin CS, Dubinsky T, Fleischer AC: Ultrasonography examination review and study guide. Los Altos, Appleton & Lange, 1987, p 144.
8. Siegel ML: Neck. In Siegel, ML, ed., Pediatric Sonography. New York, Raven Press, 1991, pp 63–87.
9. Schorzman L: High-resolution ultrasonography of superficial structures. In Ansert-Hagen SL, ed., Textbook of Diagnostic Ultrasonography, 3rd ed. St. Louis, CV Mosby, 1989, pp 320–326.
10. Barton T: The thyroid gland: a review for sonographers. Med Ultrasound 4:127–134, 1980.
11. Gavin AG: Thyroid physiology and testing of thyroid function. In Clark OH, ed., Endocrine Surgery of the Thyroid and Parathyroid Glands. St. Louis, CV Mosby, 1985, pp 1–34.
12. Guyton AC: The thyroid metabolic hormones. Textbook of Medical Physiology, 7th ed., Philadelphia, WB Saunders, 1986, pp 897–906.
13. Gary H: Parathyroid and thyroid glands. In Clemente CD, (ed). Gray's Anatomy of the Human Body, 30th ed. Philadelphia, Lea & Febiger, 1984, pp 1596–1615.
14. Healy JE, Seybold WD: The neck. A Synopsis of Clinical Anatomy. Philadelphia, WB Saunders, 1969, pp 10–39.
15. Cole-Beuglet, C. New high-resolution ultrasound evaluation of diseases of the thyroid gland. JAMA 249: 2941–2944, 1983.
16. Leisner B: Ultrasound evaluation of thyroid diseases. Horm Res 26: 33–41, 1987.
17. Higgins CB, Auffermann W: MR imaging of thyroid and parathyroid glands: a review of current status. Am J Radiol 151: 1095–1106, 1988.
18. Clark OH: In Clark OH, ed., Endocrine Surgery of the Thyroid and Parathyroid Glands. St. Louis, CV Mosby, 1985, pp 56–90.
19. Corbett, JV: Laboratory Tests and Diagnostic Procedures with Nursing Diagnoses, 2nd ed. Los Altos, Appleton & Lange, 1987, pp 347–391.
20. Anderhub B: Superficial Parts: Manual of Abdominal Sonography. Baltimore, University Park Press, 1984, pp 188–204.
21. Anderson K: High-resolution water-path scanning of the parathyroid glands. Med Ultrasound 6: 11–17, 1982.
22. Anthony CP. The endocrine system. In Anthony CP, ed., Textbook of Anatomy and Physiology, 10th ed. St. Louis, CV Mosby, 1979, pp 318–347.
23. Randel SB, Gooding AW, Clark OH, et al: Parathyroid variants: US evaluation. Radiology 165: 191–194, 1987.
24. Simeone JF, Mueller PR, Ferrucci JT, et al: High-resolution real-time sonography of the parathyroid. Radiology 141: 745–751, 1981.
25. Gooding GAW, Clark OH: Use of Color Doppler Imaging in the distinction between thyroid and parathyroid lesions. Am J Surg 164:51, 1992.
26. Gooding GAW, Clark OH, Stark DD, et al: Parathyroid aspiration biopsy under US guidance in the post-operative patient. Radiology 155: 193–196, 1985.
27. Gooding GAW, Okerlund MD, Stark DD, Clark OH: Parathyroid imaging: comparison of double-tracer (T1-210, TC-99m) scintigraphy and high-resolution US. Radiology 161: 57–64, 1986.
28. Oates E: Improved parathyroid scintigraphy with TC-99m MIBI, a superior radiotracer. Applied Radiol March 37–40, 1994.

Chapter 20

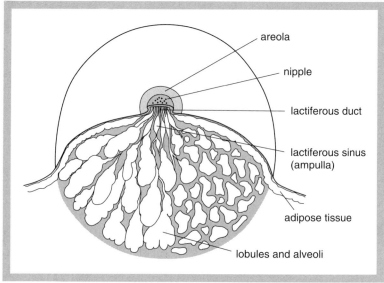

areola

nipple

lactiferous duct

lactiferous sinus
(ampulla)

adipose tissue

lobules and alveoli

BREAST SONOGRAPHY

(From Guyton AC: Textbook of Medical Physiology, 8th ed. Philadelphia, WB Saunders, 1991, p 925.)

FELICIA M. JONES

Objectives:

Describe the function of the breast.

Define the location of anatomy related to the breast.

Describe the size relationships of normal breast anatomy.

Describe the sonographic appearance of normal breast anatomy.

Describe the associated physicians, diagnostic tests, and related laboratory values.

Define the key words.

Key Words:

Acinus
Anterior pituitary gland

Areola
Breast
Breast parenchyma
Connective tissues
Cooper's ligaments
Cortisol
Estrogen
Exocrine
Hypothalamus
Insulin
Lactation
Lactiferous ducts
Mammogram
Montgomery's glands
Pectoralis major muscle
Progesterone
Prolactin
Thyroxine

INTRODUCTION

The mammary glands are modified sweat glands. They are **exocrine** organs whose main function is the secretion of milk during pregnancy (**lactation**). (See Figure 20–1.)

PRENATAL DEVELOPMENT

The mammary glands develop along two strips of ectoderm, the **mammary ridges**, which run along each side of the developing embryo. These are visible by 6 weeks' gestational development. (See Figure 20–2.)

By 8 weeks' gestation, a bud has developed in the ectoderm along the mammary ridges which extends into the underlying connective tissue. This bud will continue to develop and by the fourth month of gestation, it will begin to extend outward into secondary buds. These will further develop into the **lactiferous ducts** during puberty. Further development will occur during pregnancy due to hormonal stimulation. (See Figure 20–3.)

In the early fetus, the nipple site on the mammary gland externally is recessed slightly. This is called the **mammary pit**. By birth, this will be slightly raised on the skin surface. Further development of breast tissue will not continue until puberty.

LOCATION

The breast is anterior to the pectoralis major, serratus, and external oblique muscles and the sixth rib. It is bounded medially by the sternum and is bordered laterally by the margin of the axilla. The superior border consists of the second and third ribs. The inferior border is the seventh costal cartilage. The breast is bordered laterally by the axilla. (See Figure 20–4.)

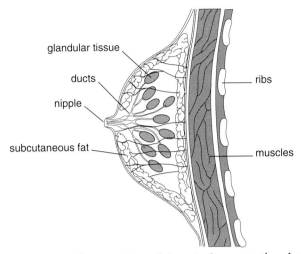

Figure 20–1. Cross-section of breast demonstrating basic anatomy.

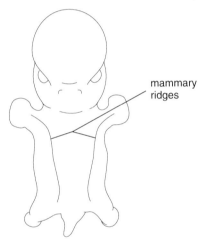

Figure 20–2. Mammary ridges seen during the prenatal development of the fetus.

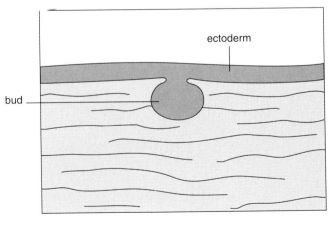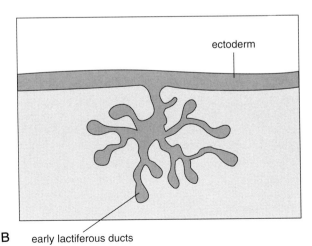

Figure 20–3. *A*, Connective tissue bud seen at approximately 10 weeks' gestational age; *B*, Outward extensions into lactiferous ducts seen at approximately 4 months' gestational age.

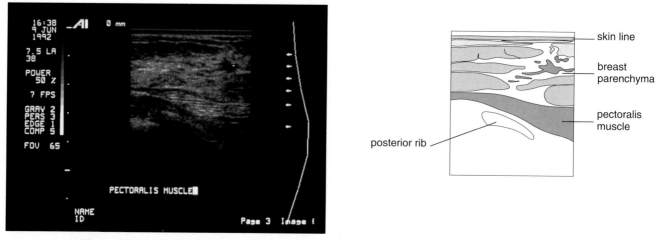

Figure 20–4. Breast anatomy showing posterior pectoralis muscle. (Image courtesy of Acoustic Imaging, Inc. Phoenix, AZ.)

SIZE

The size of the normal breast varies depending on the age, functional state, and the amount and arrangement of stromal and parenchymal elements of the individual.

There is an increase in development of breast tissue owing to stimulation by estrogen during puberty and, later, during the childbearing years and pregnancy. With the decrease in hormonal stimulation after menopause, the normal breast will atrophy to some degree.

GROSS ANATOMY

Anatomically, the breast is composed of parenchymal and stromal elements. The **parenchymal elements** in-clude the lobes, lobules, ducts, and acini. The **stromal elements** include all of the connective tissue and fat.

The breast has three layers. The **subcutaneous layer** contains the skin and all of the subcutaneous fat; the **mammary layer** contains the glandular tissues, ducts, and connective tissues; and the **retromammary layer** contains the retromammary fat, muscle, and deep connective tissues.

The normal breast is composed of 15 to 20 lobes separated by adipose tissue. Each lobe has an external drainage pathway into the nipple. The lobes are further divided into lobules, each of which contains glandular tissue elements (**alveoli**).

Support of breast tissue is provided by the **suspensory ligaments of Cooper**, which run between each two lob-ules from the deep muscle fascia to the skin surface. (See Figure 20–5.)

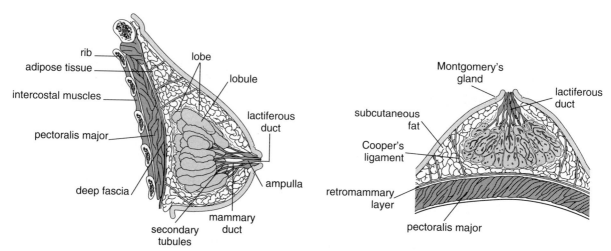

Figure 20–5. Normal breast anatomy.

PHYSIOLOGY

Breast development is stimulated by estrogen, as stated above. This stimulation causes the development of stromal and parenchymal elements throughout the breast. The glandular tissues of the breast become active due to hormonal stimulation present during pregnancy. Increased levels of progesterone stimulate the development of the breast lobules and alveoli.

Both the production of milk and its absence are controlled by hormones produced within the **hypothalamus** and **anterior pituitary gland**. The hypothalamus produces **prolactin-inhibiting factor**, which prevents the release of prolactin until milk production becomes necessary following childbirth. At this time, the anterior pituitary gland will secrete **prolactin**, which stimulates development of the secretory system of the breast.

After the placenta has been expelled and estrogen levels have decreased, the prolactin levels will begin to increase to a level which allows the production of milk. The infant's suckling stimulates the secretion of **oxytocin** from the posterior pituitary gland. This causes contraction of the lactiferous ducts, and lactation begins.

The function of the alveoli is to secrete milk into the secondary tubules. All secondary tubules from each lobule converge to form a **lactiferous duct**. Each lactiferous duct has an ampulla or expanded region called Montgomery's glands near the nipple, where milk can be stored until released during suckling. Secretions from the areolar glands keep the nipple area pliant.

SONOGRAPHIC APPEARANCE

The sonographic appearance of the breast depends on several factors, primarily the age of the woman and the functional state of the breast.

Breast tissue is visualized as three distinct layers. The most anterior layer is the subcutaneous layer, which contains the skin, the most anterior connective tissue components, and fat lobules. The middle layer is the mammary layer, which contains the breast parenchyma. Fat is seen between the parenchymal elements. This layer varies according to maternal age and breast function. The most posterior layer is the retromammary layer, which contains fat lobules and the deeper connective tissue components. This layer is bordered posteriorly by the pectoralis major muscle. (See Figure 20–6.)

Although all three layers of breast tissue are affected by natural processes, the mammary layer demonstrates the greatest changes sonographically. The younger breast has a higher percentage of parenchyma compared with the percentage of fat within the breast. This higher percentage causes the younger breast to be more dense. Dense parenchyma is difficult to visualize with mammography; therefore, younger patients presenting with possible masses are often first evaluated by sonography.

With age, the breast parenchyma becomes replaced by fatty tissues. This causes the anterior subcutaneous layer to become more prominent as the mammary layer atrophies and occupies a smaller percentage of overall breast size.

The fat components appear less echogenic than surrounding parenchymal breast tissue. Breast ducts and ductules appear as echolucent tubular structures. The fibrous components, such as Cooper's ligaments, demonstrate increased echogenicity and are seen as bright, linear echoes. The glandular or parenchymal tissues tend to appear homogeneous in texture, with medium to low level echogenicity. When scanning is done directly anterior to the nipple, posterior shadowing is visualized. (See Figure 20–7.)

The overall sonographic appearance should be consistent throughout each breast and between the two breasts. When the sonographic appearance is not homogeneous throughout the breast, it allows for easy identification of gross pathology.

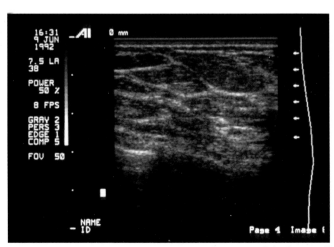
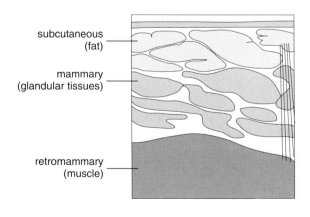

Figure 20–6. The anatomic layers of the breast. (Image courtesy of Acoustic Imaging, Inc. Phoenix, AZ.)

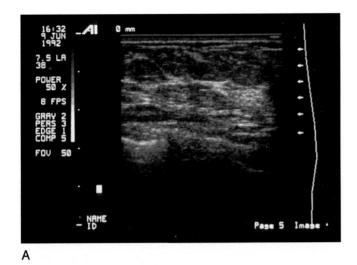

A

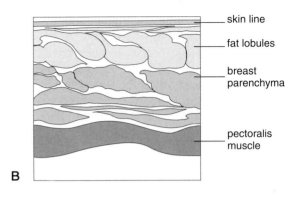

B

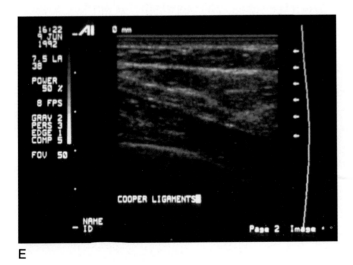

C

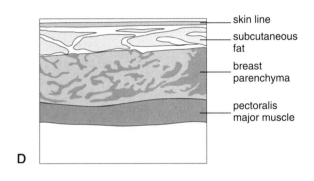

D

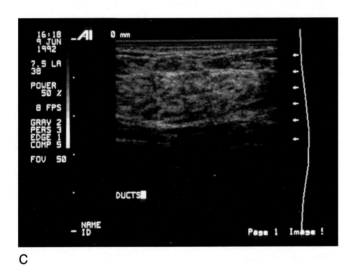

E

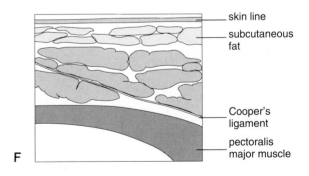

F

Figure 20–7. *See legend on opposite page.*

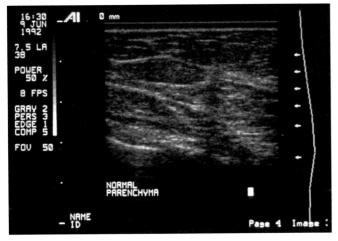

G

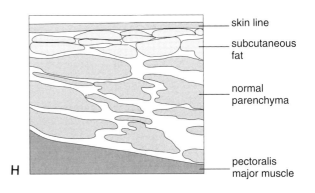

H

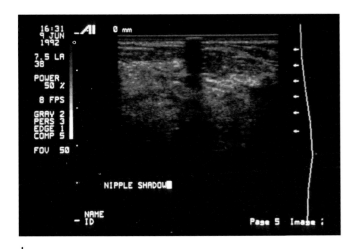

I

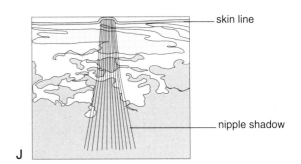

J

Figure 20–7. *A, B,* The fatty component of the breast; *C, D,* Ducts of the breast; *E, F,* The fibrous component of the breast (Cooper's ligament); *G, H,* The glandular components of the breast; *I, J,* Posterior nipple shadow. (All images in Figure 20–7 courtesy of Acoustic Imaging, Inc., Phoenix, AZ.)

SONOGRAPHIC APPLICATIONS

Sonography can be used to evaluate several aspects of breast structure. The most common application is to determine whether an identified mass is solid or cystic. The presence of large collections of calcifications may be determined sonographically, but, again, each collection or individual calcification must be fairly large, at least a few millimeters in diameter.

It is important to remember that ultrasound is not capable of detecting the very small (approximately 1 mm) calcifications that are visible with mammog-

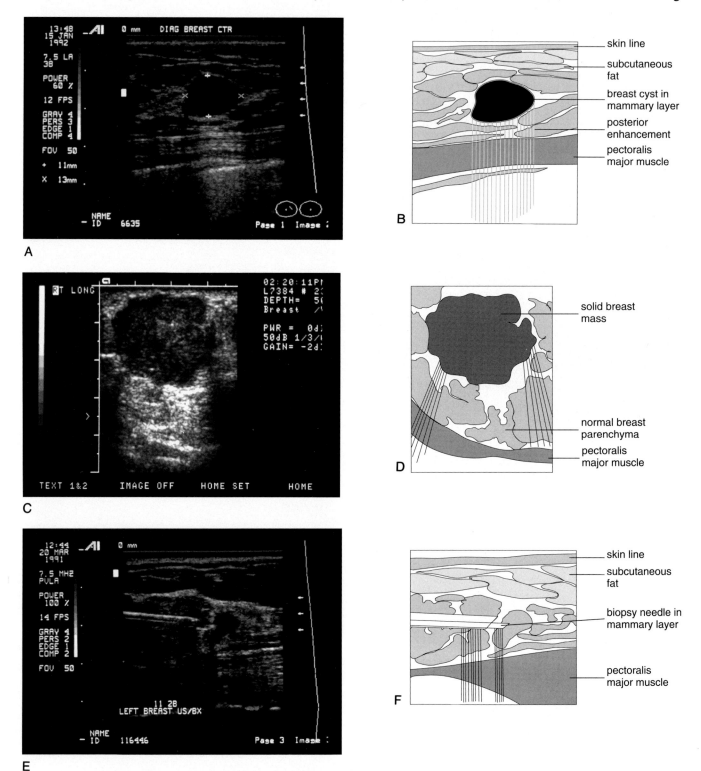

Figure 20–8. *A, B,* A breast cyst. (Image in *A* courtesy of Acoustic Imaging, Inc. Phoenix, AZ.); *C, D,* A solid breast mass. (Image in *C* courtesy Acuson Corp., Mountain View, CA.); *E, F,* Biopsy needle within breast parenchyma. (Image courtesy of Acoustic Imaging, Inc., Phoenix, AZ.)

raphy and often represent the first warning of breast cancer.

Ultrasound can also be used to determine the presence of lymph node masses and for special procedures such as guided cystic aspiration or biopsy. (See Fig. 20–8.)

NORMAL VARIANTS

Several normal variants can be appreciated sonographically. A variant very common in women of childbearing age is the fibrocystic breast. Various fibrotic components and cystic areas may be distributed throughout the entire breast.

Another variation is the fatty breast, in which the fatty components are increased, with decreased echogenicity throughout the breast. Deposition of fat increases with age and parity. Breasts often appear more fatty after menopause because the fat components become more prominent as the mammary ducts begin to atrophy. Fatty breasts may demonstrate areas of bright echogenicity due to the connective tissues surrounding the mammary ducts.

The fibrous breast has increased amounts of connective tissue and, therefore, increased echogenicity. Compression sonography is most helpful in assessing this breast as it eliminates some of the posterior shadowing resulting from the increase in dense connective tissues. (See Fig. 20–9).

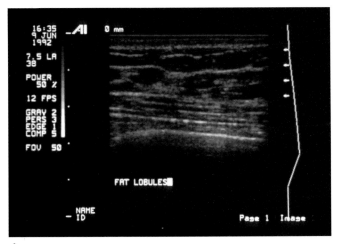

A

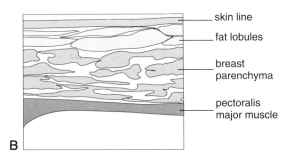

B

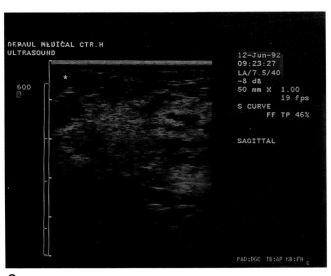

C

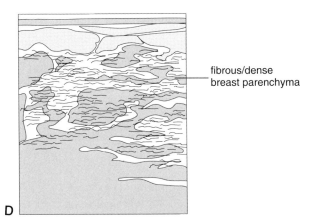

D

Figure 20–9. *A, B,* A fatty breast. (Image in *A* courtesy of Acoustic Imaging, Inc., Phoenix, AZ.); *C, D,* A fibrous breast; (Image in *C* courtesy of DePaul Medical Center, Norfolk, VA.)

REFERENCE CHARTS

Associated Physicians

Gynecologist/Obstetrician: Specializes in the examination and treatment of women, including pregnancies. The physician often performs yearly breast examinations as part of a physical examination. Diagnostic tests based on the breast examination may be ordered. Often a referral to a surgeon will be made if follow-up is necessary.

Internist: Specializes in general health care. The physician may be involved in diagnostic testing or in referrals for further follow-up. The physician may be involved in surgical follow-up, if necessary.

Surgeon: Specializes in decision making and in surgical procedures, as well as follow-up made necessary by pathologic findings. This physician is generally responsible for performing surgical procedures such as biopsies, mastectomies, and lumpectomies.

Radiologist: Specializes in interpreting the diagnostic tests used to image the breast. The radiologist may perform procedures such as fine needle biopsies if questionable areas are seen on mammography.

Pathologist: Determines the presence of pathology through typing tissue obtained at biopsy or other surgical procedures, by means of microscopic cellular analysis.

Common Diagnostic Tests

Self-Examination: This test should be performed regularly by all women more than 30 years of age, or by any woman whose family physician has determined that she is at risk for development of breast cancer. Changes of any sort should be reported and assessed by a physician as soon as possible. (See Figure 20–10.)

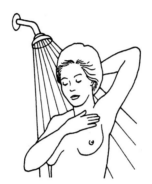

HOW TO EXAMINE
YOUR BREASTS

1 In the shower:

Examine your breasts during bath or shower; hands glide easier over wet skin. Fingers flat, move gently over every part of each breast. Use right hand to examine left breast, left hand for right breast. Check for any lump, hard knot or thickening.

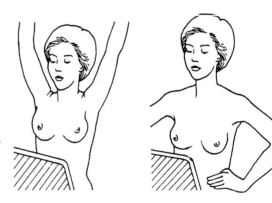

2 Before a mirror:

Inspect your breasts with arms at your sides. Next, raise your arms high overhead. Look for any changes in contour of each breast, a swelling, dimpling of skin or changes in the nipple.

Then, rest palms on hips and press down firmly to flex your chest muscles. Left and right breast will not exactly match – few women's breasts do.

Regular inspection shows what is normal for you and will give you confidence in your examination.

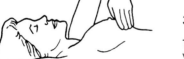

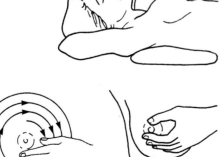

3 Lying down:

To examine your right breast, put a pillow or folded towel under your right shoulder. Place right hand behind your head – this distributes breast tissue more evenly on the chest. With left hand, fingers flat, press gently in small circular motions around an imaginary clock face. Begin at outermost top of your right breast for 12 o'clock, then move to 1 o'clock, and so on around the circle back to 12. A ridge of firm tissue in the lower curve of each breast is normal. Then move in an inch, toward the nipple, keep circling to examine every part of your breast, including nipple. This requires at least three more circles. Now slowly repeat procedure on your left breast with a pillow under your left shoulder and left hand behind head. Notice how your breast structure feels.

Finally, squeeze the nipple of each breast gently between thumb and index finger. Any discharge, clear or bloody, should be reported to your doctor immediately.

Figure 20–10. The correct procedure for self-examination of the breast. (Courtesy of the American Cancer Society.)

Mammography: This is a compression x-ray test used to visualize breast tissue. It easily demonstrates the small clusters of calcification which often indicate early breast cancer. It is recommended that women receive a baseline study at between 35 and 40 years of age, then according to their physician's guidelines. The test is performed by a radiologic technologist and interpreted by a radiologist.

Sonography: Sonography is a nonionizing imaging modality which uses sound waves to obtain diagnostic information. It is often done in conjunction with mammography. It is performed by a sonographer and interpreted by a radiologist.

Thermography: This test assesses breast tissue by indicating skin temperature, but is rarely used in the United States. It is based on the theory that the presence of cancerous tumors will cause the overlying skin to have a different temperature from normal areas. This test would be performed by a technologist and interpreted by a physician, most likely a radiologist.

Laboratory Values

Carcinoembryonic Antigen (CEA): This antigen level is used following breast cancer. It is secreted by the liver, and may be elevated in cancer removal to rule out tumor recurrence. A decrease in the antigen level represents tumor removal. Antigen levels are then monitored to detect an increase in baseline levels which would indicate tumor recurrence.

Alkaline Phosphatase: This enzyme may help rule out tumor metastasis in patients with identified breast cancer. It is secreted by the liver, and may be elevated in liver diseases as well as in bone, lung, and pancreatic carcinomas. Alkaline phosphatase is normally elevated during pregnancy and during the first year of life.

Normal Measurements

Lactiferous Ducts: Nonpregnant women—2 mm; nursing women—8 mm.

Vasculature

Arterial blood is supplied through the internal thoracic or the internal mammary artery. The internal mammary artery originates off the subclavian artery and enters the breast through the second, third, and fourth intercostal spaces medially and through the lateral thoracic artery. That artery becomes the superficial mammary artery and supplies the more superficial breast structures.

Venous drainage from the breast occurs through a combination of superficial and deep venous systems. The veins course parallel to the arteries.

Lymph drainage from the breast originates in the connective tissues of the breast and follows three main pathways. The breast's lymphatic system originates in lymph capillaries within breast connective tissues.

Seventy-five percent of lymph drainage occurs through the axillary lymph nodes. These nodes are in close proximity to the axillary tail of the breast which extends superolaterally to border the axilla. Twenty percent of lymph drainage occurs medially through the thoracic nodes, and 5 percent is subcutaneous through the intercostal nodes.

Affecting Chemicals

Prolactin: This hormone, secreted by the anterior pituitary gland, stimulates development of the breast's secretory system. Prolactin secretion is controlled by prolactin-inhibiting hormone, which is produced by the hypothalamus. After the decrease in estrogen that follows childbirth, prolactin levels increase and lactation becomes possible.

Estrogen: Estrogen, produced in the ovaries, stimulate the development of breast tissues and duct systems during puberty.

Oxytocin: This hormone, produced in the hypothalamus and stored in the posterior pituitary gland, causes duct contraction and allows for the flow of milk during nursing.

Progesterone: Progesterone is produced by the placenta. It stimulates development of the breast lobules and alveoli during pregnancy.

Insulin: Normal amounts of insulin, which is produced by the pancreas, are necessary for breast development during pregnancy.

Cortisol: This hormone, produced by the adrenal cortex, is necessary for breast development during pregnancy.

Thyroxin: Thyroxine is produced by the thyroid gland and is necessary for breast development during pregnancy.

Caffeine: A reduction in the level of caffeine may bring about a reduction in breast lumps, swelling, and soreness, especially in women with fibrocystic breast changes. Such a reduction will not affect risk factors for breast cancer.

Vitamin E: This vitamin affects the levels of fat and hormones in the blood and may help relieve pain and swelling of breast tissues.

Danazol: Danazol is a male hormone which may help to decrease pain and swelling of the breast. It suppresses activity of the anterior pituitary gland, and is used to treat women with endometriosis. The hormone may be associated with side effects.

SECTION VII

INTRODUCTION TO SPECIALTY SONOGRAPHY

Chapter 21

THE NEONATAL BRAIN

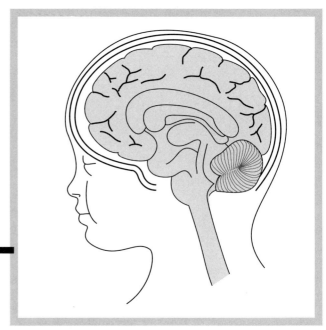

(From Tempkin BB: Ultrasound Scanning: Principles and Protocols. Philadelphia, WB Saunders, 1993.)

BRIAN SCHLOSSER

Objectives:

Describe the basic prenatal development of the human brain.

Identify the major structures in the neonatal brain.

Describe basic brain function.

Describe the sonographic appearance of the neonatal brain.

Describe normal structural variants seen sonographically.

Describe associated physicians, diagnostic tests, laboratory values, and normal measurements.

Identify the vasculature of the human brain.

Define the key words.

Key Words:

Anterior fontanelle
Aqueduct of Sylvius
Basal ganglia
Brain stem

Calcarine fissure
Caudate nucleus
Caudothalamic groove
Cavum septum pellucidum
Cavum septum vergae
Centrum semiovale
Cerebellum
Cerebral peduncle
Cerebrospinal fluid (CSF)
Cerebrum
Choroid plexus
Choroidal fissure
Cingulate gyrus/sulcus
Circle of Willis
Cisterna magna
Corpus callosum
Falx cerebri
Foramen of Monro
Fourth ventricle
Frontal lobe
Germinal matrix
Globus pallidus
Glomus

Gyrus/gyri
Interhemispheric fissure
Interpeduncular cistern
Lateral ventricle
Massa intermedia
Medulla oblongata
Midbrain
Occipital lobe
Parietal lobe
Pons
Putamen
Quadrigeminal plate cistern
Sulcus/sulci
Sylvian fissure
Temporal lobe
Tentorium cerebelli
Thalamus
Third ventricle
Trigone
Vermis

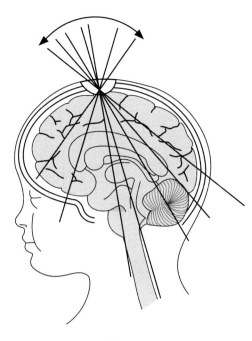

coronal

Figure 21–1. Coronal survey from the fulcrum of the anterior fontanelle. (Redrawn from Tempkin BB: Ultrasound Scanning: Principles and Protocols. Philadelphia, WB Saunders, 1993, p. 238.)

INTRODUCTION

With the significant advances in the image quality and resolution of ultrasound seen in the 1980's, sonography has become the primary imaging study in evaluation of the neonatal brain. Currently, intracranial ultrasound imaging is performed exclusively using compact, high-resolution, real-time transducers. Its portability, low cost, and relative ease of performance make ultrasound particularly advantageous, especially when evaluating unstable premature infants.

Sonographic cross-sectional anatomy of the neonatal brain is best depicted with a series of both modified coronal and sagittal planes. In the past, axial scanning was also utilized, especially for obtaining accurate ventricular dimensions. However, now it is used primarily in Doppler imaging to investigate the **circle of Willis.** Because the **anterior fontanelle** is used as the primary acoustic window, sonographic planes are different from those provided by computed tomography (CT) or magnetic resonance imaging (MRI). Therefore, both coronal and sagittal ultrasound scans are angled from the fulcrum of the anterior fontanelle. (See Figures 21–1 and 21–2.)

This chapter stresses especially the normal anatomy and sonographic appearance of the neonatal brain. Standard views and their anatomic landmarks have been described elsewhere and are not discussed here.[1] However, a routine protocol should always be followed which allows for comparable examinations.

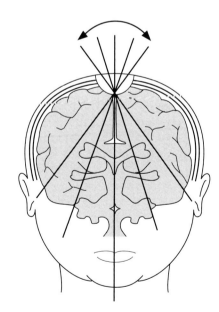

sagittal

Figure 21–2. Sagittal survey from the fulcrum of the anterior fontanelle. (Redrawn from Tempkin BB: Ultrasound Scanning: Principles and Protocols. Philadelphia, WB Saunders, 1993, p. 238.)

PRENATAL DEVELOPMENT

Brain development occurs in three specific stages, progressing from cytogenesis—the development of cells—to histogenesis—the formation of cells into tissues—to organogenesis—the formation of tissues into organs. Congenital malformations frequently result from an alteration of the normal events of organogenesis.

Organogenesis can be divided into several specific developmental events. The first major event, neural tube formation, has a peak occurrence at 3 to 4 weeks of gestation.[2] The evolving neural plate folds in on itself and closes dorsally to form the embryonic neural tube, which gives rise to the early brain and spinal cord. By the end of this time period, three primary brain vesicles are apparent: the forebrain (prosencephalon), the midbrain (mesencephalon), and the hindbrain (rhombencephalon). (See Figure 21–3.)

At 5 to 6 weeks of gestation, the most anterior brain vesicles, the prosencephalon, diverticulates (ie, folds) to form the separate telencephalon (ie, endbrain) and the diencephalon (in-between brain). (See Figure 21–4.) The telencephalon gives rise to the large cerebral hemispheres, the basal ganglia, and the lateral ventricles, while the diencephalon forms the thalamus and hypothalamus. The paired olfactory bulbs and optic tracts and unpaired pineal and pituitary glands also arise from the diverticulation of the forebrain (ie, prosencephalon).[3]

Another major event involves the proliferation of the developing brain's neurons (ie, nerve cells). This occurs between the second and fourth months of gestation. All of the neurons are located in subependymal locations and thereby proliferate from both ventricular and subventricular areas.[4] Unfortunately, very little is known about the quantitative aspects of this event. Disorders of neuronal proliferation can result in either microencephaly or macroencephaly.

Neuronal migration occurs from primarily the third to fifth months of gestation. During this time, a remarkable series of occurrences takes place. Millions of neurons in their original ventricular and subventricular sites migrate

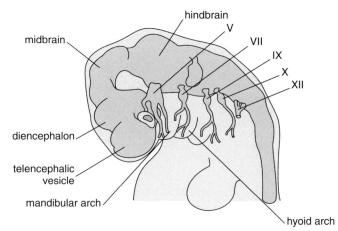

Figure 21–4. Developing brain at 5½ weeks.

to new locations within the central nervous system where they will reside permanently.[5] Again, disorders in this major event result in severe neurologic disturbances.

From approximately the sixth month of gestation to several years after birth, major organizational events occur. These events settle the elaborate circuitry that distinguishes the human brain. One example of an organizational event is the proper alignment, orientation, and layering of the neurons of the cerebral cortex.[6]

Finally, myelination, the laying down of a highly specialized myelin membrane, takes place.[7] This event takes a very long time, continuing from the second trimester of pregnancy into adult life.

LOCATION

The location of the structures of the neonatal brain are discussed under the section "Sonographic Appearance."

SIZE

Nonapplicable.

GROSS ANATOMY

The gross anatomy of the neonatal brain is identified and discussed under the section "Sonographic Appearance."

PHYSIOLOGY

The human brain, the body's largest and most complex mass of nervous tissue, functions with remarkable abilities. It can be considered in terms of four major regions: cerebral hemispheres, diencephalon, brain stem, and cerebellum.

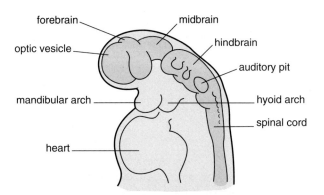

Figure 21–3. First stage in the early development of the brain at 3½ weeks.

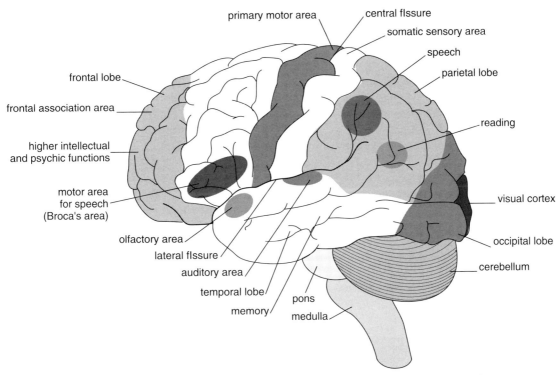

primary motor area
central fissure
somatic sensory area
speech
frontal lobe
parietal lobe
frontal association area
reading
higher intellectual
and psychic functions
motor area
for speech
(Broca's area)
visual cortex
olfactory area
occipital lobe
lateral fissure
cerebellum
auditory area
temporal lobe
pons
memory
medulla

Figure 21–5. Lateral view of the brain. Some functional areas of the cerebral hemispheres.

The brain's largest and most superior region, the paired cerebral hemispheres, exhibits elevated folds of tissue called **gyri**, and grooves called **sulci**, or fissures, which serve as important anatomical landmarks. The single deep **interhemispheric fissure**, for example, separates the hemispheres. Other fissures divide each hemisphere into four lobes. The cerebral cortical neurons (ie, the outermost gray matter) are responsible for such functions as speech, memory, voluntary movement, logical reasoning, and emotional response.[8] The **parietal lobe** contains the body's sensory receptors, which interpret the impulses that allow one to recognize such sensations as pain, cold, or a light touch.[9] (See Figure 21–5.) Importantly, because the sensory pathways are crossed pathways, the impulses from the body's right side are received by the left hemisphere's sensory cortex. This somatic sensory area is located posterior to the central fissure. Other cortical areas are responsible for interpreting impulses from the special sense organs. For example, the auditory area is adjacent to the sylvian fissure in the **temporal lobe**, while the olfactory area is deeper in the same lobe. The posterior part of the **occipital lobe** interprets visual impulses. (Refer to Figure 21–5.)

The primary motor area is located anterior to the central fissure in the **frontal lobe**. This area controls the movements of the conscious skeletal muscles, such as those in the face, mouth, and hands.[10] The motor pathways are crossed pathways as in the somatic sensory cortex.

The anterior part of the frontal lobes is believed to house the higher intellectual reasoning function. Complex memories are probably stored in both the temporal and frontal lobes. The speech function is located at the junction of the temporal, parietal, and occipital horns. (Refer to Figure 21–5.)

The diencephalon (ie, interbrain) rests superior to the brain stem and is enclosed by the cerebral hemispheres. Three distinct structures make up the diencephalon: the thalamus, hypothalamus, and epithalamus. The **thalamus** serves as a relay station for upward-moving sensory impulses. As a result, we can experience a crude recognition of both pleasant and unpleasant sensations. The hypothalamus, lying under the thalamus, plays a role in regulating body temperature, fluid balance, and metabolism. Additionally, it functions as the center for such drives as thirst, appetite, and sex.[11]

The structures of the **brain stem**, the **midbrain, pons**, and **medulla oblongata** provide a pathway for ascending and descending fiber tracts. Additionally, they have small areas (ie, nuclei) that are involved in such vital activities as swallowing and blood pressure. The pons, for example, contains nuclei involved in the control of breathing, while the medulla oblongata helps control heart rate, breathing, and vomiting, among others.[12]

The **cerebellum** functions to provide balance and equilibrium to the body by adjusting the timing of skeletal muscle activity. As a result, body movements are coordinated and smooth.

SONOGRAPHIC APPEARANCE

When the neonatal brain is examined, the relative echogenicity of various intracranial structures, along with their locations, can be described. Appreciation of the normal anatomic structures becomes essential when ruling out intracranial pathology.

Sonographically, the bones comprising the cranial vault appear highly echogenic. The parenchyma of the large cerebral hemispheres reveals a mostly homogeneous texture of relatively low echogenicity. Interspersed throughout the cerebral cortex are thin echogenic lines representing various sulci and/or fissures which separate the cerebral folds (ie, gyri).

When the neonatal brain is viewed in a modified coronal plane, the normal frontal horns and bodies of the **lateral ventricles** appear as thin, crescentic, fluid-filled bilateral spaces. The hypoechoic **corpus callosum** forms their superior margin in the midline. The longitudinal echogenic line seen extending from the superior edge of the brain in the midline marks the **falx cerebri** within the interhemispheric fissure. (See Figure 21–6.)

Anterior to the frontal horns, in the frontal cerebral cortex, a symmetric, echogenic area can be noted. Commonly referred to as the normal periventricular "blush" or "halo," this area corresponds to the frontal periventricular white matter area. The echogenic orbital cones can be seen inferiorly. (See Figure 21–7.)

The frontal horns of the lateral ventricles are separated by the septum pellucidum, which forms their medial margins in the midline. The anechoic **cavum septum pellucidum** is a normal variant sometimes noted here in the neonate. The moderately hyperechoic head of the **caudate nucleus** forms the inferolateral margin of the anterior horns. (See Figure 21–8.) It represents the more superior aspect of the gray matter of the **basal ganglia**.

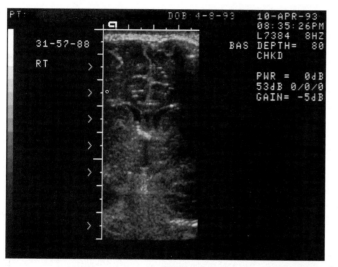

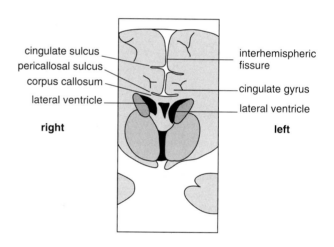

Figure 21–6. Coronal image of the bodies of the lateral ventricles.

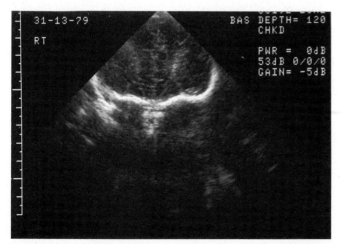

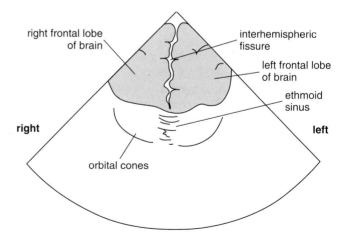

Figure 21–7. Coronal image in the frontal cerebral cortex. (Redrawn from Tempkin BB: Ultrasound Scanning: Principles and Protocols. Philadelphia, WB Saunders, 1993, p. 239.)

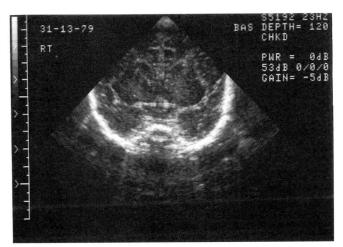
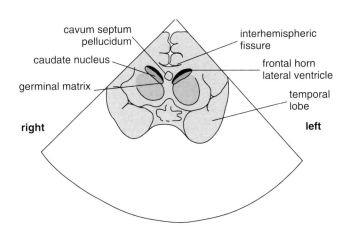

Figure 21-8. Coronal image of the frontal horns of the lateral ventricles showing the head of the caudate nucleus. (Redrawn from Tempkin BB: Ultrasound Scanning: Principles and Protocols. Philadelphia, WB Saunders, 1993, p. 240.)

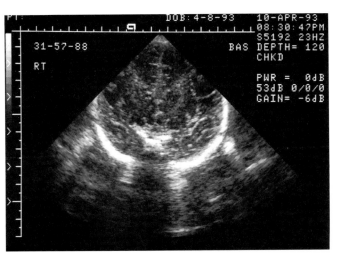
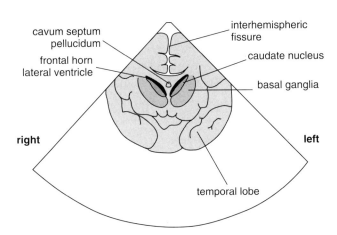

Figure 21-9. Coronal image in the area of the basal ganglia. (Redrawn from Tempkin BB: Ultrasound Scanning: Principles and Protocols. Philadelphia, WB Saunders, 1993, p. 240.)

Immediately lateral and inferior to the caudate nucleus, the **putamen** and **globus pallidus** of the basal ganglia can be noted as areas of increased echogenicity relative to the surrounding parenchyma. (See Figure 21–9.) The hypoechoic anterior corpus callosum forms the superior margin of the frontal horns. The superior margin of the corpus callosum is marked by the echogenic pericallosal sulcus. Superior to this is the hypoechoic **cingulate gyrus** and then the hyperechoic **cingulate sulcus**. (Refer to Figure 21–6.)

The area of the **foramen of Monro** can be shown just posterior to the frontal horns. The bilateral foramina lie inferomedial to the bodies of the lateral ventricles and mark the communication between the lateral and third ventricles. (See Figure 21–10.) The **third ventricle**, filled with **cerebrospinal fluid (CSF)**, lies inferior to the foramina in the midline. It can be difficult to visualize in its transverse dimension when normal in size; however, it is

clearly noted as an anechoic structure when dilated. The moderately hyperechoic body of the **caudate nucleus** marks the inferolateral margin of the bodies of the lateral ventricles. Also noted at this level are the lateral echogenic **sylvian fissures**, which divide the frontal and temporal lobes of the cerebral cortex. The middle cerebral arteries lie here and are frequently seen pulsating on a real-time image. The echogenic **interpeduncular cistern** is also noted inferiorly. Near this cistern, the pulsations of the basilar artery are also frequently seen during the real-time examination. (Refer to Figure 21–9.)

Another coronal view shows the homogeneous **thalami**, which can be seen lying inferior to the bodies of the lateral ventricles. The posterior aspect of the slit-like third ventricle lies between them. The anterior extent of the highly echogenic **choroid plexus** can be noted in the groove between the lateral ventricles. Choroid plexus also lies in the roof of the third and fourth ventricles. A

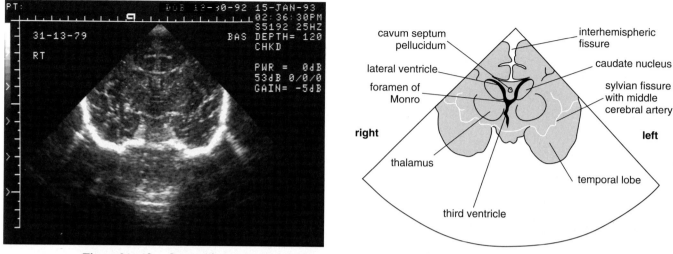

Figure 21–10. Coronal image in the area of the foramen of Monro. (Redrawn from Tempkin BB: Ultrasound Scanning: Principles and Protocols. Philadelphia, WB Saunders, 1993, p. 240.)

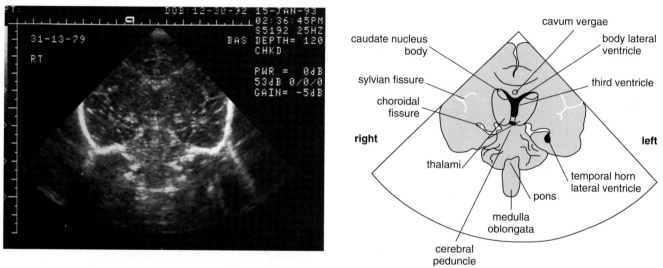

Figure 21–11. Coronal image at the level of the bilateral thalami. (Redrawn from Tempkin BB: Ultrasound Scanning: Principles and Protocols. Philadelphia, WB Saunders, 1993, p. 241.)

pair of hypoechoic structures can be shown inferior to the thalami and just above the highly echogenic **tentorium cerebelli** and **choroidal fissures**. These represent the **cerebral peduncles**. The tent-shaped tentorium cerebelli separates the cerebellum from the more superior structures. (See Figure 21–11.) This view also reveals the moderately echogenic pons and medulla oblongata of the brain stem (seen inferiorly).

A coronal view through the **quadrigeminal plate cistern** reveals an echogenic, star-shaped structure inferior to the lateral ventricular bodies. The lateral extensions meet with the choroidal fissures, the brightly echogenic curving arcs, while the tentorium is noted inferiorly. Sometimes evident at this level is the **fourth ventricle**, a rectangular anechoic space in the midline. (See Figure 21–12.) It lies just anterior to the vermis of the

cerebellum in the posterior fossa. Sonographically, the **vermis**, the midline portion of the cerebellum, is quite echogenic, while the lateral cerebellar hemispheres are noticeably less echogenic. The anechoic **cisterna magna** is seen in the space between the inferior vermis and the occipital bone. (Refer to Figure 21–12.)

Scanning more posteriorly reveals the **trigone** region of the lateral ventricles, where the bodies, occipital horns, and temporal horns converge. Most noticeable is the highly echogenic **glomus** of the choroid plexus within the trigones, which should generally demonstrate smooth margins. (See Figure 21–13.) The lateral ventricles diverge laterally at this level and are divided by the posterior corpus callosum, which appears as an echogenic line between the ventricles. The area of increased periventricular echogenicity appears lateral to the trigones and

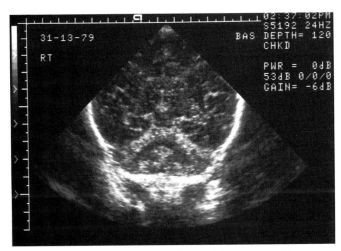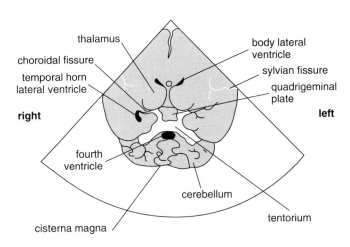

Figure 21–12. Coronal image revealing the anechoic fourth ventricle. (Redrawn from Tempkin BB: Ultrasound Scanning: Principles and Protocols. Philadelphia, WB Saunders, 1993, p. 241.)

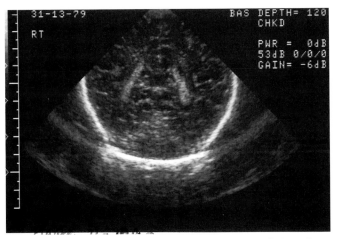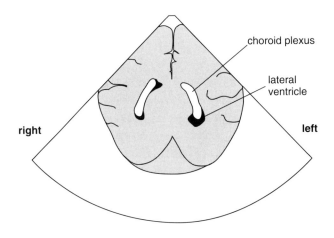

Figure 21–13. Coronal image of the trigone region of the lateral ventricles. (Redrawn from Tempkin BB: Ultrasound Scanning: Principles and Protocols. Philadelphia, WB Saunders, 1993, p. 242.)

should be less echogenic than the adjacent choroid plexus. (Refer to Figure 21–13.)

Viewing the neonatal brain posterior and cephalad to the trigones reveals the symmetric, moderately echogenic "blush" of the posterior periventricular white matter (ie, **centrum semiovale**). This area is visible on either side of the echogenic interhemispheric fissure. Also noted is the echogenic **calcarine fissure** coursing perpendicular from the interhemispheric fissure. A number of echogenic superficial cortical sulci extend from the lateral margins of the brain. (See Figure 21–14.)

Viewing the neonatal brain in sagittal sections from the fulcrum of the anterior fontanelle also reveals several important anatomic landmarks. The hypoechoic, crescent-shaped **corpus callosum**, for example, can be clearly recognized in the midline. It lies just superior to the anechoic cavum septum pellucidum and **cavum septum vergae**, when they are present. The echogenic pericallosal sulcus surrounds the corpus callosum and contains

the pericallosal arteries. The thin, hyperechoic curved line superior to the pericallosal sulcus represents the cingulate sulcus, which separates the hypoechoic cingulate gyrus from the more superficial gyri. Pulsations from the anterior cerebral arteries are often seen just anterior to the corpus callosum during real-time scanning. Lying inferior to the cavum septum pellucidum and vergae (when present) is the normal slit-like third ventricle. The **massa intermedia**, a homogeneous, soft tissue structure, can be noted in a dilated third ventricle. The echogenic band lying posterior to the third ventricle represents the quadrigeminal plate cistern. Marking the inferior end of this cistern is the highly echogenic cerebellar vermis. Again, the anechoic cisterna magna arises just inferior to the vermis. Indenting the anterior vermis is the anechoic fourth ventricle, which appears triangular in this plane. The moderately echogenic pons and medulla oblongata of the brain stem occupy the area anterior to the fourth ventricle. (See Figure 21–15.)

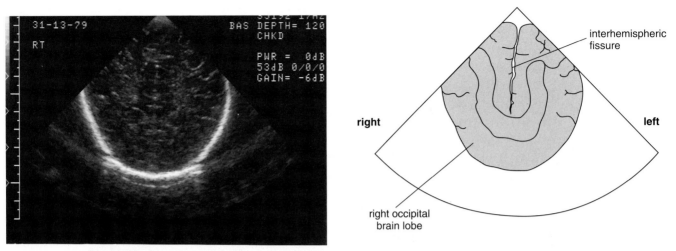

Figure 21–14. Coronal image posterior and cephalad to the trigones. (Redrawn from Tempkin BB: Ultrasound Scanning: Principles and Protocols. Philadelphia, WB Saunders, 1993, p. 242.)

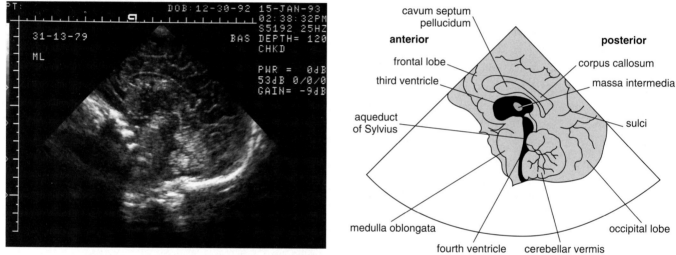

Figure 21–15. Sagittal image in the midline of the brain. (Redrawn from Tempkin BB: Ultrasound Scanning: Principles and Protocols. Philadelphia, WB Saunders, 1993, p. 243.)

Another important anatomic landmark, the **caudothalamic groove**, is clearly shown on a sagittal view. This groove is seen as a thin, brightly echogenic arc positioned between the head of the caudate nucleus and the thalamus. (See Figure 21–16.) It marks the area of **germinal matrix**, which is found more anterosuperiorly. Being composed of a fine network of blood vessels and neural tissue, the germinal matrix is highly susceptible to hemorrhage in the premature infant. (Pressure and metabolic changes can lead to rupture of these small vessels.) Although the germinal matrix lies in the subependymal layer of the ventricular system in early fetal life, it regresses to the area over the head of the caudate nucleus by 6 months' gestation. It cannot be seen as a distinct structure at term by ultrasound. The caudate nucleus, lying more anteriorly, is normally slightly more echogenic than the thalamus.

A sagittal view can also simultaneously reveal all the horns of the lateral ventricles. The amount of CSF present in them varies greatly; however, the normal anechoic ventricles are often seen as slit-like structures. This area can also be characterized by the highly echogenic glomus of the choroid plexus present in the trigone region of the lateral ventricles. (See Figure 21–17.) The normal choroid tapers as it courses anteriorly toward the foramen of Monro and should display a smooth contour. Surrounding the lateral ventricles are the frontal, parietal, temporal, and occipital lobes of the **cerebrum**. The echogenic periventricular "blush" should again be noted posterior to the occipital horns. This corresponds to an area of the posterior periventricular white matter.

A sagittal view to the far lateral left or right reveals the echogenic sylvian fissure and the temporal lobe of the cerebral cortex. (See Figure 21–18.) Again, the middle cerebral arteries can commonly be seen pulsating in the sylvian fissures. Numerous echogenic linear and curvi-

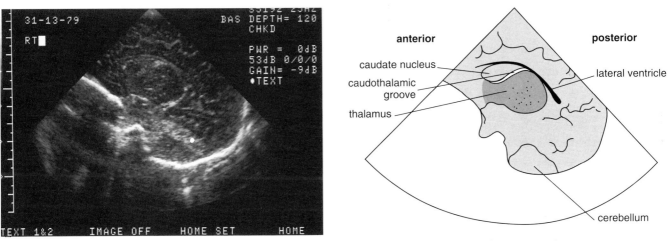

Figure 21–16. Sagittal image showing the caudothalamic groove. (Redrawn from Tempkin BB: Ultrasound Scanning: Principles and Protocols. Philadelphia, WB Saunders, 1993, p. 243.)

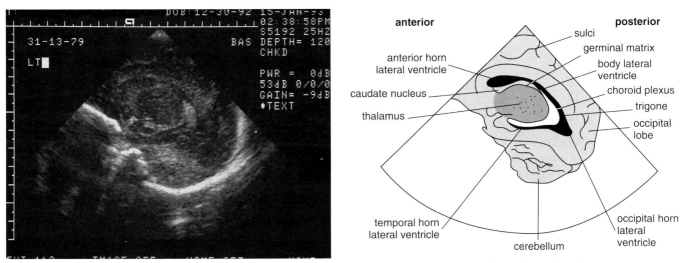

Figure 21–17. Sagittal image at the level of a lateral ventricle. (Redrawn from Tempkin BB: Ultrasound Scanning: Principles and Protocols. Philadelphia, WB Saunders, 1993, p. 244.)

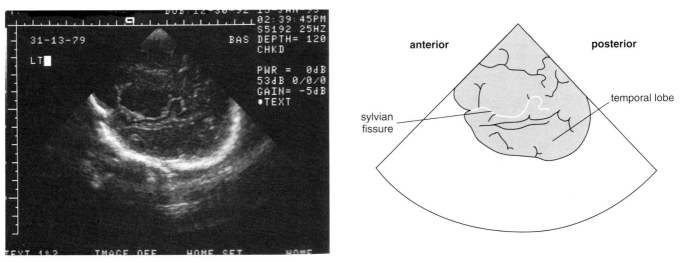

Figure 21–18. Sagittal image revealing a lateral sylvian fissure. (Redrawn from Tempkin BB: Ultrasound Scanning: Principles and Protocols. Philadelphia, WB Saunders, 1993, p. 244.)

linear sulci can be seen in the term infant at this level. The echogenic "blush" from the periventricular area is again noted.

SONOGRAPHIC APPLICATIONS

Common considerations when performing sonography of the neonatal brain include those listed below. Detection of:

1. Congenital anomalies
2. Intracranial hemorrhage
3. Intracranial masses
4. Venous malformations
5. Hydrocephalus (ie, ventricular size)
6. Intracranial infections
7. Infarction and/or edema

Doppler evaluation of cerebral blood flow abnormalities.

NORMAL VARIANTS

Normal variants of the neonatal brain are typically associated with gestational immaturity.

Lateral Ventricles

Asymmetry in the size of the lateral ventricles is a common normal variant. Approximately 40 percent of premature infants and less than 20 percent of term infants reveal some asymmetry. The left lateral ventricle is generally larger than the right. The occipital horns are particularly susceptible. (See Figure 21–19.) Interestingly, ventricular size varies with the age of the infant. As the infant matures, the lateral ventricular size decreases in relation to the size of the cerebral cortex.

Cavum Septum Pellucidum and Cavum Septum Vergae

Two common variants frequently noted in the normal infant are the cavum septum pellucidum and the cavum

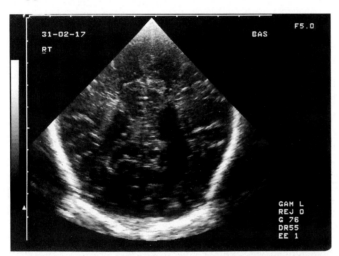
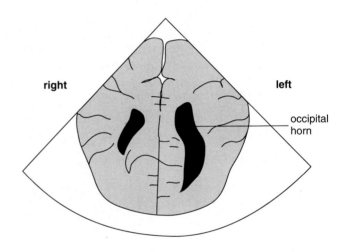

Figure 21–19. Coronal image showing asymmetry in the size of the occipital horns.

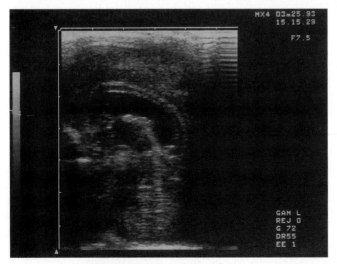
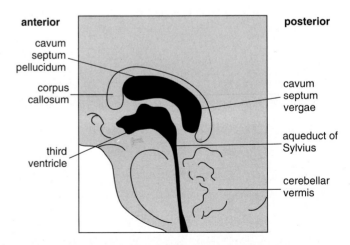

Figure 21–20. Sagittal image of a normal brain with a cavum septum pellucidum and cavum septum vergae. (Redrawn from Tempkin BB: Ultrasound Scanning: Principles and Protocols. Philadelphia, WB Saunders, 1993, p. 243.)

septum vergae. The cavum septum pellucidum is seen as an anechoic, fluid-filled space between the anterior horns of the lateral ventricles, while the cavum septum vergae lies most posterior, between the bodies. (See Figure 21–20.) Although these structures communicate with each other, they do not connect with the ventricular system.

The cavum septum vergae closes from posterior to anterior beginning in the sixth month of gestation. So, while this structure can be seen in a premature infant, it is infrequently seen in the term infant. On the other hand, the cavum septum pellucidum begins to close near term. Therefore, it can be noted alone until approximately 2 months of postnatal life.

REFERENCE CHARTS

Associated Physicians

Radiologist: Specializes in the diagnostic interpretation of imaging modalities that assess central nervous system pathology.
Neurologist: Specializes in the diagnosis and treatment of disorders of the nervous system.
Neonatologist: Specializes in the diagnosis and treatment of disorders of the newborn infant.

Common Diagnostic Tests

Computed Axial Tomography (CT Scan): Provides cross-sectional (ie, axial) x-ray images of the brain to assess anatomy. A contrast medium is often administered to differentiate between pathology and normal anatomy. This test is performed by a radiologic technologist or radiologist. Interpretation of the test is by the radiologist.

Magnetic Resonance Imaging (MRI): Provides valuable information about the body's biochemistry when the patient is placed in a magnetic field. Provides axial, sagittal, and coronal images of the brain directly. This diagnostic imaging technique does not require exposure to ionizing radiation. The test is performed by a radiologic technologist or radiologist and interpreted by the radiologist.

Electroencephalography (EEG): Records changes in electric potential (ie, activity) in various locations of the brain by means of electrodes placed on the scalp. This test is performed by a technologist and interpreted by a neurologist.

Laboratory Values

Hematocrit: This laboratory test measures the percentage of blood that is composed of red blood cells, expressed as volume percent. A decreasing hematocrit can be an indication of a possible intracranial hemorrhage.

Normal Measurements

Ventricular Size

Ventricular Depth: In a coronal plane at the level of the foramen of Monro, the bodies of the lateral ventricles are measured from wall to wall. (See Figure 21–21.) This measurement is the widest line perpendicular to the longest axis of the ventricles.[13]
NORMAL MEASUREMENT: 4 mm or less.
Midline to Lateral Dimension: In the same coronal plane, this measurement is the horizontal distance from the midline (ie, falx) to the most lateral aspect of the lateral ventricles. (Refer to Figure 21–21.)[13]
NORMAL MEASUREMENT: 12 mm or less.

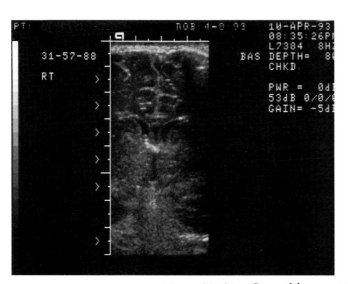

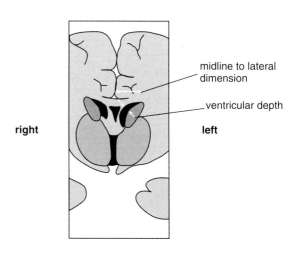

Figure 21–21. Coronal image at the level of the foramen of Monro.

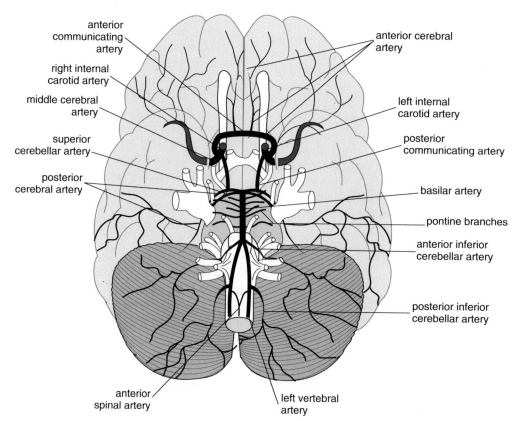

Figure 21–22. The arterial supply to the brain as seen from the inferior surface.

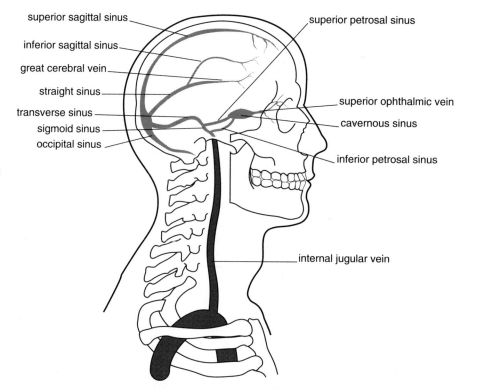

Figure 21–23. Lateral view of the head showing the major venous drainage of the brain.

Vasculature

The internal carotid and vertebral arteries supply blood to the brain. (See Figure 21–22.)

A) Aorta—brachiocephalic (rt.)—common carotid artery—INTERNAL CAROTID ARTERY—anterior cerebral artery—anterior communicating artery—middle cerebral artery—posterior communicating artery.

B) Aorta—brachiocephalic (rt.)—rt. subclavian artery—VERTEBRAL ARTERY—anterior spinal artery—basilar artery—posterior inferior cerebellar artery—anterior inferior cerebellar artery—superior cerebellar artery—posterior cerebral artery.

Large veins, called sinuses, found in the brain's tough covering (ie, the dura mater), drain the brain (see Figure 21–23.)
Superior sagittal sinus—inferior sagittal sinus—great cerebral vein of Galen—straight sinus—occipital sinus—transverse sinus—sigmoid sinus—superior ophthalmic vein—cavernous sinus—superior petrosal sinus—inferior petrosal sinus—internal jugular vein.

Affecting Chemicals

Nonapplicable.

References

1. Dykstra-Downey K: Neonatal brain scanning protocol. *In* Tempkin BB: Ultrasound Scanning: Principles and Protocols. Philadelphia, WB Saunders, 1993, 234–245.
2. Volpe, JJ: Neurology of the Newborn, 2nd ed. Philadelphia, WB Saunders, 1987, 3–5.
3. Volpe, JJ: Neurology of the Newborn, 2nd ed. Philadelphia, WB Saunders, 1987, 20.
4. Volpe, JJ: Neurology of the Newborn, 2nd ed. Philadelphia WB Saunders, 1987, 33–34.
5. Volpe, JJ: Neurology of the Newborn, 2nd ed. Philadelphia, WB Saunders, 1987, 39–42.
6. Volpe, JJ: Neurology of the Newborn, 2nd ed. Philadelphia, WB Saunders, 1987, 49–51.
7. Volpe, JJ: Neurology of the Newborn, 2nd ed. Philadelphia, WB Saunders, 1987:55–56.
8. Marieb EN: Essentials of Human Anatomy and Physiology, 3rd ed. Redwood City, CA, Benjamin/Cummings Publishing Co., 1991, 183.
9. Marieb EN: Essentials of Human Anatomy and Physiology, 3rd ed. Redwood City, CA, Benjamin/Cummings Publishing Co., 1991, 183–184.
10. Marieb EN: Essentials of Human Anatomy and Physiology, 3rd ed. Redwood City, CA, Benjamin/Cummings Publishing Co., 1991, 185.
11. Marieb EN: Essentials of Human Anatomy and Physiology, 3rd ed. Redwood City, CA, Benjamin/Cummings Publishing Co., 1991, 187.
12. Marieb EN: Essentials of Human Anatomy and Physiology, 3rd ed. Redwood City, CA, Benjamin/Cummings Publishing Co., 1991, 187–188.
13. Sauerbrei EE, Digney M, Harrison PB, Cooperberg PL: Ultrasonic evaluation of neonatal intracranial hemorrhage and its complications. Radiology 139:677–685, 1981.

Bibliography

Grant EG (ed): Neurosonography of the Pre-Term Neonate. New York, Springer-Verlag, 1986.
Marieb EN: Essentials of Human Anatomy and Physiology. 3rd ed. Redwood City, CA, Benjamin/Cummings Publishing Co.; 1991.
Naidich TP, Quencer RM, (eds.): Clinical Neurosonography: Ultrasound of the Central Nervous System. New York, Springer-Verlag, 1987.
Rumack CM, Wilson SR, Charboneau JW (eds.): Diagnostic Ultrasound. St. Louis, Mosby-Year Book, 1991.
Siegel MJ (ed.): Pediatric Sonography. New York, Raven Press, 1991.
Teele RL, Share JC: Ultrasonography of Infants and Children. Philadelphia, WB Saunders, 1991.
Tempkin BB: Ultrasound Scanning: Principles and Protocols. Philadelphia, WB Saunders, 1993.
Volpe, JJ: Neurology of the Newborn. 2nd ed. Philadelphia, WB Saunders, 1987.

Chapter 22

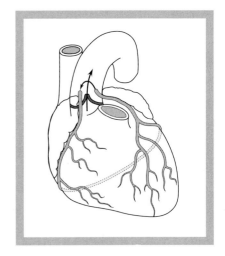

The pediatric heart. (From Guyton AC: Textbook of Medical Physiology, 8th ed. Philadelphia, W. B. Saunders, 1991, p 237.)

PEDIATRIC ECHO-CARDIOGRAPHY

VIVIE M. MILLER

Objectives:

Describe the function of the heart.

Describe the size and position of the heart in the normal child.

Name the chambers, great veins, and great arteries of the heart.

Describe the flow of blood through the heart of a fully developed fetus including the fetal shunts and their purpose.

Describe the flow of blood through the heart of a normal neonate after closure of the fetal shunts.

Describe the sonographic appearance of the pediatric heart.

Describe the associated physicians.

Describe the associated diagnostic tests.

Define the key words.

Key Words:

Aorta (ascending, transverse, descending)
Aortic valve
Apex
Atrioventricular node (A-V node)
Atrium (left, right)
Base
Bundle of His
Cardiac veins
Chordae tendineae
Common carotid artery (left, right)
Coronary arteries
Coronary sinus
Diastole
Ductus arteriosus
Ductus venosus
Endocardium

Foramen ovale
Inferior vena cava
Innominate artery
Interatrial septum
Interventricular septum
Mitral valve
Myocardium
Papillary muscles
Pericardium (parietal, visceral)
Pulmonary artery (main, left, right)
Pulmonary valve
Pulmonary veins
Purkinje fibers
Semilunar valves
Sinoatrial node (SA node)
Subclavian artery (left, right)
Superior vena cava
Systole
Tricuspid valve
Ventricle (left, right)

INTRODUCTION

The structures of the heart include four chambers, four main valves, two great veins, four smaller veins, two great arteries, septa, and muscle.

The heart is the muscular pump of the body's cardiovascular system, providing the force that propels blood through all the vessels. The heart and vessels are a "distribution and collection system in general, providing transportation for the distribution of nutrients, gases, minerals, vitamins, hormones, and blood cells to the tissues and collection of waste products for excretion from the body."[1]

"1. The tissues of the body receive oxygen and nutrients.

2. The tissues of the body have a disposal service for the collection and excretion of waste products such as carbon dioxide and other toxic materials.

3. The tissues of the body can release secretory materials or hormones that can quickly exert an influence on body parts distant from the source.

4. Medications injected into the body are distributed quickly throughout all areas of the body.

5. The body's defense system such as antibodies and white blood cells are moved to areas of infection and inflammation."[2]

PRENATAL DEVELOPMENT

In the 3-week-old embryo, the heart arises as two cords, called cardiogenic cords. These cords will canalize to form two heart tubes. The heart tubes will gradually move toward each other and fuse to form a single heart tube. (See Figure 22–1.) The tube elongates and develops alternative dilatations and constrictions which indicate the development to come. The bulbus cordis and ventricle grow faster than other regions, causing the heart tube to bend upon itself and forming a bulboventricular loop. Normal looping is toward the right. The result is that the atrium and the sinus venosus (which will later form right and left horns) come to lie posterior and superior to the bulbus cordis, truncus arteriosus, and ventricle.

Beginning in the fourth week and by the end of the seventh week, the heart is completely partitioned into two atria, two ventricles, two great arteries, and veins.

Partitioning of the atrioventricular canal begins during the fourth week of embryologic development. (See Figure 22–2.) Swellings called endocardial cushions form on the dorsal and ventral walls of the atrioventricular canal. These cushions develop and grow toward each other, fusing during the fifth week. The heart is now divided into a right and a left atrioventricular canal.

The partitioning of the common atrium is accomplished by the formation of two septa, the septum primum and the septum secundum. (See Figure 22–3.) A thin crescent-shaped membrane called the septum primum (the first septum) grows toward the fused endocardial cushions, beginning at the dorsocranial wall of the primitive atrium. As this curtain-like septum grows toward the endocardial cushions, a large opening, the foramen primum forms. This opening eventually closes as the septum primum continues to grow toward and fuse with the endocardial cushions. However, before the foramen primum is closed, perforations, or fenestrations, appear in the dorsal part of the septum primum and form another, second, opening called the foramen secundum. At about this time, the septum primum joins or fuses with the left side of the endocardial cushions to completely close the foramen primum. By the end of the fifth week, another crescentic membrane grows from the ventrocranial wall of the atrium, immediately to the right of the septum primum. This is the septum secundum or second septum. As it grows, it covers or overlaps the foramen secundum that formed in the septum primum to form an oval opening, the **foramen ovale**. The cranial part of the septum primum gradually disappears. The remaining part of the septum attaches to the endocardial cushions to form the flap of the foramen ovale. This is one of three fetal shunts.

Partitioning of the primitive ventricle begins with a muscular ridge in the floor of the single ventricle near the apex. (See Figures 22–4 and 22–7.) This foramen is subsequently closed with ridges extending from the right and left sides of the bulbus cordis, called bulbar ridges, and the endocardial cushions. (See Figure 22–5.) The thin, small membranous interventricular septum is de-

Text continued on page 360.

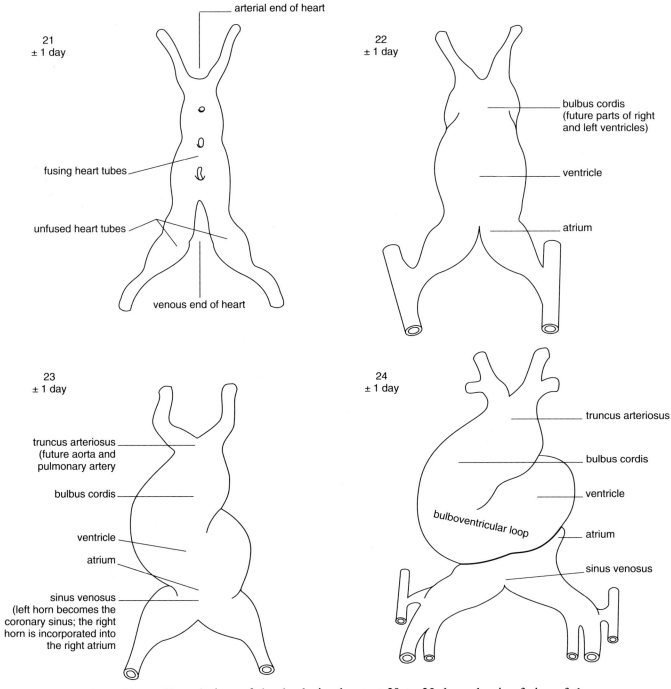

Figure 22-1. Ventral views of the developing heart at 20 to 25 days, showing fusion of the endocardial heart tube to form a single tube. Note bending to form the bulboventricular loop.

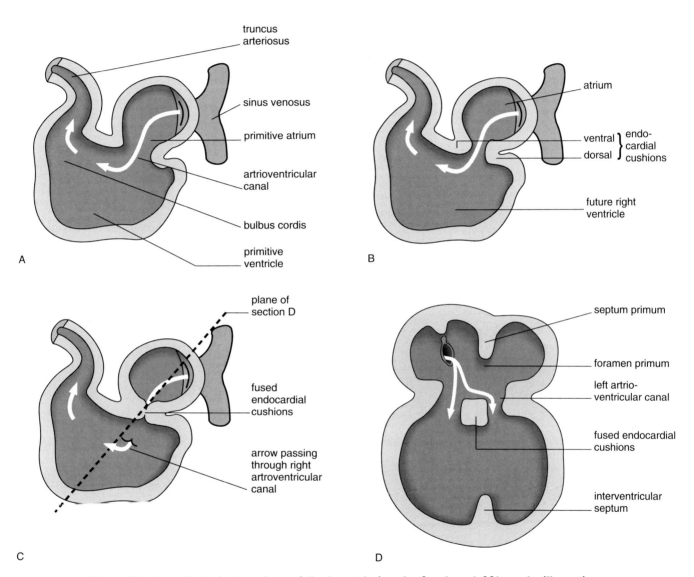

Figure 22-2. *A-C,* Sagittal sections of the heart during the fourth and fifth weeks illustrating division of the atrioventricular canal. *D,* Coronal section of the heart at the plane shown in *C.* Note that the interatrial and interventricular septa have also begun to develop.

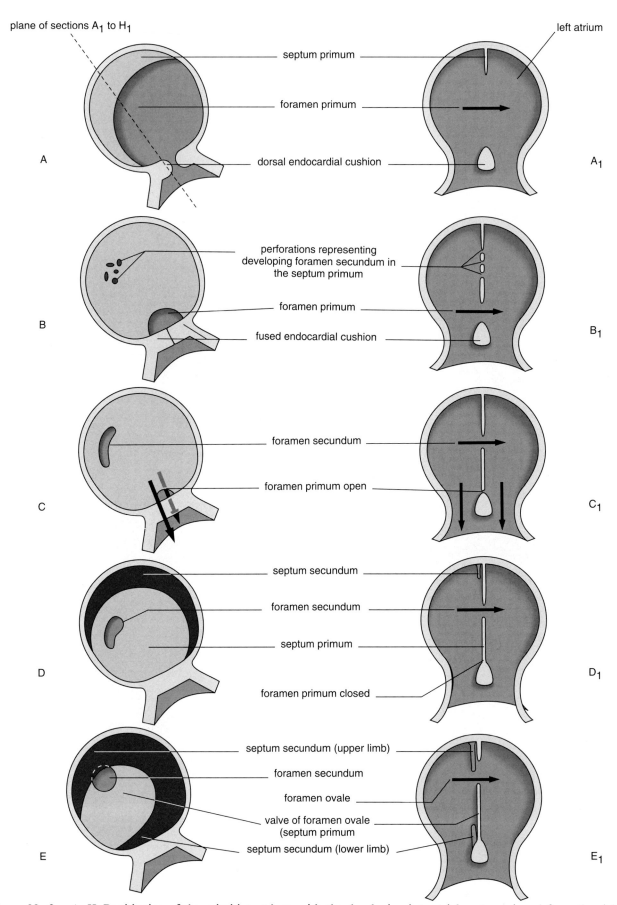

Figure 22-3. *A-H*, Partitioning of the primitive atrium, with the developing interatrial septum viewed from the right side. *A₁-H₁*, Coronal sections of the developing interatrial septum at the plane shown in *A*. Note that as the septum secundum develops, it overlaps the opening in the septum primum (foramen secundum). The valve-like nature of the foramen ovale is illustrated in *G* and *H*. When pressure in the right atrium exceeds that in the left atrium (as in the fetus), blood passes from the right to the left side of the heart. When the pressures are equal or higher in the left atrium (as is normal after birth), the septum primum closes the foramen ovale.

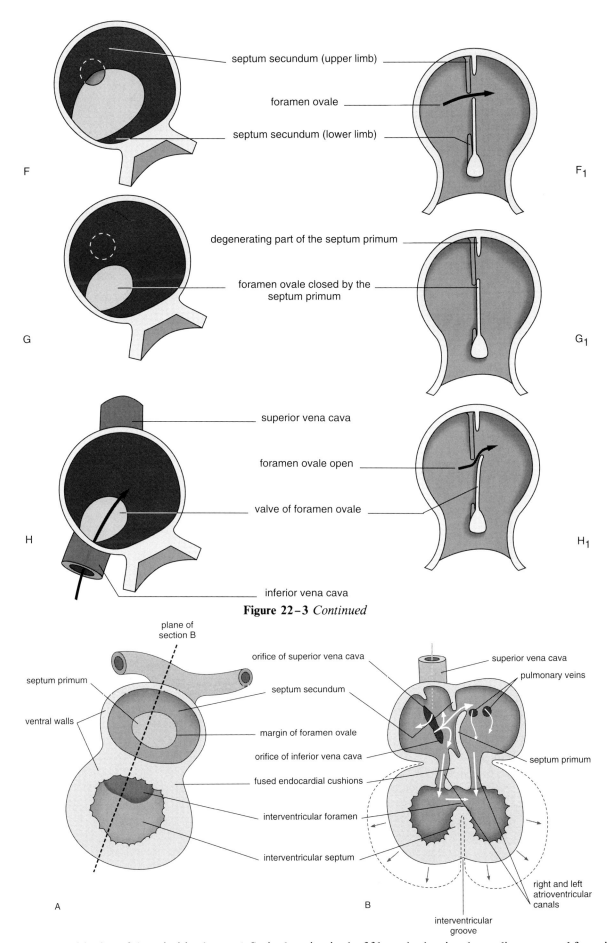

F

septum secundum (upper limb)

foramen ovale

septum secundum (lower limb)

F₁

G

degenerating part of the septum primum

foramen ovale closed by the septum primum

G₁

H

superior vena cava

foramen ovale open

valve of foramen ovale

H₁

inferior vena cava

Figure 22-3 *Continued*

plane of section B

orifice of superior vena cava

superior vena cava

septum primum

septum secundum

pulmonary veins

ventral walls

margin of foramen ovale

orifice of inferior vena cava

septum primum

fused endocardial cushions

interventricular foramen

septum secundum

interventricular septum

right and left atrioventricular canals

A

B

interventricular groove

Figure 22-4. Partitioning of the primitive heart. *A*, Sagittal section in the fifth week, showing the cardiac septa and foramina. *B*, Coronal section at a slightly later stage, illustrating the direction of blood flow through the heart and expansion of the ventricles. Note the formation of the interventricular septum and the interventricular foramen in both diagrams.

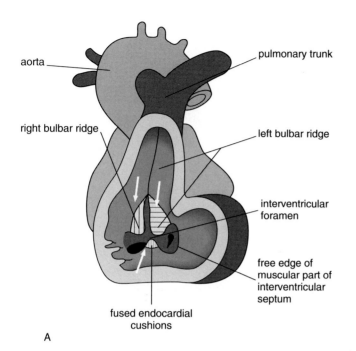

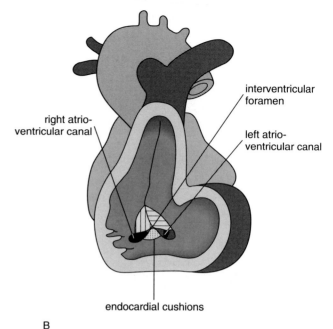

A

B

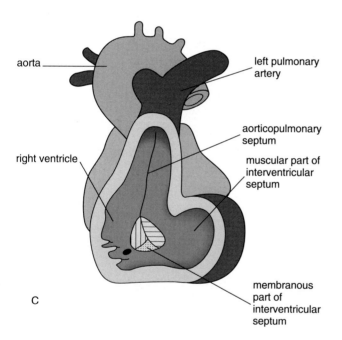

C

Figure 22–5. Closure of the interventricular foramen and formation of the membranous part of the interventricular septum. The walls of the truncus arteriosus, bulbus cordis, and right ventricle have been removed. *A*, At 5 weeks, showing the bulbar ridges and the fused endocardial cushions. *B*, At 6 weeks, showing that proliferation of subendocardial tissue diminishes the interventricular foramen. *C*, At 7 weeks, showing the fused bulbar ridges and the membranous part of the interventricular septum formed by extensions of tissue from the right side of the endocardial cushions.

rived from an extension of tissue from the right side of the fused endocardial cushions. This tissue merges with the aorticopulmonary septum (fused bulbar ridges) and the thick muscular interventricular septum. After closure of the interventricular septum, the aorta communicates with the left ventricle, and the pulmonary trunk communicates with the right ventricle. There is now no direct communication between the newly formed right and left ventricles.

The bulbus cordis and truncus arteriosus begin partitioning into the aorta and pulmonary artery during the fifth week. The growth of cells in the wall of the bulbus cordis results in bulbar ridges. Truncal ridges form in the truncus arteriosus and are continuous with the bulbar ridges. (See Figure 22–6.) The spiral formation of these ridges results in a spiral aorticopulmonary septum. In Figures 22–6B and 22–6F, this septum is shown oriented right/left at level 3. At level 2, it is oriented dorsoventrally or anterior/posterior. It twists again and at level 1 it is again oriented right/left. In Figure 22–6E and 22–6H, the septum has divided the bulbus cordis and truncus arteriosus into the aorta and pulmonary trunk. Because of the spiraling of the aorticopulmonary septum, the pulmonary trunk twists around the aorta.

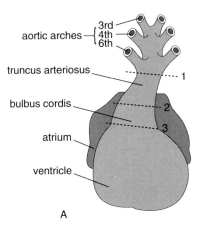

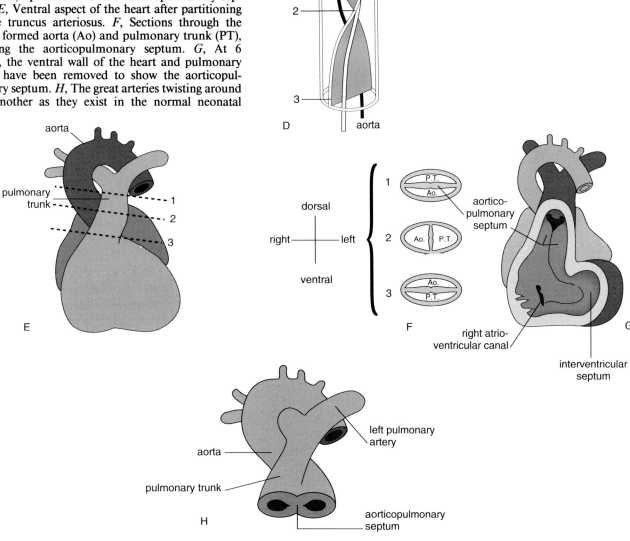

Figure 22–6. Partitioning of the bulbus cordis and truncus arteriosus. *A*, Ventral aspect of the heart at 5 weeks. *B*, Transverse sections through the truncus arteriosus and bulbus cordis illustrating the truncal and bulbar ridges. Note that the orientation is of looking down into the truncus arteriosus from above, keeping in mind the dorsal and ventral aspects of the truncal tube as the aorticopulmonary septum spirals within it. *C*, The ventral wall of the heart and truncus arteriosus has been removed to demonstrate these ridges. *D*, Spiral form of the aorticopulmonary septum. *E*, Ventral aspect of the heart after partitioning of the truncus arteriosus. *F*, Sections through the newly formed aorta (Ao) and pulmonary trunk (PT), showing the aorticopulmonary septum. *G*, At 6 weeks, the ventral wall of the heart and pulmonary trunk have been removed to show the aorticopulmonary septum. *H*, The great arteries twisting around one another as they exist in the normal neonatal heart.

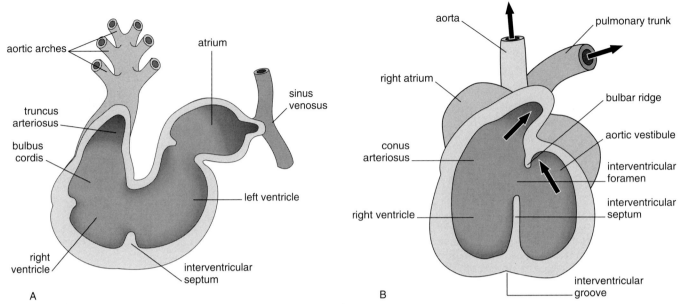

Figure 22–7. Incorporation of the bulbus cordis into the ventricles and partitioning of the bulbus cordis and truncus arteriosus into the aorta and pulmonary trunk. *A*, Sagittal section at 5 weeks, showing the bulbus cordis as one of the five primitive chambers of the heart. *B*, Coronal section at 6 weeks, after the bulbus cordis has been incorporated into the ventricles to become the conus arteriosus (infundibulum) of the right ventricle and the aortic vestibule of the left ventricle.

The bulbus cordis is absorbed into the ventricles. (See Figure 22–7.) It becomes the conus arteriosus or infundibulum of the right ventricle. In the left ventricle it is called the aortic vestibule, the part just proximal to the aortic valve.

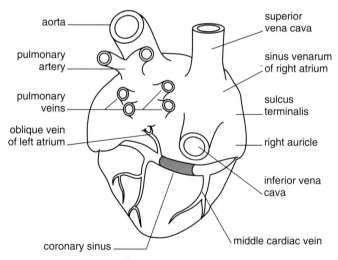

Figure 22–8. Dorsal view at 8 weeks showing the positions of the superior and inferior venae cavae with respect to the right atrium. The pulmonary veins, each with separate openings into the left atrium, are also shown.

Another fetal shunt, the **ductus arteriosus**, is a connection between the dorsal aorta and the left pulmonary artery. Both the ductus arteriosus and the left pulmonary artery are derivatives of the left sixth aortic arch. (See Figures 22–6*A* and 22–9.)

The **inferior vena cava** is derived from four segments of the primitive veins of the embryonic trunk. It enters the inferior posterior part of the right atrium. The superior vena cava is derived from two primitive veins of the embryo, the right anterior cardinal vein and the right common cardinal vein. It enters the posterior superior part of the right atrium.

The four **pulmonary veins** are derived from the primitive pulmonary vein and its four main branches. (See Figure 22–8.) As the primitive vein is incorporated into the left atrium, the four main branches remain, each one entering the left atrium separately.

Fetal Circulation

Circulation through the fully developed normal fetal heart is shown in Figure 22–9. Oxygenated blood from the mother, via the placenta, enters the umbilical vein and passes through the ductus venosus to the inferior vena cava and into the right atrium of the fetal heart. The **ductus venosus**, one of the three fetal shunts, enables oxygenated blood from the mother to pass almost di-

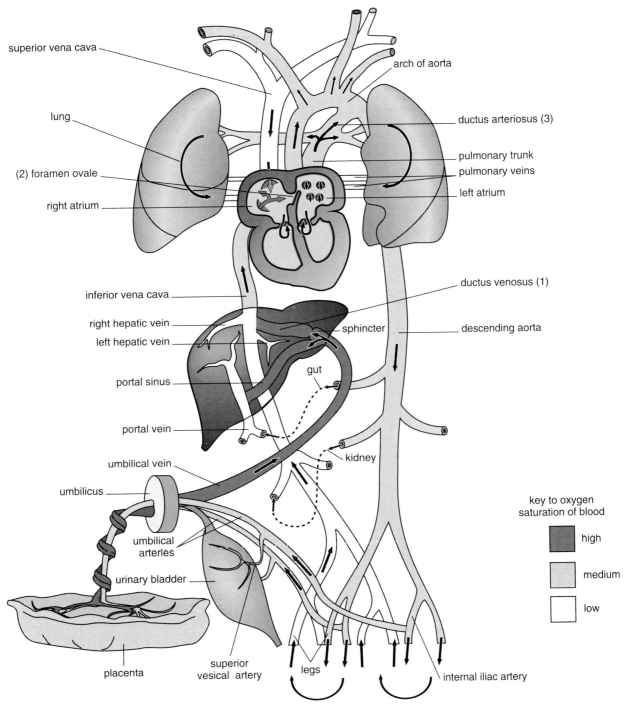

Figure 22–9. Fetal circulation. The organs are not drawn to scale. Note that the three fetal shunts permit most of the blood to bypass the liver and the lungs: (1) the ductus venosus, (2) the foramen ovale, and (3) the ductus arteriosus.

rectly into the fetal heart, bypassing the liver. After birth it will fibrose and become the ligamentum venosum.

Much of the blood from the inferior vena cava is directed across the foramen ovale, the second shunt, into the left atrium. From here the blood enters the left ventricle and then exits through the aorta.

Some blood from the inferior vena cava remains in the right atrium and mixes with blood from the superior vena cava and **coronary sinus** (the large cardiac vein draining the heart muscle) and passes into the right ventricle. This blood then exits the pulmonary trunk, some to the lungs for development, but most through the ductus arteriosus, the third shunt, to the aorta.

LOCATION

The heart, as the name implies, is roughly heart shaped. It is positioned in the lower anterior chest, posterior to the sternum and anterior to the thoracic vertebrae and esophagus. It rests on the diaphragm in the middle mediastinum bounded laterally by the right and left lungs. Two thirds of the heart lie to the left of midline and one third lies to the right. The **apex** of the heart is the bluntly pointed inferior or caudal end that is directed to the left and anteriorly. It is partially obscured by the left lung. The **base** is the broad end directed to the right posteriorly and cranially. (See Figure 22–10.)

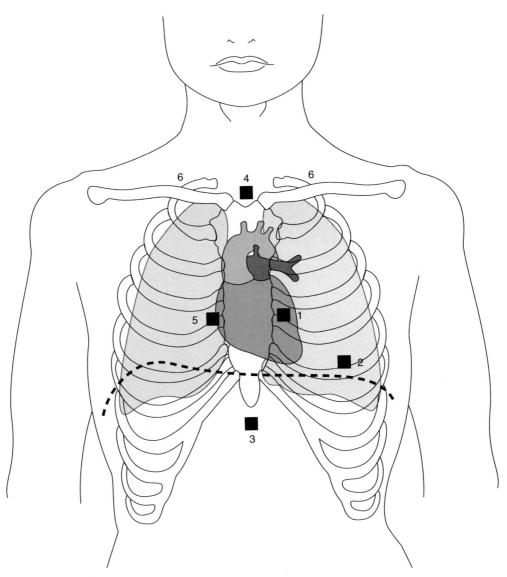

Figure 22–10. Relative position of the heart with respect to other organs within the chest cavity. Note blocks denoting transducer positions that provide "windows" for imaging the heart. (1) parasternal long axis and parasternal short axis positions; (2) apical four chamber, apical five chamber, and apical long axis; (3) subcostal or subxiphoid position; (4) suprasternal notch position; (5) right parasternal position; (6) though not indicated by dots, the supraclavicular fossa (right and/or left) is also sometimes used in obtaining echocardiographic images.

SIZE

The heart is approximately the size of a child's clenched fist. The pediatric internal dimensions of the structures vary with age and weight. Normal values for these structures are presented in Table 22–1, at the end of the chapter.

GROSS ANATOMY

Structurally, the heart is as follows: divided into upper and lower chambers, and divided into right-sided and left-sided chambers. (See Figure 22–11.)

The two upper chambers, the atria, are the filling chambers of the heart. There is a **right atrium** and a **left atrium**, of roughly equal size, thin walled, and separated by a partition called the **interatrial septum**. After birth, there is normally no direct communication between these two chambers.

The two lower chambers, the ventricles, are the pumping chambers of the heart. There is a **right ventricle** and a **left ventricle** separated by the **interventricular septum**.

The atrium and the ventricles on each side are separate; however, they communicate through openings controlled by an atrioventricular valve. The ventricles, in turn, are connected to outflow tracts with semilunar (half-moon shaped) valves controlling the exit of blood from the heart.

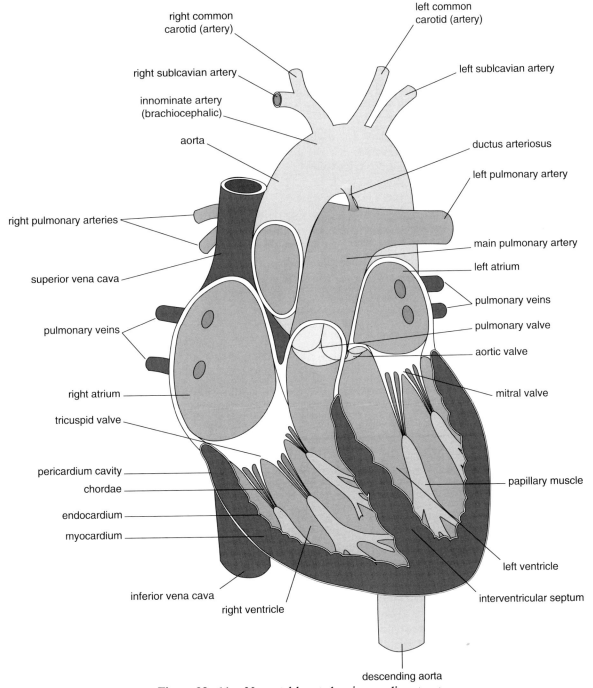

Figure 22–11. Neonatal heart showing cardiac structure.

The inner lining of the cavities of the heart is called the **endocardium**. The outer covering of the **myocardium**, or muscle of the heart, is called the epicardium. It is composed of two linings or membranes. The inner lining, the **visceral pericardium**, adheres to the myocardium. The outer lining is the **parietal pericardium**. The space between them is the pericardial cavity containing a thin, watery fluid that allowing the heat to move easily as it beats.

The beating heart makes distinctive sounds. There are two heart sounds: The first sound, S1, is caused by closure of the atrioventricular valves; the second, S2, is caused by the semilunar valves closing. There is a normal splitting of the second sound, the first being that of the aortic valve before the closure of the pulmonary valve component.

Structural differences of the chambers are very helpful in evaluating the pediatric heart. These differences help to determine situs (position), atrioventricular concordance, and ventriculoarterial concordance. The right atrium is normally connected to the two great veins, the **superior vena cava** and the **inferior vena cava**. The left atrium normally receives four pulmonary veins.

The right atrioventricular valve is called the **tricuspid valve**, having three fan-shaped leaflets connected to three sets of **chordae tendineae** which are, in turn, connected to three **papillary muscles**. The tricuspid valve has a more inferior or apical insertion point than does its counterpart on the left side. The right ventricle is triangular. It has a more heavily trabeculated endocardial surface, a moderator band in the lower third of the chamber, and an infundibular muscle band, or conus, in the right ventricular outflow tract.

On the other side, the left atrioventricular valve is called the **mitral valve**, having two fan-shaped or triangular leaflets inserted more superiorly on the septum toward the base of the heart. Normally, the mitral valve has two sets of **chordae** and two **papillary muscles**. The left-ventricular myocardium is relatively thicker than its counterpart on the right because it is pumping against higher pressures. The left ventricle has an ellipsoid shape and smooth endocardial surface. All of these characteristics help differentiate the right heart from the left heart.

The greatest volume of blood entering the right and left atria from their respective veins flows passively through the open atrioventricular valves into the ventricles. The pressure in the ventricles begin to rise. As the pressure rises, the atrioventricular valves (A-V) begin to close. The atria contract, forcing the A-V valves to reopen and the remainder of blood in the atria to be propelled into the ventricles. This is **diastole**.

The pressure in the ventricles is now greater than that in the atria. The A-V valves close, the semilunar valves open, and the cycle continues. This is **systole**. The ventricular pressure is now less than the atrial pressure as blood is continuously filling the atria. The semilunar valves close, the A-V valves open, and the cycle continues.

The right heart is concerned with the pulmonary circulation, moving blood to the lungs for oxygenation. The left heart is concerned with the systemic circulation, delivering oxygenated blood to the tissues. (See Figures 22–11 and 22–12.)

The flow of blood through the heart is as follows: Blood from the **superior vena cava**, **inferior vena cava**, and **coronary sinus** (draining the heart) empty into the right atrium. It then flows through the **tricuspid valve** into the right ventricle. From here the blood flows through the **pulmonary valve** into the main pulmonary artery. The main **pulmonary artery** branches into a right pulmonary artery to the right lung and a left pulmonary artery to the left lung. This is the pulmonary circulation.

Oxygenated blood returns to the left atrium via four **pulmonary veins**. From the left atrium it passes through the mitral valve into the left ventricle through the **aortic valve** into the ascending aorta. Blood fills the head and neck vessels and travels along the **descending aorta** to the tissues. This is systemic flow.

Cardiac Perfusion and Drainage

The **coronary arteries** perfuse the heart muscle and inner structures and are so named because they form a corona, or crown, around the heart. There are two main coronary arteries: the right coronary artery arises from the right sinus of Valsalva and the left coronary artery arises from the left sinus. (See Figure 22–13A.)

The right coronary artery courses in the atrioventricular groove separating the atria from the ventricles. It gives off a muscular branch and a marginal branch, and continues around the heart posteriorly until it anastomoses with, or joins, the left circumflex coronary artery. At this anastomosis, the right coronary artery gives off a branch called the posterior descending coronary artery, which travels along the posterior interventricular septum.

The left main coronary artery divides almost immediately into the left circumflex and the left anterior descending coronary arteries. The left circumflex extends around the heart posteriorly until it joins the right coronary artery, as mentioned. The left anterior descending coronary artery travels downward anteriorly along the interventricular septum, giving off muscular branches, or septal perforators. It curves posteriorly to meet the posterior descending coronary artery.

The veins that drain the heart do not form a corona, though they usually course with the arteries. They are simply called **cardiac veins**. (See Figure 22–13B.) Most of the veins drain into the coronary sinus, a large vein that serves as a reservoir. From here it empties into the right atrium through the thesbian valve. The veins that

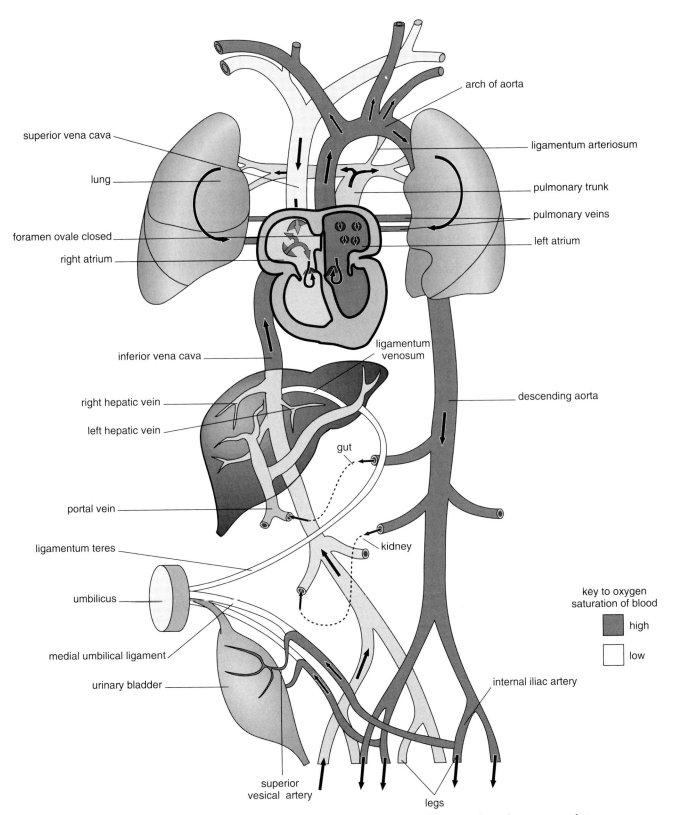

Figure 22–12. Neonatal circulation. Adult derivatives of the fetal vessels and structures that become nonfunctional at birth are also shown. Arrows indicate the course of the neonatal circulation. The organs are not drawn to scale. After birth, the three shunts that short circuited the blood during fetal life cease to function, and the pulmonary and systemic circulations become separated.

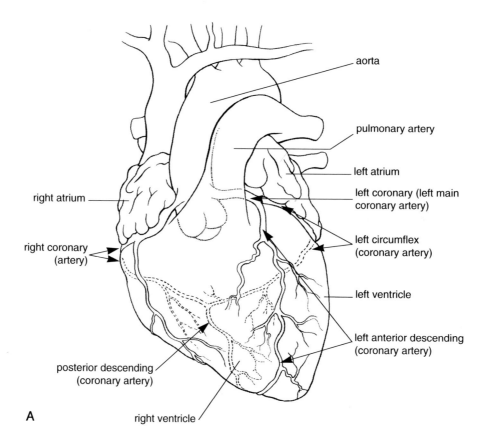

aorta

pulmonary artery

left atrium

left coronary (left main coronary artery)

left circumflex (coronary artery)

left ventricle

left anterior descending (coronary artery)

right atrium

right coronary (artery)

posterior descending (coronary artery)

right ventricle

A

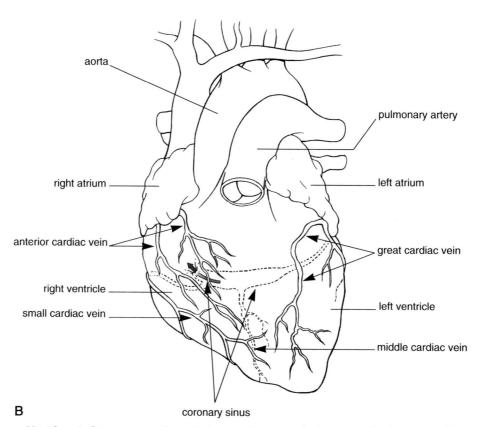

aorta

pulmonary artery

right atrium

left atrium

anterior cardiac vein

great cardiac vein

right ventricle

small cardiac vein

left ventricle

middle cardiac vein

B

coronary sinus

Figure 22-13. *A,* Coronary arteries and their positions on the heart. *B,* Cardiac veins. These are anterior or ventral views. The dashed lines indicate the position of the vessels as viewed from the posterior or dorsal surface of the heart.

do not drain into the sinus drain directly into the right atrium.

Normal variations in coronary artery anatomy and perfusion must be taken into account when an evaluation of them is needed for diagnostic purposes.

Cardiac Conduction

The cardiac conduction system is the mechanism by which the heart is made to effectively pump blood through the vessels. The muscle fibers of the heart have the inherent ability to contract without a nerve stimulus. However, if each fiber contracted independently, the heart would not be very effective in getting blood to the tissues.

The cardiac conduction system is a specialized group of cardiac muscle, nodes, tracts, and fibers which can generate and conduct electrical impulses through heart muscle, causing a synchronous, coordinated contraction or heartbeat. (See Figure 22–14.)

Figure 22–14. Cardiac conduction system and an ECG tracing. The numbers on the ECG corresponding with the numbers indicated on the heart diagram relate the electrical activity of the heart to the waveform of the ECG.

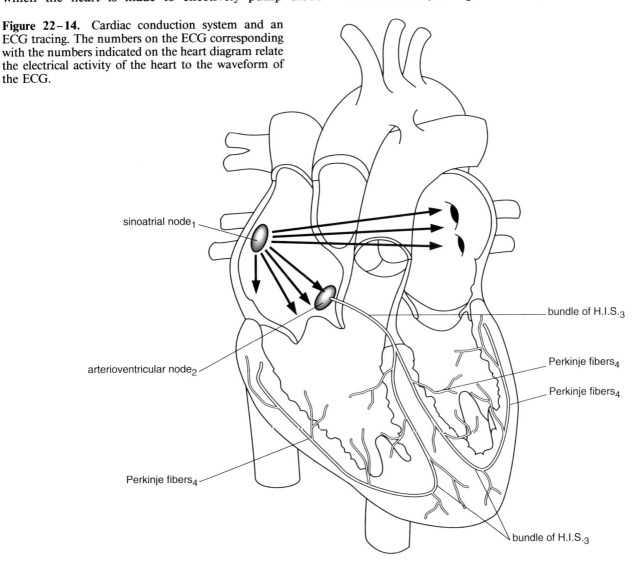

sinoatrial node₁

bundle of H.I.S.₃

Perkinje fibers₄

Perkinje fibers₄

arterioventricular node₂

Perkinje fibers₄

bundle of H.I.S.₃

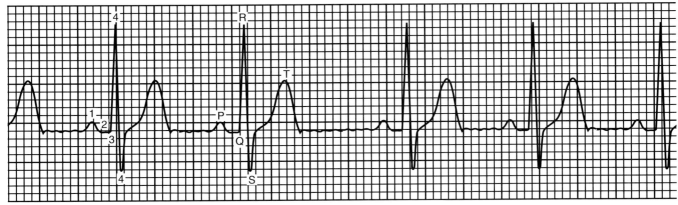

The **sinoatrial node**, or **SA node**, sets the pace of the heart. It is therefore called the pacemaker of the conduction system. The electrocardiogram (ECG or EKG) measures the electrical activity of the conduction system and indirectly myocardial activity. As the SA node fires, electrical impulses travel through internodal tracts to both atria, SA_1. On the ECG this is reflected by the P-wave signaling that atrial contraction is about to take place. Contraction occurs at once.

At the same time that impulses are passing through the atria, they also travel to the **atrioventricular**, or **A-V node**, located in the medial wall of the right atrium. There is a very brief delay in the activation and transmission of the A-V node. This is reflected on the ECG as the end of the P-wave, labelled 2 and $A-V_2$, on the heart diagram. After this delay the A-V node fires, sending impulses along the **bundle of His** located superficially on the interventricular septum. From here the impulses travel through the **Purkinje fibers** into the myocardium. The ventricles contract at once from above downward. The QRS deflection on the ECG reflects this transmission and is numbered 3 and 4. BH_3 and Pf_4 reflect this electrical activity.

The T-wave indicates a recovery of electrical charge in the ventricles or return of the myocardium to a resting state. The next cycle begins with another P-wave.

Normal pacemaker (SA node) rates (beats/min) at various ages are as follows[3]:

SA node rate	100–180	110–180	60–120	55–110	50–100
Age	0–1 mo	1 yr	5 yrs	10 yrs	Adult

Cardiac muscle, as mentioned earlier, has the inherent ability to contract without a nerve stimulus. However, stimulation by the autonomic nervous system (ANS) affects the rate of SA node firing and also the coronary arteries.

The sympathetic fibers of the ANS cause an increase in the heart rate. The parasympathetic division, specifically the vagus nerve, or tenth cranial nerve, causes the heart rate to slow down.

The semilunar valves, aortic and pulmonary, have three leaflets or cusps so named because they are "half-moon" shaped. The aorta has a right coronary cusp, a left cusp, and a noncoronary cusp. Immediately distal to these cusps are recessed pockets or outpouchings of the aorta called sinuses of Valsalva. These sinuses house the openings, or ostia, of the coronary arteries. There are three sinuses, each of which is associated with one cusp of the aortic valve. The right sinus is related to the coronary cusp where the ostium of the right coronary artery is located. The left sinus is behind the left cusp and houses the ostium of the left coronary artery. The noncoronary cusp is so named because no coronary artery is associated with its sinus.

PHYSIOLOGY

The heart is the primary organ of the circulatory system, providing the force that propels blood through all the vessels of the body.

The basic function of the heart is to receive deoxygenated blood from the head and body for transportation to the lungs and distribution of oxygenated blood to all parts of the body.

SONOGRAPHIC APPEARANCE

The heart muscle (myocardium) has a soft, homogeneous, even-textured echogenicity. The appearance ranges from medium to low intensity. The valves and chordae appear more echogenic than the myocardium. The valves will appear as thin, flexible lines that are freely mobile. The pericardium is the most echogenic structure, having a smooth, fluid-like, linear appearance.

Figure 22–15 shows the plane of sound through the heart in the parasternal long axis view. Figure 22–16 shows echocardiographic images in the parasternal long axis view and their schematic representations, respectively. Note the structures and their positions relative to one another. Also note that the left ventricular apex is not seen in this view.

Basic M-mode (for time-motion mode) includes measurements taken at the aortic valve level, the mitral valve level, and the chordal level in the left ventricle. (See Figure 22–17.)

Figure 22–18 shows an M-mode tracing of the left ventricle. Note the chordae on the inner surface of the left ventricular posterior wall. Figure 22–19 is a tracing at the mitral valve level. The echogenic areas seen in the right ventricle after each QRS complex are artifacts caused by inspiration of air into the lungs. The tracing of the aortic valve is shown in Figure 22–20 taken from the short axis view.

The planes of the short axis views through the heart are shown in Figure 22–15.

Figure 22–21 shows the echocardiographic image in the parasternal short axis view at the aortic valve level. Note that the commissure, or closure line, between the noncoronary and left coronary cusp of the aortic valve is not well visualized. This occurs because of the orientation of the plane of sound, which strikes the structure parallel rather than perpendicularly.

The mitral valve level is seen in Figure 22–22. The left ventricle should appear as a concentric circle; the anterior and posterior mitral valve leaflets should appear with the circle toward the posterior aspect of the cavity. In real time, the leaflets should open symmetrically and appear unrestricted in their movement. The left ventricular outflow tract is seen anterior to the mitral valve. The left ventricular walls should contract and relax concen-

Text continued on page 377.

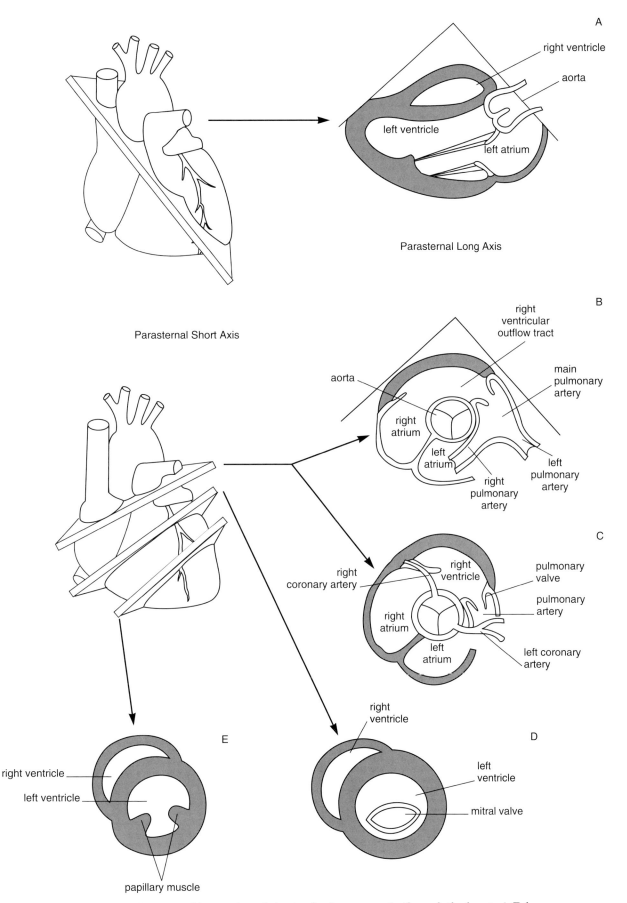

A

right ventricle

aorta

left ventricle

left atrium

Parasternal Long Axis

B

right
ventricular
outflow tract

main
pulmonary
artery

aorta

right
atrium

left
atrium

left
pulmonary
artery

right
pulmonary
artery

Parasternal Short Axis

C

right
coronary artery

right
ventricle

pulmonary
valve

pulmonary
artery

right
atrium

left
atrium

left coronary
artery

E

right ventricle

left ventricle

right
ventricle

D

left
ventricle

mitral valve

papillary muscle

Figure 22–15. Parasternal long axis and short axis planes, or cuts, through the heart. *A,* Echocardiographic sketch of the parasternal long axis view. *B,* Parasternal short axis view at the level of the aortic valve. *C,* Short axis view showing the coronary arteries. *D,* Short axis view at the level of the mitral valve and *E,* At the level of the papillary muscles.

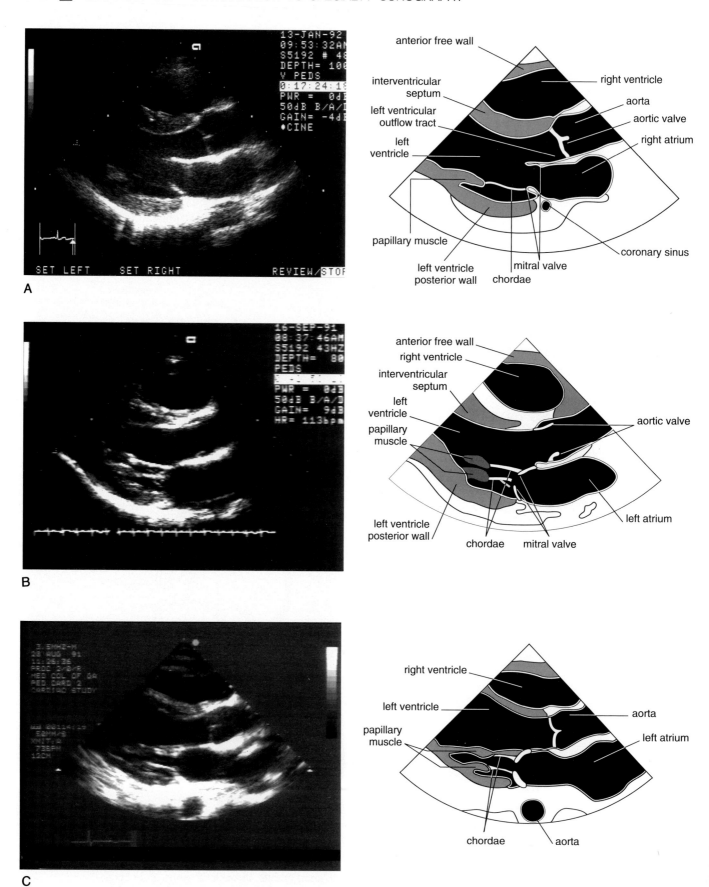

Figure 22–16. Echocardiographic images in the parasternal long axis view. *A*, Diastolic frame, *B*, Systolic frame, and *C*, Late diastolic frame.

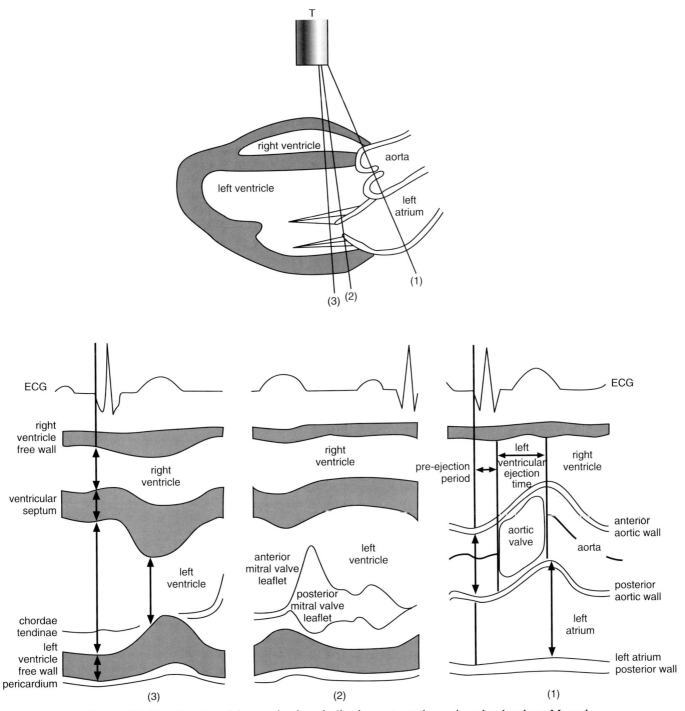

Figure 22-17. Parasternal long axis view, indicating cuts at the various levels where M-mode tracings will be recorded. The lower diagram is a schematic of an M-mode tracing at the various levels shown in the upper diagram. (From Park MK: Pediatric Cardiology for Practitioners, 2nd ed. Chicago, Year Book, 1988.) Currently, M-mode tracings are also being done in parasternal short axis views.

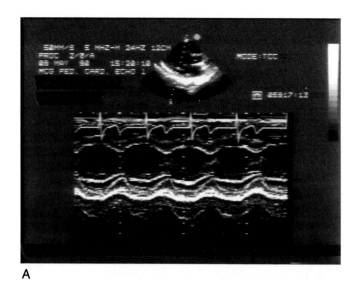

A

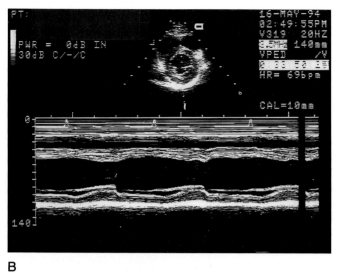

B

Figure 22–18. *A*, M-mode of the left ventricle in the parasternal long axis view. *B*, M-mode of the left ventricle in the parasternal short axis view.

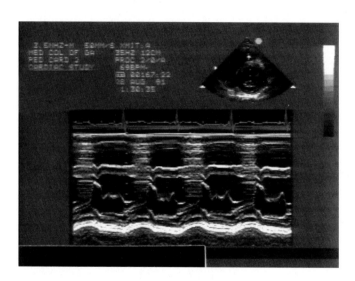

Figure 22–19. M-mode tracing of the mitral valve in the parasternal short axis view.

Figure 22–20. M-mode tracing of the aorta and left atrium from the parasternal short axis view.

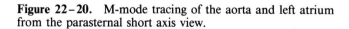

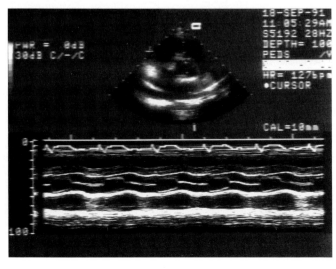

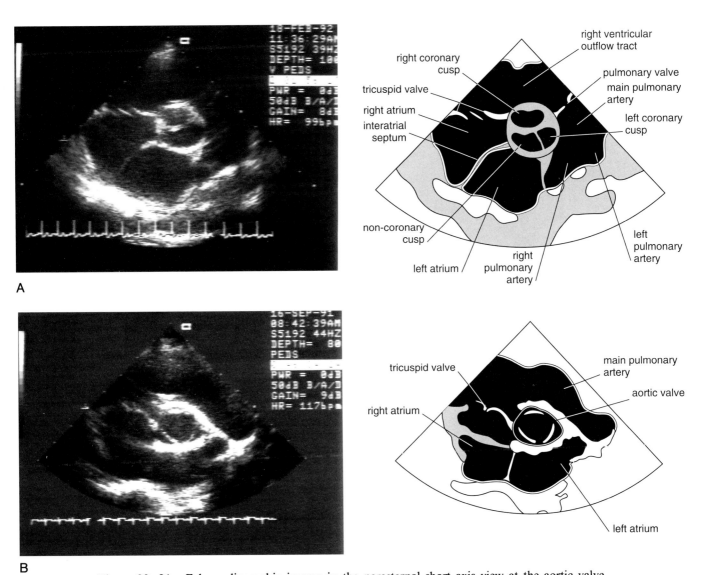

Figure 22–21. Echocardiographic images in the parasternal short axis view at the aortic valve level. *A*, with the valve closed and *B*, with the valve open.

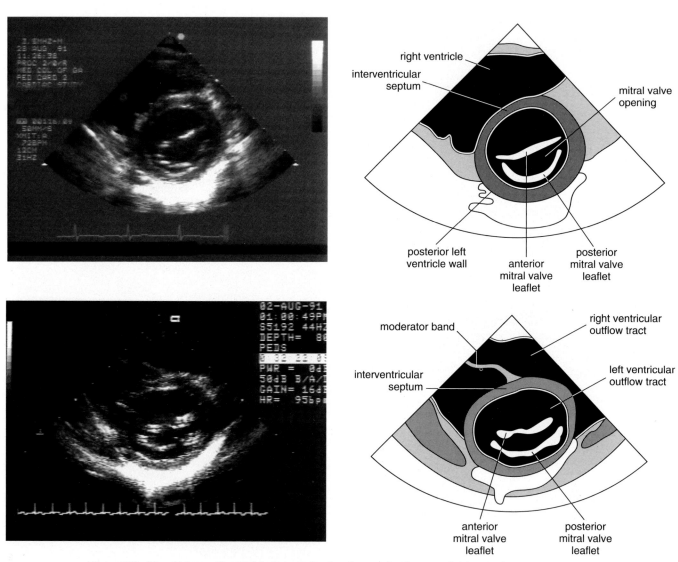

Figure 22–22. Echocardiographic images in the short axis plane at the level of the mitral valve.

trically and smoothly. The right ventricle is often seen in this view. It should look like a half-moon, adjacent to the interventricular septum. The moderator band may also be visualized.

The echocardiographic image and schematic of the papillary muscle level are shown in Figure 22-23. Again, the left ventricle should appear as a concentric circle. The anterolateral papillary muscle is seen at its usual position, 3 or 4 o'clock. The posteromedial papillary muscle is most often positioned at 8 o'clock. Note the areas of the interventricular septum, the anterior and anterolateral walls, the posterior lateral wall, and the inferoposterior wall of the left ventricle.

The apical views include the apical four chamber, the apical five chamber and the apical long axis. (See Figure 22-24.) There is also an apical two chamber view, not shown, visualizing the left atrium and ventricle only.

Echocardiographic images of the four chamber view are shown in Figure 22-25. All four cardiac chambers are visualized as well as the tricuspid and mitral valves. There may be an artifactual dropout of echoes in the midportion of the interatrial septum. The interventricular septum in usually seen in its entirety. It is usually possible to visualize the four pulmonary veins entering the left atrium. However, confirmation can be realized only by Doppler examination.

In the apical long axis view, note the left atrium, mitral valve, left ventricle, left ventricular outflow tract, the aortic valve, and the ascending aorta. (See Figure 22-26.)

Text continued on page 381.

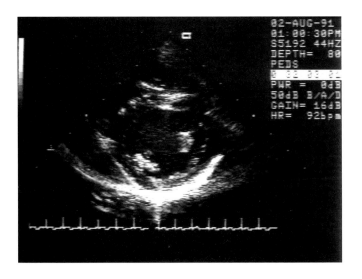

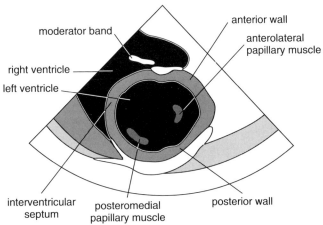

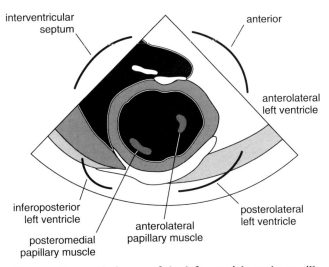

Figure 22-23. Echocardiographic image of the left ventricle at the papillary muscle level.

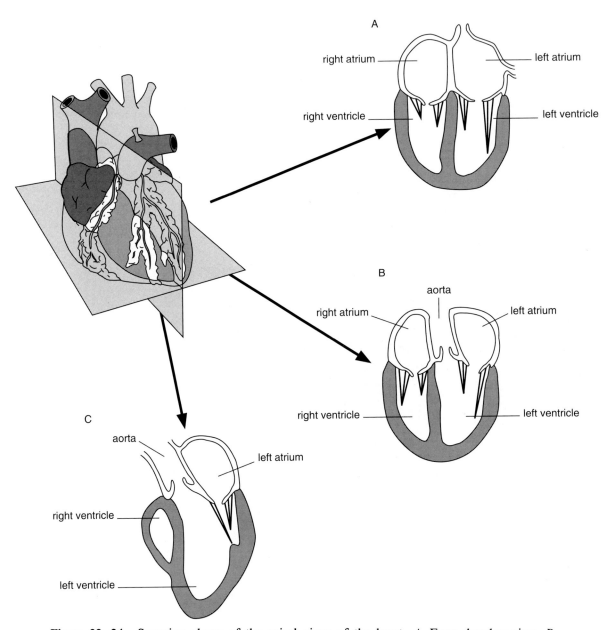

A
right atrium
left atrium
right ventricle
left ventricle

B
aorta
right atrium
left atrium
right ventricle
left ventricle

C
aorta
left atrium
right ventricle
left ventricle

Figure 22–24. Scanning planes of the apical views of the heart. *A*, Four chamber view, *B*, Five-chamber view, and *C*, Apical long axis view. (From Park MK: Pediatric cardiology for Practitioners. Chicago, Year Book, 1988.)

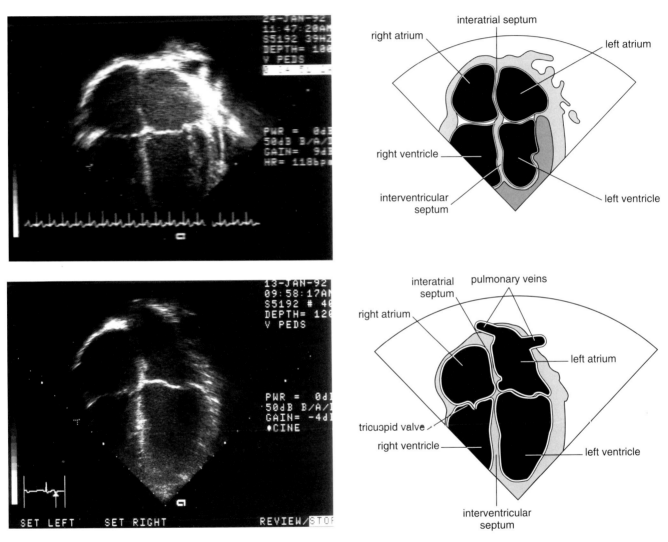

Figure 22-25. Echocardiographic images of the apical four chamber view.

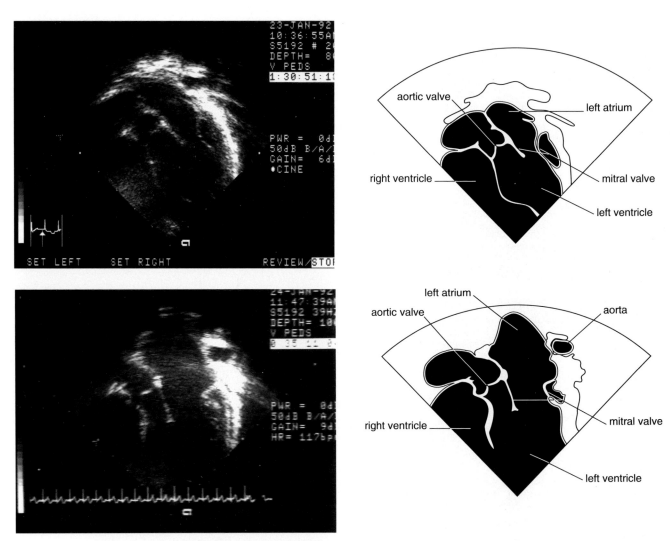

Figure 22-26. Echocardiographic images in the apical long axis view of two patients. Both are shown in the anatomically correct position.

Subcostal views provide a wealth of information. (See Figure 22–27.)

The subcostal four chamber view is used mainly to interrogate the interatrial septum. In this view the septum is perpendicular to the plane of sound giving the best possible image of the structure. (See Figure 22–28.) The entire heart and surrounding area can be seen very well in this view, making it excellent for determining situs and optimum for detecting pericardial efusions. (See Figure 22–29.)

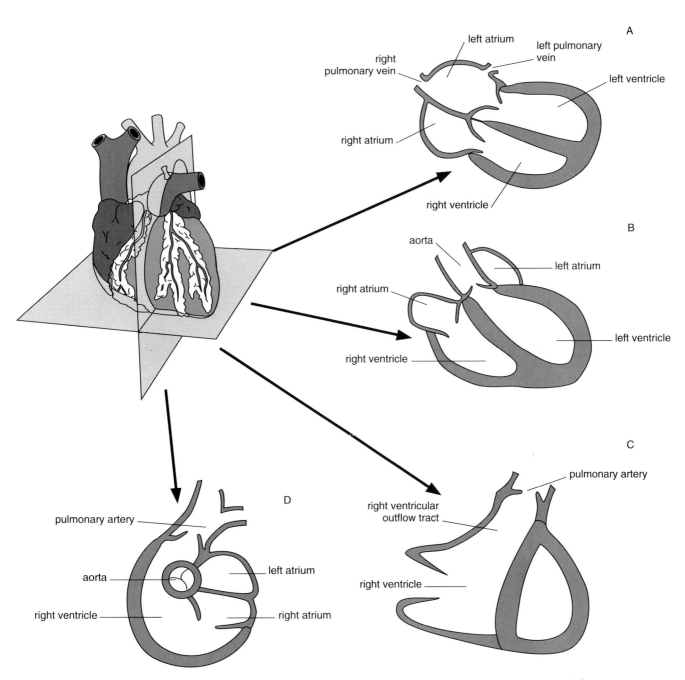

Figure 22–27. Four planes in the subcostal position are shown. *A,* Four chamber, *B,* Five chamber, *C,* Long axis of right ventricular outflow tract, and *D,* Short axis at aortic valve level. (Adapted from Park MK: Pediatric Cardiology for Practitioners, Chicago, Year Book, 1988.)

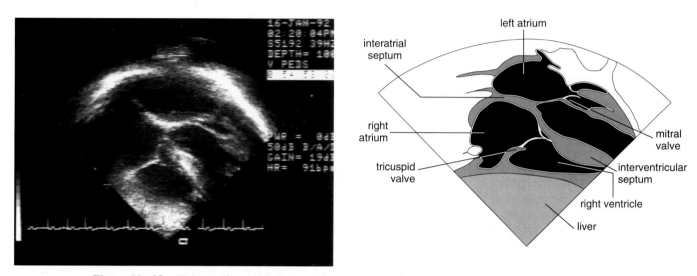

Figure 22-28. Echocardiographic image in the subcostal four chamber view for interrogation of the interatrial septum.

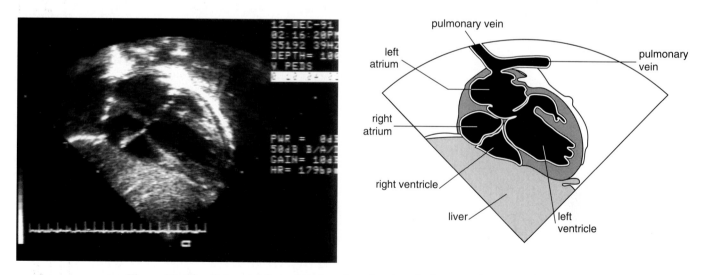

Figure 22-29. Subcostal four chamber view showing the heart and surrounding area.

See Figure 22–30 to visualize the suprasternal planes, particularly Figure 22–30A, for the long axis view of the aorta.

Figure 22–31 shows echocardiographic images and simplified diagrams, respectively, of the long axis of the aorta. The **ascending aorta, transverse arch,** and **descending aorta** are shown. The **innominate artery, left common carotid artery,** and **left subclavian artery** are visualized leaving the arch. The right pulmonary artery is cut in cross-section and is seen as a circular structure in the inner curvature of the arch.

The long axis of the right ventricular inflow tract is shown in Figure 22–32. It offers an excellent image of the right ventricular inflow tract. In some patients all three papillary muscles and chordae may be seen. Note the eustachian valve in the right atrium marking the entrance of the inferior vena cava.

The long axis view of the right ventricular outflow tract is shown in Figure 22–33. It includes the right ventricular outflow tract, pulmonary valve, main pulmonary artery, and the right and left pulmonary artery branches.

Views of the coronary arteries from the parasternal, short axis view, aortic valve level are shown in Figure 22–34.

Text continued on page 388.

A

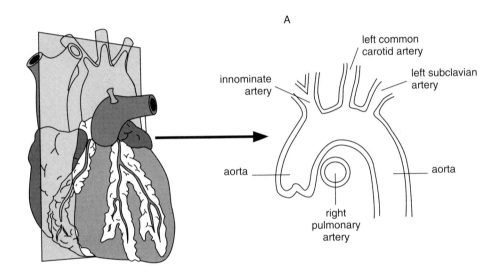

B

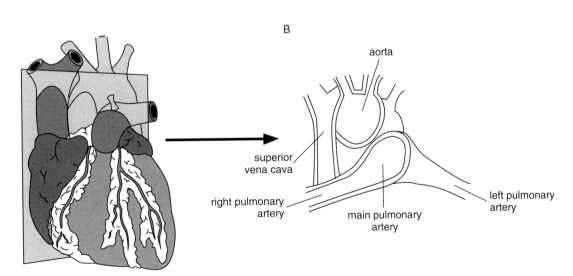

Figure 22–30. Schematic of the planes of sound through the heart in the suprasternal position. *A,* Long axis view and *B,* Short axis view. (From Park MK: Pediatric Cardiology for Practitioners. Chicago, Year Book, 1988.)

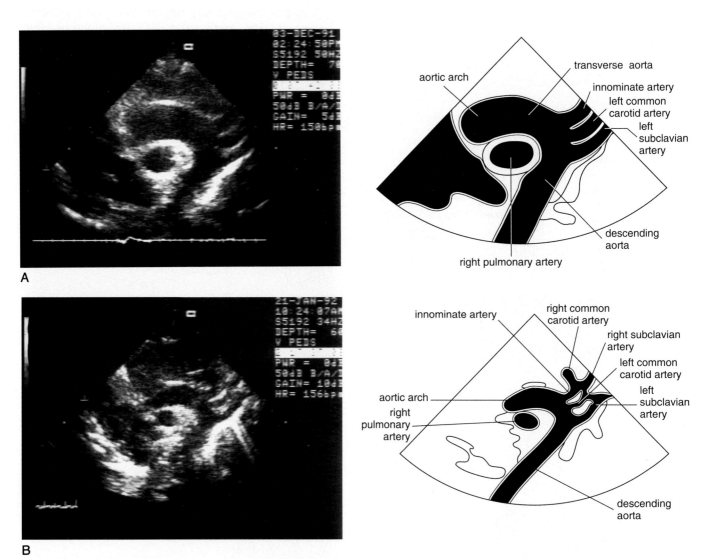

Figure 22–31. *A, B,* Echocardiographic images of the aortic arch in long axis. *B,* Note the bifurcation of the innominate artery into the right subclavian and right common carotid arteries.

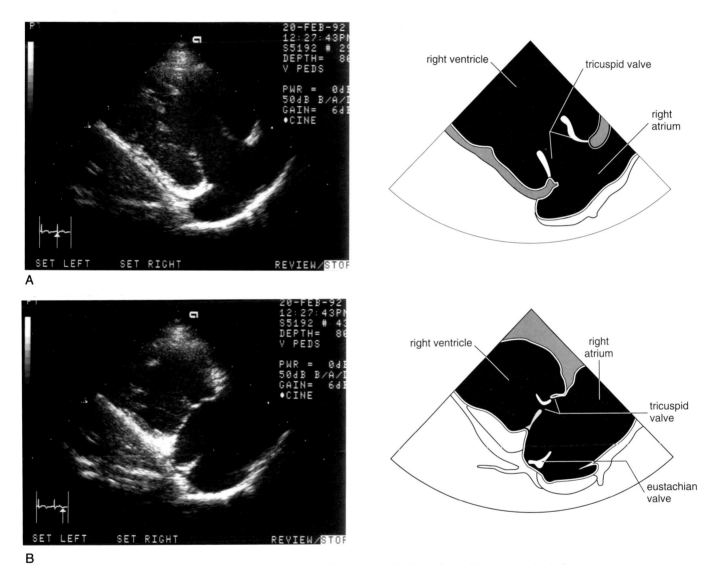

Figure 22-32. Echocardiographic image of the long axis view of the right ventricular inflow tract. *A*, Diastolic image, and *B*, Systolic frame.

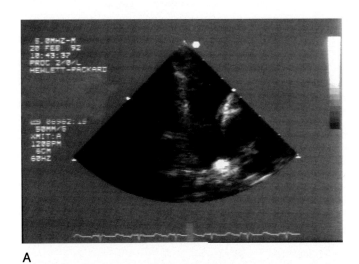
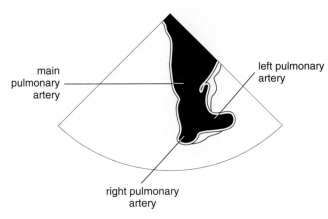

A

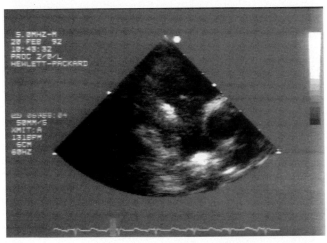
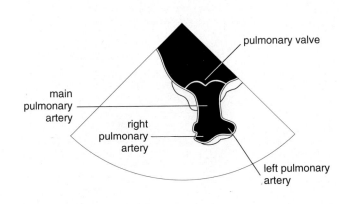

B

Figure 22-33. Echocardiographic image of the parasternal long axis of the right ventricular outflow tract. *A*, Systolic frame with the pulmonary valve open, and *B*, Diastolic frame with the pulmonary valve closed.

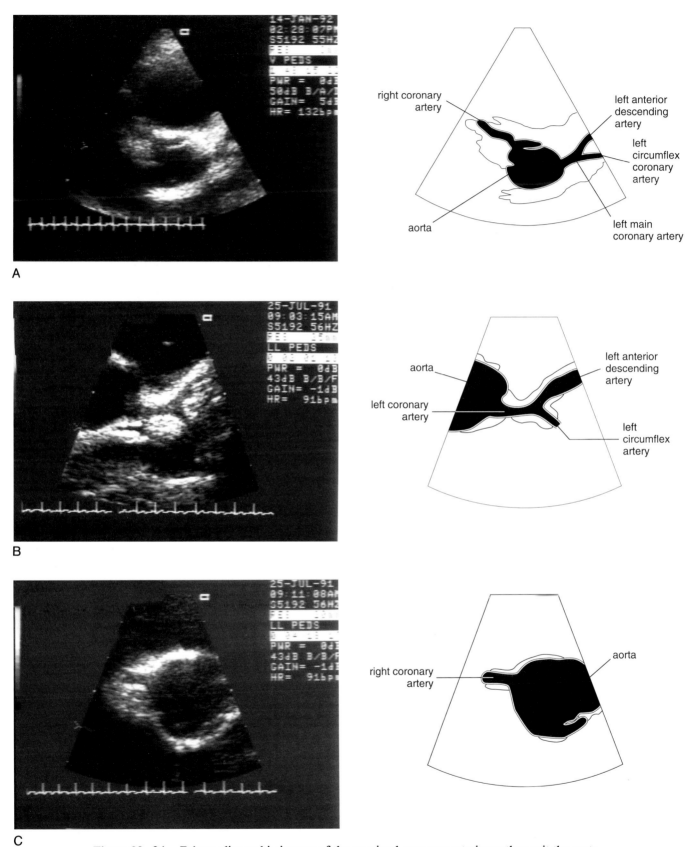

Figure 22–34. Echocardiographic images of the proximal coronary arteries as they exit the aorta. *A*, View of the RCA, LCA and bifurcation, LAD, and LCX. Part of the aortic valve leaflets are seen within the aorta. *B*, Image of the LCA and branches, and *C*, RCA. (RCA, right coronary artery; LCA, left coronary artery, LAD, left anterior descending coronary artery; LCX, left circumflex coronary artery.)

The long axis of the coronary sinus as it empties into the right atrium is seen in Figure 22–35.

Figures 22–36 are sagittal cuts. "A" is at the level of the long axis view of the left ventricular outflow tract, aortic valve, and ascending aorta. "B" is of the right ventricular outflow tract and the pulmonary valve. "C" is a short axis view of the heart at the aortic valve level.

The long axis of the superior and inferior venae cavae entering the right atrium is shown in Figure 22–37.

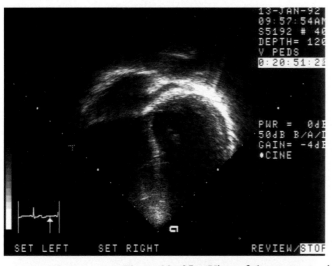
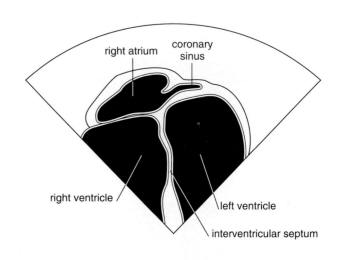

Figure 22–35. View of the coronary sinus from the apical four chamber position.

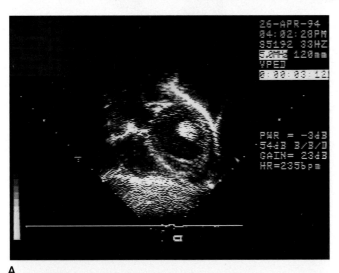
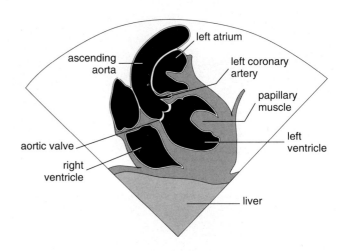

A

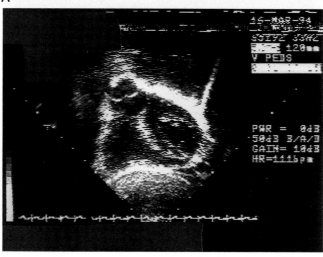
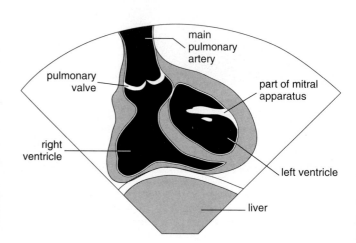

B

Figure 22–36. *A and B. See Legend on the following page.*

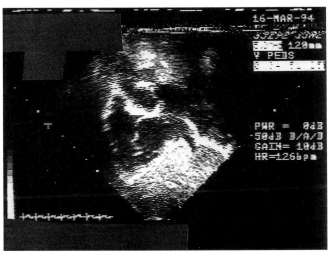
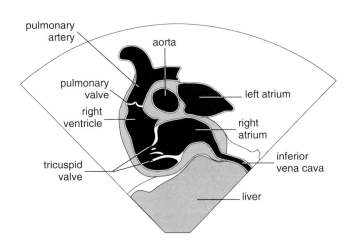

C

Figure 22–36. *A,* Subcostal short axis or sagittal view of the heart showing the left ventricular outflow tract, aortic valve, and ascending aorta. Note the left main coronary artery. *B,* Subcostal or subxiphoid short axis view demonstrating the right ventricular outflow tract, pulmonary valve, and main pulmonary artery. *C,* Subxiphoid short axis, aortic valve level showing left and right atrium, tricuspid valve, right ventricular outflow tract, and main pulmonary artery.

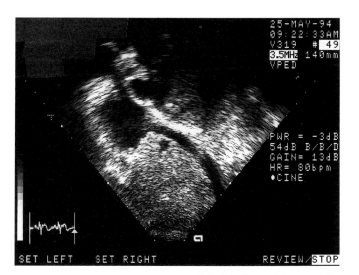
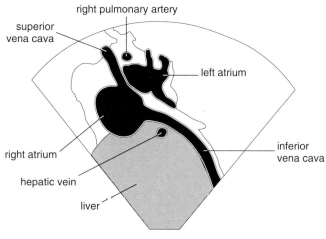

Figure 22–37. Subxiphoid view of the superior and inferior venae cavae entering the right atrium.

SONOGRAPHIC APPLICATIONS

Sonography is an aid in diagnosing congenital structural and flow abnormalities in the heart such as ventricular septal defect, patent ductus arteriosus, tetralogy of Fallot, transposition of the great arteries, and others. It helps in ruling out intracardiac masses and tumors. Sonography is helpful in assessing and monitoring heart size and function in patients on continual medical therapy which may affect the heart, such as chemotherapeutic drugs. Echocardiography is used to evaluate and monitor patients with conditions that directly or indi-

rectly affect the heart such as sickle cell anemia and Kawasaki disease. Sonography is used to evaluate the results of medical treatment and surgical repair of diseases of the heart.

NORMAL VARIANT

Dextrocardia

Dextrocardia is a condition in which the heart is located *to the right of the sternum* as a mirror image of its normal position on the left.

REFERENCE CHARTS

Associated Physicians

Radiologist: Specializes in the diagnostic interpretation of imaging modalities that aid in the diagnosis of heart disease.

Cardiologist: Specializes in the diagnosis and treatment of the diseases of the heart and related vessels.

Thoracic Surgeon: Specializes in the structural modification of the heart in the treatment of heart disease.

Common Diagnostic Tests

Chest X-ray Study: This record on photographic film, provides a picture of the ribs, lungs, and heart. If the possibility of congestive heart failure is considered, this study aids in determining whether the heart is abnormally enlarged and there is fluid in the lungs. The test is performed by a radiologic technologist and interpreted by a radiologist.

Electrocardiogram (EKG or ECG): This test monitors or measures the electrical activity of the heart and indirectly the heart muscle. Electrodes are placed on various positions on the chest and on each wrist and ankle. The electrodes are connected to a machine that amplifies the electrical impulses of the heart and records them on graph paper. A stress ECG may be done to measure the electrical activity of the heart during exertion, such as exercise on a treadmill. This test is usually performed by an ECG technician or a cardiologist and interpreted by a cardiologist.

Cardiac Scan: This scan involves the injection of a radioactive substance while a special camera traces its movement, through the heart. "Hot spot" imaging shows areas of heart muscle damage due to an infarct by increased activity in the area. A thallium scan will indicate areas where heart muscle is not receiving oxygen. A blood pool scan will reveal how efficiently blood is moving through the heart. This test is performed by a nuclear medicine technologist and interpreted by a radiologist or cardiologist.

Electrophysiologic Study (EPS): A catheter with electrodes attached to the end are placed through the femoral vein and guided to the heart. One electrode is placed near the sources of electrical activity, the SA node, and the bundle of His. Another electrode may be guided through the subclavian vein into the right ventricle. This study maps the electrical activity of the heart and is used to help diagnosis patients with various arrhythmias. It is more accurate than an ECG because the electrodes are closer to the source of the electrical activity. This test is performed by an EPS technician and cardiologist and interpreted by a cardiologist. It is a sterile procedure.

Cardiac Catheterization: Catheterization is a sterile procedure in which one or more catheters are introduced into a vein or artery and guided to the heart. The catheter can be used to assess intracardiac pressures, retrieve samples of blood for testing (oxygen content) and injecting contrast agent to render the heart visible on film. This test is used to evaluate chambers, valves, and coronary arteries. Cardiac catheterization is performed by cardiologists assisted by radiologic/cardiac technicians. The exam is interpreted by the cardiologist.

Laboratory Values

The laboratory values for the heart are shown in Figure 22-38. Note that the oxygen content in the pulmonary

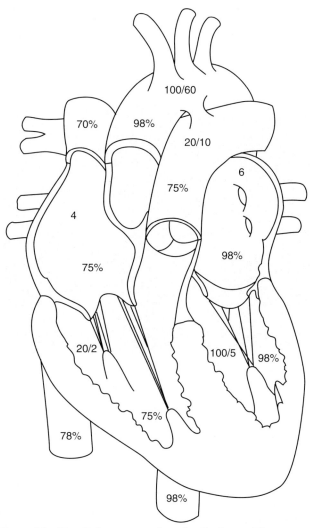

Figure 22-38. Laboratory values for the heart. The percentages show the relative oxygen saturations of the blood in the various vessels and cavities of the heart. The numbers with the slash between them show the normal systolic and diastolic pressures respectively. The pressure values in the atria are diastolic since they have no systolic pressure.

circuit is lower than in the systemic circuit. Normal oxygen content on the right side is usually between 65 percent and 80 percent. Oxygen content on the left side ranges between 95 percent and 100 percent.

The pressures on the left side are normally higher than those on the right side, with right-sided systolic pressures being about one fourth to one fifth of those on the left.

TABLE 22-1. Normal Values for Children Arranged by Weight[3]

	Weight (lbs.)	Mean (cm.)	Range (cm.)	Number of Subjects
RVD	0-25	.9	.3-1.5	26
	26-50	1.0	.4-1.5	26
	51-75	1.1	.7-1.8	20
	76-100	1.2	.7-1.6	15
	101-125	1.3	.8-1.7	11
	126-200	1.3	1.2-1.7	5
LVID	0-25	2.4	1.3-3.2	26
	26-50	3.4	2.4-3.8	26
	51-75	3.8	3.3-4.5	20
	76-100	4.1	3.5-4.7	15
	101-125	4.3	3.7-4.9	11
	126-200	4.9	4.4-5.2	5
LV and IV septal wall thickness	0-25	.5	.4-.6	26
	26-50	.6	.5-.7	26
	51-75	.7	.6-.7	20
	76-100	.7	.7-.8	15
	101-125	.7	.7-.8	11
	126-200	.8	.7-.8	5
LA dimension	0-25	1.7	.7-2.3	26
	26-50	2.2	1.7-2.7	26
	51-75	2.3	1.9-2.8	20
	76-100	2.4	2.0-3.0	15
	101-125	2.7	2.1-3.0	11
	126-200	2.8	2.1-3.7	5
Aortic root	0-25	1.3	.7-1.7	26
	26-50	1.7	1.3-2.2	26
	51-75	2.0	1.7-2.3	20
	76-100	2.2	1.9-2.7	15
	101-125	2.3	1.7-2.7	11
	126-200	2.4	2.2-2.8	5
Aortic valve opening	0-25	.9	.5-1.2	26
	26-50	1.2	.9-1.6	26
	51-75	1.4	1.2-1.7	20
	76-100	1.6	1.3-1.9	15
	101-125	1.7	1.4-2.0	11
	126-200	1.8	1.6-2.0	5

From Rudolph AM, et al: Rudolph's Pediatrics, 19th ed. East Norwalk, Appleton and Lange, 1991, p. 1340. Used with permission.

Normal Measurements

Normal measurements are presented in Table 22-1 below.

Vasculature

Aorta—Right and Left Coronary Arteries—Right and Left Coronary Artery Branches—Heart Muscle and Structures—Capillaries—Cardiac Veins—Right Atrium or Coronary Sinus—to Right Atrium.

Affecting Chemicals

Epinephrine: A hormone secreted by the adrenal medulla that causes an increase in the heart rate and an increase in the blood pressure.

References

1. Mallett M: Handbook of Anatomy and Physiology for Students of Medical Radiation Technology, 3d ed. Mankato, Burnell, 1981, 129-137.
2. Elson M: It's Your Body. New York, McGraw-Hill. 1975, 479.
3. Rudolph AM, et al: Rudolph's Pediatrics, 19th ed. East Norwalk, Appleton and Lange, 1991, 1340.

Bibliography

Feigenbaum H: Echocardiography, 4th ed. Philadelphia, Lea & Febiger, 1986.
Fink BW: Congenital Heart Disease a Deductive Approach to its Diagnosis, 2nd ed. Chicago, Year Book, 1985.
Monaghan MJ: Practical Echocardiography and Doppler, Chichester, Wiley, 1990.
Moore KL: The Developing Human, 4th ed. Philadelphia, WB Saunders, 1988, 286-333.
Snider A, Serwer GA: Echocardiography in Pediatric Heart Disease. Chicago, Year Book, 1990.
Williams G, et al: Echocardiographic Diagnosis of Cardiac Malformations. Boston, Little, Brown, 1986.

Chapter 23

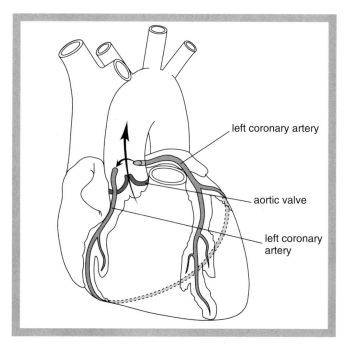

The adult heart. (From Guyton AC: Textbook of Medical Physiology, 8th ed. Philadelphia, WB Saunders, 1991, p 231)

ADULT ECHO-CARDIOGRAPHY

MAUREEN E. MCDONALD

Objectives:

Describe the location of the heart in the chest.

Describe the sonographic appearance of the heart.

Describe the imaging planes of the heart.

Identify cardiac anatomy in the various imaging planes.

Describe cardiac hemodynamics and physiology.

Describe the phases of the cardiac cycle, and relate them to intracardiac events.

Learn the normal values for heart chamber sizes, wall thickness, and Doppler flow velocities.

Identify normal Doppler flow patterns.

Define the key words.

Key Words:

Aortic valve

Apex

Apical

Appendage

Atrioventricular node (AV)

Atrioventricular valves

Atrium(a) (left and right)

Base

Bundle of His

Chordae tendineae

Continuous wave (CW)

Coronary arteries

Coronary sinus

Diastole

Doppler

Electrocardiogram

Endocardium

Epicardium

Eustachian valve

Inferior vena cava

Interventricular septum

Mitral (bicuspid) valve

M-mode echocardiogram

Moderator band

INTRODUCTION

The heart is the center of the cardiovascular system. It is a muscular organ, about the size of your fist, that beats over 100,000 times every day.

The heart's main function is to pump unoxygenated blood to the lungs and oxygenated blood to the vessels and tissues of the body.

The echocardiogram is a noninvasive diagnostic test used to evaluate the structural and hemodynamic relationships within the heart. It is an important tool used to assess overall cardiac function.

PRENATAL DEVELOPMENT

See Chapter 22, Pediatric Echocardiography pp. 355 to 364.

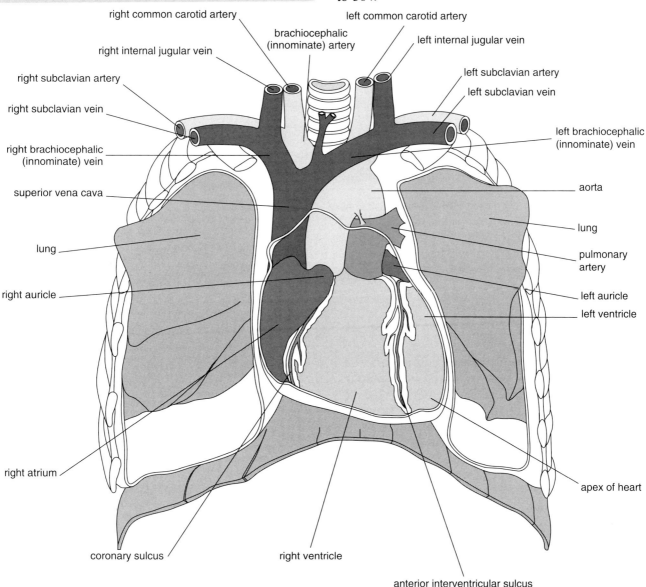

Figure 23–1. The external structures and location of the heart in the thoracic cavity.

LOCATION

The heart lies within the thoracic cavity, obscured by bone and lung. Located posterior to the sternum, the heart is situated between the right and the left lung within a space called the middle mediastinum. (See Figure 23–1.) The heart lies at a 45 degree angle, between the third and fifth intercostal spaces.

The heart sits within a sac called the **pericardium**. This sac contains a small amount (10 to 20 mL) of serous fluid that lubricates the heart as it beats.

The lower border of the heart forms a blunt point called the **apex**. The apex is formed by the tip of the left ventricle. It is directed to the left of the midline and sits more inferiorly and anteriorly than the **base** of the heart, where the great vessels arise.

The superior border of the heart is formed by the atria. The inferior portion is almost entirely right ventricle and only a small portion of the left ventricle.

The anterior surface of the heart is composed almost entirely of right ventricle, though a small portion of the right atrium and left ventricle can be seen. The left heart covers the posterior surface.

The right atrium makes up the right border of the heart, and the left ventricle, along with a small portion of the left atrium, covers the left border.

SIZE

The size of the heart is dependent on a person's age, weight, and sex. The American Society of Echocardiography has set standards by which the heart should be measured. These measurements will be discussed further in the section on M-mode echocardiography.

GROSS ANATOMY

The heart is a muscular four chambered pump located in the center of the chest. Internally it is divided into two collecting chambers (atria) and two pumping chambers (ventricles). A system of connecting arteries and veins allows the heart to move blood from systemic to pulmonary circulation and back. (See Figure 23–2.)

The walls of the heart consists of three layers: (1) the **epicardium**, the smooth, thin outer layer; (2) the **myocardium**, the thick layer of contractile muscle; and (3) the **endocardium**, the thin layer of endothelial tissue lining the internal surface.

The two upper cavities of the heart are the **right and left atria**. From the superior portion of each atrium is a small triangular extension called an **appendage**. The appendages are also called auricles (because they resemble ears). Within the appendages and extending out to the anterior surfaces of the atria are the pectinate muscles. The remaining endocardial surfaces of the atrial walls are smooth.

The atria are separated medially by the interatrial septum. Along this septum is a thinner oval region known as the fossa ovalis. This corresponds to the foramen ovale in the fetal heart.

The right atrium receives deoxygenated blood from all parts of the body including itself. The blood returning from the peripheral tissues enters the heart via the inferior and superior venae cavae. The coronary sinus also enters the right atrium and drains the vessels that had supplied the heart. The left atrium, on the other hand, receives blood from the lungs via four pulmonary veins.

The two inferior chambers are the **right and left ventricles**. The ventricles are thicker walled than the atria, with the left ventricle being almost three times thicker than the right. This is because the pressure is greater in the left heart than in the right. The right ventricle is also more trabeculated than the left and contains four prominent muscular bands; (1) parietal band, (2) crista supreventricularis, (3) septal band, (4) **moderator band** (often seen with ultrasound). Medially, the ventricles are separated by the **interventricular septum (IVS)**.

On the external surface of the heart, the ventricles are separated by the anterior and posterior interventricular sulci. The ventricles are then separated from the atria by the coronary sulcus. The sulci are grooves that contain the coronary vessels, all of which are embedded in fat. The fat serves to protect the vessels.

Located within the heart are four one-way valves. Their function is to maintain a uniform direction of blood flow. These valves are divided into two groups; atrioventricular and semilunar. The **atrioventricular valves** are located between the atria and the ventricles, and are anchored at one end to the annulosus fibrosus. **Chordae tendineae** attach the tips of the leaflets to **papillary muscles** located in the ventricles. Normally this arrangement keeps blood flowing in one direction only.

The **semilunar valves** are located at the junction where the ventricles meet the great vessels. They are called semilunar because each of the three leaflets is shaped like a half moon. The pocket shape of the leaflets, as well as the pressure exerted during diastole, closes the semilunar valves and prevents blood from moving backward.

The right-sided atrioventricular valve is called the **tricuspid valve** because it has three leaflets: anterior, posterior, and septal. The left-sided atrioventricular valve is called the **mitral (or bicuspid) valve** because of its similar appearance to a bishop's miter. It has two leaflets: anterior and posterior.

The two semilunar valves are the **aortic valve** and the **pulmonic valve**. The aortic valve is located at the junction of the left ventricle and the aorta. Its three cusps are the right coronary cusp, left coronary cusp, and the non-

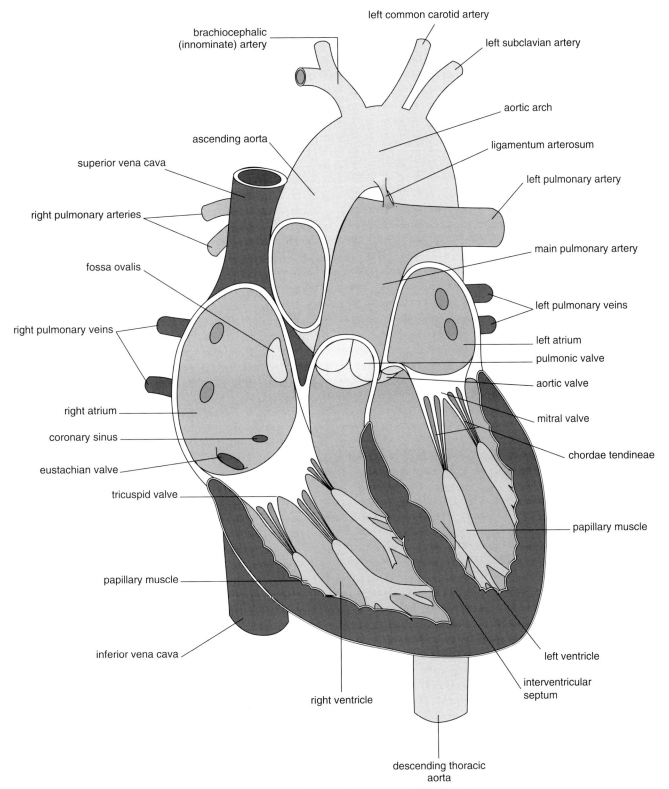

Figure 23-2. The internal structures of the heart.

coronary cusp. The pulmonic valve is located at the junction of the right ventricle and the pulmonary artery. It has three cusps: anterior, right, and left.

Just distal to the aortic valve in the proximal aortic root are outpouchings known as the sinuses of Valsalva.

Just as there are three cusps to the valve, there are three sinuses. This is where the **coronary arteries** originate. The right and left coronary arteries arise from the right and left sinuses of Valsalva. The noncoronary sinus has no artery associated with it.

PHYSIOLOGY

Circulatory System

As blood circulates throughout the body, it carries valuable nutrients and the oxygen required for survival of the tissues. Circulation of the blood is controlled by the heart.

Right heart circulation begins in the right atrium, which collects deoxygenated blood from the entire body. (See Figure 23–3.) Blood returning from the upper portion of the body enters the right atrium via the **superior vena cava**. Deoxygenated blood from the lower body enters the right atrium by way of the **inferior vena cava**. The heart also drains deoxygenated blood from itself through the **coronary sinus**. This blood also enters the right atrium.

Once the right atrium is full, the oxygen-depleted blood flows through the tricuspid valve and into the right ventricle. The right ventricle then pumps the blood past the pulmonic valve and into the **main pulmonary artery**. The main pulmonary artery shortly thereafter bifurcates into the **right and left pulmonary arteries**. These in turn enter each of the lungs where the blood is reoxygenated in the pulmonary circuit.

Once the blood has passed through the pulmonary-capillary circuit and reoxygenated, it needs to be collected and distributed to the heart and the rest of the body. This is the function of the left heart. Freshly oxygenated blood is returned from the lungs to the left atrium through the four **pulmonary veins**. The blood then passes from the left atrium, through the mitral valve, and into the left ventricle. The left ventricle then pumps the blood past the aortic valve and into the aorta. From here, the oxygenated blood is distributed to the heart and the rest of the body through the arterial system. This is the start of systemic circulation.

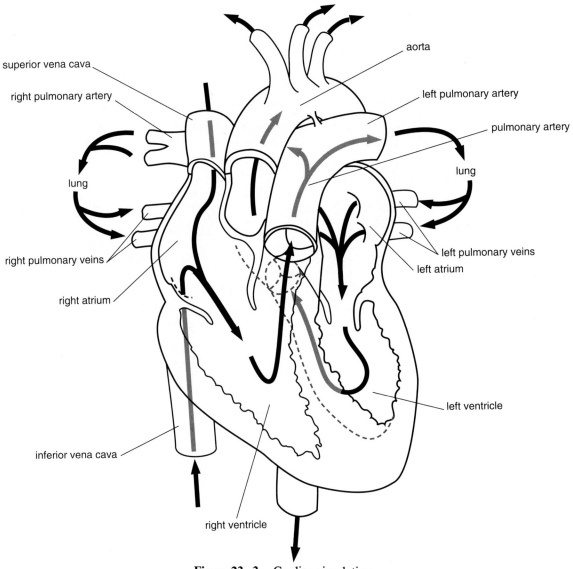

Figure 23–3. Cardiac circulation.

Cardiac muscle tissue needs a constant supply of fresh blood to remain viable. It accomplishes this through the coronary arterial system. There are two major coronary arteries: the right and the left main coronary arteries. The origin of the coronaries is the aortic root just posterior to the valve in the region of the right and left sinuses of Valsalva.

The left coronary artery differs from the right in that shortly after its origin, the left main artery bifurcates, forming the left anterior descending artery, which usually supplies the anterior left ventricular (LV) wall, apex, and a portion of the interventricular septum with oxygenated blood. The other branch is the left circumflex coronary artery, which mainly supplies the left atrium and the lateral and posterior walls of the left ventricle.

The right coronary artery also branches into the posterior descending artery, which supplies portions of the right and left ventricles with oxygenated blood, and the marginal artery, which supplies the right atrium and some of the right ventricle.

The heart also has a venous system which courses over its surface and drains into the coronary sinus. The specific pattern of the arteries and veins may vary from individual to individual.

The Conduction System

The heart has an intricate electrical system composed of highly specialized cardiac muscle tissue. The conduction system is designed to provide continuous electrical stimulation to the heart, assuring that the various segments of the cardiac cycle progress in the normal, sequential manner.

The conduction system is composed of four major sections; the **sinoatrial (SA) node**, the **atrioventricular (AV) node**, the **bundle of His** (pronounced hiss), and the **Purkinje fibers**. (See Figure 23–4.) Each section has a specific task to perform in regulating the cardiac cycle. In addition to its specific tasks, each portion of the conduction system has its own intrinsic rate of discharge. This allows the different sections of the conduction system to regulate the cardiac cycle in the event of a primary pacemaker failure. The dominant pacemaker of the heart is going to be the one discharging at the highest rate.

Normally, the SA node is the pacemaker. It therefore sets the basic pace for the heart rate with a discharge rate of between 60 and 100 beats per minute. Located in the upper portion of the right atrium, near the entrance of the superior vena cava, the SA node receives input from both the sympathetic and parasympathetic nervous systems. Electrical impulses from the SA node spread over both atria by way of internodal pathways, causing them to contract at the same time (atrial systole). This impulse is responsible for the P wave of the electrocardiogram and, in turn, causes the AV node to depolarize.

The AV node is the second section of the conduction system. It is located near the inferior portion on the right side of the interatrial septum. Its primary task is to delay transmission of the SA nodal impulse long enough to give the ventricles time to repolarize and fill completely. The AV node is responsible for the P-R interval of the electrocardiogram, with an intrinsic discharge rate of 55 beats per minute. In the event of SA node failure, the AV node is the backup pacemaker for the heart.

The impulse is then delivered to the final segments of the conduction system, the bundle of His and the Purkinje fibers. The bundle of His divides into the right and left bundle branches which run down the interventricular septum. The Purkinje fibers innervate the ventricular myocardium. Together they are responsible for distributing the electrical impulse to the ventricular muscle fibers, thereby causing mechanical contraction. This transmission is responsible for the QRS complex noted on the electrocardiogram. The bundle of His and the Purkinje fibers (with discharge rates of 40 to 30 respectively), are next in line in the event of pacemaker failure, with the ventricular myocardium (discharge rate of 20 beats per minute) acting as a final backup in the event of total pacemaker failure.

The Electrocardiogram

The **electrocardiogram** (ECG, EKG) is composed of a number of different waveforms that represent the electrical impulses of the cardiac cycle. These impulses can be detected on the surface of the body; when electrodes are placed on the skin, the change in the electrical field can be measured. Three distinct waves are recognized and labeled, with letters P, Q, R, S, and T. (Refer to Figure 23–5.)

The P wave and the P-R interval represent the final portion of the cardiac cycle, known as diastole. The P wave appears as a small upward bump. This reflects atrial depolarization caused by the SA node, as the electrical impulse travels through atrial muscle tissue. The atria contract, resulting in atrial systole. The P-R interval reflects the delay in transmission caused by the AV node.

The next downward deflection represents the beginning of the QRS complex, which continues in an upward direction and ends in a downward motion. This reflects the electrical stimulation of the ventricular myocardium, caused by the distribution of the electrical impulse through the bundle of His and the Purkinje fibers. The QRS complex represents the beginning of the portion of the cardiac cycle known as systole.

The T wave of the electrocardiogram represents the ventricular repolarization (relaxation) phase of the cardiac cycle, and marks the start of the diastolic portion of the cardiac cycle. The S-T segment is a refractory period and begins at the end of ventricular systole to the time of repolarization.

By study of the variations in the sizes of the deflections and the time intervals of the ECG, abnormal cardiac rhythms and conduction patterns can be diagnosed.

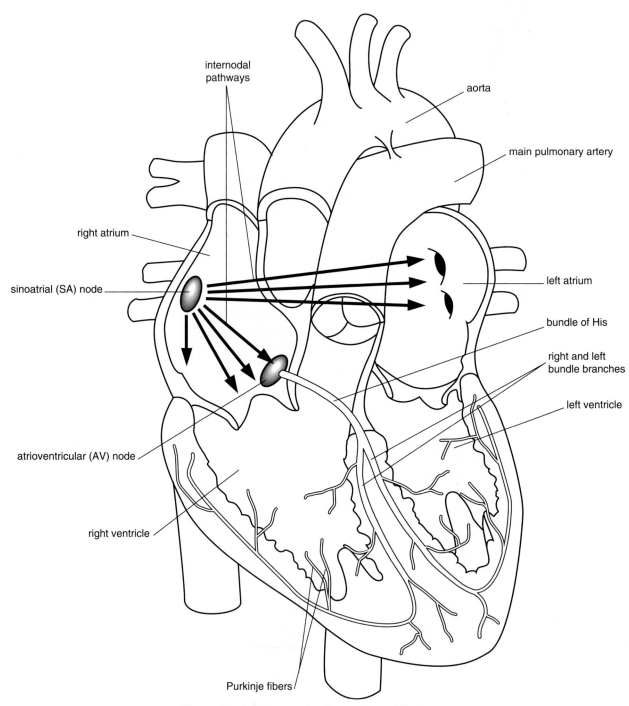

Figure 23–4. The conduction system of the heart.

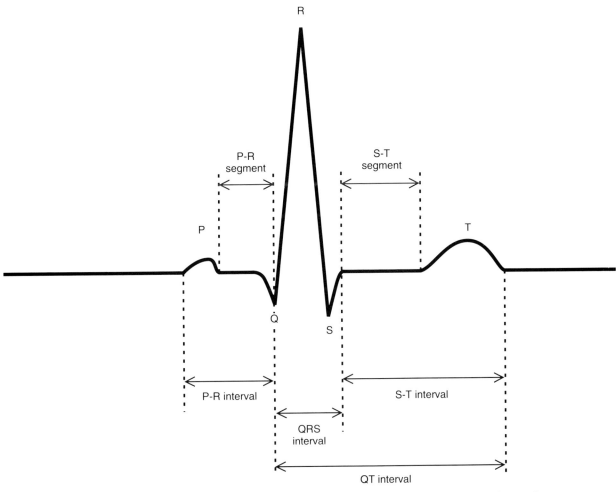

Figure 23–5. Single beat on a normal electrocardiogram demonstrating the QRS complex.

Systole/Diastole

The cardiac cycle is categorized into two separate and distinct segments: systole and diastole. Both segments contribute significantly to maintaining the cardiac output. A thorough understanding of the systolic and diastolic phases of the cardiac cycle as well as the hemodynamics (the movement of blood) associated with them will allow the sonographer to think through the echocardiographic examination.

Diastole is the left ventricular relaxation and filling phase of the cardiac cycle. Diastole occurs from the end of the T wave, until the beginning of the next QRS complex. During this portion of the cardiac cycle the atria are filling with blood. The AV valves are closed and the ventricular pressures are at or near 0 mmHg. As pressure in the atria rises to a point above the ventricular pressures, the AV valves open to eject the volume of blood into the ventricles. This is known as the rapid filling phase of the cardiac cycle. At that point, ventricular myocardium is relaxed. As pressures rise in the ventricle and fall in the atria, the AV valves begin to drift shut. Just prior to ventricular systole, the atria contract (corresponding to the P wave on the ECG) to eject their

final volumes of blood into the ventricles. This increases the amount of stretch on ventricular muscle fibers, thereby increasing the force of muscle contraction. During this period of time, the semilunar valves are closed and pressure in the ventricles increases just as the volume of blood increases, prior to systole.

Systole is the ventricular ejection phase of the cardiac cycle and occurs from the onset of the QRS complex to the end of the T wave. The ventricular muscle fibers contract. The increase in pressure causes the AV valves to close, preventing backflow of blood and the semilunar valves to open. The blood is ejected from the ventricles and enters the aorta and pulmonary artery. As the blood is ejected, the pressure in the ventricles starts to decrease and, in turn, pressure in the atria starts to increase. This sets the stage for the next cardiac cycle.

SONOGRAPHIC APPEARANCE

Two Dimensional Echocardiography

Sonographically, the pericardium is the most echogenic structure of the heart and is often seen as bright or white in color. Blood or any other fluids appear anechoic or black. The myocardium and papillary muscles are homogeneous and appear sonographically to be composed of medium-gray shades. The thin, mobile leaflets, or valve cusps, have a slightly increased echogenicity when compared to heart muscle, depending on the angle of the ultrasound beam.

A parasternal long axis view transects the heart from the base to the apex. (See Figure 23–6.) Most anteriorly, the right ventricle will be visualized. This is separated from the left ventricle by the interventricular septum (IVS). The IVS is continuous with the anterior portion of the aortic root. Only two of the aortic valve leaflets are visualized from this view. The more anterior leaflet is the right coronary cusp and the more posterior leaflet is the noncoronary cusp. Posterior to the aortic root is the left atrium. The posterior portion of the aortic root is continuous with the anterior mitral valve leaflet. The posterior mitral valve leaflet attaches to the valve annulus, near the atrioventricular groove. Attached to the posterior wall of the left ventricle, the posteromedial papillary muscle may be visualized. The chordae tendineae can be seen to extend from this muscle to the tips of the mitral valve leaflets. The area from the tips of the mitral valve leaflets to the aortic valve is considered the left ventricular outflow tract (LVOT). At the level of the atrioventricular groove a small echofree area may be noticed. This represents the coronary sinus. Posterior to the heart another anechoic area is seen. This represents a cross-section of the descending thoracic aorta.

During diastole, the mitral valve is in the open position, allowing the left ventricle to fill with blood, and the aortic valve is closed. (See Figure 23–7A.) As the ventricle fills with blood, the distance between the septal and posterior walls increases. During systole, the left ventricle contracts and the walls squeeze closer together. The mitral valve is now closed and the aortic valve is open, allowing blood to leave the left ventricle and enter the aortic root. (See Figure 23–7B.) The patient is connected to an EKG monitor which runs simultaneously along the image. This helps to assist in timing the cardiac cycle.

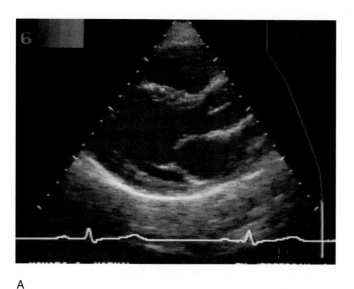

A

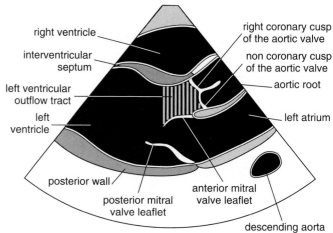

B

Figure 23–6. Two dimensional image (*A*), and illustration (*B*), including plane of section (*C*) of the parasternal long axis view.

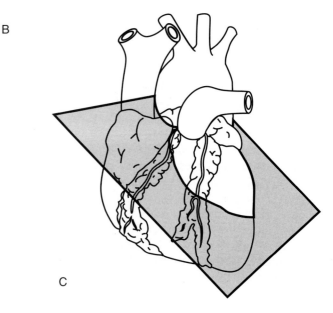

C

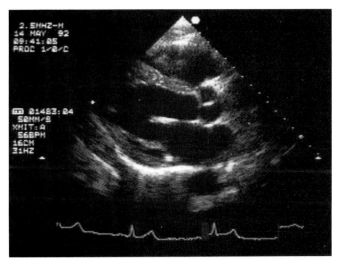

A

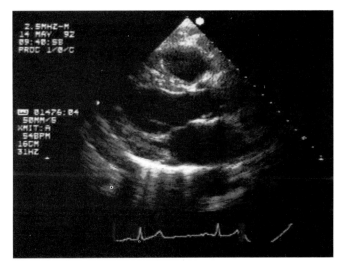

B

Figure 23–7. Two dimensional images of the parasternal long axis view in diastole (*A*) and systole (*B*).

In a parasternal short axis view at the level of the aortic valve the great arteries of the heart are visible. (See Figure 23–8.) Centrally located in this view is the aortic valve. This should appear as a circle with a Y in the middle, representing the aortic valve cusps in the diastolic phase of the cardiac cycle, when the leaflets are normally closed. At this point in the cardiac cycle one can easily visualize the right, the left, and the noncoronary cusps. During systole, the valve leaflets open to form a triangle. (See Figure 23–9.) The origin of the coronary arteries may be seen at this level near the right and left coronary cusps. Posterior to the aorta, the left atrium (LA) can be seen. In some instances, the left atrial appendage may be seen jutting off to the right of the screen. The right atrium can be seen on the left side of the screen separated from the left atrium by the interatrial septum (IAS). Moving anteriorly along the left side of the screen, the next structure noted is the tricuspid valve, which separates the right atrium from the right ventricle. The right ventricle is most anterior and can be seen wrapping around the aorta. The right ventricle is separated from the pulmonary artery, which is seen on the right side of the screen, by the pulmonic valve.

The mitral valve can be visualized from a parasternal short axis view. The heart appears as a circle with the anterior and posterior valve leaflets seen in the center of the image. (See Figure 23–10.) As the leaflets open and close during the cardiac cycle, they look somewhat like a fish's mouth. Anterior to the left heart is the right ventricle. These structures are separated by the interventricular septum.

At the level of the papillary muscles the left ventricle again appears as a circular structure and the papillary muscles protrude from the inner surface of the ventricular wall. Two papillary muscles are visible. (See Figure 23–11.) The posteromedial muscle is seen on the left of the screen and the anterolateral is seen on the right of the screen. The anechoic area within the left ventricle then takes on the shape of a mushroom. The right ventricle is again anterior to the left ventricle and separated by the IVS.

Figure 23–12 is an apical four chamber view displaying all four chambers of the heart. The ventricles are displayed at the top of the screen and the atria are displayed at the bottom of the two dimensional sector image. The left ventricle and left atria are displayed on the left side of the screen. The right ventricle and right atria are displayed on the right side of the screen. Wall motion can be evaluated from the apical view by further subdividing the left ventricle into basal (proximal), mid, and apical (distal) walls (Refer Figure 23–13.)

The interventricular septum separates the left from the right ventricle. Deep in the right ventricle, near the apex, the moderator band can be seen to cross from the right ventricular free wall to the interventricular septum. The interatrial septum separates the left from the right atria. The pulmonary veins can be seen entering the inferior portion of the left atrium. Both the anterior and posterior mitral valves can be seen in the left heart, while only two of the tricuspid leaflets can be seen in the right heart. The septal leaflet of the tricuspid valve is situated slightly closer to the apex of the heart (normally no more than 1 cm) than the anterior leaflet of the mitral valve.

Text continued on page 407.

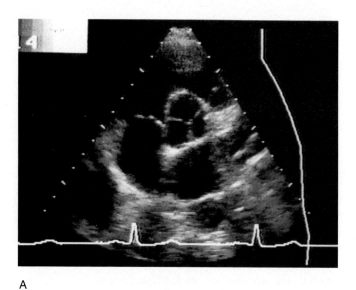

A

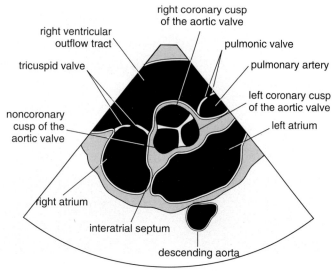

right coronary cusp
of the aortic valve

right ventricular
outflow tract

pulmonic valve

tricuspid valve

pulmonary artery

left coronary cusp
of the aortic valve

noncoronary
cusp of the
aortic valve

left atrium

right atrium

interatrial septum

descending aorta

B

Figure 23–8. Two dimensional image (*A*), and illustration (*B*) including plane of section (*C*) of the parasternal short axis view at the level of the aortic valve during diastole.

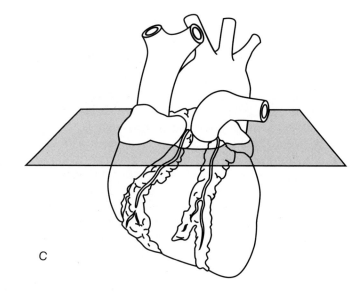

C

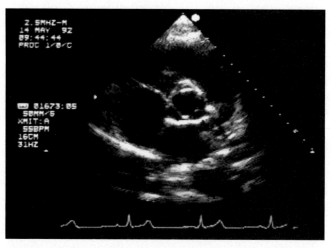

Figure 23–9. Two dimensional image of the parasternal short axis at the level of the aortic valve during systole.

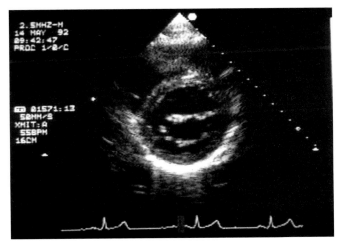

A

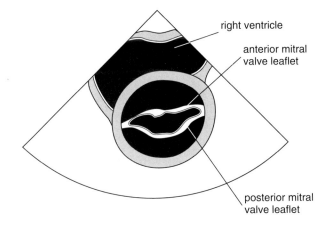

right ventricle

anterior mitral
valve leaflet

posterior mitral
valve leaflet

B

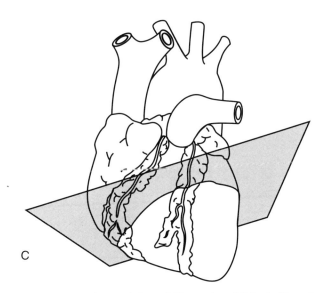

C

Figure 23-10. Two dimensional image (*A*), and illustration (*B*) including plane of section (*C*), of the parasternal short axis view at the level of the mitral valve.

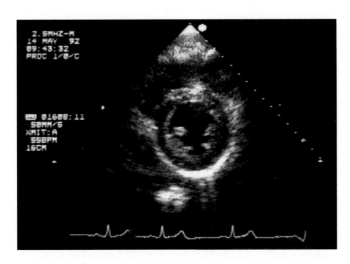

A

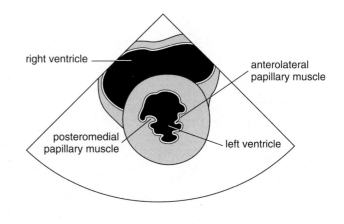

B

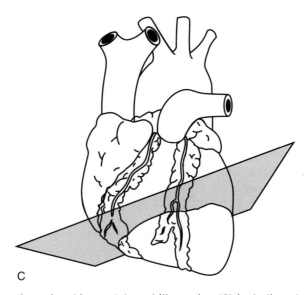

C

Figure 23–11. Two dimensional image (*A*), and illustration (*B*) including plane of section (*C*), of the parasternal short axis view at the level of the papillary muscles.

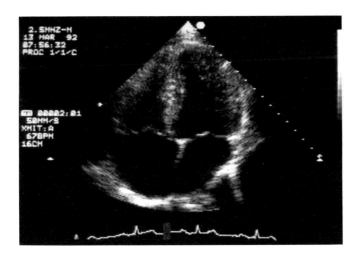

A

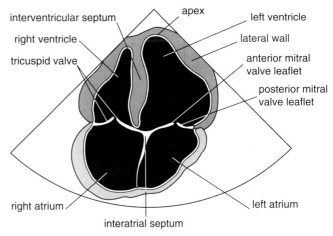

B

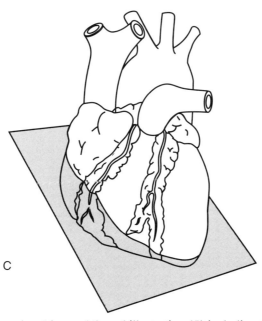

C

Figure 23-12. Two dimensional image (*A*), and illustration (*B*) including the plane of section (*C*) of the apical four chamber view.

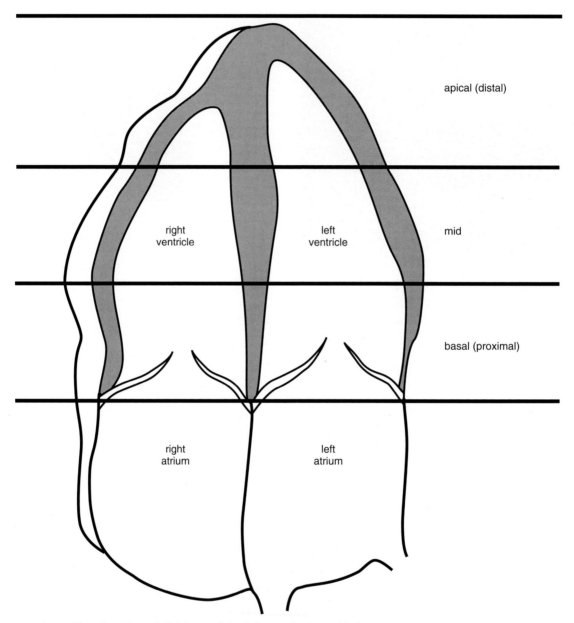

Figure 23–13. The subdivisions of the left ventricular walls from an apical four chamber view.

The aortic root can be imaged along with the other four chambers. This is referred to as an apical five chamber view. (See Figure 23–14.)

An image of the ascending and descending aorta and the aortic arch, as well as the vessels that arise from it, can be visualized from a suprasternal orientation. (See Figure 23–15). The vessels in descending order are (1) brachiocephalic (or innominate) artery, (2) left common carotid artery, (3) left subclavian artery.

Posterior to the arch, a cross-sectional view of the right pulmonary artery can be seen. In some instances, the left atrium can be seen posterior to this.

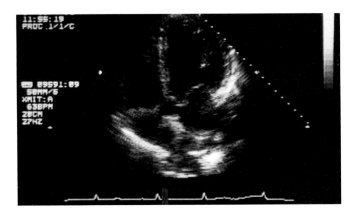

A

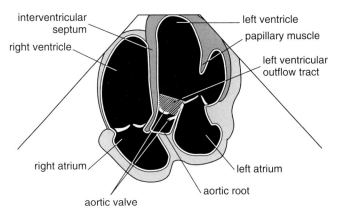

B

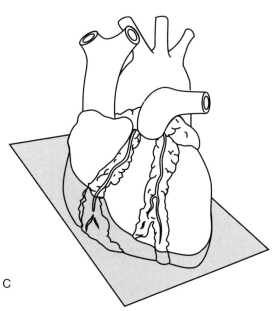

C

Figure 23–14. Two dimensional image (A), and illustration (B) including plane of section (C), of the apical five chamber view.

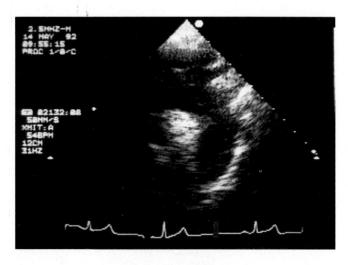

A

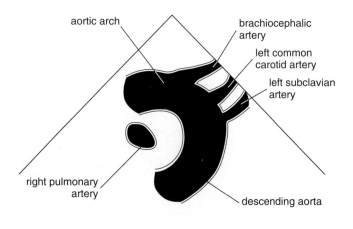

aortic arch

brachiocephalic artery

left common carotid artery

left subclavian artery

right pulmonary artery

descending aorta

B

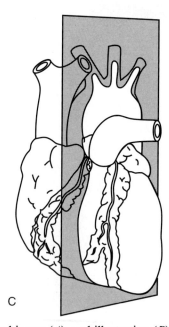

C

Figure 23–15. Two dimensional image (*A*), and illustration (*B*) including plane of section (*C*), of the aortic arch from the suprasternal notch.

M-Mode Echocardiography

Two dimensional imaging is a very powerful diagnostic tool and has superseded the qualitative role of M-mode in the echocardiographic examination. Yet M-mode is still an important supplement to the cardiac examination. It provides a quantitative system through which measurements of cardiac structures can be obtained. Where a structure should be measured and what is considered normal is based on the recommendations of the American Society of Echocardiography. This makes the practice of assessing an M-mode consistent.

M-mode is also a tool for evaluating subtle changes or rapid movements of the heart that the eye may not see during the real time examination.

Simply put, the M in M-mode stands for motion. Imagine drawing a line through the heart. Everything along that line is portrayed on a graph, creating a one-dimensional reproduction of the cardiac structures.

An M-mode is a measure of distance over time. Distance is presented on the x axis and is calibrated by a series of dots that are 1 cm apart. Time is displayed across the y axis. Here a series of dots 0.5 second apart are used for calibration (See Figure 23–16.)

The M-mode is most commonly scrolled on paper from a strip chart and appears as a black tracing on a white background.

The anatomy seen at the level of the aortic valve includes the right ventricle anteriorly, the anterior wall of the aortic root, the posterior wall of the aortic root, and the left atrium. The aortic valve is seen within the aortic root. Only two cusps are seen from this view: the right coronary cusp, anteriorly, and the noncoronary cusp, posteriorly. (See Figure 23–17.) These cusps can be seen to form a sort of box during systole as blood is ejected from the left ventricle. The closed valve appears as a straight line during diastole.

The mitral valve is a biphasic valve caused by the rapid filling phase of the LV and the atrial "kick" in the latter part of the cardiac cycle. (See Figure 23–18.) The valve is open during diastole and closed during systole. Its biphasic quality causes the motion of the anterior leaflet to appear in the shape of an M. The posterior leaflet mirrors the anterior and appears as a W.

The anterior leaflet of the mitral valve is labeled alphabetically to correspond with the various phases of diastole. (See Figure 23–19.) To begin with, the D point represents the opening of the valve during diastole and the E point represents the maximum excursion of the leaflet. This occurs during the passive filling phase. The anterior leaflet then begins to close. The point where it stops moving posteriorly is the F point. The next peak anterior motion of the mitral valve is the A wave. This corresponds to atrial contraction and the P wave on the

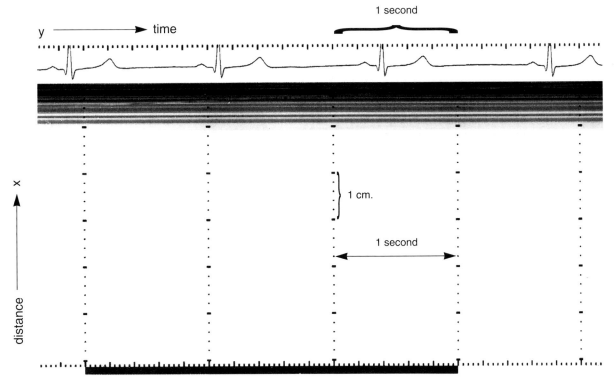

Figure 23–16. Proper calibration for an M-Mode.

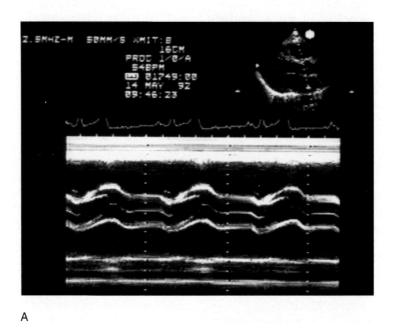

A

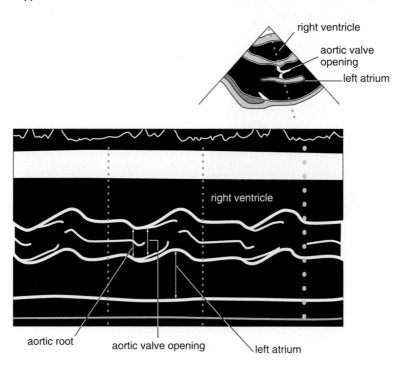

right ventricle

aortic valve
opening

left atrium

right ventricle

aortic root   aortic valve opening   left atrium

B

Figure 23–17. Two dimensional image (*A*), and illustration (*B*) of an M-mode at the level of the aortic valve.

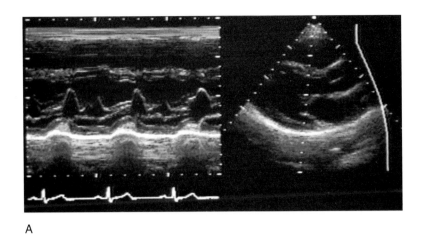

A

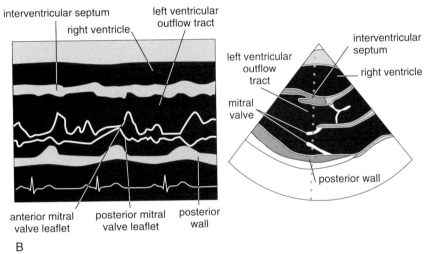

interventricular septum

left ventricular outflow tract

right ventricle

interventricular septum

left ventricular outflow tract

right ventricle

mitral valve

anterior mitral valve leaflet

posterior mitral valve leaflet

posterior wall

posterior wall

B

Figure 23–18. Two dimensional image (*A*), and illustration (*B*) of an M-mode at the level of the mitral valve.

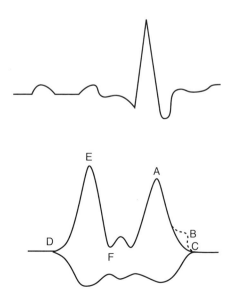

Figure 23–19. Proper labeling of the mitral valve.

ECG. Valve closure is appropriately represented by the C point. In some situations, such as diastolic dysfunction of the left ventricle, an additional bump may occur between the A and C points. This abnormal closure of the valve creates what is known as a B notch.

M-mode sampling from the left ventricle is seen in Figure 23–20. Starting anteriorly, the anatomy seen is the right ventricle, the interventricular septum, the left ventricle, and the posterior wall of the left ventricle.

Other areas of the heart can be evaluated by M-mode. Generally, the only other structures seen are the valve leaflets from the tricuspid and pulmonary valves. Normally, only one tricuspid valve leaflet is seen with M-mode. (See Figure 23–21.) The pulmonic valve is most difficult to visualize, but can be especially helpful in patients with pulmonary stenosis or hypertension. (See Figure 23–22.) The pulmonic valve is also labeled using letters A through F.

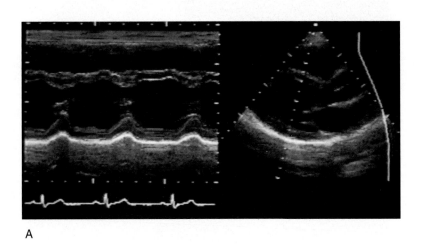

A

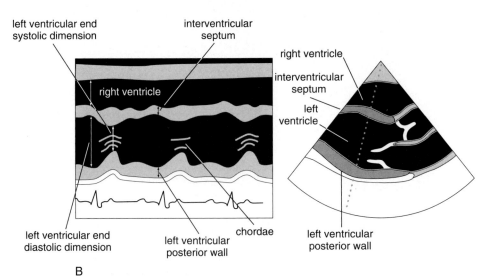

B

Figure 23–20. Two dimensional image (*A*) and illustration (*B*) of an M-mode at the level of the left ventricle.

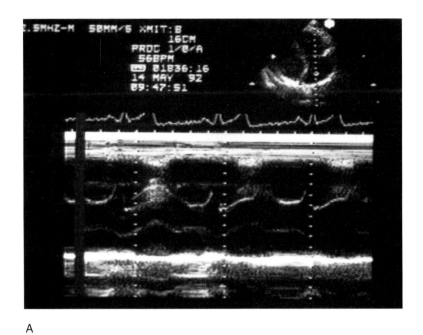

A

B

Figure 23–21. Two dimensional image (*A*) and illustration (*B*) of an M-mode through the tricuspid valve.

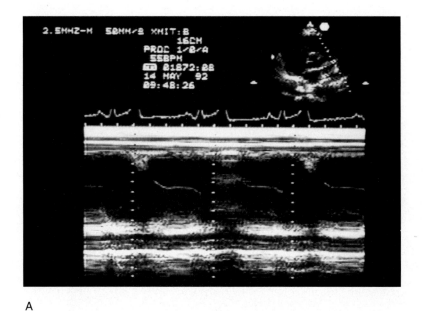

A

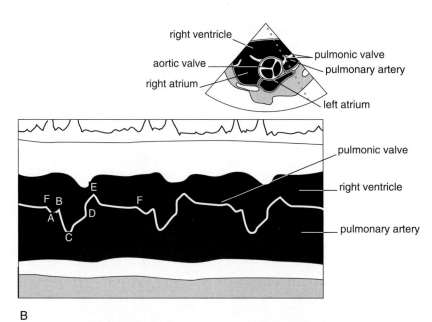

B

Figure 23–22. Two dimensional image (*A*) and illustration (*B*) of an M-mode through the pulmonic valve with its proper alphabetical labels.

Doppler Echocardiography

Spectral Doppler and color flow mapping are two forms of Doppler used to derive hemodynamic information about the heart. Spectral Doppler is divided into two forms: pulsed wave and continuous wave. Each has its advantages and disadvantages but should be used in conjunction to realize their full potential.

Normal Doppler Waveforms

Normal flow within the heart has a characteristic appearance. When interrogating each valve it is important to recognize these normal patterns so that any type of disturbance can be fully evaluated. Abnormal flow within the heart indicates increased velocities, regurgitation, and turbulence.

It is also important to note the direction of flow. Blood moving toward the transducer will be represented above the baseline on the Doppler strip and flow moving away from the transducer will fall below the baseline. When evaluating a profile, it is important to look at the pattern, velocity, direction of flow, and timing, in accordance with the cardiac cycle.

Doppler is best evaluated when flow is parallel to the transducer. This is not necessarily where the best two-dimensional image was obtained.

The Mitral Valve. Normal mitral flow is biphasic, taking the shape of an M. Like the M-mode tracing, the E wave is higher than the A wave. In the apical four chamber view, flow moves toward the transducer from the left atrium to the left ventricle. Mitral flow, therefore, is above the baseline and occurs during diastole. (See Figure 23–23.)

The Aortic Valve. Normal aortic flow is systolic and is shaped like a bullet. When sampled from the apical five chamber view, blood moves away from the transducer; from the left ventricle to the aortic root. Here the profile would appear below the baseline. (See Figure 23–24.)

The Aortic Arch. Either the ascending or the descending aorta may be evaluated from the suprasternal notch. Depending on how the transducer is angled, flow will appear above the baseline within the ascending aorta and below the baseline within the descending aorta. Flow will be systolic and bullet shaped. (See Figure 23–25.)

The Tricuspid Valve. Normal tricuspid flow is also shaped like an M. It occurs during diastole and appears above the baseline. The velocity range is lower than that for the mitral valve. This is due to lower pressures found in the right heart. (See Figure 23–26.)

The Pulmonic Valve. The systolic flow of the pulmonic valve appears below the baseline and has a bullet shape. (Refer to Figure 23–27.)

In addition to a duplex Doppler evaluation, which provides an image of the heart along with the Doppler waveform, a dedicated continuous wave Doppler probe may be used. (See Figure 23–28.) This specialized probe provides only the spectral waveform, without the two-dimensional image.

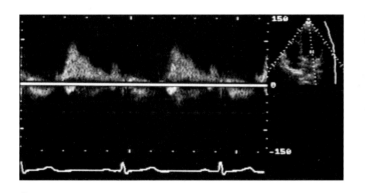

A

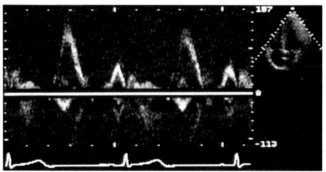

B

Figure 23–23. Doppler flow profiles of the mitral valve in both continuous wave (*A*) and pulsed wave (*B*).

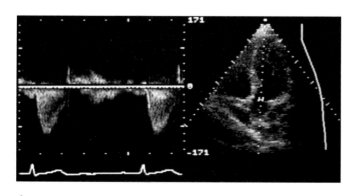

A

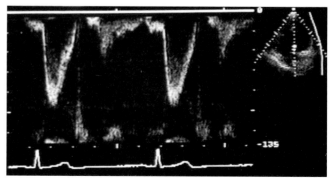

B

Figure 23–24. Doppler flow profiles of the aortic valve in both continuous wave (*A*) and pulsed wave (*B*).

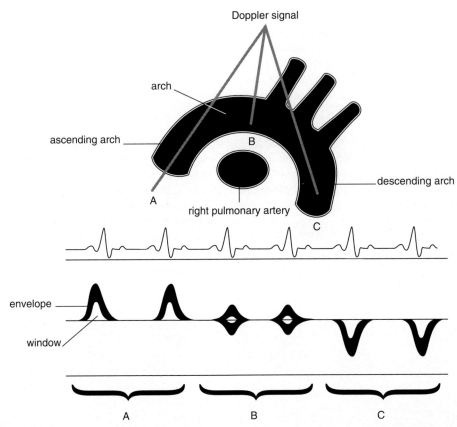

Figure 23–25. Doppler flow in the aortic arch. As flow moves toward the transducer in the ascending aorta, it appears above the baseline; as the flow moves away in the descending aorta, it falls below the baseline.

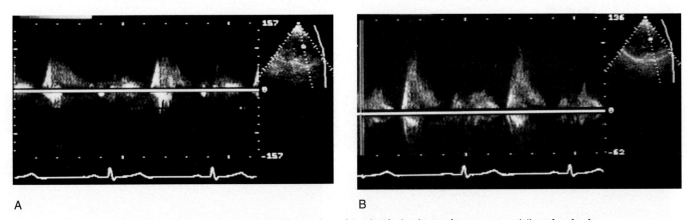

A

B

Figure 23–26. Doppler flow profiles of the tricuspid valve in both continuous wave (*A*) and pulsed wave (*B*).

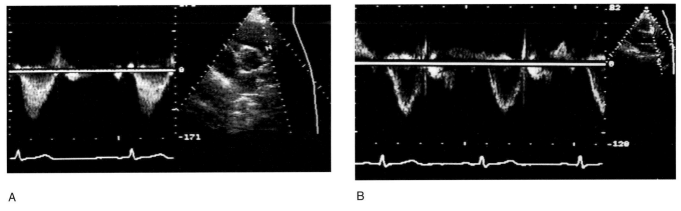

A   B

Figure 23–27. Doppler flow profiles of the pulmonic valve in both continuous wave (*A*) and pulsed wave (*B*).

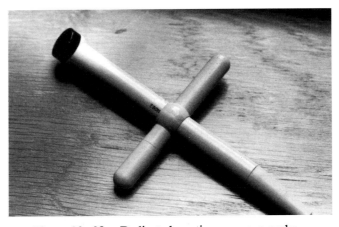

Figure 23–28. Dedicated continuous wave probe.

SONOGRAPHIC APPLICATIONS

Echocardiography is commonly used in the evaluation of the following: cardiac anatomy, cardiac size, acquired heart disease (stenosis, valve replacement), congenital heart disease, coronary heart disease, pericardial diseases, cardiac tumors/thrombi, diseases of the aorta, cardiomyopathies, and hemodynamic information.

NORMAL VARIANTS

Eustachian Valve

The **eustachian valve** can be seen in the right atrium near the entrance of the inferior vena cava. In the fetus, it was a functional valve covering the IVC. Only a remnant of the valve is now seen. It is best visualized in the right ventricular inflow view.

Moderator Band

The moderator band is a normal tissue structure that extends from the anterior free wall of the right ventricle to the interventricular septum. It provides a quick path for the conduction system to reach the ventricular wall. The moderator band is best visualized in the apical four chamber view.

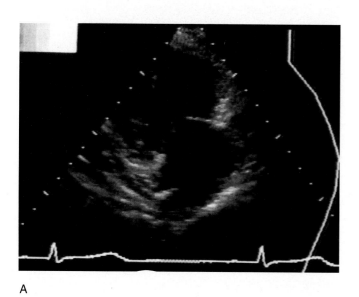

A

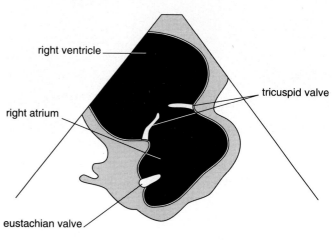

B

Two dimensional image (*A*) and illustration (*B*) of the eustachian valve as seen in the right ventricular inflow view. Found in the right atrium, it is a normal variant.

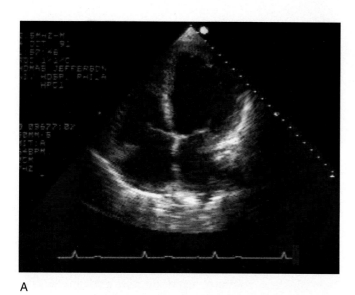

A

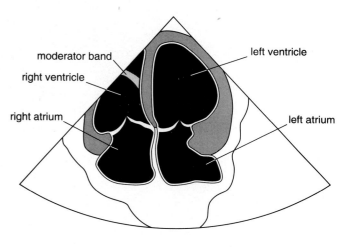

B

Two dimensional image (*A*) and illustration (*B*) of the moderator band as seen in the apical four chamber view. It is a normal structure found in the right ventricle.

Chiari Network

The Chiari network appears as a fine mobile fiber within the right atrium that originates near the entrance of the inferior vena cava and often extends to the crista terminalis. This can be seen in any of the views in which the right atrium is pictured.

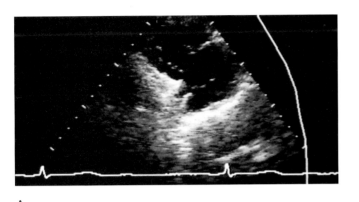
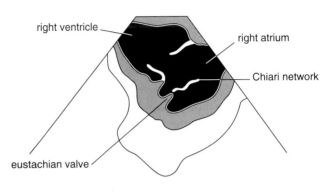

A

B

Two dimensional image (*A*) and illustration (*B*) of a Chiari network as seen in the right ventricular inflow view. It is a normal variant found in the right atrium.

Ectopic Chordae

Ectopic chordae are thin fibrous strands that extend from one ventricular wall to another. They can be found in either ventricle and are best visualized in the apical views.

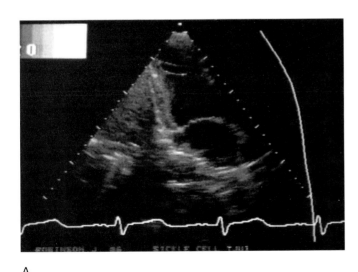
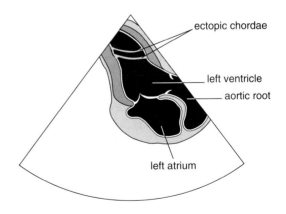

A

B

Two dimensional image (*A*) and illustration (*B*) of ectopic chordae as seen in the left ventricle of the apical long axis view. These are normal variants and can be found in either ventricle.

Interatrial Septal Aneurysm

An interatrial septal aneurysm appears as a bulge in the atrial septum that moves to and fro with respiration.

This is best seen in either the apical four chamber view or the subcostal four chamber view.

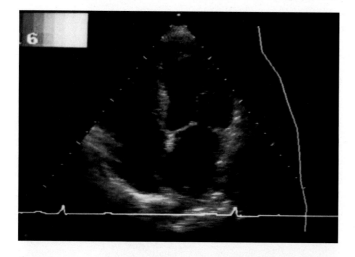

A

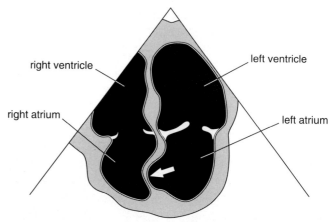

B

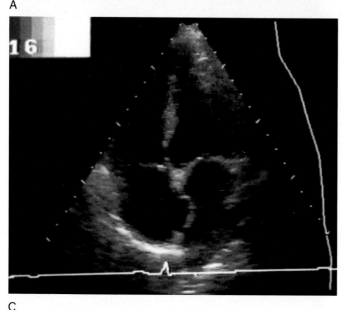

C

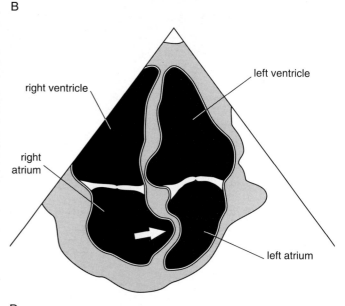

D

Two dimensional image (*A,C*) and illustrations (*B,D*) of an interatrial septal aneurysm as seen in the apical four chamber view. This is considered a normal variant and moves to and fro with respiration.

REFERENCE CHARTS

Associated Physicians

Cardiologist: Specializes in the medical treatment of patients with heart disease.

Radiologist: Specializes in the diagnostic interpretation of imaging modalities; therefore, some radiologists may also read echocardiograms.

Common Diagnostic Tests

History and Physical Examination: The cardiologist questions the patient to gather a good history and performs a full physical examination. This can help determine the diagnosis.

Auscultation: Listening to the sounds of the heart with the aid of a stethoscope.

Chest X-ray Study: This provides information on the size and structure of the heart. At times the cardiac silhouette is diagnostic for specific abnormalities. The test is performed by a technician but is interpreted by either the radiologist or the cardiologist.

Electrocardiogram (ECG): Provides information on the electrical behavior of the heart during the cardiac cycle. A technician performs the test, which is then interpreted by a cardiologist.

Exercise Stress Test: The patient may be exercised on a bicycle or treadmill when coronary artery disease is suspected. During the stress test an ECG is done. This provides information on functional changes in the heart and determines the degree of stimulus that will provoke an adverse reaction. Thallium can also be used. It is a radionuclide that traces the path of the blood as it flows through arteries and perfuses the myocardial cells. A stress test is not performed when valvular disease is suspected. The technician performs the test in the presence of a cardiologist, who then interprets the results.

Transesophageal Echocardiography (TEE): A semi-invasive procedure in which a specialized ultrasound probe is swallowed by the patient. The heart is then viewed from the esophagus. This allows the heart to be visualized without interference from lung, bone, or body habitus. The study can be done on either an inpatient or an outpatient basis. In addition, TEE can be used during surgery to monitor cardiac function. The cardiologist performs and interprets the study. The role of the technician is to assist the cardiologist with the operation of the machine and to help monitor the patient's status.

Computed Axial Tomography (CT) and Magnetic Resonance Imaging (MRI): These are two other imaging studies that can be used in the evaluation of heart disease. They are most useful in evaluating cardiac masses, tumors, or effusions. They are often performed by a technician but may be done in the presence of a physician. These tests are interpreted by a radiologist.

Cardiac Catheterization: An invasive technique in which the tip of a long catheter is introduced into either an artery or a vein through an arm or leg. The catheter is then threaded into the heart. This is an important clinical test used to evaluate coronary artery disease, ventricular and valvular function, pressures within the chambers and across the valves, and the oxygen content of the blood (important in cases of septal defects). The test is performed and interpreted by a cardiologist.

Laboratory Values

Creatine Phosphokinase (CPK): An enzyme found in all muscle tissue. The MB fraction of CPK helps in assessing the presence of myocardial infarction. Elevation of CK-MB indicates that an infarct is present. The CK-MB should peak within 24 hours.

Lactic Dehydrogenase (LDH): LDH is also found throughout the body and a certain percentage is used to assess myocardial infarction. LDH usually peaks within 24 to 48 hours and when elevated indicates the presence of an infarct.

Normal M-Mode Measurements

Aortic root dimension: 1.9–4.0 cm
Aortic cusp separation: 1.5–2.6 cm
Left atrial dimension: 1.9–4.0 cm

Mitral valve excursion: 1.6–3.0 cm
Mitral valve EF slope: 70–150 mm/sec
Left ventricular end diastolic dimension: 3.5–5.7 cm
Left ventricular ejection fraction: >55%
Left ventricular fractional shortening: >25%
Interventricular septal thickness: 0.6–1.2 cm
Posterior left ventricular wall thickness: 0.6–1.2 cm
Right ventricular dimension: 0.7–2.7 cm

Normal Doppler Velocities in Adults

Mitral valve: 0.6–1.3 m/sec
Aortic valve: 1.0–1.7 m/sec
Tricuspid valve: 0.3–0.7 m/sec
Pulmonic valve: 0.6–0.9 m/sec
Left ventricular: 0.7–1.1 m/sec

Affecting Chemicals

Epinephrine: Produced by the adrenal medulla, it increases the excitability of the SA node, thereby increasing the heart rate and the strength of the contractions.

Potassium: Can interfere with nerve impulse generation; therefore, it decreases heart rate and the strength of the contractions.

Sodium: Also may decrease heart rate and contraction strength since it tends to interfere with calcium participation in muscular contraction.

Calcium: As with sodium, a high amount of calcium can increase the heart rate and the strength of its contractions.

References

1. Felner JM: Echocardiography and Doppler Techniques. In Hurst JW, et al., eds., The Heart, 6th ed. vol. 2. New York, McGraw-Hill, 1986, 1926–1973.
2. Feigenbaum H: Echocardiography. In Braunwald E, ed., Heart Disease. A textbook of Cardiovascular Medicine, 2nd ed. Philadelphia, WB Saunders, 1984, 88–105.
3. Feigenbaum H: Echocardiography, 5th ed. Philadelphia, Lea & Febiger, 1994.
4. St. John Sutton M, Plappert T, Oldershaw P: Normal Doppler echocardiographic examination. In St. John Sutton M, Olderstrom P, eds., Textbook of Adult and Pediatric Echocardiography and Doppler. Boston, Blackwell Scientific, 1989, 47–75.
5. Sahn DJ, DeMaria A, Kisslo J, Weyman A: The Committee on M-mode Standardization of the American Society of Echocardiography. Recommendations regarding quantitation in M-mode echocardiographic measurements. Circulation 58:1072–1082, 1978.
6. Hatle L: Dopplier ultrasound in cardiology. In Hatle L, Angelsen B, eds., Physical Principles and Applications, 2nd ed. Philadelphia, Lea & Febiger, 1985.
7. Henry WL, et al: Report of the American Society of Echocardiography Committee on Nomenclature and Standards in Two-dimensional Echocardiography. Circulation 62:212–217, 1980.
8. Netter FH, Yonkman FF, eds., The Ciba Collection of Medical Illustrations, vol. 5, The Heart. Summit, NJ, Ciba Pharmaceutical, Division of CIBA-GEIGY, 1978, 2–14; 48–50.
9. Weyman AE: Cross Sectional Echocardiography. Philadelphia, Lea & Febiger, 1982, 98–136.
10. Schuster AH, Nanda NC: Doppler Exam of the Heart, Great Vessels and Coronary Arteries. In Nanda NC (ed.) Doppler Echocardiography. Tokyo, Igaku-Shoin Ltd, 1985, 93–129.

Chapter 24

VASCULAR TECHNOLOGY

MARSHA M. NEUMYER

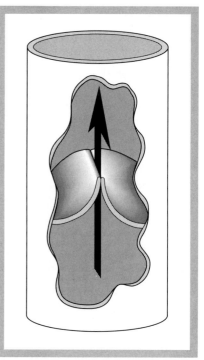

Venous valves of the leg. (From Guyton AC: Textbook of Medical Physiology, 8th ed. Philadelphia, WB Saunders, 1991, p 166.)

Objectives:

Define the role of indirect and direct noninvasive techniques used for the evaluation of vascular disease.

Describe the anatomy of the extracranial carotid and vertebral arteries and the peripheral arterial, venous, and visceral vascular systems.

Describe the function of the cerebrovascular, peripheral arterial, venous, and visceral vascular systems.

Describe the sonographic appearance of the carotid and vertebral vessels, lower extremity peripheral arteries and veins, and the visceral vasculature.

Define the hemodynamic patterns and spectral waveforms found in the normal vasculature.

Define the key words.

Key Words:

Boundary layer separation
Direct/indirect noninvasive vascular tests
Doppler color flow imaging
Doppler time-velocity waveform
Duplex scanning
Laminar flow
Linear reflectivity
Low-/high-resistance vascular bed

Spectral bandwidth/spectral broadening
Systolic window
Transmural pressure
Triphasic Doppler spectral waveform

INTRODUCTION

Noninvasive vascular diagnostic technology has evolved rapidly over the past two decades from the use of the simple hand-held continuous wave Doppler velocimeter to the sophisticated and complex technology found in duplex and triplex ultrasound systems. Vascular laboratory evaluations complement the clinical impression by providing information about the location and severity of cerebrovascular, peripheral arterial, venous, and visceral vascular disease.

Noninvasive vascular diagnostic tests are divided into two types: **indirect** and **direct**. The indirect physiologic test procedures indicate the presence of significant occlusive disease by demonstrating pressure or volume changes downstream from the area of disease. They are an integral part of vascular laboratory evaluations. The direct procedures, in contrast, evaluate the flow patterns in vessels at the location of disease. This is most often accomplished with the use of B-mode ultrasound imaging of the vessel with Doppler velocity spectral analysis of blood flow patterns. These technologies may be complemented by **Doppler color flow imaging**, which color encodes the Doppler-shifted frequencies within the gray scale image of the surrounding tissues.

This presentation focuses on the direct ultrasound examination of the cerebrovascular, peripheral arterial, venous, and visceral vascular systems.

EXTRACRANIAL CEREBROVASCULAR SYSTEM

Common Carotid Arteries, Internal Carotid Arteries, External Carotid Arteries, and Vertebral Arteries

The extracranial cerebrovascular system comprises the common carotid arteries, the internal carotid arteries, the external carotid arteries, and the vertebral arteries. The system is symmetric on each side of the neck. (See Figure 24–1.)

The carotid arteries supply blood flow principally to the anterior cerebral hemispheres, the eye, and muscles of the face, forehead, and scalp. The vertebral arteries carry blood to the posterior cerebrum, meeting to form the basilar artery at the level of the foramen magnum. Intracranially, the carotid arterial system anastomoses with the vertebral-basilar system to form the circle of Willis, an arterial ring around the base of the brain. (See Figure 24–2.)

Each extracranial carotid system has a common carotid artery which bifurcates, most often at the level of the superior thyroid cartilage, into an internal and an external carotid artery.

On the right side of the body, the common carotid artery arises from the innominate, or brachiocephalic,

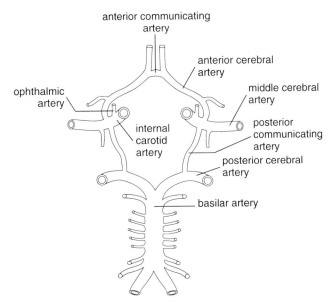

Figure 24–2. Circle of Willis.

artery, which also branches into the subclavian artery. On the left, the subclavian and common carotid arteries arise separately from the aortic arch. Variations may include absence of the innominate artery with the right subclavian and common carotid originating from the arch, or the presence of a left innominate artery; or the aorta may arch to the right with the normal arterial arrangement reversed.

The common carotid arteries pass cephalad into the anterolateral aspect of the neck slightly behind the thyroid gland. The level of the carotid bifurcation and the arrangement of the internal and external carotid arteries may vary. In most patients, the internal carotid artery (ICA) is posterior and lateral to the external carotid artery (ECA). The internal carotid artery has no branches in the neck but intracranially gives rise to the ophthalmic artery, which supplies blood flow to the eye, and to the middle and anterior cerebral arteries. The external carotid artery has branches that supply blood flow to the neck, face, and scalp. These branches sonographically help to distinguish the ECA from the ICA. Anatomic variations may include the absence of the common carotid artery, with the internal and external carotid artery arising directly from the aortic arch, or the absence of a carotid bifurcation.

The vertebral arteries arise as the first branch of the subclavian arteries and pass cranially through the foramina of the transverse processes of the upper six cervical vertebrae. The vertebrals pass superiorly to the atlas, winding around the lateral mass of the atlas, and enter the vertebral canal anterior to the spinal cord. The two vertebral arteries enter the skull through the foramen magnum and join to form the basilar artery, which supplies structures in the posterior fossa.

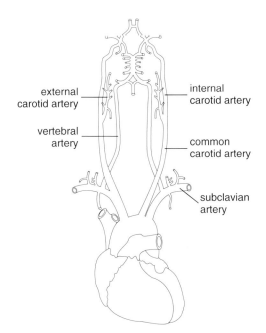

Figure 24–1. The extracranial cerebrovascular system.

Size of the Extracranial Cerebrovascular Vessels

The normal common carotid artery is approximately 5 to 6 mm in diameter. This vessel may decrease in transverse diameter due to atherosclerotic occlusive disease, which prevents antegrade blood flow.

The extracranial portion of the internal carotid artery measures approximately 4 to 5 mm in width. The vessel decreases in diameter as it enters the brain.

The external carotid artery is usually of smaller diameter than the internal carotid, measuring approximately 3 to 4 mm.

The vertebral arteries are approximately 2 to 3 mm wide at their origin, decreasing in diameter as they course cephalad.

Sonographic Appearance of the Extracranial Carotid and Vertebral Arteries

Using an anterior oblique or posterior oblique longitudinal scan plane, the skin, platysma, and fascia will lie between the probe and the carotid artery.

The lateral lobe of the thyroid gland is identified posterior to the common carotid artery. The jugular vein lies lateral to the common carotid and displays characteristic movement varying with respiration and cardiac activity. (See Figure 24–3.) Transverse pulsatility of the carotid artery will be noted to be in phase with the cardiac cycle.

At the level of the carotid bifurcation, the dilatation (carotid sinus) of the carotid bulb can be identified and the division into the internal and external carotid arteries noted. (See Figure 24–4.) The relationship between these two vessels is variable and may depend on whether an antero- or a postero-oblique plane has been used. The vessels can be further identified by their signature Doppler waveform.

The sonographic evaluation of the normal arterial wall will document the **linear reflectivity** associated with the echogenic properties of the collagen fibers that are found in the intima and media of arteries. (See Figure 24–5.)

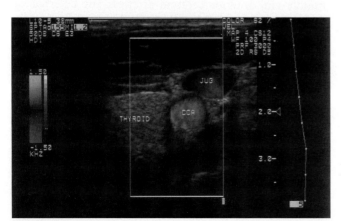

Figure 24–3. Transverse Doppler color flow image of the common carotid artery, jugular vein, and thyroid gland. (See Color Plate 8 at the back of this book.)

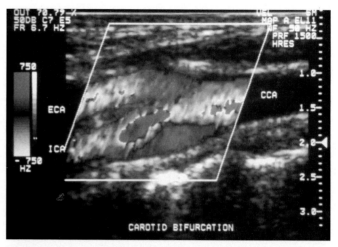

Figure 24–4. Long axis Doppler color flow image of the carotid bifurcation showing the common carotid artery, external carotid artery, and internal carotid artery. Note the zone of retrograde flow in the carotid bulb caused by boundary layer separation. (See Color Plate 9 at the back of this book.)

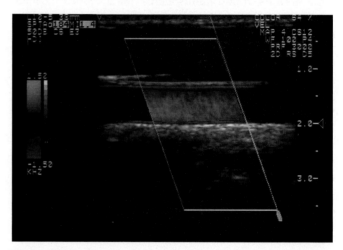

Figure 24–5. Long axis image of the common carotid artery. Arterial wall definition reveals linear reflectivity resulting from the echogenicity of collagen found in the intima and media. (See Color Plate 10 at the back of this book.)

Examination of the walls of the jugular vein will fail to reveal these properties.

The vertebral arteries may be visualized using an anteroposterior approach in the midcervical segment of the neck as they course through the fossae of the transverse vertebral processes. The origin of the vertebral vessels can be documented using a transverse approach to the subclavian artery at the level of the common carotid origin. (See Figure 24–6.)

Hemodynamic Patterns of the Extracranial Carotid and Vertebral Arteries

The common carotid artery supplies approximately 80 percent of its flow to the internal carotid artery and about 20 percent to the external carotid artery.

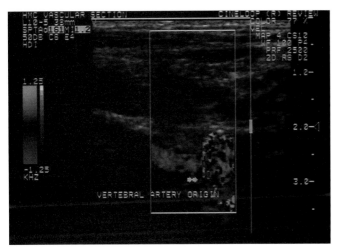

Figure 24-6. Doppler color flow image of the vertebral artery origin. The subclavian artery is seen in the transverse plane just distal to the origin of the right common carotid artery. (See Color Plate 11 at the back of this book.)

As the internal carotid artery supplies the **low-resistance vascular bed** of the brain and eye, the flow will be cephalad throughout the cardiac cycle. In contrast, the external carotid artery supplies the **high-resistance vascular bed** of the face and scalp. The flow pattern for this vessel is characterized by forward flow in systole, and a low or reverse diastolic flow component.

A pressure gradient develops as a result of dilatation of the carotid bulb resulting in separation of the flow stream into central forward flow entering the internal carotid artery and reversed flow near the posterolateral wall. (See Figure 24-7.)

The vertebral arteries supply blood flow, by way of the basilar artery, to the posterior cerebral hemispheres. Therefore, their flow patterns will be similar to those seen in the internal carotid artery with constant forward diastolic flow.

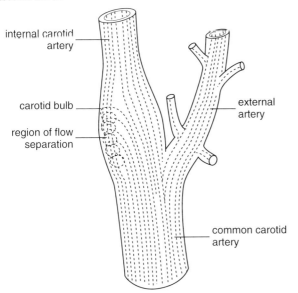

internal carotid artery

carotid bulb

region of flow separation

external artery

common carotid artery

Figure 24-7. Carotid bifurcation demonstrating boundary layer separation in the carotid bulb.

The red blood cells move through the arteries in layers or laminae. The laminae slide over each other, impeded by friction from within the fluid or from movement against the arterial wall. Velocity profiles will, in general, be influenced by tapering or curvature of the vessel, entrance and exit effects on inertia of blood as the vessel widens and dilates, and the presence of turbulence caused by anatomic abnormality or disease.

The velocity spectral information must be collected at an angle of insonation of 60° with respect to the blood flow vector in order to accurately evaluate the hemodynamic patterns. Remember the Doppler equation:

$$F = \frac{2VF_0\cos\Theta}{c}$$

Where
- F = Doppler shifted frequency
- V = Velocity of red cell movement
- F_0 = Carrier Doppler frequency
- cos Θ = Angle of insonation with respect to blood flow vector
- c = Constant for speed of sound in soft tissue (1,540 m/sec)

Doppler Velocity Spectral Waveforms

The common carotid artery has a Doppler velocity spectral waveform that mimics both the internal carotid and external carotid waveforms. The blood flow pattern is characterized by a sharp systolic upstroke, a rapid systolic deceleration, and constant forward diastolic flow. There is a "window," an area absent of Doppler shifts, under the systolic component. During systole, the red blood cells will move at a uniform velocity with an undisturbed flow profile in a normal common carotid artery. This flow pattern is characterized by a very narrow Doppler velocity spectrum. (See Figure 24-8.)

During the deceleration phase of systole, the velocity will decrease, and the viscous drag on the cells nearest the wall will result in the movement of the cells over a slightly broader range of velocities. This is manifested by

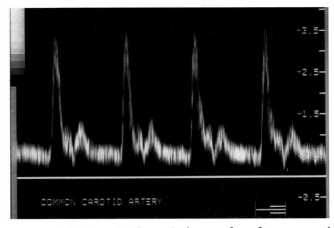

Figure 24-8. Doppler time-velocity waveform from a normal common carotid artery.

TABLE 24-1. Diagnostic Doppler Velocity Criteria for Determining Degree of Carotid Artery Diameter Reduction

DIAMETER STENOSIS (CATEGORY)	PEAK SYSTOLIC VELOCITY (cm/sec)	END DIASTOLIC VELOCITY (cm/sec)
0% (Normal)	<110	<40
1-39% (Mild)	<110	<40
40-59% (Moderate)	<130	<40
60-79% (Severe)	>130	>40
80-99% (Critical)	>250	>100
100% (Occlusion)	N/A	N/A

N/A = not applicable

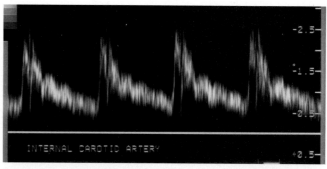

Figure 24-9. Doppler time-velocity waveform from a normal internal carotid artery demonstrating constant forward diastolic flow.

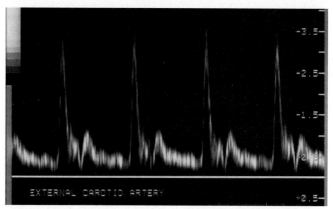

Figure 24-10. Doppler time-velocity waveform from a normal external carotid artery. Note the low diastolic flow component.

a thickening of the velocity spectral envelope. This **spectral broadening** becomes more evident during diastole.

If frequency information is desired, the carrier Doppler frequency and angle of insonation (60°) must be known. The normal velocity in the carotid artery is approximately 100 cm per sec, but a wide range of normal velocities from 30 to greater than 110 cm per sec has been documented. (See Table 24-1.)

The internal carotid artery is characteristically a high flow, low-resistance vessel. The Doppler velocity waveform from this artery demonstrates quasi-steady flow with a blunt systolic peak and constant forward diastolic flow. (See Figure 24-9.) A systolic window is present in the absence of disease or vessel tortuosity.

In contrast, the external carotid artery is a low flow, high-resistance vessel. The Doppler velocity waveform exhibits multi-phasicity with a sharp systolic upstroke, rapid deceleration, and low diastolic flow. (See Figure 24-10.) In the presence of internal carotid artery occlu-

sion, the external carotid artery may mimic the internal carotid waveform due to collateral potential for blood flow to the brain offered by the ECA.

The **Doppler time-velocity waveform** from the carotid bulb will vary with position of the sample volume. (See Figure 24-11.) If the sample volume is placed in the

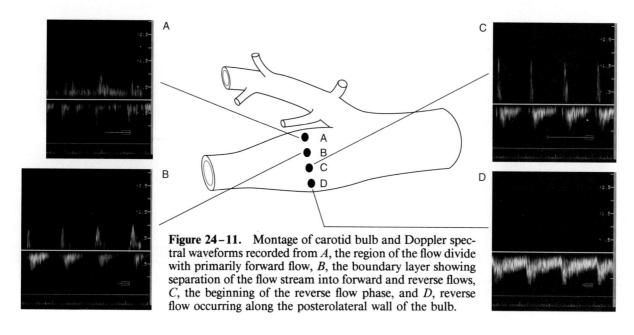

Figure 24-11. Montage of carotid bulb and Doppler spectral waveforms recorded from *A*, the region of the flow divide with primarily forward flow, *B*, the boundary layer showing separation of the flow stream into forward and reverse flows, *C*, the beginning of the reverse flow phase, and *D*, reverse flow occurring along the posterolateral wall of the bulb.

region of the flow divide, the wave form will demonstrate forward diastolic flow. As the sample volume is stepped across the lumen of the carotid bulb to the posterior wall, the waveform will exhibit reverse flow in the region of the **separation of the boundary layers**.

The spectral display from the normal vertebral arteries should resemble that recorded from the ICA with constant forward flow demonstrated during diastole. The vertebrals are high flow, low-resistance vessels.

THE LOWER EXTREMITY ARTERIAL SYSTEM

Common Iliac, External Iliac, Common Femoral, Superficial Femoral, Popliteal, and Tibial Arteries

The lower extremity peripheral arterial vessels can be divided into three systems: aortoiliac (inflow), femoropopliteal (outflow), and tibioperoneal (run-off). (See Figure 24–12.)

The aortoiliac system begins at the aortic bifurcation and ends at the level of the inguinal ligament. It comprises the distal abdominal aorta and the common iliac, external iliac, and internal iliac (hypogastric) arteries. Blood flow through this system supplies the buttocks, pelvis, and thighs. The aortoiliac system is the second most common site for lower extremity arterial occlusive disease.

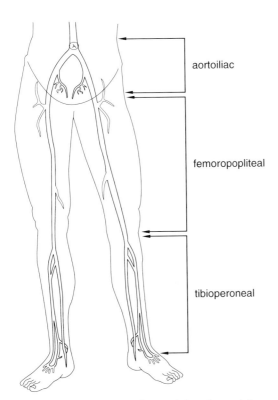

Figure 24–12. Lower extremity peripheral arterial tree demonstrating the aortoiliac, femoropopliteal, and tibioperoneal systems.

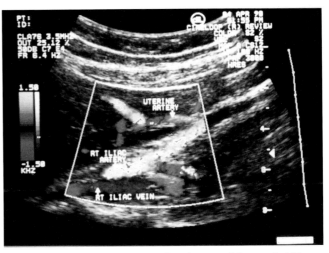

Figure 24–13. Doppler color flow image of the aortic bifurcation. (Courtesy of Advanced Technology Laboratories.) (See Color Plate 12 at the back of this book.)

The femoropopliteal system begins at the level of the inguinal ligament and ends at the trifurcation of the popliteal artery in the popliteal fossa behind the knee. This system comprises the common femoral, superficial femoral, deep femoral (profunda femoris), and popliteal arteries. The thighs and calves receive blood flow through these major vessels. This system is the most common site for atherosclerotic occlusive disease of the lower extremities.

The tibioperoneal system begins at the termination of the popliteal artery in the popliteal fossa and ends at the ankle where these vessels anastomose with the plantar and metatarsal vessels of the foot. These arteries make up the supply system for blood flow to the calves and feet.

Sonographic Appearance of the Lower Extremity Peripheral Arterial Vessels

The bifurcation of the abdominal aorta takes place on the left side of the body of the fourth lumbar vertebra. The common iliac arteries pass posterolaterally from the termination of the aorta to the margin of the pelvis and divide opposite the last lumbar vertebra and the sacrum into the external and internal iliac arteries. (See Figure 24–13.)

The peritoneum, small intestine, and ureter lie anterior to the right common iliac artery. The common iliac veins and the psoas magnus muscle lie posteriorly with the inferior vena cava sharing a lateral relationship.

The left common iliac artery lies posterior to the ureter and peritoneum. It is anterior to the left common iliac vein. The psoas magnus muscle borders the left common iliac artery laterally. The location of the aortic bifurcation is subject to variation as is the point of division of the common iliac arteries. On occasion, the common iliac artery may be absent, with the external and internal iliac arteries arising directly from the aorta.

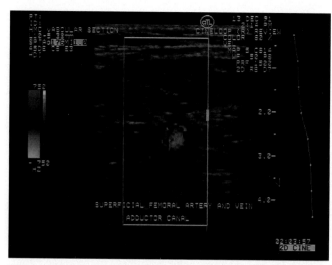

Figure 24–14. Transverse Doppler color flow image of the superficial femoral artery and vein in Hunter's canal. (See Color Plate 13 at the back of this book.)

The external iliac artery is larger than the internal iliac artery. This vessel passes obliquely posterolateral to the inner border of the psoas muscle from the bifurcation of the common iliac to Poupart's ligament, where it enters the thigh and becomes the common femoral artery.[1] The common and external iliac arteries are frequently difficult to image due to overlying bowel gas.

The common femoral artery commences posterolateral to Poupart's ligament between the anterior superior spine of the ilium and the symphysis pubis and courses down the medial aspect of the thigh through Scarpa's triangle as the superficial femoral artery, where it is contained in Hunter's canal.[1] This vessel terminates in the lower third of the thigh at the opening of the adductor magnus, where it becomes the popliteal artery. (See Figure 24–14.) It is bordered on its medial side by the superficial femoral vein and laterally by the adductor muscle. On rare occasions the superficial femoral artery may divide into two trunks below the origin of the profunda femoris, reuniting in the adductor canal to form the popliteal artery.

The popliteal artery commences at the termination of the superficial femoral artery in Hunter's canal and passes obliquely behind the knee joint to the lower border of the femur, where it divides into the anterior and posterior tibial arteries. It is bordered medially by the inner head of the gastrocnemius and posteriorly by the popliteal vein. Occasionally the popliteal artery divides prematurely into its branch vessels. (See Figure 24–15.)

The anterior tibial artery commences at the bifurcation of the popliteal and passes through the interosseous membrane to the deep part of the front of the leg lying close to the inner side of the neck of the fibula. At the lower third of the limb, it lies on the tibia and on the anterior ligament of the ankle joint, where it moves superiorly to become the dorsalis pedis artery. The ante-

rior tibial artery is accompanied by the anterior tibial veins lying on each side of the artery.

The posterior tibial artery extends obliquely downward along the lateral (tibial) side of the leg, lying posterior to the deep transverse fascia. It is accompanied by the two posterior tibial veins. (See Figure 24–16.)

The peroneal artery lies along the posteromedial side of the fibula. It arises from the posterior tibial trunk about an inch below the border of the popliteus muscle passing obliquely outward to the fibula. (See Figure 24–16.) The peroneal veins lie on either side of the artery.

In the absence of disease, the lumen of the peripheral arteries will be anechoic with linear reflectivity apparent along both the anterior and posterior walls of the vessels. Transverse pulsation of the arteries is notable and may become quite pronounced in tortuous segments of the lower extremity arterial tree.

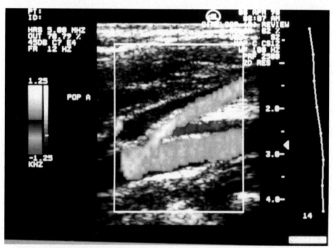

Figure 24–15. Long axis color flow image of the popliteal artery. (See Color Plate 14 at the back of this book.)

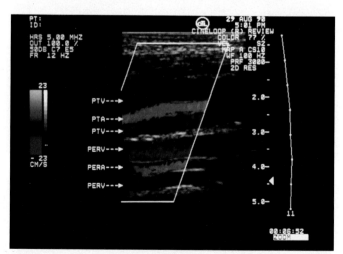

Figure 24–16. Long axis Doppler color flow image of the posterior tibial and peroneal arteries surrounded by their companion tibial veins of the same name. (See Color Plate 15 at the back of this book.) (Courtesy of Advanced Technology Laboratories.)

Size of the Lower Extremity Arteries

External iliac artery – 0.79 cm
Common femoral artery – 0.82 cm
Superficial femoral artery (proximal) – 0.60 cm
Superficial femoral artery (distal) – 0.54 cm
Popliteal artery – 0.52 cm

Hemodynamic Patterns in the Lower Extremity Peripheral Arterial System

The pulsatile pressure wave that results from the pumping action of the heart is transmitted from the aortic root, to the feet. During systole, and left ventricular contraction, the walls of the aortic root will expand, creating a high pressure wave. This wave is transmitted down the aorta and into the lower extremity arterial system. As the high pressure wave travels peripherally, the lower extremity arterial walls will also expand and contract in a pulsatile manner.

The resistance to blood flow in the small diameter tibial vessels is greater than that in the wide diameter aorta, resulting in a pressure gradient between the aorta and the distal tibial vessels. In the absence of arterial occlusive disease, systolic pressure is greater in the tibial arteries than in the abdominal aorta.

As the primary high pressure wave from the aortic root meets the high resistance of the tibial vascular tree, a secondary reflected pressure wave is created. The blood flow pattern to this high resistance vascular bed is therefore triphasic. There is forward flow in systole, then early reverse diastolic flow, and a forward diastolic component in vessels with normal arterial wall compliance.

Doppler Velocity Spectral Waveforms

A **triphasic Doppler spectral waveform** is normally found in arteries from the level of the abdominal aorta to the tibial arteries at the ankle. (See Figure 24–17.) In

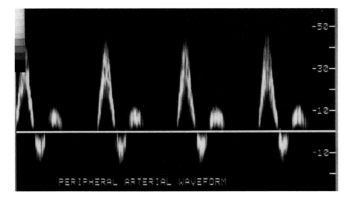

Figure 24–17. Doppler time-velocity waveform recorded from a lower extremity peripheral artery. Note the triphasic pattern of flow.

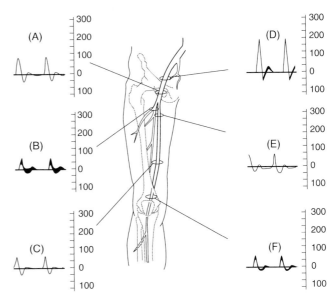

Figure 24–18. Normal velocity spectral waveforms from the *A*, common femoral artery, *B*, profunda femoris artery, *C*, distal superficial femoral artery, *D*, external iliac artery, *E*, proximal superficial femoral artery, and *F*, popliteal artery. Note the decreases in peak systolic velocity between the external iliac artery and proximal superficial femoral artery and between the proximal superficial femoral artery and the popliteal vessel. (From Neumyer MM, Thiele BL: The evaluation of lower extremity occlusive disease with Doppler ultrasonography. In Taylor KJW, Burns PN, Wells PNT (eds.): Clinical Applications of Doppler Ultrasound. New York, Raven Press, 1988.)

healthy, young adults with marked elasticity of the vessel wall, an additional reverse flow component may be recorded. Vessel wall compliance may decrease with advancing age, and the peak systolic forward velocity and peak diastolic forward velocity may diminish slightly resulting in a biphasic waveform. Velocity waveforms recorded from peripheral arteries of women will generally demonstrate lower peak diastolic velocities than those from men of the same age.

The **spectral bandwidth** will be narrow throughout the systolic and early reversed diastolic flow cycles. Spectral broadening may occur at bifurcations because of boundary layer separation and the presence of disturbed flow.

In the absence of proximal disease, the reverse flow component will be present and a systolic window will be noted.

The peak systolic velocity decreases in the normal lower extremity arterial tree from the central to the peripheral vessels.[2] (See Figure 24–18.) In the normal abdominal aorta, the velocity averages 90 cm per sec and decreases between the external iliac artery and the proximal superficial femoral artery and again between the superficial femoral and popliteal arteries to average 60 cm per sec in the popliteal artery.

THE LOWER EXTREMITY VENOUS SYSTEM

The veins of the lower extremity are divided into the deep, superficial, and perforating veins. The deep veins accompany the arteries and share the same names.

The Deep Venous System

The paired anterior tibial veins arise in the dorsal venous arch and accompany the anterior tibial artery up the calf. (See Figure 24–19A.) The anterior tibial veins pass posteriorly from the anterior compartment of the leg to penetrate the interosseous membrane and course between the tibia and fibula to meet the popliteal vein.

The posterior tibial veins arise from the plantar venous arch of the foot. They accompany the posterior tibial artery through the leg and join the peroneal veins. The posterior tibial veins unite with the anterior tibial veins at the distal border of the popliteus muscle to form the popliteal vein.

The peroneal veins arise medial to the lateral malleolus. These veins follow the medial surface of the fibula in the lower half of the calf and then course medially to form the posterior tibial trunk in the upper third of the calf.

The popliteal vein is formed by the posterior tibial and anterior tibial trunks at the level of the knee. From this location, the popliteal vein extends cephalad to the me-dial aspect of the femur, lying 1 to 2 cm from the posterior surface of the distal femur, and then passes through the adductor hiatus to become the superficial femoral vein. The popliteal vein accompanies the popliteal artery lying within a fascial sheath. The popliteal vein will course posterior and superficial to the popliteal artery. At the distal popliteal fossa, the vein lies slightly medial to the artery but crosses the artery to lie lateral to it as it ascends into the proximal part of the fossa. This vessel normally contains two valves.

The superficial femoral vein is the continuation of the popliteal vein. It accompanies the superficial femoral artery as it courses up the medial aspect of the thigh to the level of the inguinal ligament to form the common femoral vein. The superficial femoral vein normally contains two to five valves along its course.

Anatomic variations are common in the deep venous system. The most common anomalies seen include duplication of the popliteal and/or superficial femoral veins, duplication of the distal segment of the superficial femoral vein subsequently uniting to form a single vein in the mid- to proximal thigh, and the presence of three or more popliteal or superficial femoral veins.

The Superficial Venous System

The major superficial veins are the greater saphenous and the lesser saphenous veins. (See Figure 24–19B and

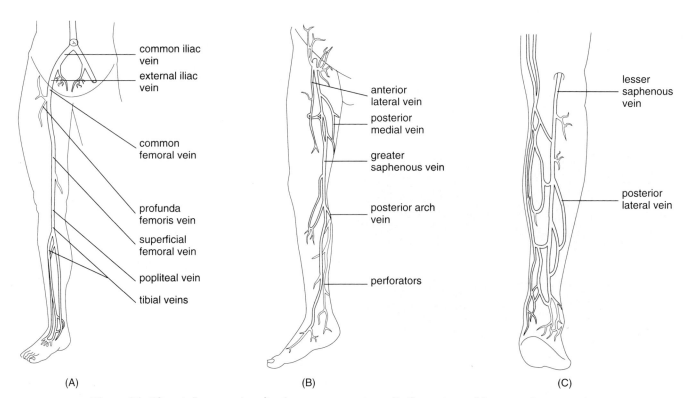

(A)   (B)   (C)

Figure 24–19. *A*, Lower extremity deep venous system; *B, C*, greater and lesser saphenous veins.

C.) These veins lie in subcutaneous tissue and are superficial to the deep fascia.

The greater saphenous vein arises from the medial aspect of the dorsal venous arch, continuing in the foot, and ascends in the ankle anteromedial to the medial malleolus. It then moves posteriorly to cross behind the medial condyle of the femur at the level of the knee. It courses up the medial aspect of the thigh to drain into the common femoral vein about 3.5 cm below the inguinal ligament. There are usually four valves in the greater saphenous vein in the lower leg and up to six valves in the thigh.

The lesser saphenous vein begins at the lateral end of the dorsal venous arch and ascends in the ankle posterior to the lateral malleolus. This vein extends up the back of the calf to the distal popliteal fossa where it perforates the deep fascia, passing between the heads of the gastrocnemius muscle, and drains into the popliteal vein. The greater and lesser saphenous veins may communicate through the femoropopliteal vein.

The Perforating Veins

The deep venous system and the superficial venous systems are connected by the perforating or communicating veins.

The posterior group of perforators connects the lesser saphenous vein with the greater saphenous vein. The medial perforating veins connect the greater saphenous vein with the posterior tibial veins, and the lateral perforators join the greater saphenous vein with the anterior tibial and peroneal veins. There are up to six perforating veins in the medial thigh connecting the superficial femoral vein with the greater saphenous vein.

Size of the Deep and Superficial Veins

Average diameter of the deep veins:

Tibial veins – approximately 5 mm
Popliteal veins – 0.9 to 1.5 cm
Superficial femoral vein – 0.9 to 1.0 cm
Common femoral vein – 1.2 to 1.9 cm

Average diameter of the superficial veins:

Greater saphenous vein – 2 to 3 mm (calf)
– 4 to 6 mm (thigh)
Lesser saphenous vein – 4 to 7 mm

Sonographic Appearance of the Deep and Superficial Venous Systems

Every deep vein is accompanied by an artery that courses in close proximity to it.

The common femoral vein lies midway between the pubis and the iliac spine at the level of the inguinal crease. It should be found medial to the common femoral artery and slightly deeper than this vessel. The lumen of the normal common femoral vein is anechoic and the walls of the vein will coapt entirely with gentle transducer pressure applied to the anterior vein wall from the transverse image plane.

The greater saphenous vein arises medially from the common femoral vein and courses superficially to the fascia of the thigh and calf to the dorsum of the foot.

The common femoral vein bifurcates into the superficial femoral vein and deep femoral vein (profunda femoris) about 2 to 4 cm distal to the takeoff of the greater saphenous vein. The profunda femoris vein courses laterally and deep to the superficial femoral vein. It will lie in the same scan plane as the profunda femoris artery.

The superficial femoral vein will accompany the artery of the same name, lying deep to this vessel and medial to the profunda femoris. Both the superficial femoral vein and artery enter the adductor canal, crossing beneath the adductor fascia in the lower third of the thigh. The superficial femoral vein is duplicated, over at least a short length, in 15 to 20 percent of patients.

The superficial femoral vein becomes the popliteal vein at the level of the adductor canal. The vein will remain posterior to the popliteal artery; however, the vein is most easily interrogated from the popliteal fossa. From this image plane, the popliteal vein will appear superficial to its companion artery. The popliteal vein will be duplicated in approximately 35 percent of patients.

The lesser saphenous vein normally arises from the popliteal vein proximally at about midknee level. The vessel courses posterolaterally down the leg, terminating anterior to the lateral malleolus. The paired gastrocnemius veins also arise from the popliteal vein, originating from the distal segment of the vein, and run parallel to the popliteal artery.

The popliteal vein can be imaged to the proximal calf where it bifurcates into the anterior tibial trunk and the tibioperoneal trunk, which lies deep to the gastrocnemius and soleus muscles. At this point, the veins duplicate. For each tibial artery there are at least two tibial veins.

The anterior tibial veins can be imaged from the anterior aspect of the leg as they emerge after crossing the interosseous membrane. They remain on top of the membrane as they course down the leg to cross the region of the angle.

The posterior tibial veins can be imaged from the medial aspect of the calf at about midcalf to the level of the medial malleolus. They will lie superficially.

The peroneal veins can also be imaged from midcalf level, lying deeper than the posterior tibial veins and adjacent to the fibula.

Hemodynamic Patterns of the Lower Extremity Deep Venous System

The movement of blood in the lower extremity veins is influenced by respiratory variation, which causes changes in intra-abdominal pressure, the calf muscle pump, and the presence of competent venous valves.

As one inhales, the diaphragm descends and blood flow return from the lower extremities is impeded due to an increase in intra-abdominal pressure. With expiration, the diaphragm rises, intra-abdominal pressure decreases, and venous return is possible.

As much as 20 percent of the body's total blood volume may be pooled in the leg veins within 15 minutes of standing still. When a person is at rest, the energy for transport of venous blood from the legs to the heart is supplied by contraction of the left ventricle. This cardiac contraction alone is insufficient to move blood from the legs and is complemented by the calf muscle pump, which is activated with exercise. The calf muscle pump helps to control the hydrostatic pressure in the leg veins by continuously pumping blood out of these veins. The venous pressure in the feet of an exercising adult will therefore usually be less than 25 mm Hg.

The cephalad movement of blood in the lower extremities is a complex function of the calf muscles and the venous valves. With each step taken during walking, there are periods of relaxation and contraction of the calf muscles. When the calf muscles are relaxed, the blood flows into the lower pressure deep venous system from the high-pressure superficial venous system. As the muscle contracts, the blood moves from the deep calf veins into the deep thigh veins. Valves in the deep veins prevent the flow of blood toward the feet, and valves in the perforating veins prevent blood from flowing from the deep to the superficial system.

One of the most remarkable characteristics of veins is the capacity to undergo tremendous volume changes with little change in **transmural pressure**. (See Figure 24–20A.) The venous wall is about one tenth as thick as the arterial wall with little elastin present in the media of the vein. The percentage of smooth muscle found in the media will vary depending on the location of the vein,

A

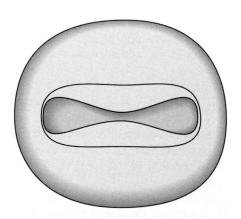

B

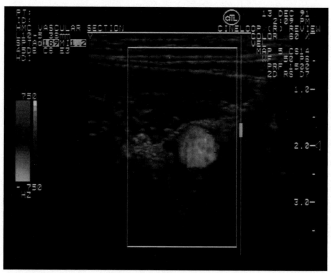

C

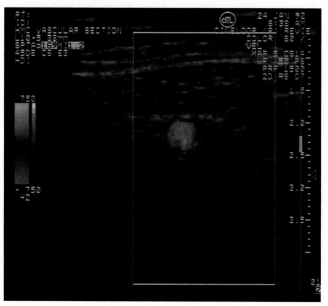

Figure 24–20. *A,* Cross-sectional vein demonstrating collapse of the vein wall with low transmural pressure; *B,* transverse Doppler color flow imaging of the superficial femoral artery and vein; *C,* Doppler color flow image of the superficial femoral artery and vein demonstrating coaptation of the venous walls that occurs with gentle transducer pressure. (See Color Plate 16 at the back of this book.)

with about 60 percent muscle being found in the veins of the foot—the veins subjected to the greatest hydrostatic pressure. The walls of a normal vein can be coapted with gentle transducer pressure during transverse imaging of the vein. (See Figure 24-20B and C.)

Doppler Spectral Analysis

Blood flow in the lower extremity veins is spontaneous and phasic with respiration, ceasing with inspiration and augmenting with expiration. (See Figure 24-21.) Pulsatility of flow may be caused by increased central venous pressure due to fluid overload or tricuspid insufficiency or may be related to the proximity of the veins to the heart.

Flow can be augmented by compressing the limb proximally and impeded by distal compression. (See Figure 24-22.) A Valsalva maneuver often will enlarge a vein, dramatically aiding in identification and localization of the vessel.

Because they lie deep in the pelvis and are noncompressible, veins proximal to the inguinal ligament cannot be reliably studied using **duplex technology** alone. The

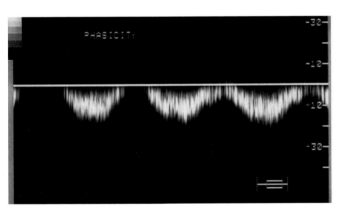

Figure 24-21. Doppler spectral waveform recorded from the normal common femoral vein. Note phasicity of flow, which varies with the respiratory cycle.

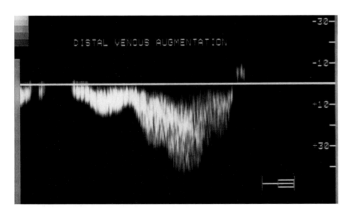

Figure 24-22. Doppler spectral waveform demonstrating augmentation of venous flow with manual compression of the limb proximal to the transducer position.

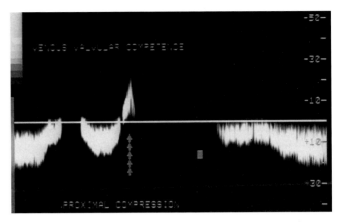

Figure 24-23. Doppler spectral waveform demonstrating the absence of retrograde venous flow when the limb is manually compressed distal to the transducer position. The valve is competent, preventing reflux of blood with distal compression.

addition of Doppler color flow imaging to confirm luminal filling has complemented the examination procedure.

Valvular competence may be confirmed by noting the absence of retrograde venous flow with distal compression of the limb. (See Figure 24-23.)

In general, the following flow characteristics should be examined in each limb: spontaneity, phasicity, augmentation, competence, and absence of pulsatility.

THE VISCERAL ARTERIAL SYSTEM

The visceral arterial system consists of the abdominal aorta from the level of the diaphragm to the aortic bifurcation; the celiac axis, common hepatic, splenic, superior mesenteric, inferior mesenteric, and renal arteries; and the vessels of the renal parenchyma. (See Figure 24-24.)

The celiac, superior mesenteric, and inferior mesenteric arteries all arise from the anterior wall of the aorta. (See Figure 24-25.) The celiac axis is located 1 to 3 cm below the diaphragm. This vessel bifurcates into three major branches, the common hepatic, splenic, and left gastric arteries, 1 to 2 cm from its origin. The celiac and its branches supply blood to the stomach, liver, spleen, and small intestine.

The superior mesenteric artery (SMA) originates from the aorta 1 to 2 cm distal to the origin of the celiac axis. This artery anastomoses to the celiac artery by way of the superior and inferior pancreaticoduodenal arteries, which serve as major collateral pathways in the presence of arterial occlusive disease of the SMA or celiac artery. The superior mesenteric artery supplies blood to the small intestine, cecum, and ascending and transverse colons.

The inferior mesenteric artery arises from the anterolateral aortic wall approximately 4 cm proximal to the aortic bifurcation. This vessel lies in close proximity to the aorta along the first several centimeters of its course and it is difficult to interrogate with Doppler ultrasound. The artery supplies blood to the descending and sigmoid flexures of the colon and the greater part of the rectum.

The renal arteries arise from the lateral wall of the aorta below the superior mesenteric artery just posterior to the left renal vein. The right renal artery is longer than the left as it must pass behind the inferior vena cava to enter the hilum of the right kidney. The left renal artery originates from the aortic wall somewhat higher than the right. (See Figure 24–26.)

Before entering the hilum of the kidney, each renal artery divides into four or five branches, the greater number of which most often will lie between the renal vein and the ureter. The vessels further branch to form

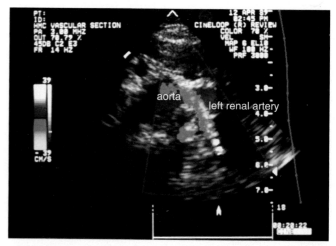

Figure 24–26. Transverse color flow image of the abdominal aorta showing the origin of the left renal artery. (See Color Plate 18 at the back of this book.)

the interlobar and arcuate arteries, which pass between the medullary pyramids of the renal parenchyma. (See Chapter 8.)

Occasionally, accessory renal arteries are noted arising from the aortic wall. These may enter the upper or lower pole of the kidney rather than entering the organ at the hilum.

Size of the Visceral Arteries

Average diameter:

Aorta–2.0 to 2.5 cm
Celiac–0.70 cm
Superior mesenteric–0.60 cm
Inferior mesenteric–0.30 cm
Renal arteries–0.40 to 0.50 cm

Sonographic Appearance of the Visceral Arteries

The abdominal aorta commences at the aortic opening of the diaphragm, lying slightly to the left of the vertebral column. It terminates on the body of the fourth lumbar vertebra at which point it bifurcates into the common iliac arteries. The vessel diameter tapers slightly from its proximal to distal segments.

The abdominal aorta is bordered anteriorly by the stomach, pancreas, celiac axis, splenic vein, and superior mesenteric artery and vein, and on its right by the inferior vena cava. It lies anterior to the vertebral column.

The celiac artery lies anterior to the abdominal aorta. It is bordered on its left side by the cardiac end of the stomach and rests on the upper border of the pancreas.

The superior mesenteric artery lies anterior to the aorta, being covered at its origin by the splenic vein and pancreas. In its proximal segment it lies between the pancreas and the transverse portion of the duodenum.

The inferior mesenteric artery lies anterolateral to the distal abdominal aorta at its origin. It then descends to the left iliac fossa, anterior to the left common iliac

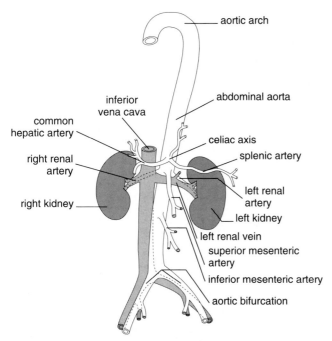

Figure 24–24. Diagram of the visceral arterial system.

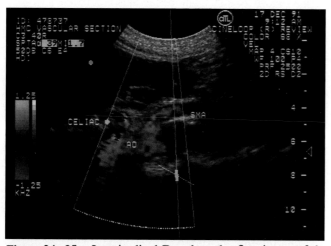

Figure 24–25. Longitudinal Doppler color flow image of the abdominal aorta and the origins of the celiac and superior mesenteric arteries from the anterior wall of the aorta. (See Color Plate 17 at the back of this book.)

artery, to enter the pelvis as the superior hemorrhoidal artery.

The renal arteries originate from the lateral wall of the aorta immediately below the superior mesenteric artery. In their proximal segment, the renal arteries follow the crus of the diaphragm. On the right, the renal artery is posterior to the right renal vein and inferior vena cava in its mid- to distal segments. On the left, the renal artery lies posterior to the left renal vein.

Hemodynamic Patterns

The suprarenal abdominal aorta supplies the largest portion of its blood flow to branch vessels, which feed low resistance vascular beds. The liver, spleen, and kidneys all have high metabolic rates and demand constant forward blood flow. The superior mesenteric artery, in contrast, supplies the high resistance vascular bed of the stomach and small intestine in the fasting state. Blood flow through the suprarenal aorta will, therefore, meet little resistance to runoff and forward flow will be noted throughout the cardiac cycle. We have noted that the peak aortic systolic velocity decreases with age, perhaps as a result of loss of vessel wall compliance. The infrarenal aortic blood supply is principally to the high resistance peripheral arterial system of the lower extremities and lumbar arteries. The pressure wave noted in this segment of the aorta will, therefore, resemble the velocity waveforms recorded from peripheral arteries.

The celiac axis supplies the low resistance end organs, the liver and spleen, through its branch vessels, the hepatic, gastric, and splenic arteries. Like the flow patterns seen in the suprarenal aorta, constant forward flow is documented throughout the vascular tree supplied by the celiac artery.

The superior mesenteric artery supplies the tissues of the stomach and small intestine. Flow in the superior mesenteric artery will vary depending on the activity of these organs and their metabolic status. In the fasting state, there is relatively high resistance to arterial flow to the tissues of the gut. Following ingestion of a meal, remarkable changes occur in the flow patterns in the superior mesenteric artery, reflecting the metabolic demands imposed by the digestive process. There is an increase in the diameter of the SMA, the peak systolic and end-diastolic velocity increases, the volume flow to the small bowel increases, and constant forward flow is documented.

The kidneys, like the brain, eye, liver, and spleen, are low resistance organs, which demand constant blood flow to moderate their metabolic activity. Hemodynamic flow patterns in the normal renal arteries supplying nondiseased kidneys will demonstrate high diastolic flow. In the presence of chronic renal disease, the vascular resistance of the kidney increases. This increase in renovascular resistance of the end organ may be expressed in the flow patterns from the renal artery as a decrease in the diastolic flow component.

Doppler Velocity Spectral Analysis

The Doppler time-velocity waveform from the suprarenal abdominal aorta demonstrates an absence of reversed diastolic flow, reflecting the low vascular resistance of its end organs. (See Figure 24–27A.) In contrast, the signals from the infrarenal abdominal aorta will be triphasic, consistent with a vessel feeding a high resistance peripheral arterial tree. (See Figure 24–27B.)

Time-velocity waveforms from the celiac, hepatic, and splenic arteries demonstrate forward diastolic flow compatible with the high-flow demands of the liver and spleen. (See Figure 24–28.) The splenic artery is frequently tortuous, and spectral broadening may be noted in the quasi-steady waveform recorded from this vessel.

In the fasting state, the Doppler spectral waveform from the superior mesenteric artery demonstrates low or reversed flow during the diastolic portion of the cardiac cycle. (See Figure 24–29A.) Postprandially, the peak systolic velocity increases in the normal artery, and a two- to three-fold increase in end-diastolic flow may be documented. (See Figure 24–29B.) Due to the collateral potential expressed in the mesenteric arterial system, disease in one of the three major arteries may result in increased flow and velocity in the others.

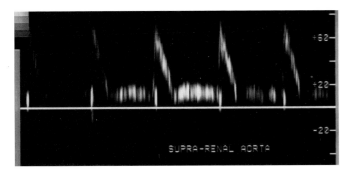

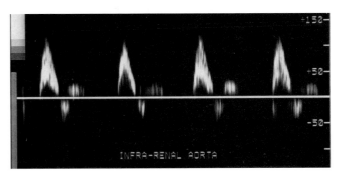

A

B

Figure 24–27. *A*, Doppler time-velocity waveform from the suprarenal abdominal aorta. Note forward diastolic flow. *B*, Doppler spectral waveform from the infrarenal aorta demonstrating the triphasic velocity waveform consistent with a vessel feeding a high-resistance vascular bed.

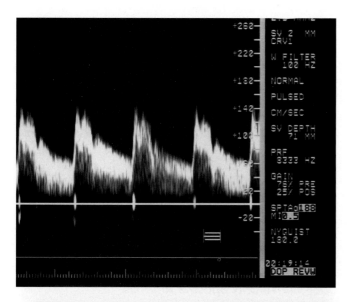

As the inferior mesenteric artery is difficult to accurately identify by duplex or Doppler color flow imaging technology, this vessel is not included in the routine evaluation of patients.

The signature Doppler velocity waveform from the renal arteries resembles that from other vessels feeding organs with a high flow demand. (See Figure 24–30.) The normal waveform from the proximal renal artery usually demonstrates a clear **systolic window** with spectral broadening evident in the mid- to distal segments of the vessel. This increase in spectral bandwidth is due to

Figure 24–28. Doppler velocity waveform from the celiac axis. Note constant forward diastolic flow.

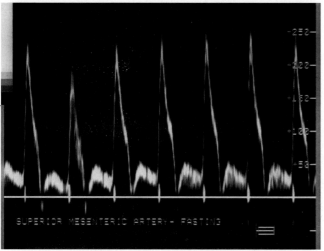

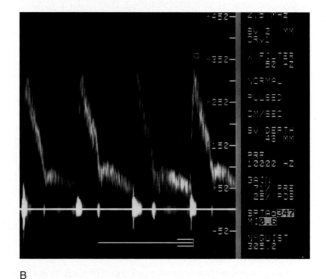

A   B

Figure 24–29. *A*, Velocity spectral waveform recorded from the fasting superior mesenteric artery; *B*, postprandially, the superior mesenteric artery diastolic flow component increases two- to three-fold in response to the metabolic demands imposed by digestion.

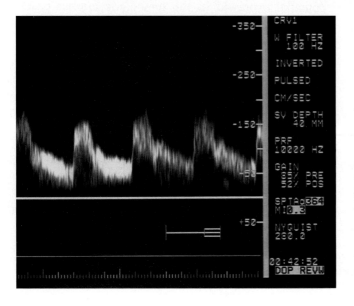

the fact that the sample volume size used to monitor the flow is normally large in relation to the lumen of the vessel, or increased in size to encompass the entire lumen of a poorly visualized artery during the study.

As the normal kidney has high metabolic demands and low vascular resistance, the Doppler velocity waveform from the interlobar and arcuate arteries of the renal medulla and cortex should demonstrate high diastolic flow. (See Figure 24–31*A*.) With increase in renovascular resistance due to intrinsic renal pathology, the end-diastolic flow component will decrease throughout the vascular tree of the organ and the velocity waveform will become markedly pulsatile. (See Figure 24–31*B*.)

Figure 24–30. Doppler time-velocity waveform from the normal renal artery. The high diastolic flow component is consistent with a vessel feeding a low-resistance end organ.

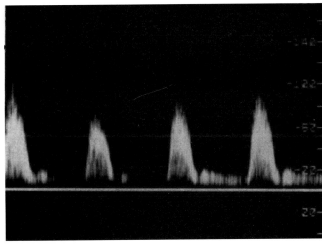

A

B

Figure 24-31. *A,* Doppler velocity waveform recorded from the normal renal parenchyma. *B,* Diastolic flow component of the renal parenchymal Doppler velocity signal decreases as renovascular resistance increases due to intrinsic renal pathology.

SUMMARY

Noninvasive vascular diagnostic methods have shown tremendous advancement over the past two decades with the development of sophisticated instrumentation and technology. Thus, a large armamentarium of direct and indirect test procedures is available for the identification and evaluation of cerebrovascular, peripheral arterial, venous, and visceral vascular disease. The laboratory staff must not only be skilled in performance of each test, but must also recognize the capabilities and limitations of these test procedures and understand the pathophysiology of vascular disease. The goal of the vascular diagnostic laboratory is to provide accurate, cost-effective, noninvasive diagnostic procedures which will answer the following questions:

Is vascular disease present? Where is it located? How severe is the vascular disorder? What is the prognosis? And, are therapeutic results being obtained?

REFERENCE CHARTS

Associated Physicians

Vascular Surgeon: Specializes in the surgical treatment of cerebrovascular, peripheral arterial, venous, and visceral vascular disorders.

Common Diagnostic Tests

Vascular Angiography: A contrast medium is injected into an artery or vein and x-ray films are taken at specific intervals to observe blood flow patterns in vessels and organ vasculature. Performed by angiographers (radiologists) and radiologic technologist, and interpreted by radiologists and vascular surgeons.

Laboratory Values

Nonapplicable.

Normal Measurements

Nonapplicable.

Vasculature

Nonapplicable.

Affecting Chemicals

Nonapplicable.

References

1. Pick TP, Howden R (eds.): Gray's Anatomy. New York, Bounty Books, 1977.
2. Neumyer MM, Thiele BL: Evaluation of lower extremity occlusive disease with Doppler ultrasound. In Taylor KJW, Burns PN, Wells PNT (eds.): Clinical Applications of Doppler Ultrasound. New York, Raven Press, 1988, 317–337.

Bibliography

Bernstein EF (ed.): Noninvasive Diagnostic Techniques in Vascular Disease, 3rd ed. St. Louis, CV Mosby, 1985.
Kremkau FW: Doppler Ultrasound: Principles and Instruments. Philadelphia, WB Saunders, 1990.
Strandness DE Jr: Duplex Scanning in Vascular Disorders. New York, Raven Press, 1990.
Zweibel WJ (ed.): Introduction to Vascular Ultrasonography, 2nd ed. Orlando, Grune & Stratton, 1986.

Chapter 25

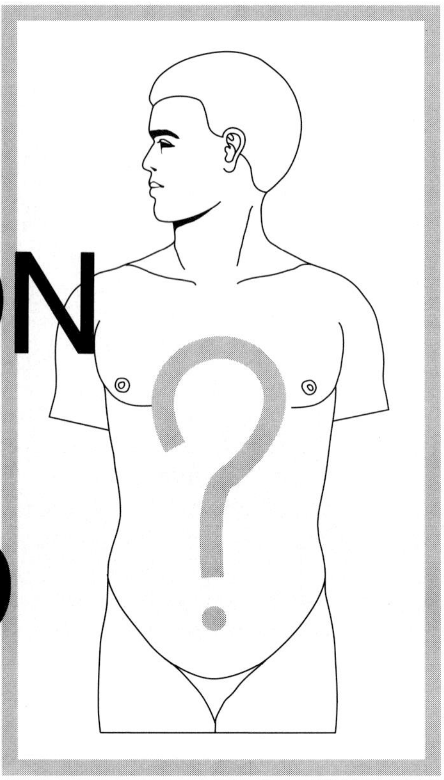

INTRODUCTION TO ULTRASOUND OF HUMAN DISEASE

FELICIA M. JONES

Objectives:

Describe the sonographic terms used to describe pathology.

Aids in the identification of pathology.

Demonstrate the basic types of pathology commonly seen with ultrasound.

Demonstrate the proper method for documenting pathologic findings.

Demonstrate the proper way to present pathologic findings to the interpreting physician.

Define the key words.

Key Words:

Attenuation
Complex
Cyst(ic)
Degenerating
Echogenic
Echolucent
Enhancement
Homogeneous
Isoechoic
Mass
Neoplasm
Nonhomogeneous
Parenchyma
Septations
Shadowing
Solid
Texture
Universal precautions

INTRODUCTION

Ultrasound is based on the concept that every soft tissue organ visualized by ultrasound has an individual normal **textural** appearance. This appearance is highly consistent person-to-person, with only small variations seen. The textural patterns help the sonographer to detect changes in the tissue **parenchyma** and the pathologic conditions that those changes might represent. All pathology visualized by ultrasound in some way disrupts the normal textural pattern of the organ involved. The more common changes are briefly discussed, as is the correct sonographic terminology.

The primary responsibility of the sonographer is to fully view all areas of interest and identify the textural patterns seen as part of the examination documentation process. By performing this function in a responsible and consistent manner, the sonographer is able to aid the interpreting physician in identifying any area of pathology. This approach allows a full description of the pathologic process to be presented to the referring physician in order to determine the best follow-up for the patient.

PRENATAL DEVELOPMENT

Some pathologic states arise due to a fault in prenatal development while others arise as **neoplasms** (new, abnormal growth of existing tissues; this may be benign or malignant). Still other pathologic states arise having no identified etiology.

The development of pathologic states, prenatal or otherwise, is not discussed. The purpose of this chapter is to aid the sonographer in the ability to describe and report the pathology seen to the interpreting physician without offering a diagnosis.

LOCATION

Pathology can arise anywhere in the body. The sonographer's goal is to report and describe the findings as consistently and accurately as possible without actually stating a diagnosis. This goal is reached through performing a thorough survey with careful examination and documentation, which includes correct labeling.

SIZE

The size of the pathology can vary. There are too many variables to permit a discussion of all of them in detail. Extensive pathology will disrupt the normal anatomy and be observed as changes in parenchymal appearance. All changes must be noted during the survey and then documented accordingly.

GROSS ANATOMY

A discussion of pathologic gross anatomy is not within the scope of this chapter.

PHYSIOLOGY

Pathology can arise from several pathways. The pathway of most concern to health care workers is bloodborne, as occurs with hepatitis. Such pathologies are spread by direct contact of diseased body fluids through open cuts or other skin tears. These pathologies may remain undetected for long periods of time. Therefore there is increased emphasis on **universal precautions** against such disease states. Precautions include wearing gloves, masks, or protective clothing when dealing with patients identified as being at high risk for such pathologies. This often means wearing gloves when scanning a patient with a possible skin tear. Thus gloves should be worn when scanning every patient.

Other pathologic states, such as cancerous tumors, arise internally and cannot be transmitted through body or fluid contact. Universal precautions are still to be followed, however, as much to protect the patient as to protect the sonographer.

SONOGRAPHIC APPEARANCE

All soft tissue organs possess a normal textural appearance, which varies very little person-to-person. Most soft tissue organs have a smooth, or **homogeneous**, texture composed of low to medium level shades of gray. Many examples of normal textural appearances have already been presented in this text. See Figure 25–1, which demonstrates the normal textural pattern of the liver and the right kidney. Note the difference in echogenicities between the outer renal cortex, inner renal medulla, and the liver parenchyma.

It is especially important to assess all segments of each organ during the survey part of the sonographic examination. This allows detection of pathologic states before image documentation is begun, and therefore allows the sonographer to proceed with image documentation in an orderly manner.

When the normal homogeneous texture of an organ becomes disrupted, the parenchyma assumes an irregular or **nonhomogeneous** pattern. In other words, the parenchyma is no longer smooth and uniform. There are several key findings that can be utilized to help detect any parenchymal changes. The changes may be diffuse (spread generally throughout the organ) or localized (found in one specific area). A localized change in par-

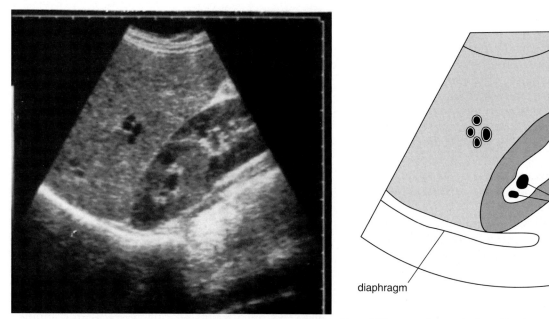

Figure 25–1. Normal liver and right kidney. Note differences in parenchymal echogenicities.

enchyma represents a **mass**. Further description is often necessary and will be presented according to the terminology used in this chapter.

The first key change to look for in assessing tissue parenchyma is the presence of a **cyst** or cystic area within the organ borders. To be considered a true cyst, the area in question must meet three criteria. The first criterion is that it contain no internal echoes. This means that the central area of a cyst is the same color as the background color of the screen. It is possible to observe anterior cystic noise within a true cyst; that is, low level echoes located near the anterior wall of the cyst. Echoes never occur in the posterior portion of a true cyst. The second criterion is that the walls of the cyst must be well defined,

thin, and smooth. Any irregularities in the cystic border must be noted. The final criterion is that there be posterior through transmission, or **enhancement**. Posterior through transmission refers to an area immediately posterior to the cyst which appears brighter or more echogenic than the adjacent tissues. (See Figure 25–2.)

There are two situations in which the enhancement criterion may be difficult to meet: (1) a cyst located very deep in the body: if the cyst is located beyond the focal zone, not enough sound remains to create the enhancement effect; (2) a cyst located immediately anterior to a bony structure: in such a case, the bone absorbs the extra sound and eliminates the enhancement effect.

If any one of these three criteria is not met, the struc-

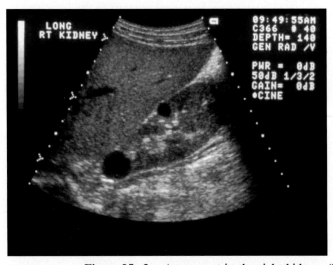
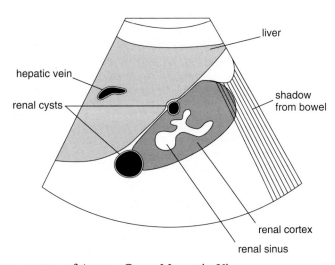

Figure 25–2. A true cyst in the right kidney. (Image courtesy of Acuson Corp., Mountain View, CA.)

ture is not a true cyst. A structure which meets one or more of these criteria, but not all three, is said to be cystic in nature, although not a true cyst. An example of a cystic area which does not meet the requirements for a true cyst would be ascites in the abdominal cavity, or a pleural effusion. Both ascites and pleural effusion are echolucent areas with no internal echoes, and demonstrate posterior though transmission, but neither fluid collection has well-defined smooth walls.

A cystic structure that contains thin membranous inclusions is said to be **septated**.

A cyst that contains solid or echogenic components is said to be **complex**. Complex masses may be primarily cystic or primarily solid. It is the combination of both appearances within the same structure which gives rise to the term complex.

The internal composition of a mass may vary with time. This is especially true of vascular masses, which may be echolucent when the internal blood is fresh, but become complex and even solid as the blood forms clots. Another example is a solid mass which **degenerates** over time. An example of this occurrence may be seen with uterine fibroids. These benign tumors may remain very stable for years and then, due to various hormonal changes, begin to change internally. This type of degenerating process usually means that a solid mass has begun to liquefy and thereby assume a more complex appearance. (See Figure 25–3.)

The second key finding in assessing the parenchymal patterns of soft tissue organs is the presence of **solid** masses. A solid area is said to be **echogenic**. These areas may be composed of various shades of gray, but there are always internal echoes present. Image processing and/or gain manipulation may be necessary in order to highlight

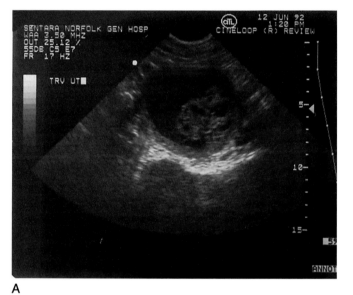

A

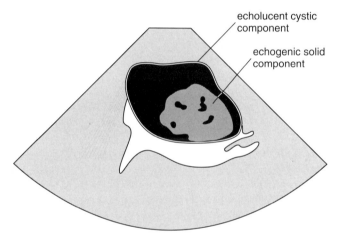

B

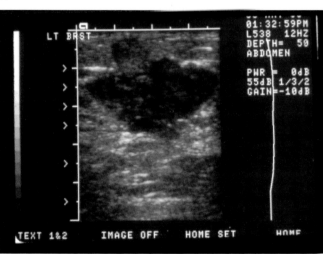

C

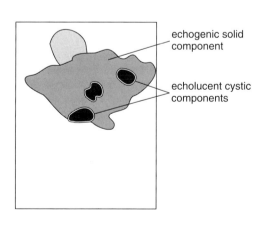

D

Figure 25–3. *A, B,* A primarily cystic complex mass. (Image courtesy of Sentara Norfolk General Hospital, Norfolk, VA.) *C, D,* A primarily solid complex mass. (Image courtesy of Acuson Corp., Mountain View, CA.)

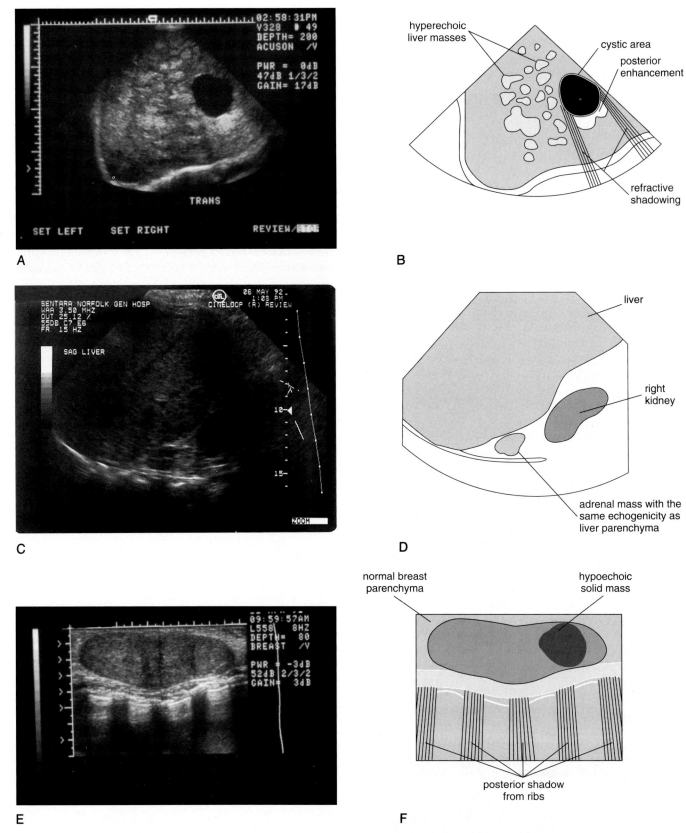

Figure 25-4. *A, B,* A hyperechoic solid mass. Note the separate cystic area. (Image courtesy of Acuson Corp., Mountain View, CA.) *C, D,* An isoechoic mass in the adrenal gland compared to liver parenchyma. (Image courtesy of Sentara Norfolk General Hospital, Norfolk, VA.) *E, F,* A solid hypoechoic mass. (Image courtesy of Acuson Corp., Mountain View, CA.)

these echoes. Solid masses are described on the basis of the levels of echogenicity within them.

A mass that is more echogenic than normal tissue parenchyma is said to be hyperechoic. A mass having the same echogenicity as the surrounding tissue is said to be **isoechoic**. Border differentiation may be the only clue to the presence of this type of solid mass. A solid mass which is less echogenic than the surrounding tissues is said to be hypoechoic. This type of mass will have a darker appearance on the screen, and gain manipulation or processing techniques may be necessary to differentiate it from a cystic mass. (See Figure 25–4.)

The third finding that will help in identifying the presence of pathology is the assessment of the borders of the mass. It is very important to convey the appearance of mass borders to the interpreting physician. This means describing whether the borders are smooth or irregular in contour, whether the borders are thin or thick, and whether the borders are uniform throughout the circumference of the mass. (See Figure 25–5.)

The final finding to aid in identifying pathology is the presence of posterior **shadowing**. Shadowing may be present under two sets of circumstances. The first is shadowing posterior to a calcified structure. The posterior shadow is **echolucent**. Thus there are no echoes within the area of the shadow. Posterior shadows will have fairly clean, well-defined edges. This type of shadowing occurs because the anterior calcific structure absorbs the bulk of the sound and there is no sound remaining to continue along the beam path. An example of a structure which causes this type of shadowing is a gallstone. The calcified structure itself will appear brightly echogenic with variable border definition. (See Figure 25–6.)

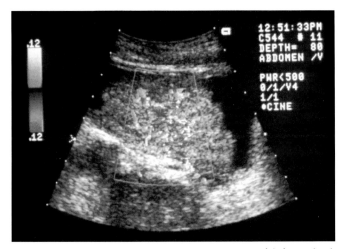

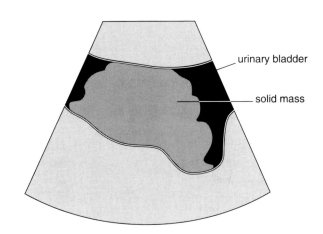

Figure 25–5. A bladder mass with irregular borders. (Image courtesy of Acuson Corp., Mountain View, CA.) (See Color Plate 19 at the back of this book.)

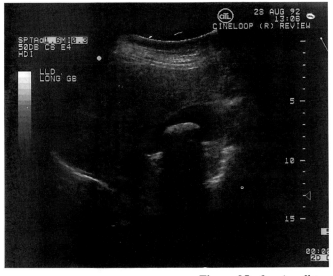

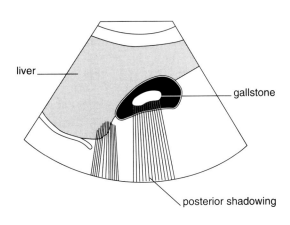

Figure 25–6. A gallstone with posterior shadowing.

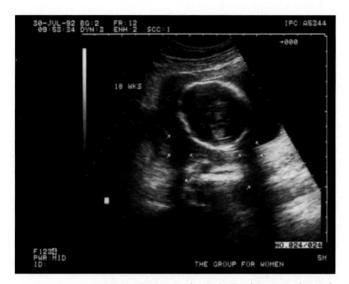
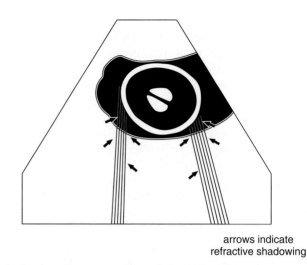

arrows indicate
refractive shadowing

Figure 25–7. A fetal skull with posterior refractive shadowing. (Image courtesy of the Group for Women, Norfolk, VA.)

Shadowing does not always mean that pathology is present. The second type of shadowing is refractive. Refractive shadowing may occur at edge margins, especially on rounded structures. This often occurs at large, smooth targets which are located within a structure that has a different propagation velocity. An example of this is a fetal skull surrounded by amniotic fluid. Refractive shadowing occurs because a target acts as a partial specular reflector and the sound changes the propagation angle. The sound beam becomes more perpendicular to the beam path and the sound is bent or refracted and refocused. This creates the area of shadowing. An example of this type of shadowing commonly seen is the shadows at the edges of a fetal skull. (See Figure 25–7.)

Both shadowing and posterior through transmission are forms of posterior **attenuation**. In the case of enhancement there is less attenuation through the fluid within the cystic structure than there is through the adjacent soft tissue path. Therefore, more sound remains posterior to the cyst and that area appears more echogenic.

With shadowing, the opposite occurs. The calcific structure anteriorly is highly attenuating and there is much less sound available to continue along the beam path. Therefore, an area of decreased echogenicity is seen.

SUMMARY OF PATHOLOGIC FINDINGS

Internal echogenicity
  Cystic
    True cysts
    Cystic structures
    Septated
  Complex
    Primarily cystic
    Primarily solid
  Solid
    Hyperechoic
    Isoechoic
    Hypoechoic
Posterior attenuation
  Enhancement
  Shadowing
    Calcific structures
    Refractive shadowing
Border definition
  Smooth and regular
  Irregular

SONOGRAPHIC APPLICATIONS

One of the responsibilities of the sonographer is to report variations in tissue appearance which represent the presence of pathology. This should be reported utilizing correct sonographic terms. The following are two examples of how this might be stated: (1) *a solid echogenic mass is seen in the right posterior lobe of the liver. The mass has irregular borders;* (2) *a single cystic area with smooth borders and posterior enhancement is seen within the left ovary.*

Although these may represent very common, easily

identifiable pathologies, the definition of the pathology present is a decision the interpreting physician must make. The goal of the sonographer is to provide all the information necessary in a nonbiased manner.

It is important to remember that the presentation of findings by the sonographer often leads to a detailed discussion of pathologic possibilities between the sonographer and the interpreting physician. A properly trained, experienced sonographer can provide the physician with a great deal of information which can aid in the interpretation process. This is a common practice which reflects the degree of experience many sonographers posses. The final decision still falls to the interpreting physician.

The goal of this chapter is to provide the sonographer with the knowledge base necessary to relay the sonographic finding to the interpreting physician without directly stating a diagnosis.

NORMAL VARIANTS

The many aspects of pathologic variants are not within the scope of this chapter and are not discussed.

REFERENCE CHARTS

Associated Physicians

Radiologist: Specializes in the diagnostic interpretation of imaging modalities that are used to determine the presence of pathologic processes. The physician may utilize invasive maneuvers to determine the exact nature of the demonstrated pathology, such as biopsies.

Pathologist: Specializes in determining the nature of pathologic tissues. This is usually done through biopsies and cellular examination.

Obstetrician/Gynecologist: Specializes in treating female patients, whether pregnant or not. The physician often performs and/or interprets the ultrasound examinations and may perform whatever follow-up is necessary.

Cardiologist: Specializes in the interpretation of cardiac testing methods, including the echocardiogram (ultrasound of the heart).

Common Diagnostic Tests

Computed Axial Tomography (CT Scan): This test utilizes x-rays to demonstrate a cross-sectional image of the body. A contrast medium is often injected to help differentiate pathology from normal anatomic variants. The test is performed by a radiologic technologist and interpreted by a radiologist.

Magnetic Resonance Imaging (MRI): This imaging modality utilizes changes in magnetic fields to assess anatomy. The test may also require the injection of a contrast medium. An MRI is performed most often by a specially trained radiologic technologist and is interpreted by a radiologist.

Laboratory Values

The laboratory findings vary from case to case and organ to organ. Some have been mentioned in previous chapters and further review is not presented in this chapter.

Normal Measurements

All pathology should be imaged and measured in two planes, including the longest axis of the mass.

Vasculature

It is extremely important to determine the lie of pathology relative to adjacent vasculature. Normal vasculature can be very helpful in stating the correct location of pathology for the interpreting physician. Adjacent vasculature must be assessed to determine if pathologic involvement or changes are present due to the pathologic state.

Affecting Chemicals

The chemicals affecting the potential for pathologic development, as well as those which can affect existing pathologies, vary from organ to organ and are not discussed further in this chapter. Refer to previous chapters for relevant information.

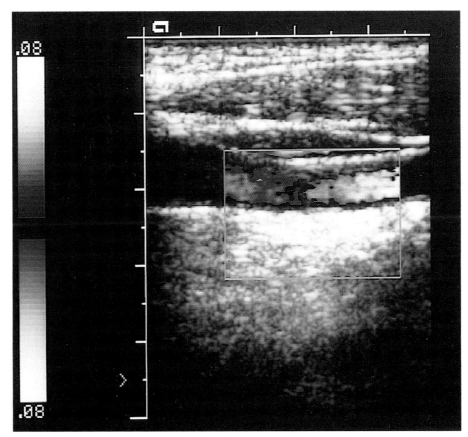

PLATE 1. Color flow Doppler image.

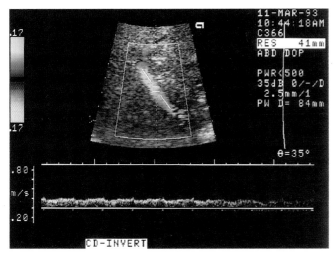

PLATE 2. Color flow Doppler image showing the characteristic waveform of a normal portal vein. Note that the blood flow is in the direction of the liver toward the transducer.

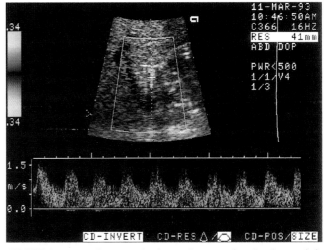

PLATE 3. Color flow Doppler image demonstrating the characteristic arterial waveform of the normal hepatic artery.

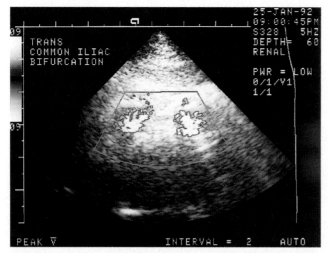

PLATE 4. Color Doppler sonogram demonstrating the common iliac arteries.

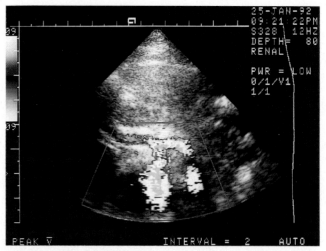

PLATE 5. Color Doppler sonogram demonstrating flow within the aorta, celiac artery, splenic artery, and common hepatic artery.

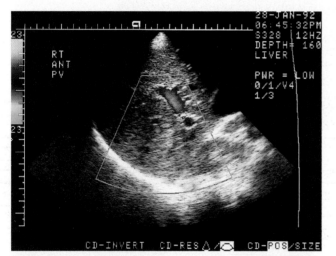

PLATE 6. Longitudinal section of the right lobe of the liver demonstrating normal color flow Doppler. Note that flow toward the transducer is indicated in red. Thus, the flow is toward the transducer (into the liver) in this case.

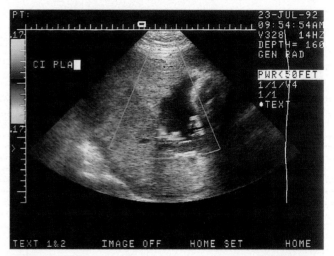

PLATE 7. Color flow demonstration of the placental cord insertion site.

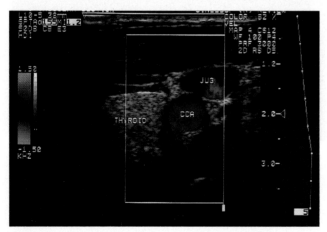

PLATE 8. Transverse Doppler color flow image of the common carotid artery, jugular vein, and thyroid gland.

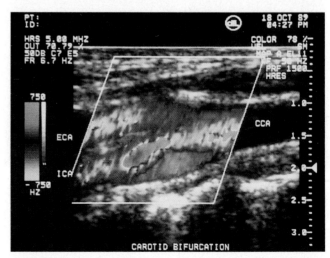

PLATE 9. Long axis Doppler color flow image of the carotid bifurcation showing the common carotid artery, external carotid artery, and internal carotid artery. Note the zone of retrograde flow in the carotid bulb caused by boundary layer separation.

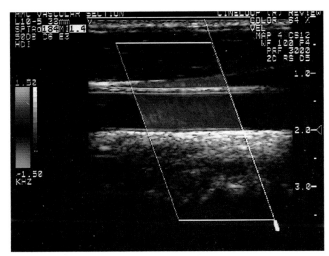

PLATE 10. Long axis image of the common carotid artery. Arterial wall definition reveals linear reflectivity resulting from the echogenicity of collagen found in the intima and media.

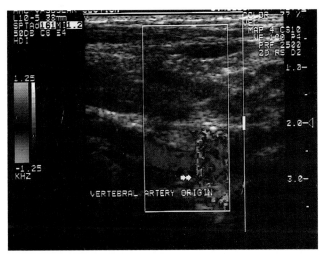

PLATE 11. Doppler color flow image of the vertebral artery origin. The subclavian artery is seen in the transverse plane just distal to the origin of the right common carotid artery.

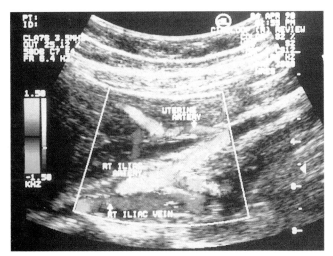

PLATE 12. Doppler color flow image of the aortic bifurcation. (Courtesy of Advanced Technology Laboratories.)

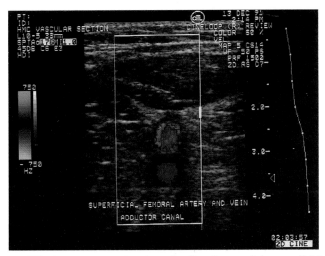

PLATE 13. Transverse Doppler color flow image of the superficial femoral artery and vein in Hunter's canal.

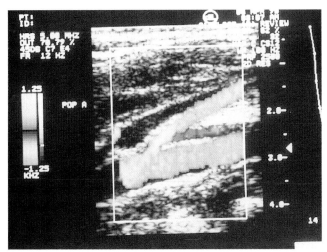

PLATE 14. Long axis color flow image of the popliteal artery.

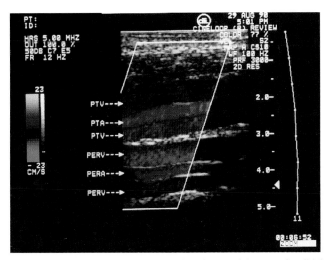

PLATE 15. Long axis Doppler color flow image of the posterior tibial and peroneal arteries surrounded by their companion tibial veins of the same name. (Courtesy of Advanced Technology Laboratories.)

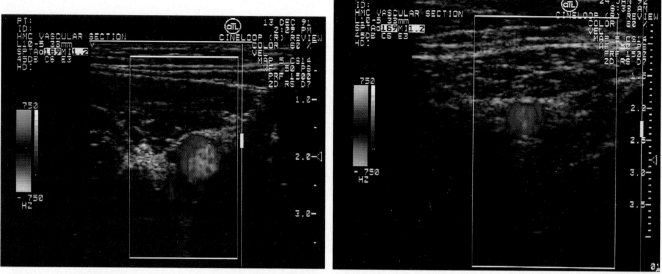

PLATE 16. *Left,* Transverse Doppler color flow imaging of the superficial femoral artery and vein; *right,* Doppler color flow image of the superficial femoral artery and vein demonstrating coaptation of the venous walls that occurs with gentle transducer pressure.

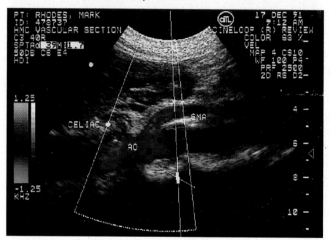

PLATE 17. Longitudinal Doppler color flow image of the abdominal aorta and the origins of the celiac and superior mesenteric arteries from the anterior wall of the aorta.

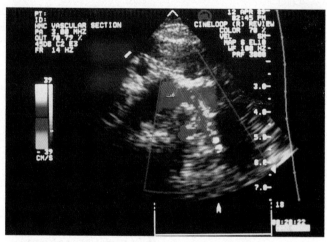

PLATE 18. Transverse color flow image of the abdominal aorta showing the origin of the left renal artery.

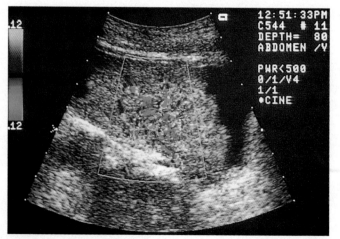

PLATE 19. A bladder mass with irregular borders. (Courtesy of Acuson Corp., Mountain View, CA.)

SECTION VIII

APPENDICES

I

ULTRASOUND DOCUMENTS RELATED TO PATIENT EXAMINATION

HEATHER LEVY
REVA ARNEZ CURRY

The ultrasound request form, patient chart, and final report are essential documents for ultrasound examinations. The following explanation should assist the entry level sonographer in utilizing these materials.

ULTRASOUND REQUEST FORM AND PATIENT CHART

The ultrasound request form and patient chart are usually reviewed by the sonographer before the ultrasound examination is performed. A request should include patient identification data, clinical symptoms, and the type of examination requested.

A sample request form is shown in Figure 1. This form has four main sections (each institution uses a different type of request, dependent upon the information it requires). The top right corner of this request is used to record patient identification. Adjacent to this section is the information needed to report preliminary results. To the far left is a check box for stat or portable procedures. Immediately beneath this area is a check box for patients who require isolation precautions.

The next section contains the referring physician or clinic's name, address, and essential clinical data which explain the reason that the examination has been requested.

The following section contains space for additional patient history, a bar code for computerized entry into the department's data system, and space for the referring physician's signature and beeper number.

ULTRASOUND REQUEST
THOMAS JEFFERSON UNIVERSITY HOSPITAL
DEPARTMENT OF RADIOLOGY
DIVISION OF DIAGNOSTIC ULTRASOUND

		MEDICAL RECORD #
		NAME

☐ STAT

☐ PORTABLE

CALL PRELIMINARY REPORT TO;		
DOCTOR		ADDRESS
LOCATION		AGE
		BIRTH DATE
PHONE NO		PHONE NO.

ISOLATION PRECAUTION   ☐ YES

REFERRING PHYSICIAN/CLINIC (NAME & ADDRESS)	PHONE NO.

ESSENTIAL CLINICAL FACTS • (MUST BE COMPLETED BEFORE EXAM IS PERFORMED)

REASON FOR EXAMINATION

RELEVANT MEDICAL HISTORY

A 3 4 1 4 7 6

PHYSICIAN'S SIGNATURE & BEEPER #   DATE

ABDOMEN
- ☐ **ABDOMEN COMPLETE**
- ☐ LIVER
- ☐ GALLBLADDER
- ☐ SPLEEN
- ☐ ASCITES
- ☐ PALPABLE MASS
- ☐ DOPPLER

RETROPERITONEUM
- ☐ **RETROPERITONEUM COMPLETE**
- ☐ PANCREAS
- ☐ KIDNEYS
- ☐ ADRENALS
- ☐ AORTA/IVC
- ☐ LYMPH NODES
- ☐ DOPPLER

CHEST
- ☐ MEDIASTINUM
- ☐ PLEURAL EFFUSION
- ☐ THORACENTESIS

EXAM.		
TECH.		
ROOM		
DATE		

PELVIS
- ☐ **RENAL TRANSPLANT**
- ☐ URINARY BLADDER
- ☐ PROSTATE
- ☐ RECTUM
- ☐ SCROTUM
- ☐ DOPPLER

HEAD AND NECK
- ☐ BRAIN
- ☐ URINARY BLADDER
- ☐ URINARY BLADDER

HEART
- ☐ **COMPLETE ECHOCARDIOGRAM**
- ☐ M-MODE & 2D ECHOCARDIOGRAM
- ☐ DOPPLER ECHOCARDIOGRAM

VASCULAR
- ☐ CEREBROVASCULAR COMPLETE
- ☐ PERIPHERAL VASC. (ARTERIAL)
- ☐ PERIPHERAL VASC. (VENOUS)
  - ☐ IMAGING
  - ☐ IPG

NOT LISTED
- ☐ (SPECIFY)

GYNECOLOGY
- ☐ **PELVIS COMPLETE**
- ☐ UTERUS
- ☐ OVARIES
- ☐ FOLLICLE SIZE
- ☐ IUD LOCALIZATION
- ☐ DOPPLER

OBSTETRICAL
- ☐ **FETAL COMPLETE**
- ☐ FETAL COMPLETE (INTERNAL GROWTH)
- ☐ OBSTETRIC DOPPLER
- ☐ AMNIOCENTESIS
- ☐ SPECIAL (SPECIFY)

SUPERFICIAL
- ☐ BREAST
- ☐ PALPABLE
- ☐ JOINT/TENDON/MUSCLE

INTERVENTIONAL
- ☐ BIOPSY (SPECIFY AREA BELOW)
- ☐ ASPIRATION (SPECIFY AREA BELOW)
- ☐ ABSCESS DRAINAGE
- ☐ INTRAOPERATIVE GUIDANCE

AREA:

Figure 1. Department request form. (Courtesy of Thomas Jefferson University Hospital, Philadelphia, PA.)

The last section of the form contains check-off boxes for the type of examination ordered. The lower left corner of the form contains space for sonographer identification and where the procedure was performed.

This request form stresses information needed in this particular tertiary care center. Notice the emphasis on providing assistance to referring physicians through preliminary reporting and listing the types of procedures which can be ordered.

Another document that sonographers review before an inpatient examination is the patient's chart. Refer to the accompanying list, in Section IV of the appendices, of the different information which may be included in a chart. The most important items for sonographers are any type of assessment notes (the results of the physical examination, a listing of patient's symptoms, and the like) and laboratory test results. Most charts will contain labelled sections for easier reference.

Since outpatient charts are kept in the referring physician's office, it is essential that the ultrasound request contain the patient's clinical symptoms and the reason the ultrasound study was ordered. In addition to this, many ultrasound departments require sonographers to take a brief medical history of the patient before conducting the examination. In lieu of a detailed history written on the request, this may be the only means that information can be obtained for some outpatient examinations.

INTERPRETIVE REPORT (THE FINAL REPORT)

After the ultrasound examination has been completed, the sonologist (usually a radiologist) will dictate a report interpreting the ultrasound findings. This report usually lists differential diagnoses (possible pathologic conditions which were indicated by the ultrasound examination). This final report is sent to the referring physician, a copy is put in the inpatient's chart, and a copy is kept in the patient's ultrasound file.

Figure 2 shows a sample report on a fetal age study. Note that the report presents the final diagnosis first. NOTE: More than one diagnosis may be indicated by the ultrasound examination. Several likely diagnoses (called differential diagnoses) may therefore be listed in the report.

The next section of the report explains the ultrasound findings in detail. The report concludes with the most likely diagnoses based on the ultrasound findings.

FETAL AGE

DIAGNOSIS:

Findings compatible with complete spontaneous abortion, ectopic pregnancy, or very early intrauterine pregnancy.

COMMENT:

Real-time ultrasound of the pelvis was performed using transabdominal and endovaginal technique. No previous studies are available for review. The patient has a positive urine pregnancy test by history.

The uterus measures 10.2 x 4.2 x 5.0 cm. No intrauterine gestational sac is identified on transabdominal or endovaginal scan.

The left ovary is enlarged, measuring 4.2 x 2.9 x 3.6 cm. A cystic structure measuring less than 1 cm is seen in the left ovary.

The right ovary measures 2.6 x 1.1 x 2.8 cm. There are no right adnexal masses.

There is no free fluid in the cul de sac.

In light of the history of positive urine pregnancy test, the differential diagnosis for the above findings includes complete spontaneous abortion, ectopic pregnancy, or, less likely, very early intrauterine pregnancy. Correlation with serial beta-HCGs is advised.

Survey views of both kidneys reveal no hydronephrosis.

Figure 2. Sonologist's final report on a fetal age study. (Courtesy of Thomas Jefferson University Hospital, Philadelphia, PA.)

THE SONOGRAPHER'S TECHNICAL IMPRESSION

The sonologist's final report differs significantly from the sonographer's "technical impression." Some institutions require sonographers to write a technical impression after the examination is completed. This impression should describe the location, shape, size, and echogenicity of any abnormal findings. The sonographer should **not** write a diagnosis or differential diagnoses (eg, "The patient has pancreatitis"). This complies with standards developed by the Society of Diagnostic Medical Sonographers (SDMS) and the American Institute of Ultrasound in Medicine (AIUM). To obtain further information about technical impressions, please contact either professional organization.

ULTRASOUND INSTRUMENTATION

HEATHER LEVY

This section describes the ultrasound system controls and explains how to operate them. Ultrasound systems are software-based systems and need to be configured correctly before some controls will appear on the touch panel or others will function as expected. Configuration is performed at installation by an ultrasound customer support representative.

Although hospitals around the world employ different types of ultrasound equipment, the basic "knobology" is the same. Here are a few of the common control buttons and their functions which may be used by an experienced professional performing the ultrasound examination.[1]

KEYBOARD CONTROLS

Keyboard controls (alphanumeric) allow user to enter patient's name, ID number, and provide full screen annotation; they may also include specific function keys, eg:

1. **Annotation on/off**, which allows annotation to be entered from the keyboard onto the screen.
2. **Erase screen** will erase all user-entered annotations from the screen where the cursor is located.
3. **Backspace** will erase the last user-entered character to the left of the cursor.

Some systems employ a **HELP** menu to access and provide a quick reference manual to the system usage.

PRIMARY CONTROLS

Trackball. The basic functions of the trackball are to guide the cursor on the screen and position the measurement cursors during the freeze mode. In systems with cineloop, this control allows 2-D image review to be scrolled in real time. Depending upon the system, the trackball may serve various other functions.

Time Gain Compensation (TGC). TGC is used to equalize the differences in received echo amplitudes due to reflector depth. This is accomplished because the TGC provides a gradual increase in amplification with depth by compensating for attenuation of the signal strength over depth. This control adjusts the shape of the TGC curve. The TGC curve is displayed vertically to the right of the ultrasound image on the screen.

2-D/M Overall Gain. This controls the overall amplification or gain applied to the signals produced by the echoes returning from the body.

Focal Zone Position. This control positions the focal zone to the desired scan depth.

Focal Zone Depth. The depth range of the display is controlled by this function. Adjusting this will either increase or decrease the number of focal zones; however, the maximum allowed depth is dependent upon the scanhead selected.

Freeze Frame Key. Once the desired ultrasound image has been obtained, it may be stored in the system's memory by activating the freeze key. After the image is stored, measurements and calculations may be performed. Freezing automatically enables cineloop image review or Doppler review when applicable. Depress button when finished to restore frozen image to real time.

Print Key. Activates the resident multi-image camera to record the frozen image. The system will remain in freeze until the image is recorded. If the system was scanning before the print, it will resume scanning after the image is captured. If it was frozen before the print was taken, it will remain frozen.

Calc Key. Activates the appropriate calculations package.

Transducer Button (XCTR). This allows the operator to select different transducers and scan heads.

Image Direction. Depressing this button electronically reverses the scan direction of the displayed image.

Body Pattern. Used to display the body pattern to indicate patient positioning during the scan session.

New Patient Key. Will clear current patient ID, graphics, and comments so that new information may be entered.

Measurement Keys

1. **Distance**–place cursor for distance measurements.
2. **Trace**–outline for curve or circumference measurements.
3. **Measure**–to complete above measurements and display results.
4. **Off**–to erase cursors, outlines, and measurement results.

Monitor Controls. Allows user to adjust the amount of detail in the ultrasound image.

Brightness. Adjusts the light output of the entire image.

Contrast. Adjusts the difference in light output between the light and dark parts of the image. CAUTION: Maintaining a very high display contrast level can damage your screen. Avoid using high contrast settings for an extended period of time.

BASIC OPERATIONS

1. Enter patient name and ID. (Some machines may require depressing "new patient" soft key.)
2. After entering the information, press RETURN key to store patient information.
3. Place transducer on the patient with a generous amount of coupling gel.
4. Adjust TGC until desired image is obtained.
5. Adjust focal zones to cover the area of interest in the image.
6. Adjust image size by utilizing depth control.

Proper use of the above controls must be coupled with appropriate transducer selection. Below is a list of the basic types of transducers available with most modern machinery:

1. Flat linear array
2. Curved linear array
3. Electronic phases array
4. Annular array

Once the images have been stored, the next task is in the recording. Currently, there are a variety of ways in which images can be documented. Polaroid film makes it possible to record hard copies in black and white and even color. X-ray film can provide transparent or opaque hard copy images. Also, x-ray film can be used with a multi-image camera to record multiple images on a single sheet of film or photographic paper. More recently, fiberoptic recorders using light-sensitive paper to produce black and white hard copy frozen images have been employed. Videotape recorders and video disk recorders are also being utilized to store information using a magnetic medium. The videotape recorder can store live or frozen images, and the newer video disk recorders are designed to store frozen images on mini-diskettes.[2]

FILM PROCESSING

HEATHER LEVY

However competent the sonographer is, adequate visibility of necessary structures will not occur unless the film is properly developed. The individual developing the film must initially familiarize himself or herself with the darkroom layout upon entering the darkroom. First locate the processor and make sure it is on. If it is not, there is usually a button about 5 inches under and to the left of the feeding tray that will turn the machine on. Next, locate the film bin but DO NOT OPEN. Doing so will expose the film inside and make it unusable. Before turning the lights out, orient the cassette so that changing the film will occur as rapidly and efficiently as possible. Turn on the safety light (usually red), and then turn off the overhead lights.

Lay the cassette on the counter. Begin to unload the cassette by pulling out the protective sheet on top of the cassette. This will slide right out if the tab is pulled. Turn down the safety strip located on the bottom of the cassette and slide the film out. (See Figure 3A.) You will notice that the film has two different textured sides, a shiny side and a dull side (the emulsion side). Place the film on the feeding tray of the processor with the shiny side down and push forward until the film is taken in by the processor's rollers. To avoid jamming the processor, a low level bell will sound, indicating that the processor is now ready to accept another film. To reload the cassette, reach into the film bin for a single sheet of film. Place the shiny side down and slip it into the cassette, making sure the film is wedged between the two grooves along the length of the cassette. Flip up the safety strip and replace the protective sheet with the white border facing outward to show that the cassette contains unexposed film. (See Figure 3B.) If both sides of the cassette are exposed, repeat this process. Before turning the lights

back on, make sure the film bin is closed and that your film in the processor is secured from light exposure (the low level bell will ring). Once this is checked, turn the lights on. Your film will drop into the receiving bin when it is fully developed.

The type of system described above is known as automatic processing and was developed in the 1950's. It increased efficiency and improved image quality compared to the old way of developing film by hand. As film is fed into the film tray the transport system begins to process the film. Excluding the entering rollers at the feed tray, most of the rollers in the transport system are positioned on a rack assembly. These racks are easily removable and provide for convenient and efficient maintenance of the processor. Completing this process is the dryer system, which thoroughly extracts all residual moisture from the processed film and drops it into the receiving bin either inside or outside the darkroom. This entire process takes 90 seconds.[3]

Another type of processing system employed at some hospitals is commonly known as daylight processing. There is no manual loading or unloading of film necessary and therefore the concept of a darkroom is eliminated. Instead, the system is divided into a modular dispenser and a modular unloader with automatic identification.[4]

The dispenser is divided into two basic parts. The upper half is for unexposed film storage and dispensing, while the lower half accepts and lifts the empty cassette for loading one sheet of film. When an empty cassette is placed in the cradle of the dispenser and pressed against a pair of interlock switches, the cassette is automatically lifted to the load position. It is recommended that the cassette be inserted with the white side out; however, this

453

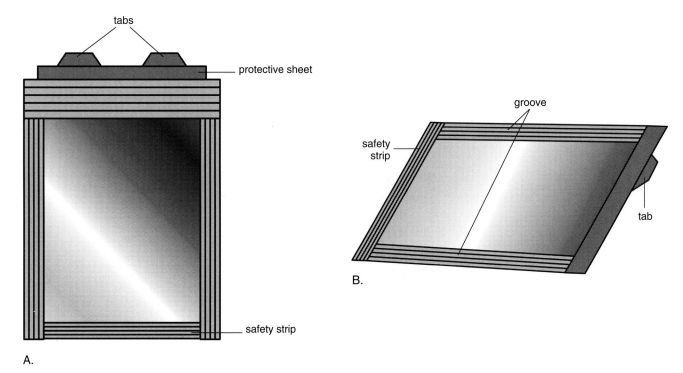

Figure 3. *A*, 8 × 10 film cassette. *B*, Side view.

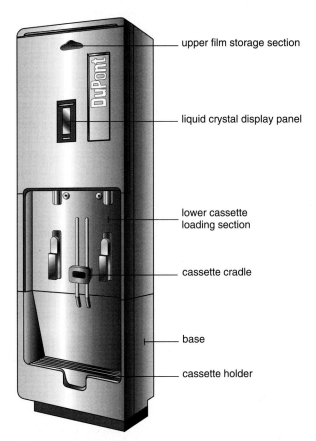

Figure 4. Modular dispenser. (Courtesy of E. I. Dupont Co. Inc., Wilmington, DE.)

switch will not close if the cassette is upside down. The arrow on the display panel appears as an indication that a film is being dispensed. The cassette is then lowered and ready for use. In addition to these features, a base for dispenser support and cassette storage is provided. (See Figure 4.)

To use the modular unloader, first observe on the display panel that the green power light is on. Insert the patient identification card into the slot provided with the image side down. Next, insert a cassette with the green colored side toward the operator. A spring-loaded movable guide block adjusts automatically to match the width of the cassette. Press down on the cassette and observe the display panel to see an image of the film leaving the cassette. This will not occur if the cassette is upside down. When the above process is complete, remove the cassette and wait for your image to be processed. (See Figure 5.)

With either automatic processing or daylight processing systems, the sequence of events when processing a film is as follows[3]:

1. **Wetting** – This step swells the emulsion to permit subsequent chemical penetration.

2. **Development** – This is the production of the manifest image from the latent image. The temperature during this stage is most critical and should remain constant at around 93° F.

3. **Stop Bath** – During this time, the developmental process is finished and excess chemicals are removed from the film's emulsion.

identification cardholder shelf

cassette entrance port

movable guide block

liquid crystal display panel

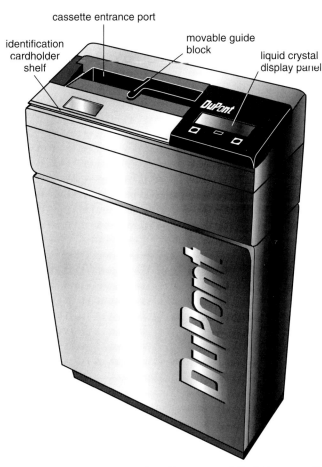

Figure 5. Modular unloader. (Courtesy of E. I. Dupont Co. Inc., Wilmington, DE.)

4. **Fixing**–The fixer removes the remaining silver halide from the emulsion and hardens the gelatin covering the film.

5. **Washing**–This is the final removal of any excess chemicals before the ultimate step occurs.

6. **Drying**–It is during this step that excess water is removed and the film is prepared for viewing.

Film development is a chemical reaction, and it is governed by three physical properties: time, temperature, and concentration of the developer.[3] Manufacturers of film and developing chemicals have carefully selected the conditions for these parameters to work optimally. Deviation from these recommendations will result in loss of image quality, possibly due to chemical or developmental fog.

As with any electromechanical device, maintenance is crucial. If the equipment is not properly maintained, it will malfunction when least expected, causing serious delays in providing optimal images by decreasing film quality.

References

1. Acuson XP: Acoustic Imaging AI 5200, ATL Ultramark 9, and General Electric Operator's Instrumentation Manuals.
2. Pickney N: A Review of the Concepts of Ultrasound Physics and Instrumentation. West Point, PA, Sonicor Inc., 1991.
3. Bushong SC: Radiologic Science for Technologists, 4th ed. St. Louis, CV Mosby, 1988, 225–240.
4. E. I. Dupont De Nemours Co. Inc.: Dupont Modular Daylight System Operations Manual: Modular Dispenser and Modular Unloader: Auto ID. Wilmington, 1987.

IV

PATIENT CHART INFORMATION: MEDICAL/SURGICAL ASSEMBLY ORDER

Lists of documents which comprise patient charts. (Courtesy of Thomas Jefferson University Hospital, Philadelphia, PA.)

HEATHER LEVY
REVA ARNEZ CURRY

The following lists the type of information found in inpatient charts. Items of particular importance to sonographers are in boldface type.

ROUTINE INPATIENT CHART

Diagnosis worksheet
Admission form
Consent for routine examination and treatment
Patient authorizations
Consent for operations, procedures, etc.
Consent for anesthesia
Release form

Living will
Preadmission forms
Physician's orders for admission
Discharge summary
Discharge summary sheet
Emergency room record
Patient care plan
Acute dialysis unit patient care plan
Patient problem list
Nursing transfer summary
History, physical progress notes
Social work evaluation and social work notes go in date order within progress notes

Respiratory care department, patient care record
Patient teaching record
Discharge planning record
Discharge planning assessment
Home IV therapy performance checklist
Instructions to patient
Discharge summary note
Consultations
Cardiac catheterization reports
   Preoperative nursing record
   Cardiac catheterization nursing
   Preliminary catheterization report
   Catheterization report
Operative reports: Perioperative nursing record
Preoperative anesthesia summary
Operative notes
Pathology
OR sponge/instrument count
Postanesthesia record
Recovery room record
Cardiopulmonary perfusion record
Endoscopy report
Fibroscopic bronchoscopy
Data mount
Clinical laboratory summary sheets
MRICU blood gas laboratory report
Radiology reports
Ultrasound reports
EKG rhythm strips
EEG
Nuclear medicine
Pulmonary function test
Request for blood components and testing
Antibody ID report
Blood component–ID tag
Miscellaneous
Energy expenditure–Nutrition department
Cardiopulmonary resuscitation record
Transfer order sheet
Adult total nutrient admixture physician's treatment sheet
Acute dialysis unit treatment sheet
Physician's treatment sheets
   Precatheterization orders
   Postanesthesia physician's treatment sheets
Physician's order sheet for antimicrobial agents
Assessment notes
   Assessment guidelines/falls risk potential
   Assessment guidelines/pressure sore potential
   Nursing assessment
   Daily assessment
Medication administration record
Nursing Kardex
Nursing care record
Critical care flow sheet
Flow sheet
Neurologic assessment sheet

Neurologic checklist
Diabetes control chart
Intake-output chart
Graphic record

OB CHART

Diagnosis worksheet
Admission form
Consent forms
Obstetric discharge summary
Prenatal
   Initial pregnancy profile
   Health history summary
   Prenatal flow record
Perinatal data base
Patient care plan
Progress notes
Discharge instruction sheet
Operative notes
Delivery room count record
Labor unit prep room assessment
Holister forms
   Obstetric admitting record
   Labor progress chart
   Labor and delivery summary
   Postpartum progress notes
Labs
Radiology
EKG
Obstetric ultrasound
Antenatal evaluation center form
Physician's treatment sheets
Medication sheets
Nursing Kardex
Nursing care record
(Antenatal unit) pad count
Intake-output chart
Graphic record

NOTE: Newborn identification/footprints to be kept with birth certificate on mother's chart.

BABY CHART

Diagnosis worksheet
Admission form
Birth certificate
Consent forms
Newborn discharge summary
Pediatric admission nursing assessment and discharge planning
Patient care plan

Progress notes
Discharge instructions
Holister forms
  Obstetric admitting record
  Labor and delivery summary
  Labor progress chart
  Initial newborn profile
  Newborn flow record
Footprints
MicroBase
Labs
Newborn maturity rating and class
Growth record for infants
Audiologic record–1
Impedance measurement
Neonatal neurosonography
Pulmonary evaluation and diagnostic system neonatal test report
Physician's treatment sheets
Nursing Kardex
Flow sheets
IV therapy record
Apnea and bradycardia record

REHAB CHART

Same order as medical chart except for the following forms:

1. Patient discharge/readmission form–before discharge summary

2. Assessment/treatment/plan/goals form–before progress notes
Department of Rehabilitation Medicine progress note sheet–behind progress notes

3. Interdisciplinary conference summary and discharge plan form–after progress notes

The following forms are placed in the miscellaneous section of the chart in the order listed:

4. Neurological examination
5. Record of patient visits
6. Occupational therapy section form
7. Physical therapy section, general rehab in patient summary form

PSYCHIATRY ASSEMBLY ORDER

1. Application for involuntary emergency examination and treatment forms are placed behind consent forms
2. Psychiatric data base form–after ER sheets
3. 12-Hour treatment plan–after psychiatric data base
4. Creative arts therapies form–after 72-hour treatment plan
5. Psychiatric data base, corresponds to admissions
6. Crisis medication sheet–before medication administration sheets
7. Seclusion/restraint observation record–behind flow sheets
8. Observation checklist for patients in seclusion or on suicide precautions form–behind seclusion/restraint observation record

INDEX

Note: Page numbers in *italics* refer to figures; page numbers followed by t indicate tables; page numbers followed by n indicate footnotes.